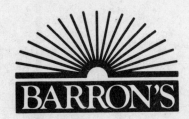

HOW TO PREPARE FOR THE MEDICAL COLLEGE ADMISSION TEST

MCAT

SEVENTH EDITION

by

Hugo R. Seibel, Ph.D.

Professor of Anatomy
Associate Dean of Medicine for Student Activities
School of Medicine and
School of Basic Health Sciences
Medical College of Virginia, Virginia Commonwealth University

Kenneth E. Guyer, Ph.D.

Associate Professor of Biochemistry
School of Medicine, Marshall University
Huntington, West Virginia

Anthony B. Mangum, Ph.D.

Associate Professor of English
Virginia Commonwealth University

C. M. Conway, Ph.D.

Assistant Professor of Biology
Virginia Commonwealth University

Arthur F. Conway, Ph.D.

Associate Professor of Biology
Randolph-Macon College
Ashland, Virginia

Wesley L. Shanholtzer, Ph.D.

Professor and Chairman
Department of Physics and Physical Sciences
Marshall University

BARRON'S EDUCATIONAL SERIES, INC.
New York • London • Toronto • Sydney

All inquiries should be addressed to:
Barron's Educational Series, Inc.
250 Wireless Boulevard
Hauppauge, New York 11788

Library of Congress Catalog Card No. 90-27731

International Standard Book No. 0-8120-4646-3

Library of Congress Cataloging in Publication Data
  Barron's how to prepare for the medical college admission test,
  MCAT/ by Hugo R. Seibel . . . [et al.].—7th ed.
     p. cm.
  ISBN 0-8120-4646-3
  1. Medical colleges—United States—Entrance examinations—
Study guides. I. Seibel, Hugo R. II. Title: How to prepare for the
medical college admission test, MCAT.
R838.5.B36 1991
610′.76—dc20
                                                  90-27731
                                                  CIP

PRINTED IN THE UNITED STATES OF AMERICA

1234   100   987654321

Contents

Preface   iv

Introduction   v
    Timetable for the MCAT   vi
    Role of the MCAT   vii

Science Review   1
    Review Outline   1
    Biology   8
    Chemistry   103
    Physics   138

Mathematics Review   181

Verbal Reasoning—Test-Taking Strategies   203

Writing the Essay   225

Model Examination A   227
    Answer Key   267
    Answer Explanations   268

Model Examination B   287
    Answer Key   327
    Answer Explanations   328

Model Examination C   345
    Answer Key   384
    Answer Explanations   385

Model Examination D   403
    Answer Key   445
    Answer Explanations   446

Appendix   464
    Logarithms and Exponents   464
    Table of Common Logarithms   465
    Periodic Table of the Elements   467
    List of Elements with Their Symbols   468
    Reference Tables for Chemistry   469

Preface

Can you prepare for the Medical College Admission Test (MCAT)? Some students are hesitant to utilize a book of this sort to assist in preparation for the medical college admission test, perhaps believing there is something dishonest about this method of preparation. Other students may believe that they can utilize this book or a similar one just before the test to prepare themselves.

In our estimation both of these viewpoints are incorrect. These practice materials should provide experience in timed tests of this type and point out areas of weakness for additional study in appropriate textbooks. By proper and careful preparation utilizing all possible modes, the individual is simply presenting his or her true potential for the study of medicine. For maximum benefit we would suggest that students begin their preparation two or three months before the examination. This will allow time to take some of the practice examinations, review the areas of weakness, and retake some of the practice examinations without having the pressure of time to produce undue frustration and a feeling of hopelessness.

Obtaining admission to medical school is a very difficult task today. We hope that, in preparing this volume, we have been able to offer you a greater chance of success. Good luck!

We wish to ackowledge the help we have received from many of our colleagues; a special thank you should be extended to H. Meetz; G. D. Meetz; J. Gregorek; J. D. Reynolds; W. M. Reams; C. Kirksey; R. J. Krieg; J. H. Johnson; S. S. Craig; J. D. Povlishock; W. Seibel; L. Crane; L. P. Gartner; L. M. Sawyer; G. J. Somori; W. J. McIntyre; J. Washburn; J. L. Poland; S. L. Quattropani; M. P. Golka; F. M. Bush; R. L. Salisbury; M. M. Sholley; G. Miller; C. H. Fowlkes; R. B. Brandt; P. L. Szabo; N. Whisner; J. Wood; J. P. Guyer; J. Kass; Lester Schlumpf; B. P. Dezzutti; S. Falzone; I. K. Schneider; L. S. Costanzo; S. C. Dudley; J. Pettit; W. M. Grogan; S. G. Bradley; A. N. Avakian; C. P. Ruch; S. M. Ayers; J. J. Mc Govern; W. J. Borowy; J. Astruc, Jr.; J. F. Snyder; J. I. Townsend; J. Perlin; W. L. Banks; W. E. Blake, Jr.; L. Padilla; S. E. Kennedy; J. M. Messmer; S. A. Messmer; J. A. Rosecrans; M. N. De Pillars; B. Owen; R. G. Bass; R. S. Vacca; J. Mundie; E. Pollard; D. James; P. F. H. Campbell; T. Fleet; H. Tuttle; M. Ripley; R. Perry; R. Dale; S. V. Doud; L. Graham; D. J. Vick and Robert Lehrman. Particular gratitude is extended to Mrs. Marilyn P. Bertrand for her cheerful and spirited assistance and the typing of the manuscript. We are indebted to Dr. Edith E. Seibel for her contributions and the proofreading of the book. Dr. Erwin E. Seibel deserves a special commendation since he contributed the bulk of the physics review.

Introduction

The present MCAT was first administered to prospective medical students in the spring of 1977. The new MCAT will first be administered in April of 1991. It represents an attempt to evaluate (1) the student's knowledge and ability to solve problems in the areas of biology, chemistry, and physics, (2) the student's skill in analysis of paragraphs, tabular material, graphs, etc., and (3) the ability to write two first draft compositions in correct English. Separate scores will be reported for Verbal Reasoning, Physical Sciences, Writing Sample, and Biological Sciences.

It is expected that those taking the test will have the equivalent of one year of college study in each of the following scientific areas: biology, general and/or inorganic chemistry, organic chemistry, and physics. Although advanced study in one or more of these disciplines may give a better understanding of concepts, it is not intended that the questions will require a knowledge of concepts not taught in basic courses.

A mathematics background including one year of college mathematics should suffice for the science questions; calculus is not required. Indeed, it has been suggested that high school courses including two years of algebra, use of trigonometric functions, memorization of sine and cosine of 0°, 90°, and 180°, facility in use of metric and English units and conversion from one set of units to another (when conversion factors are given); experimental error; statistics to include the concepts of arithmetic mean, range, variability, and significant figures; and vector addition and subtraction would represent adequate preparation in mathematics.

It is our suggestion that you begin preparation by studying the review sections of this book. Areas that are particularly difficult for you may require some review of your college texts. When you begin taking the practice tests, try to pace yourself to allow completion of each section within the allotted time. (If it is necessary to omit some questions because of time limitations, you may wish to go back after you have scored the test and try to answer them without the pressure of time.)

After taking your first practice test and correcting the answers, you should score your test as it will be done after the actual test. First count the number of correct answers in (1) Verbal Reasoning, (2) Physical Sciences, and (3) Biological Sciences. In each case this will represent the number of correct answers in that discipline.

The number of correct answers is the raw score and must then be converted into a 15-point scaled score *approximated by* the following tables. The approximation exists because raw score to scaled score tables may vary from test to test due to slight differences in degree of difficulty.

Although individual medical schools will vary with respect to the scores they require, a standard score of 11 or greater will probably be considered to be quite competitive. A standard score of 7 or less would indicate an area requiring substantial additional preparation. Before taking the next practice test, you should concentrate on areas of low score.

The Science area may be remediated by additional study and working problems. The area of Verbal Reasoning, however, may require a slightly different approach. Try going back over this part of the examination, reading carefully, and answering the questions again without a time limit. Read the paragraph again and try to determine why you missed certain questions. Be sure to use only the information in the paragraph. Then go on to additional practice examinations. One additional suggestion: Read the questions carefully before answering. Sometimes students answer the question they *expected* rather than the question that was asked. Try to avoid this pitfall.

If you are unable to read at the required rate and comprehension level, then your problem may be more serious. After studying the Verbal Reasoning section of this book, you may want to review some reading selections from your Freshman English course.

Verbal Reasoning		Physical Sciences		Biological Sciences	
Raw Score	Scaled Score	Raw Score	Scaled Score	Raw Score	Scaled Score
0–7	1	0–8	1	0–8	1
8–14	2	9–16	2	9–16	2
15–20	3	17–28	3	17–28	3
21–26	4	29–33	4	29–33	4
27–31	5	34–39	5	34–39	5
32–36	6	40–44	6	40–44	6
37–41	7	45–49	7	45–49	7
42–46	8	50–55	8	50–55	8
47–50	9	56–60	9	56–60	9
51–53	10	61–64	10	61–64	10
54–57	11	65–67	11	65–67	11
58–60	12	68–70	12	68–70	12
61–62	13	71–73	13	71–73	13
63–64	14	74–75	14	74–75	14
65	15	76–77	15	76–77	15

As you progress through the other practice tests, you should develop facility in working faster to allow completion of each section. Although wild guessing is of no value, it is to your advantage to guess among a select number of answers if you have ruled out some answers.

Remember: we cannot hope to present everything you should have learned in years of study. We can only help you to identify areas of weakness, give some review of important concepts and provide experience and confidence in taking a test having the format of the Medical College Admission Test. We hope that this will allow you to reach your own potential on this test.

Four sections will comprise the MCAT examination; they are: Biological Sciences, Physical Sciences, Verbal Reasoning, and Writing Sample.

The Biological Sciences test will concentrate on basic biology and biologically-related chemistry, whereas the Physical Sciences examination will focus on physics and physically-related chemistry areas.

TIMETABLE FOR THE MCAT

TOTAL TIME: Approximately 5 hours and 45 minutes, plus 1 hour for lunch, 20 minutes for breaks

85 minutes	Verbal Reasoning (65 questions)	9 passages 6–10 questions/passage
10 minutes	REST PERIOD	
100 minutes	Physical Sciences (77 questions)	10 problem sets 5–10 questions/set 15 problems 1 question/set
60 minutes	LUNCH	
60 minutes	Writing Sample (2 essays)	2 topics 30 minutes/topic
10 minutes	REST PERIOD	
100 minutes	Biological Sciences (77 questions)	10 problem sets 5–10 questions/set 15 problems 1 question/set

Verbal Reasoning

Typically this section will be composed of 9 passages from the humanities, social sciences, and natural sciences; each passage will be followed by 6–10 questions. These questions will be based on, and can be answered from, the information presented.

Physical Sciences

Typically this section will be composed of a series of problems upon which the subsequent multiple-choice questions are based. There usually will be 10 problem sets that will be followed by 5–10 questions each and 15 problems to be followed by a single question.

Writing Sample

Typically this section will be composed of two topics; 30 minutes will be allowed for each. The student will be asked to develop a central theme, synthesize material, separate major from minor issues, propose alternative solutions, present a theme in a logical manner, and write in correct English.

Biological Sciences

Typically this section will be composed of a series of problems upon which the subsequent multiple-choice questions are based. There usually will be 10 problem sets that will be followed by 5–10 questions each and 15 problems to be followed by a single question.

ROLE OF THE MCAT

The MCAT, in combination with college grades (overall and science GPA), types and quality of courses, letters of recommendation, extracurricular activities, major undergraduate institution attended, the interview, SAT, etc., is a screening device. The test is an objective measure and high scores will help an individual with average grades. Average or slightly lower MCAT scores probably do not significantly affect a superior college record. The literature points to a positive correlation between high MCAT scores (especially science subtests) and future success in the basic medical sciences (preclinical phase) and National Board of Medical Examiners Part I examination scores.

MCAT Science Review

The purpose of this section is to help the student review some key material quickly, to place some of his or her information in perspective and to help identify areas of weakness and strength. No attempt has been made to cover all of the material in the subject matter; but it is hoped that after the student has worked through the practice examinations and has studied the explanations to the questions, this section will amplify for him or her the highlights and essentials that are expected baseline knowledge for all educated people. A brief presentation such as this cannot cover all areas in sufficient depth. Some areas are omitted and others are presented only in a simplified manner. The individual who is well prepared will sometimes recognize compromises that must be made for the sake of brevity. This section should not be used as a substitute for a good general text in the areas but it should be used as a guide and in conjunction with a text so that the student may efficiently prepare for the MCAT. Again, we urge the student to begin preparation for the examination early and to be conscientious and thorough.

REVIEW OUTLINE

Biology

1. The Cell—Its Structure and Function
   A. Size
   B. Composition of Protoplasm
   C. Properties of the Cell and Protoplasm
   D. Components of a Typical Cell
   E. Cell Division—Mitosis
   F. Methods of Examining the Cell
   G. Eukaryotic vs. Prokaryotic Cell Structure

2. Classification of Living Organisms

3. Organization of the Human Body
   A. Organ System
   B. Four Basic Tissues

4. Skeletal System
   A. Axial Skeleton
   B. Appendicular Skeleton
   C. Characteristics of Bone
   D. Joints

5. Muscular System
   A. Classification
   B. Skeletal Muscles
   C. Muscle Attachment and Function
   D. Terms to Describe Movement
   E. Muscle Names
   F. Structural Organization of a Muscle Fiber
   G. Myofilaments
   H. Sarcoplasm

      I.   Excitation
     J.   Contraction
    K.   Muscle Twitch
     L.   Tetanus
    M.   Energy Sources
    N.   Types of Muscle Fibers

6. Circulatory System
    A.   Functions
    B.   General Components and Structure
    C.   Course of Circulation
    D.   The Heart
    E.   Blood

7. Respiratory System
    A.   Removal of Inhaled Particles
    B.   Pulmonary Ventilation
    C.   Inspiration and Expiration
    D.   Positive and Negative Pressure Breathing
    E.   Neuronal Control and Integration of Breathing
    F.   Gas Exchange in the Alveoli
    G.   Oxygen Transport
    H.   Carbon Dioxide Transport
     I.   Chemical Regulation of Respiration

8. Urinary System
    A.   Structure of the Kidney
    B.   Tubular Passageways
    C.   Functions of the Kidney and Uriniferous Tubules
    D.   Hormonal Control of Secretion and Resorption

9. Integumentary (Skin) System
    A.   Skin
    B.   Glands
    C.   Hair
    D.   Nails

10. Digestive System and Nutrition
    A.   Nutrition
    B.   The Digestive System
    C.   The Major Digestive Glands
    D.   General Functional Schema of the Digestive Tube
    E.   Intestinal Motility
    F.   Innervation of the Intestinal Tract
    G.   Summary of Digestive Juices
    H.   Hormones of the Digestive Tract
     I.   General Digestion of the Major Food Groups

11. Nervous System
    A.   Nervous Tissue
    B.   The Neuron
    C.   Classification of Neurons
    D.   Groups of Neurons
    E.   Supportive Elements

    F. The Central Nervous System
    G. The Peripheral Nervous System
    H. Reflex Arc

12. Organs of Special Sense
    A. The Eye
    B. The Ear
    C. The Olfactory System
    D. The Gustatory System

13. Endocrine System
    A. The Pituitary Gland (Hypophysis)
    B. The Thyroid Gland
    C. The Parathyroid Glands
    D. The Pancreas
    E. The Adrenal Glands
    F. The Testes
    G. General Function Scheme of Both Sexes
    H. The Ovaries
    I. Menstrual Cycle
    J. Female Contraception
    K. The Placenta
    L. The Pineal
    M. The Prostaglandins
    N. The Small Intestine

14. Reproductive System
    A. Reproductive Organs
    B. Hormonal Control
    C. Gametogenesis and Meiosis
    D. Mature Gametes
    E. Other Modes of Reproduction

15. Development
    A. Fertilization
    B. Cleavage
    C. Blastocyst Formation
    D. Implantation in the Uterus
    E. Second Week
    F. Second Month
    G. Fetal Membranes and Placenta
    H. Fetal and Neonatal Circulation
    I. Multiple Pregnancy

16. Genetics
    A. Mendelian Characteristics
    B. Polygenic Traits
    C. Paternity Exclusion and Reassignment of Misassigned Infants

17. The Animal Kingdom
    A. Distribution of Living Organisms
    B. Interrelationships of Animals
    C. Population Dynamics
    D. Major Environment–Habitats
    E. Learning, Conditioning, Rhythms

18. Evolution
    A. Key People and Concepts
    B. Process of Evolution
    C. Adaptive Radiation
    D. Extinction
    E. Analogy and Homology

Chemistry

1. General Chemistry
    A. The Atom
    B. Components of the Atom
    C. Placement of Electrons—Energy Levels
    D. Periodic Table
    E. Gases
    F. Liquids and Solids
    G. Phase Changes
    H. Chemical Compounds
    I. Balanced Chemical Equations
    J. Solutions
    K. Acids and Bases, pH, and Buffers
    L. Electrochemistry
    M. Thermodynamics
    N. Rate Processes in Chemical Reactions

2. General Principles
    A. Characteristics of Mixtures and Compounds
    B. Reactions
    C. Role of Enzymes in a Reaction
    D. Temperature Conversion Factors
    E. Formulas and Laws

3. Organic Chemistry
    A. General Considerations
    B. The Alkanes
    C. The Cycloalkanes
    D. The Alkenes
    E. The Alkynes
    F. Aromatic Compounds
    G. The Grignard Reagent
    H. Alcohols
    I. Amines
    J. Amides
    K. Aldehydes and Ketones
    L. Carboxylic Acids
    M. Esters
    N. Ethers
    O. Final Remarks

4. Biochemistry
    A. Areas of Biochemistry
    B. pH and Buffers
    C. Amino Acids, Peptides, and Proteins
    D. Enzymes

E. Carbohydrates
F. Lipids
G. Nucleotides and Nucleic Acids; Biosynthesis of Nucleic Acids and Proteins

Physics

1. Accelerated Motion
   A. Falling Objects—Gravity Acceleration
   B. Uniform Velocity
   C. Nonuniform Motion
   D. Uniform Deceleration
   E. Free Fall

2. Forces and Motion
   A. Forces and Acceleration
   B. Weight and Acceleration
   C. Negative Acceleration
   D. Resultant Forces
   E. Equilibrium States

3. Projectile Motion

4. Friction

5. Work and Power
   A. Work and Energy
   B. Power and Power Units

6. Energy
   A. Potential Energy
   B. Kinetic Energy

7. Momentum

8. Uniform Circular Motion
   A. Centripetal Acceleration
   B. Circular Motion
   C. Centripetal Force
   D. Centrifugal Force

9. Fluids at Rest
   A. Pressure
   B. Density
   C. Specific Gravity
   D. Buoyancy

10. Gravity

11. Temperature Calculations and Measurement

12. Heat
    A. Specific Heat
    B. Heat Lost = Heat Gained
    C. Heat of Vaporization

13. Thermodynamics
   A. Work and Heat
   B. Efficiency of a Boiler

14. Electrostatics
   A. The Electric Force
   B. The Quantum of Charge
   C. Electric Field
   D. Electric Potential Difference

15. Electricity
   A. Ohm's Law

15. Electric Circuits
   A. Electromotive Force (emf) and Internal Resistance
   B. Resistors in Series
   C. Resistors in Parallel
   D. Cells in Series
   E. Cells in Parallel

17. Electric Energy
   A. Joule's Law
   B. Power and Resistance

18. Alternating Current
   A. Effective Values

19. Machines and Mechanical Advantage
   A. Actual Mechanical Advantage
   B. Theoretical Mechanical Advantage
   C. Efficiency

20. Simple Harmonic Motion
   A. Period and Frequency
   B. Phase

21. Waves
   A. Frequency, Wavelength, and Phase
   B. Interference
   C. Standing Waves

22. Sound Waves
   A. Pitch and Frequency
   B. Intensity
   C. Speed of Sound
   D. Beats
   E. Doppler Effect

23. Light Rays
   A. Reflection
   B. Refraction
   C. Index of Refraction
   D. Refraction between Two Media
   E. Total Internal Reflection

24. Mirrors
   A. Plane Mirrors
   B. Convex Mirrors
   C. Concave Mirrors

25. Lenses
   A. Concave Lenses
   B. Convex Lenses
   C. Combinations of Lenses

26. Composition of the Atom
   A. Subatomic Particles
   B. Isotopes
   C. Nuclear Reactions

27. Radioactivity
   A. Alpha Decay
   B. Beta Decay
   C. Half-life

28. Nuclear Energy
   A. Units of Measure
   B. Fusion Reactions
   C. Nuclear Fission

29. Photons
   A. Wave Property of Light
   B. Photon Energy
   C. Photoelectric Effect

30. Atomic Energy Levels
   A. Spectra
   B. Spectrum of Atomic Hydrogen

BIOLOGY

The Cell—Its Structure and Function

The cell is the basic unit of structure and function and basis of all life; all cells come from preexisting cells.

Size

Most cells are between 10 and 100μ (microns) in diameter. Measurements are made utilizing the following units:

$$1 \text{ cm} = 10 \text{mm}$$
$$1 \text{ mm} = 1000 \mu$$
$$1 \mu = 10,000 \text{ Å (angstrom units)}$$

Average sizes of structures may be listed as follows:

cells about	10μ	(100,000 Å)
mitochondria about	1μ	(10,000 Å)
bacteria about	1μ	(10,000 Å)
viruses about	0.1μ	(1,000 Å)
macromolecules about	0.01μ	(100 Å)
molecules about	0.001μ	(10 Å)
hydrogen ion about	0.0001μ	(1 Å)

Resolution is commonly defined as the ability to discriminate two points and visualize them as two points, even though they are extremely close together. With the unaided eye these points might appear as one point, but the microscope can aid in resolving them as two. The resolution is dependent on the wavelength of the light source and can be calculated to be about one-half the wavelength. Examples of resolving power are:

human eye about 0.1 mm (100μ)
light microscope about 0.2μ (2000 Å)
electron microscope about 2–5 Å

Composition of Protoplasm

Protoplasm is made up mainly of proteins, carbohydrates, fats, salts and water; its average elemental composition is:

Oxygen 75+%	Potassium about 0.3%
Carbon 10+%	Chlorine about 0.1%
Hydrogen 10%	less than 0.1%—sodium
Nitrogen 2+%	calcium
Sulfur about 0.2%	magnesium
Phosphorus about 0.3%	iron, etc.

Properties of the Cell and Protoplasm

1. Irritability
2. Conductivity
3. Respiration
4. Absorption
5. Secretion
6. Excretion
7. Growth
8. Reproduction
9. Metabolism

Components of a Typical Cell

Cells are commonly recognized as having two major compartments: *cytoplasm*—includes all components within the cell membrane but outside the nucleus, and *nucleoplasm*—includes everything within the nuclear membrane.

1. Cell Membrane: The cell membrane, or unit membrane, usually is about 75–100 Å hick; it is a trilaminar structure. As described by Danielli and Davson (1935), two protein ayers sandwich a bimolecular lipid layer.

The cell membrane:

provides for a boundary resulting in a controlled environment.

is a relatively watertight barrier.

maintains a constant composition and environment resulting in homeostasis.

is semipermeable; only certain types of molecules are allowed to pass.

is composed mainly of proteins, lipids and carbohydrates; the major types of lipids found in nature are fats, phospholipids and steroids.

Structure. Electron microscopy suggests that the central region of the membrane consists of two layers of lipid molecules, mainly phospholipids and steroids. Each layer is thought to be one molecule thick. The phospholipid molecules are fairly long and have two functional poles: one exhibits lipid properties (it exhibits hydrophobic properties, repelling water); the other exhibits polar properties (it has a tendency to dissolve in water, and exhibits hydrophilic properties). The hydrophobic ends of both layers of lipid molecules associate with each other since they have affinity for one another. The hydrophilic portions face toward the protein layers; parts of proteins associate readily with water.

Electron microscopy substantiates that there is a light central layer surrounded by two denser layers. The two denser layers are thought to represent the proteins and hydrophilic portions of the lipid molecules while the light layer represents the hydrophobic portions of the lipid molecules.

Recent evidence, however, suggests that the arrangement of the protein molecules is far more complex. The protein molecules probably do not cover the entire surface but are arranged in definite, specialized, functional and structural packages throughout the entire membrane. Channels may exist where the lipid layers are interrupted and a continuous zone of hydrophilic molecules is present. This zone is thought to be occupied by a pore. A pore is only a few angstrom (Å) units in diameter and allows for the passage of water, inorganic ions and very small molecules.

Membranes vary and are highly specialized. All membranes, however, are made up of the same basic molecules and possess similar characteristics. The particular amount and arrangement of proteins, lipids and carbohydrates at the cell surface, however, impart specific properties. It is at these specific sites that different molecules are processed.

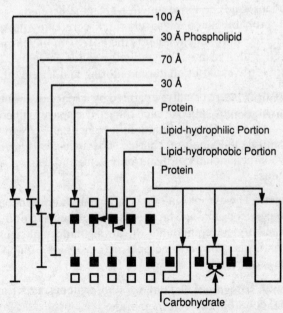

100 Å
30 Å Phospholipid
70 Å
30 Å
Protein
Lipid-hydrophilic Portion
Lipid-hydrophobic Portion
Protein
Carbohydrate

Composite representation of a lipoprotein membrane

Activities. As pointed out before, the plasma membrane is semi-permeable. It controls the passage of materials into and out of the cell. The movement of materials into and out of the cell is called *transport*.

There are two types of transport—passive, or transport that does not require the cell's energy, and active, which does require energy expenditure.

There are two types of passive transport—diffusion and osmosis.

In *diffusion* molecules pass from an area of higher concentration to that of lower concentration until the concentrations are equal on both sides of the membrane. Diffusion, in other words, follows the concentration gradient.

Osmosis is the movement of water across the semi-permeable membrane. Water will pass into a more concentrated solution and this passage of water will equalize the concentration of dissolved substances on each side of the membrane so that equilibrium is theoretically achieved.

Equilibrium implies an equal number of molecules of all dissolved material per unit volume on each side of the membrane compartment; the same applies to the concentration of each individual diffusable component.

Gases pass through the cell membrane with ease. Water and small molecules pass more readily than large molecules and lipid soluble materials enter the cell easier than nonlipid-soluble substances.

Active transport requires the cell to expend energy to allow materials to pass through the membrane. (Also called uphill transport, energy dependent transport can operate against concentration gradients.)

Electrical charge has also to be considered. The inside of the cell is usually electrically negative in comparison to the outside environment.

In active transport, materials enter the cell in membrane-bound vesicles, formed by the membrane. This process is known collectively as *endocytosis*. When it involves solid material we speak of *phagocytosis;* liquid material enters via *pinocytosis*. The process of expulsion of material is known as *exocytosis*.

Special Sites. To amplify the complexities of the cell membrane some general statements are in order at this point.

Cells must be held together and specialized structures are required. Adjacent cell membranes interdigitate and intercellular cement is utilized.

A *desmosome* is a specialized area of connection between adjacent cellular membranes (macula adherens).

A *terminal bar* is a dense area surrounding the apical cellular surface. It includes the tight junction (zona occludens) and the loose junction (zona adherens).

Layers of material (probably mucopolysaccharide) secreted by the cell are found on the surface of the cell. The most prominent layer is the *basement membrane,* or *basal lamina*. The thick cellulose cell wall of plants falls within the above category. These structures are boundaries and must be traversed by material entering and leaving the cell.

2. Intercellular Space: Cells are usually separated by a space of about 100–200 Å. Only at specialized contact points do cells appose each other. The space is filled mainly by a matrix of proteins and polysaccharides which function in cementing cells to one another. Some cells possess special extracellular polysaccharide substances: cartilage is rich in chondroitin sulfate; joints have large amounts of hyaluronic acid; and cell walls of plants are composed largely of cellulose.

3. Cytoplasmic Matrix: The cytoplasm of a cell appears homogeneous, translucent, and structureless; the homogeneous mass, which is also called cell-sap or hyaloplasm, contains inorganic substances and organic compounds of varying molecular sizes. The more peripheral layer of this matrix is also known as ectoplasm (plasmagel). It appears more rigid and seems to lack granules completely.

4. Cellular Inclusions: These may be composed of proteins, fats, carbohydrates, granules, pigments, and crystals.

a. *Secretion granules (products of cell activity)*. These are usually membrane-bound products that await extrusion by the cell (exocrine secretion into ducts or endocrine secretion into the extracellular space and capillaries). Release of secretory product from the cells is via exocytosis. Under the general term endocytosis (taking into the cell), are the more specific terms, pinocytosis (taking in of fluid) and phagocytosis (taking in of solids).

b. *Lipid droplets*. These are globular accumulations synthesized by the cell. During periods of need they may serve as a source of energy.

c. *Glycogen granules*. These are small spherical units synthesized by the cell. They serve as storage reservoirs of carbohydrates.

d. *Pigment granules*. These may be of two types: endogenous pigments derived from cell metabolism or exogenous pigments taken in by the cell. Hemosiderin is an example of an exogenous pigment, while the lipochromes and the melanins are endogenous in nature.

e. *Vacuoles*. Under this general term may be classified any membrane-bound globular structure.

f. *Plastids*. The plastids are composed of leucoplasts, chromoplasts and chloroplasts. Leucoplasts resemble chloroplasts but have no chlorophyll; they manufacture starch, oil and protein. Chromoplasts possess pigments and are responsible for the color of flower petals. Chloroplasts possess chlorophyll, which is capable of capturing light energy to produce glucose from CO_2 and H_2O.

5. Mitochondria: Mitochondria are the best known of the cellular organelles. They had been described during the 19th century, notably by Kollicker and Fleming. Altman, using Janus green, was able to stain them in 1890. Structurally, the mitochondrion is composed of an outer trilaminar membrane and an inner trilaminar membrane; the inner one forms folds which are known as *cristae*. The space between the two membranes is about 6–10 nm wide.

Mitochondria as a whole and specifically the cristae vary greatly in size, shape and number not only in different cells but also in the same cell depending on its functional state. Mitochondria are present in greater numbers in cells exhibiting high levels of activity and having more energy requirements. Muscle and glandular tissues fall in the above category.

DNA has been found in the mitochondria of animals and the chloroplasts of plants. Mitochondria are capable of division and are not generated *de novo*.

Granules have been observed in the mitochondrial matrix. Their identity is in question, however; some believe that they might be reservoirs of calcium and other divalent ions. Phosphate is taken up with Ca^{2+} and calcium phosphate deposits might be the end result.

Mitochondria are the biochemical powerplants of cells. They recover energy from foodstuffs (via Krebs cycle, or citric acid cycle; tricarboxylic acid cycle and the respiratory chain) and convert it via phosphorylation into adenosine triphosphate (ATP). In this manner they produce the energy necessary for the metabolic processes.

Enzymes. The organization of enzymes and coenzymes (especially enzymes involved in oxidative phosphorylation) in the cristae appears to be highly specific facilitating an orderly and proper sequence of reactions.

Enzymes concerned with the Krebs cycle are presumed to be either free in the mitochondrial matrix (internal medium) or loosely bound to the membranes since they are readily recovered when mitochondria are disrupted. The electron transport components involved in respiratory activity and the oxidative phosphorylation systems are presumed to be tightly bound to the inner membranous system. Electron transport and oxidative phosphorylation seem to be coupled.

Enzymes then are associated with the outer membrane, the inner membrane, the space between the outer and inner membranes, and the matrix.

DNA and Protein Synthesis. Most extranuclear DNA, if not all, can be found in mitochondria (and in plants, in the chloroplast). There is evidence that proteins are synthesized in mitochondria under the direction of mitochondrial DNA. In biochemical preparations of mitochondria the synthesizing enzymes necessary for RNA and proteins have been isolated. However, there also is considerable documentation that the code for the enzymes involved in oxidative phosphorylation originates in nuclear DNA. Therefore, it must be assumed that mitochondrial DNA is involved only in the partial coding of the proteins manufactured in the organelle.

Krebs Cycle. Mitochondria are involved in the Krebs or citric acid cycle in which organic acids are oxidized to CO_2. In each successive step oxidation of a single carbon of the chain takes place and each reaction requires a different enzyme. The Krebs cycle reactions are further described under the topic "Carbohydrates" on page 133.

The ATP produced is a small molecule and can diffuse out of the mitochondrion into the cytoplasm and participate in the *endothermic* reactions of the cell.

6. Chloroplast: For completeness sake, let us examine the homologue of the mitochondria in plants—namely, the chloroplasts. Joseph Priestley discovered photosynthesis in 1771. In 1888 Haberlandt associated chloroplasts directly with oxygen production. Just as cellular respiration takes place in the mitochondria, photosynthesis occurs in chloroplasts. Composition of chloroplasts: 56% protein, 35% lipid, 8% chlorophyll.

Chloroplasts are somewhat larger and exhibit more variability than mitochondria. They are bounded by two membranes and possess an amorphous ground substance, or *stroma,* throughout which rows of parallel membranes called *grana* are distributed. These membranes house the photosynthetic machinery.

Photosynthesis. In photosynthesis light energy (photons) is absorbed by chlorophyll in the chloroplasts and utilized in the production of sugars from water and atmospheric carbon dioxide.

The process (light dependent reaction) may be outlined as follows:

$$CO_2 + H_2O \xrightarrow[\text{radiant energy}]{\text{green plants}} (CH_2O)_n + O_2 + H_2O$$
sugars & starches

or

$$6CO_2 + 12H_2O + light \xrightarrow{\text{chlorophyll}} 6O_2 + C_6H_{12}O_6 + 6H_2O$$

The oxygen produced is returned to the air. The sugars are used by mitochondria and the energy produced joins the high energy bonds of ATP. Chloroplasts can also produce ATP independently. Broadly speaking the photosynthetic process, due to its production of water, carbohydrates and oxygen, sustains all higher forms of life. Once the sugar has been produced no distinction can be made in the biochemical processes of plants and animals.

As implied before, photosynthesis is a two reaction process: one is dependent on light while the other is known as the dark reaction. They may be summarized as follows:

Light-dependent reaction
results in production of ATP (adenosinetriphosphate) from ADP (adenosinediphosphate) via phosphorylation
results in formation of reduced NADP from NADP (nicotinamide adenine dinucleotide phosphate)
results in release of oxygen from water
results in ATP production

Dark reaction
results in carbohydrates from carbon dioxide
utilizes the ATP and reduced NADP from the light reaction

As in the mitochondrion the sequence of reactions dictates a high degree of molecular organization. During fractionation studies most of the enzymes of the dark reaction can be isolated in the supernatant. The enzymes of the light reaction are associated with the membranous structures. In general terms one can speculate that while carbohydrate synthesis occurs in the stroma, the production of ATP, reduced NADP and O_2 is associated with membranes.

7. Endoplasmic Reticulum (ER): This cellular organelle had not been observed with the ordinary light microscope; it was first described using phase microscopy by Porter, Claude and Fallam in 1945. In general terms it is an extensive network of interconnecting channels. The endoplasmic reticular membranes are unit membranes (trilaminar). When ribosomes line the outer surface, it is designated as *rough endoplasmic reticulum* (RER). The primary form of this organelle is the rough variety. The smooth is derived from the rough due to the loss of ribosomes. The amount of each depends on the cell type and the cellular activity.

The RER (rough endoplasmic reticulum) is the synthetic machinery of the cell (messenger RNA influences that machinery; it is manufactured in the nucleus). It is mainly concerned with protein synthesis. Smooth endoplasmic reticulum (SER) is mainly concerned with lipid or fat synthesis. In the liver, SER probably plays a significant role in the detoxification of potentially harmful substances.

Ribosomes (probably in the form of polysomes; a group of ribosomes, like rosettes) are located on the external surface of ER. The rough endoplasmic reticulum is highly developed in protein-secreting cells such as found in the pancreas. Autoradiographic methods have revealed that labeled amino acids first appear on the RER (polysomes); then in the cisternae of the ER, where the material is processed and transported; later in the Golgi complex, where it is chemically modified and condensed; then in secretion granules (in the case of pancreas, zymogen granules), which move towards the cell surface (secretory pole); and finally in the extracellular space (via exocytosis) as a released secretory granule.

The movement of the material from the ribosomal area on the membrane into the ER seems to require no special energy or transport enzymes. Evidence is available for transport by the ER of: lipoproteins, lysosomal hydrolases, peroxisomal enzymes, albumin, and a variety of other molecules.

The isolated microsome cell fraction contains enzymes involved in the synthesis of: phospholipids, steroids, and triglycerides.

Both RER and SER can function in lipid synthesis; however, usually we assign prominence of the RER to protein-secreting cells and to the SER to steroid-secreting cells. The steroid hormone-producing cells of the adrenal and testis are rich in SER. The SER (sarcoplasmic reticulum) is extremely extensive and specialized in cardiac and smooth muscle. It encases the myofibrils and functions in the release and sequestering of calcium ions needed during contraction. It is obvious that the membranes are very dynamic systems and are extremely adaptable to the demands and needs of the cell.

8. The Golgi Complex: This structure was well known to light microscopists and was first described by Camillo Golgi in 1898.

All eukaryotic cells, except for the red blood cell, possess a Golgi apparatus; in plants the sacs of the Golgi complex are referred to as *dictyosomes*. The Golgi apparatus is composed of numerous and diverse channels of cisternae (flattened sacs) and interspersed vesicles and granules; it is a very heterogeneous cellular organelle. It is located usually near one pole of the nucleus and in close relation to the centriole.

Generally speaking, the Golgi complex is prominent in glandular cells and is thought to function in the production, concentration, packaging, and transportation of secretory material. Important enzyme systems are associated with the membranes (flattened cisternae or round vesicles or sacs) of the Golgi complex. It is thought that substances manufactured by the endoplasmic reticulum are transferred to the Golgi cisternae, processed there, and then stored or released by the cell. The Golgi elaborates polysaccharide moieties.

The functions of the Golgi apparatus are highly diverse and complex. During the early period of elucidating the processes of this organelle a condensing role was ascribed; it has now been shown that not only does condensing of products take place but also certain factors, such as carbohydrate moieties, are contributed and added to glycoproteins. Sulfation is also carried out.

Recently, utilizing cell fractions containing Golgi material, high concentrations of glycosyl transferase were detected; these enzymes catalyze the polymerization of sugars into polysaccharides and also attach sugars to glycoproteins. Evidence shows phosphatase, thiamine pyrophosphatase (TPPase) and nucleoside diphosphatase (NDPase) activity in the Golgi zone.

As pointed out in a previous section, when radioactive tracers (tritium labelled amino acids) are utilized, they appear first over ribosomes, then in the ER, and later the protein is found in or near the Golgi complex. However, when tritium labelled sugars are employed they first make their appearance in the Golgi. This fact has fostered the idea that the Golgi complex is the site of synthesis of secretory polysaccharides.

The associations, interrelationships, and interactions of the various membranous components of the organelle are not completely elucidated. However, a certain amount of association and transformation is evidenced. The peripheral sacs of the Golgi are probably related to the endoplasmic reticulum; the central ones, however, seem to be different. The products that come from the Golgi apparatus are very complex in nature and exhibit mixtures of proteins and polysaccharides, or lipids and proteins in a variety of concentrations. Concentration or condensing is thought to be accomplished by the extrusion of water.

Lysosomes (organelles containing hydrolytic enzymes) have been linked to the Golgi membranes. Vesicles containing acid phosphatase have been shown to originate from the Golgi zone. The presence in the Golgi (a good marker) of galactosyltransferase activity which is absent from other membranes might help shed light on the complex functions.

In summary one can link the Golgi complex to:

secretion,
membrane biogenesis,
lysosome formation,
membrane recycling,
hormone modulation.

Secretory proteins undergo modifications such as: glycosylation, sulfation, proteolytic processing, and condensing and concentrating.

Lysosome: The term lysosome, denoting a membrane-bound lytic particle or body, was introduced in 1955 by Christain DeDuve. Lysosomes were described as containing proteolytic enzymes (hydrolases).

Lysosomes contain acid phosphatase and other hydrolytic enzymes. These enzymes are enclosed by a membrane and are released when needed into the cell or into phagocytic vesicles. The enzymes found in lysosomes are probably manufactured by the endoplasmic reticulum and Golgi apparatus. The membrane surrounding these enzymes confines these potentially lethal chemicals so that they can perform their functions without harming the cell. The enzymes not only digest material which the cells ingest but also function in the debridement of the cell, a process known as *autophagy*. Prominent examples of cells with conspicuous lysosomes are the granulocytic leucocytes and macrophages; these specific lysosomes are also known as *bacteriocidal lysosomes*. Acid phosphatase activity is the most widely used enzyme marker and so far over fifty hydrolases have been identified.

Related to the lysosome is the *phagosome*. The phagosome, as the lysosome, is membrane bound; it is a structure in which phagocytized bacteria or other substances that enter the cell are transported. Lysosomes come in contact and fuse with phagosomes and in this fashion a *secondary lysosome,* or *phagolysosome,* is created.

Where all lysosomes are produced is still in question. Most lysosomal enzymes, however, are produced first by ribosomes, then processed by the endoplasmic reticulum, shipped from there either to lysosomes directly or processed further via the Golgi membranes to finally enter the lysosomal pool.

Lysosomal enzymes have the capacity to hydrolyze all classes of macromolecules. A generalized list of substrates acted upon by respective enzymes is given below:

Lipids by lipases and phospholipases;
Proteins by proteases;
Polysaccharides by glycosidases;
Nucleic acids by nucleases;
Phosphates (organic-linked) by phosphatases;
Sulphates (organic-linked) by sulfatases.

9. Peroxisomes: Peroxisomes are found in virtually all mammalian cell types and probably arise from swellings of the endoplasmic reticulum. These structures are often smaller than lysosomes. The enzymes they possess are active in the production of hydrogen peroxide (urate oxidase, D-amino acid oxidase, α-hydroxyacid oxidase), and one functions in destroying hydrogen peroxide (catalase). Other oxidases have been proposed also. The peroxisomes function in purine catabolism and in the degradation of nucleic acids.

10. Nucleus: The nucleus was first described by Robert Brown in 1831. The nucleus is surrounded by a double layer of the typical trilaminar membrane which is pierced by small pores. The pores measure about 50–80 nm in diameter. The pores allow and serve in the interchange of nuclear and cytoplasmic material. For example, messenger RNA can pass into the cytoplasm to elicit its effect. The outer membrane of the nuclear envelope (exposed to cytoplasm) has ribonucleoprotein particles (ribosomes) attached to it and may also be continuous with the RER. The inner membrane (exposed to nuclear content) lacks ribosomes.

Approximate composition of the nucleus:

80% protein,
15% DNA (deoxyribonucleic acid),
5% RNA (ribonucleic acid),
3% lipid.

Functions: Simply speaking, the nucleus controls the metabolic aspects of the cell and is responsible for its structural integrity, function, survival and the passage of the hereditary material to the next generation. The nucleus is necessary for: life, growth, differentiation, and reproduction.

DNA Structure. DNA—deoxyribonucleic acid—is a nucleic acid. A nucleic acid is a polymer of nucleotides. The combination of a *purine* or *pyrimidine* base, a sugar, and phosphoric acid is called a *nucleotide. Deoxyribose* is the sugar in DNA; ribose is the other nucleic acid, ribonucleic acid, or RNA.

DNA molecules are composed of two nucleotide strands coiled together in a double helix. Watson and Crick (1953) proposed a double helix model of DNA. The two strands consist of sugar-phosphate backbones which are connected by pairs of bases. The DNA molecule may be illustrated as follows:

Single chain

Sugar-Base
/
Phosphate
\
Sugar-Base
/
Phosphate
\
Sugar-Base

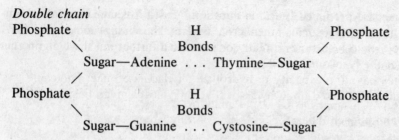

Double chain
Phosphate   H   Phosphate
       \   Bonds   /
      Sugar—Adenine . . . Thymine—Sugar
      /   \
Phosphate   H   Phosphate
       \   Bonds   /
      Sugar—Guanine . . . Cystosine—Sugar

Each strand is a chain of nucleotides. All DNA nucleotides consist of a 5-carbon sugar (deoxyribose) with a phosphate group attached at one end and a nitrogen-containing ring compound (the base) at the other. The nitrogenous bases are: adenine and guanine (*purines*); and thymine, cytosine, and uracil (*pyrimidines*). In DNA they pair specifically in the following manner:

> adenine and thymine
> guanine and cytosine

In RNA they pair as follows:

> adenine and uracil
> guanine and cytosine

The paired bases are held together chiefly by hydrogen bonds. The strands complement each other since the base sequence present on one determines the base sequence of the other. Duplication of this material involves the splitting of the unions between purines and pyrimidines; each nucleotide then acquires a new complementary nucleotide and the phosphate and pentose moieties are then joined enzymatically and the duplication process has taken place.

The phosphate groups of DNA are negatively charged. Basic dyes (hematoxylin, Feulgen stain) which are positively charged stain the DNA and RNA since positive and negative charges attract each other. The regions that attract a basic stain are referred to as *basophilic*.

DNA Functions. One of the premier functions of DNA is the production of RNA. Most RNA is produced in the nucleus. DNA and RNA are similar. They are both nucleotide chains; however, RNA differs in the following manner:

> RNA is single stranded (certain viruses are exceptions)
> the 5-carbon sugar in RNA is ribose

CHARACTERISTICS OF DNA AND RNA

DNA	RNA
double stranded sugar—deoxyribose base—thymine	single stranded (mainly) sugar—ribose base—uracil

DNA determines and acts as a template for RNA synthesis. With the help of a transcription enzyme (RNA polymerase) a complementary RNA strand is produced. The base pairings are as follows:

DNA	*RNA*
T-thymine	A-adenine
C-cytosine	G-guanine

Once RNA has been manufactured in the nucleus it moves fairly quickly into the cytoplasm.

Messenger RNA (mRNA) from the nucleus brings the coded message for protein synthesis to ribosomal RNA (rRNA). Ribosomal RNA imparts the message to *transfer* RNA (tRNA), which carries the specific amino acids coded for to the ribosomes, where protein synthesis is carried out.

Chromatin. The survival of the cell, organism, and species depends upon the chromatin material in the nucleus. Chromatin is DNA combined with protein, and stains with basic dyes. During the interphase of the cell cycle some chromosomes are visualized as tight coils and are referred to as *heterochromatin*. Heterochromatin is metabolically quite inactive and appears more electron dense. When chromosomes are active in the synthetic process, they are loosely coiled and one speaks in terms of *euchromatin*, which is more granular in appearance.

11. Ribosomes and Polysomes: Ribosomes may be free or attached to the membranes of the endoplasmic reticulum, which is then designated as rough ER. Ribosomes are the sites of protein synthesis in the cell. If ribosomes appear in clusters (rosettes) in the cytoplasm, they are commonly termed *polyribosomes* or *polysomes*.

Ribosomes are dense structures measuring about 15–25 nm in diameter. Both ribosomes attached to the endoplasmic reticulum and the free ones in the cytoplasm, form polyribosomes and perform identical functions.

Ribosomes possess RNA known as ribosomal RNA (rRNA) and both rRNA and messenger RNA (mRNA) are produced on DNA templates in the nucleus. Ribosomal RNA is very large in comparison to transfer RNA (tRNA), while the size of mRNA varies greatly.

Even though protein synthesis was discussed earlier, a brief repeat is in order since a form of RNA is an intricate part of every step. Amino acids are attached in the cytoplasm to tRNA, which consists of specific base triplets. The tRNA bonds to complimentary base triplets on the mRNA (formed on a DNA template in the nucleus). Therefore, specific base pairing and the nucleotide sequence of the mRNA determines the position of the tRNA sequence and thus the amino acid sequence. Amino acids are linked and form a polypeptide chain which eventually is released from the RNA. Transfer RNA and mRNA interaction form the ribosome mRNA complex and accomplish the synthesis of proteins.

As said earlier, ribosomes are complexed into polyribosomes; the number of ribosomes in a polyribosome seems to vary from 10 to 20. The importance of the polyribosome complex seems to lie in the fact that as amino acid sequences are laid down on the ribosome-mRNA complex in several areas, multiple chains of polypeptides are probably synthesized simultaneously on the polysomes using the same mRNA molecules.

12. Microtubules: These structures are usually associated with centrioles and basal bodies. They are also present in the cytoplasm of various cells, in particular the axons of neurons. Microtubules apparently function in the maintenance of the structural integrity (shape and rigidity) of the cell. Transport of material and movement of cilia and flagella are also ascribed to these organelles.

The microtubules are generally found to be 20–30 nm in diameter; their length is considerable. They are not membrane limited but their walls seem to be composed of regular units when observed in cross section. About a dozen units are seen and are thought to be composed of proteins called *tubulins*.

13. Microfilaments: These structures are prominent in the microvilli of the absorptive cells of the intestines. They have been shown to be associated with the regions of the terminal web and the desmosome. Their diameter is usually 5–8nm, and they are observed in groups of various sizes and distributions. They seem to work in conjunction with microtubules and function in maintaining the cytoskeletal configuration of the cell and in cellular movements.

14. Centrioles, Cilia and Flagella: The centrioles are self-reproducing organelles that play an important role in the separation of the chromosomes during mitosis. Before divi-

18 • MCAT SCIENCE REVIEW
sion of the cell the centriole splits into two and the daughter centrioles migrate to opposite sides of the nucleus. They form the center of the *spindle* and *aster* configuration during cell division; from the centriole the microtubules of the spindle radiate. Electron microscopy reveals that centrioles are composed of a peripheral cylinder which consists of 9 parallel sets of tubules in a triplet pattern. The triplets are embedded in an amorphous matrix.

Organelles almost identical in structure to the centriole are the basal bodies of cilia and flagella. A *basal body* is present at the base of each cilium and flagellum and it has the 9 + 0 configuration of the centriole. The centriole and basal bodies may, therefore, be closely related. Basal bodies control the structural makeup of cilia and flagella.

The structure and function of cilia and flagella are similar. They, like the centriole, have nine (9) sets of tubules arranged in a peripheral cylinder; the sets, however, are doublets, not triplets. And unlike centrioles, cilia and flagella have an additional pair of central tubules. Therefore we can summarize the arrangement in centrioles as 9 + 0, and cilia and flagella as 9 + 2.

There are usually two centrioles per cell (diplosome); many cilia per cell and usually only one flagellum. The two centrioles are usually arranged perpendicular to each other. Centrioles have no specific relationship or association with a membrance, but cilia and flagella are in a sense bounded by an extension of the cell membrane. Cilia and flagella participate in active movements. Cilia beat in unison and move liquid and particles on the surface of cells (ciliated epithelium of respiratory tract) while flagella move the whole cell or organism.

The nitrogenous bases can be listed as adenine, guanine, thymine, cytosine, and uracil. They pair in the following manner in DNA:

(1.) adenine and thymine
(2.) guanine and cytosine

There are four nitrogenous bases in RNA: adenine pairs with uracil and cytosine pairs with guanine.

The Watson and Crick model clearly illustrates the above pairings. Duplication of this material involves the splitting of the unions between purines and pyrimidines; each nucleotide then acquires a new complementary nucleotide and the phosphate and pentose moieties are then joined enzymatically and the duplication process has taken place.

RNA of the nucleolus provides the vehicle for the coded messages of the nuclear DNA to reach the machinery of the cell. Ribosomal RNA and RNA of the nucleolus are quite similar; ribosomal RNA probably is derived from RNA of the nucleolus. Messenger RNA from the nucleus brings the coded message for protein synthesis to ribosomal RNA. Ribosomal RNA imparts the message to transfer RNA, which carries the specific amino acids to the ribosomes, and protein synthesis is carried out.

Cell Division-Mitosis

For purposes of convenience, mitosis is divided into prophase, metaphase, anaphase, and telophase; the process, however, is a continuous one. The major events during the phases are:

1. Prophase: Chromosomes become distinct and nucleolus (nucleoli) disappear(s); centriole(s) and asters and spindle appear; nuclear membrane disappears.

2. Metaphase: Chromosomes move to the equator of the cell and duplicate.

3. Anaphase: The two chromatids split apart and start migration toward the poles of the spindle; the spindle loses its definition.

4. Telophase: Chromosomes lengthen and become less distinct; nucleoli reappear. The next period of growth and rest is known as *interphase*.

5. Interphase: Cell growth; protein synthesis; DNA synthesis; chromosome duplication.

Methods of Examining the Cell

1. Histological Methods:

a. *Microscopy.* Microscopes are usually classified according to the type of energy source. Besides the straight light microscope and the electron microscope, the researcher utilizes polarization, phase contrast, interference, ultraviolet, and X-ray microscopes.

b. *Stains.* Dyes are used in solution to stain generally the nucleus and/or cytoplasm, or specifically, particular cell components. Dyes in general are neutral salts having both acidic and basic radicals. A basic dye exhibits its coloring property because of the basic radical it possesses. Structures stained by it are designated as basophilic—the nucleus, for example. An acidic dye exhibits its staining property because of the acidic radical. Structures delineated by it are acidophilic—the cytoplasm, for example.

Examples of stains routinely employed:

1) Hematoxylin, a common histologic stain, stains nuclei blue;
2) The common histological stain eosin (H&E) and other acidic dyes, such as picric acid, stain the general cytoplasm;
3) Iron hematoxylin, which stains chromosomes, mitochondria, Golgi complex, and contractile elements of muscle cells black or dark blue;
4) Carmine, which stains nuclei red-purple;
5) Basic aniline dyes, such as toluidine blue, azure A and methylene blue, which stain mucopolysaccharides metachromatically;
6) Mallory's connective tissue (CT) stain, which stains collagen fibers bright blue, nuclei red or orange, and various cell components blue, red, orange or purple;
7) Reticular fibers, which are argyrophilic, are stained brown by silver impregnation methods.

2. Histochemical Methods:
Tissues are composed of various chemicals such as proteins, carbohydrates, lipids, inorganic salts and miscellaneous substances, and various tests are used to detect these chemicals.

Examples:

1) Proteins (with tyrosine)—yellow color;
2) Enzymes—various tests for phosphatases, lipases, oxidases, esterases, and dehydrogenases;
3) Carbohydrates—glycogen by periodic acid Schiff (PAS) test results in a magenta or purple color; glycoproteins give a positive PAS magenta color. Basal laminae and reticular fibers are strongly PAS positive;
4) Lipids—Sudan dyes or osmic acid;
5) Nucleic acids—Feulgen reaction is specific for DNA, but not for RNA, which can be detected by ribonuclease. Both DNA and RNA are basophilic (because they are both acids).

3. Fixation:
The fixative must modify the cell to resist further treatments and also to make further treatments possible. Fixatives may be classified as either coagulant or non-coagulant. Examples of each are:

1) *coagulant:* methanol, ethanol, acetone, nitric acid, hydrochloric acid, picric acid, trichloroacetic acid and mercuric chloride.
2) *non-coagulant:* formaldehyde, glutaraldehyde, osmium tetroxide, potassium dichromate, acetic acid, and potassium permanganate.

Fixatives can also be subclassified into two categories. The following are examples:

1) *additive:* osmium tetroxide, formaldehyde, and glutaraldehyde.
2) *non-additive:* methanol, ethanol, and acetone.

4. Method of Preparation

1) *Fixation:* a piece of tissue is placed in a killing (preservative) solution; processes of the cell are stopped as close to normal as possible;

2) *Dehydration:* water is usually removed from the tissues by passing it through a series of increasing strengths of alcohol solutions;

3) *Embedding:* embedding places the tissues in a solid medium;

4) *Sectioning:* tissue is cut into 5 microns or 5000 nm for light, and about 60 nm for electron microscopic evaluation;

5) *Staining:* dyes for light microscopy and heavy metals for electron microscopy enhance visualization.

Eukaryotic vs. Prokaryotic Cell Structure

Eukaryotes: All higher animals and plants, as well as protozoa, are eukaryotes, and their cells possess the following characteristics:

A nucleus surrounded by a nuclear membrane (nucleolemma)

Discrete chromosomes that are present in the nucleus and undergo reduplication.

DNA (deoxyribonucleic acid) that stores the vital information for the functioning of the cell.

DNA synthesis as the mode of duplication. Mitosis separates chromosomes which have already duplicated.

Cellular metabolites such as protein, RNA, vacuoles, ribosomes, and mitochondria in the cytoplasm.

Cilia and flagella that possess the basic structure of two inner fibrils surrounded by nine outer ones. (Flagella of eukaryotic and prokaryotic organisms are structurally different.)

In addition, most eukaryotic cells are surrounded by a lipoprotein cell membrane; some also possess a cell wall (plants).

Prokaryotes: Bacteria (and blue-green algae) are the organisms which make up this important category. They possess the following characteristics:

1) The nucleus or nucleoid consists mostly of DNA and is never enveloped by a nuclear membrane. DNA is visualized as fine fibrils and is not organized into chromosomes. Mitosis does not occur.

2) In the cytoplasm vacuoles and mitochondria are absent. Many of the reactions that take place in the mitochondrion of the eukaryotic cell are carried out by the prokaryotic cell membrane.

3) Cytoplasmic granules which store carbohydrates, lipids, or volutin (polymetaphosphate) are present.

4) Ribosomes are present.

5) A cell membrane surrounds the cytoplasm; however, unlike the eukaryotic cell membrane, it lacks sterols and is made up only of phospholipid and protein.

6) The cell membrane is a highly synthetic structure: it contains the respiratory enzymatic machinery; is the site of DNA attachment; and serves in the control of permeability.

7) A cell wall giving integrity to the organism is present. In some cells constituents such as endotoxins play a role in disease. (Cell wall structure determines susceptibility to the attack by chemotherapeutic agents.)

8) A polysaccharide-polypeptide capsule is laid down outside the cell wall. This material may play a vital role in the virulence of a pathogenic bacteria since it can interfere with the ability of the host's leukocytes to phagocytize the bacteria. The capsular material of each bacterial strain is unique.

9) Flagella, if present, have a structure different from that of eukaryotes. Each flagellum consists of a single fibril (not the typical 11 axial fibrils), which originates from a basal granule of the cytoplasmic membrane.

10) They may produce spores (endospores) which are thick-walled and protect them during unfavorable conditions. Spores exhibit greater resistance to heat, drying, freezing, chemical agents and radiation than their vegetative counterparts. Spores possess the compound dipicolinic acid; the calcium salt of this acid plays a role in resistance to heat (the higher the calcium dipicolinate concentration, the more heat resistant).

Reproduction and Genetics in Eukaryotes and Prokaryotes: Genetic stability in eukaryotes and prokaryotes is comparable. Frequency of mutations is the same. Eukaryotes introduce changes via sexual reproduction (combination of gametes). They also reproduce asexually using various methods. Sexual reproduction *per se* does not occur in prokaryotes. However, three very effective processes do result in the mixing of genetic material. They are:

a. *Transformation*. DNA released from a donor cell into a medium is taken up and incorporated by a recipient cell; it results in the replacement of part of the cell's genetic material.

b. *Conjugation*. Genetic material is transferred from one bacterium to another via a conjugation bridge.

c. *Transduction*. Genetic material is transferred from one bacterium to another via a bacteriophage (a bacterial virus).

Classification of Living Organisms

Taxonomy is the classification of living organisms based on characteristics and ancestry. Two *kingdoms*—animal and plant— are easily distinguished. In general, members of the former consume food and are mobile while those of the latter are stationary and produce their own nutrients.

Several systems have evolved to classify the great variety of living organisms. One such system divides living things into five kingdoms based on (1) the presence (eukaryotic) or absence (prokaryotic) of membrane-bound nuclei in the cells; (2) the number of cells forming the organism, and (3) the mechanism for nutrition. This five-kingdom classification system is shown in the following table.

FIVE-KINGDOM CLASSIFICATION SYSTEM

Kingdom	Characteristics	Examples
Monera	unicellular without organized nuclei; absorb or produce their own nutrients	bacteria, blue-green algae
Protista	unicellular with membrane-bound nuclei; ingest, absorb or produce nutrients via photosynthesis	protozoans, algae
Fungi	multicellular with membrane-bound nuclei; absorb nutrients	mushrooms, molds
Plants	multicellular with membrane-bound nuclei and a cell wall; possess chlorophyll and undergo photosynthesis	flowering plants and trees; evergreens
Animals	multicellular with membrane-bound nuclei; ingest nutrients	mammals, birds, amphibians, fish, reptiles, insects, crustaceans, etc.

These kingdoms can be divided into three main groups based on the mode of nutrition—photosynthetic organisms (plants and algae), organisms which absorb their nutrients (bacteria and fungi), and organisms which engulf or ingest their nutrients (protozoa and animals).

Each kingdom is further divided into phyla (sing. phylum), which are subdivided as follows: phyla → into classes → into families → into genera → into species. Each of these groups may be divided into 6 additional subgroups.

All living organisms are given a scientific name using the combination of genus and species. Under this binomial naming system, the scientific name for a human is *Homo sapiens*. To illustrate the classification system a demonstration of how one classifies a human is given below:

CLASSIFICATION OF THE HUMAN

Classification Group		Distinguishing Features
Kingdom	Animalia	Consume food and are mobile.
Phylum	Chordata	Notochord, hollow nervous system (neural tube) dorsally positioned, gill slits in pharyngeal wall, heart ventral to digestive system.
Subphylum	Vertebrata	Segmental vertebral column.
Class	Mammalia	Mammary glands for nourishment of young; hair or fur; warm-blooded; diaphragm.
Order	Primates	Large cerebral hemispheres; opposable digits; nails; highly developed sense of sight—eyes directed forward; teeth specialized for different functions.
Family	Hominidae	Walk with two limbs (bipedal locomotion); binocular color vision.
Genus	Homo	Ability to speak and most highly developed and largest brain.
Species	sapiens	Large skull, high forehead, reduced size of brow (supraorbital) ridges, prominent chin; decreased amount of body hair.

Organization of the Human Body

A multicellular organism is composed of millions of cells organized into functional units (organs and systems) which are formed by various groups of similar cells (tissues) working together. These cells are embedded in intercellular substances and tissue fluids. A *tissue* consists of a group of cells performing a similar function. Four basic tissues compose the human (mammalian) body: epithelium, connective tissue, muscle and nerve tissues. The four basic tissues may be organized to form functional units known as *organs*. Each organ has a definite function which results from the combined functions of the various tissue components. Several organs which function together as a unit for a specified purpose make up an organ *system*. The animal *organism* is composed of several interrelated organ systems. The human body is composed of the systems listed in the following table.

Organ Systems

The human body is composed of the systems listed in the following table.

ORGAN SYSTEMS IN THE HUMAN

System	Functions
Muscular	Produces motion of body parts and viscera.
Skeletal	Supports the body, protects organs and produces blood cells.
Circulatory	Transports nutrients, wastes, gases (oxygen and carbon dioxide), hormones, blood cells throughout body; also protects body against foreign organisms.
Nervous	Responds to internal and external stimuli; regulates and coordinates body activities and movements.
Integumentary	Limits and protects the body as a whole; prevents excess loss of water and functions in regulating body temperature.
Digestive	Enzymatically breaks down food materials into usable and absorbable nutrients.
Respiratory	Functions in the exchange of gases (oxygen and carbon dioxide).
Urinary	Removes body wastes from blood stream and helps regulate homeostasis of internal environment.
Reproductive	Perpetuates the living organism by the production of sex cells (gametes) and future offsprings.
Endocrine	Regulates body growth and function via hormones.

Four Basic Tissues

1. Muscle Tissue: Muscle tissue is contractile in nature and functions to move the skeletal system and body viscera.

TYPES OF MUSCLE

Type	Characteristics	Location
Skeletal	striated, voluntary	skeletal muscles of the body
Smooth	non-striated, involuntary	walls of digestive tract and blood vessels, uterus, urinary bladder
Cardiac	striated, involuntary	heart

2. Nervous Tissue: Nervous tissue is composed of cells *(neurons)* that respond to external and internal stimuli and have the capability to transmit a message *(impulse)* from one area of the body to another. This tissue thus induces a response of distant muscles or glands, as well as regulating body processes such as respiration, circulation, and digestion. Nervous tissue composes the central (brain and spinal cord) and peripheral (peripheral nerves, ganglia and receptors) nervous systems and the special sensory receptors (eye, ear, taste buds and olfactory region).

3. Epithelial Tissue: Epithelial tissue covers the external surfaces of the body and lines the internal tubes and cavities. It also forms the glands of the body. Characteristics of epithelial tissue (epithelium) are that it
  (1) has compactly aggregated cells;
  (2) has limited intercellular spaces and substance;
  (3) is avascular (no blood vessels);
  (4) lies on a connective tissue layer—the basal lamina;
  (5) has cells that form sheets and are polarized;
  (6) is derived from all three germ layers.

TYPES OF EPITHELIUM

Classification	Location(s)	Function(s)
Simple squamous epithelium	Endothelium of blood and lymphatic vessels; Bowman's capsule and thin loop of Henle in kidney; mesothelium lining pericardial, peritoneal and pleural body cavities; lung alveoli; smallest excretory ducts of glands.	Lubrication of body cavities (permits free movement of organs); pinocytotic transport across cells.
Stratified squamous keratinized epithelium	Epidermis of skin.	Prevents loss of water and protection.
Stratified squamous nonkeratinized epithelium (moist)	Mucosa of oral cavity, esophagus, anal canal; vagina; cornea of eye and part of conjunctiva.	Secretion; protection; prevents loss of water.
Simple cuboidal epithelium	Kidney tubules; choroid plexus; thyroid gland; rete testis; surface of ovary.	Secretion; absorption; lines surface.
Stratified cuboidal epithelium	Ducts of sweat glands; developing follicles of ovary.	Secretion; protection.
Simple columnar epithelium	Cells lining lumen of digestive tract (stomach to rectum); gall bladder; many glands (secretory units and ducts); uterus; uterine tube (ciliated).	Secretion; absorption; protection; lubrication.
Pseudostratified columnar epithelium	Lines lumen of respiratory tract (nasal cavity, trachea and bronchi) (ciliated); ducts of epididymis (stereocilia); ductus deferens; male urethra.	Secretion; protection; facilitates transport of substances on surface of cells.
Stratified columnar epithelium	Male urethra; conjunctiva.	Protection.
Transitional epithelium	Urinary tract (renal calyces and pelvis, ureter and urinary bladder).	Protection.

Epithelial cells may also have specializations at the cell surface. For example,

microvilli—fingerlike projections of plasma membranes. Mainly located at luminal surfaces of absorptive cells (brush border of proximal convoluted tubules and striated border of intestinal epithelium).

cilia—motile organelles extending into the luman consisting of specifically arranged microtubules. Mainly located in respiratory epithelium and part of female reproductive tract.

flagella—similar to cilia. Primary examples are human spermatozoa.

stereocilia—are actually very elongated microvilli.

4. Connective Tissue: Connective tissue is the packing and supporting material of the body tissues and organs. It develops from mesoderm (mesenchyme). All connective tissues consist of three distinct components: ground substance, cells and fibers.

a. *Ground substance*. Ground substance is located between the cells and fibers, both of which are embedded in it. It forms an amorphous intercellar material. In the fresh state, it appears as a transparent and homogeneous gel. It acts as a route for the passage of nutrients and wastes to and from the cells within or adjacent to the connective tissue. The ground substance is composed of mucopolysaccharides *(glycosaminoglycans)*, proteins, lipids and water. The primary glycosaminoglycans found in the ground substance are chondroitin sulfate and hyaluronic acid, the latter present in greater quantity.

b. *Fibers*. The fiber components of connective tissue add support and strength. Three types of fibers are present: *collagenous, elastic* and *reticular*.

Collagen fibers (white fibers) are the most numerous fiber type and are present in all types of connective tissue in varying amounts. Collagen bundles are strong and resist stretching. They are found in structures such as tendons, ligaments, aponeuroses and fascia, which are subjected to pull or stretching activities.

Elastic fibers (yellow fibers) are refractile fibers which are thinner (0.2 to 1 μm diameter) than collagen fibers. They are extremely elastic and are located in structures with a degree of elasticity, such as the walls of blood vessels (elastic arteries), true vocal cords and trachea.

Reticular fibers are thinner (0.2 to 1 μm diameter) than collagenous fibers. They are arranged in an intermeshing network (reticulum) which supports the organ. Reticular fibers are inelastic. They are found in the walls of blood vessels, lymphoid tissues (spleen and lymph nodes), red bone marrow, basal laminae and glands (liver and kidney).

c. *Cells*. The *cells* of connective tissue are primarily attached and non-motile *(fixed cells),* but some have the ability to move *(wandering or free cells)*. The typical cells found in connective tissue are:

Fibroblasts constitute the largest number of cells present in connective tissue. In an actively secreting state, they are flattened stellate-shaped cells with an oval nucleus and basophilic cytoplasm due to the numerous rough endoplasmic reticulum. In the inactive state, they appear as elongated spindles with a more basophilic oval or elongated nucleus. In this state, they are referred to as *fibrocytes*. The latter are the main cellular constituents of connective tissue structures such as tendons and ligaments. Only the nuclei of fibrocytes are observed between the fibers since the cytoplasm is indistinct. The terms fibrocyte and fibroblast are often used interchangeably.

Mesenchymal cells are undifferentiated connective tissue cells which have the potential to differentiate into other types of connective tissue cells. They are primarily found in embyronic and fetal tissues; some are thought to be present in the adult abutting the walls of capillaries. They are smaller than fibroblasts and are stellate in shape. They are capable of moving by extending their cell processes into the gel-like ground substance.

Macrophages (histiocytes) may be fixed or free. Free macrophages may wander through the connective tissue by extending their cell processes. Fixed macrophages are very numerous in loose connective tissue. They are polymorphic in shape and contain an oval nucleus. They have the ability to engulf extracellular material (foreign matter or necrotic cells). Macrophages are difficult to distinguish except when they are actively phagocytosing material and thus contain many vacuoles.

Adipocytes (fat cells) are found in most connective tissue, either singly or in groups. If the connective tissue layer is primarily composed of fat cells, it is referred to as adipose tissue. An adipocyte is a round, large cell with a distinct, dense nucleus usually located at the periphery of the cytoplasm. The majority of the cytoplasmic (cell) volume is taken up by a large lipid droplet. Due to the clear appearing cytoplasm and dark nucleus at one pole, the cell has a signet ring appearance. Fat cells do not undergo mitosis.

Mast cells are ovoid cells with small round nuclei. The cytoplasm contains numerous coarse basophilic granules which also stain metachromatically and are soluble in water. The mast cell granules are composed of *histamine* and an anticoagulant known as *heparin*. Histamine dilates blood vessels and increases the permeability of capillaries, thus increasing interstitial fluid. Mast cells take part in the allergic response of the body. Mast cells are found in most connective tissue and are numerous in the respiratory tract and near small blood vessels.

Plasma cells have a characteristic eccentric nucleus which contains chromatin arranged in a definite pattern near the nuclear envelope. This pattern gives a "cartwheel or spoke wheel" appearance. The juxtanuclear cytoplasm appears clear and less basophilic due to the Golgi complex located in this area. Plasma cells are found in the lamina propria of the gastrointestinal tract. They function in protecting the body against bacterial invasion by secreting antibodies (immunoglobulins—IgG) into the circulating blood.

Reticular cells are star-shaped cells which join via their processes to form a cellular network. They are found abutting reticular fibers in certain glands and lymphoid tissues.

Pericytes are located in the adventitia of blood vessels. They are believed to be multipotential cells which may differentiate into various connective tissue cells as well as into smooth muscle cells.

White blood cells or leukocytes. Certain white blood cells migrate out of the blood into the extracellular ground substance. The main leukocytes found in the connective tissue are lymphocytes, monocytes, eosinophils, basophils and neutrophils. The leukocytes in connective tissue are similar in structure and function to those in the blood. The agranular leukocytes migrate in large numbers under normal conditions. Lymphocytes accumulate in areas in response to chronic inflammation. Neutrophils also migrate in large numbers into the interstitium during an inflammatory response. Eosinophils occur in areas involved in allergic reactions, such as the respiratory tract.

Skeletal System

The skeletal system of vertebrates is an *endoskeleton*—that is, it is within the body—as compared to an *exoskeleton* characteristic of arthropods. The human skeletal system provides:

(1) support
(2) protection of vital organs
(3) sites for muscle attachment
(4) storage sites of body calcium and phosphates
(5) sites for blood cell formation

The *human skeleton* consists of bone and cartilage. The bones form the main rigid structure of the skeleton. The human skeleton consists of about 206 bones, some of which are fused while others are joined together at sites which permit various degrees of movement.

The sites of junction, or articulation, whether movable or immovable, are known as *joints*.

The human skelton is divided into an *axial skeleton* and an *appendicular skeleton*.

Axial Skeleton

The axial skeleton consists of 80 bones forming the trunk (spine and thorax) and skull.

Vertebral Column: The main trunk of the body is supported by the spine, or vertebral column, which is composed of 26 bones, some of which are formed by the fusion of a few bones. The vertebral column from superior to inferior consists of 7 cervical (neck), 12 thoracic and 5 lumbar vertebrae, as well as a sacrum, formed by fusion of 5 sacral vertebrae, and a coccyx, formed by fusion of 4 coccygeal vertebrae. Each vertebra consists of a body anteriorly and an arched posterior region circumscribing an inner central canal, the *vertebral canal,* which extends from the foramen magnum at the base of the skull through the sacrum. The vertebral column functions to support the trunk of the body and to protect the spinal cord located in the vertebral canal. The vertebrae of the cervical, thoracic and lumbar regions are separated from each other by round fibro-cartilaginous articular discs known as *intervertebral discs*. The entire vertebral column is held together by ligaments.

Ribs and Sternum: The axial skeleton also contains 12 pairs of *ribs* attached posteriorly to the thoracic vertebrae and anteriorly either directly or via cartilage to the *sternum* (breastbone). The ribs and sternum form the *thoracic cage,* which protects the heart and lungs. Seven pairs of ribs articulate with the sternum *(fixed ribs)* directly, and three do so via cartilage; the two most inferior pairs do not attach anteriorly and are referred to as *floating ribs*.

Skull: The *skull* consists of 22 bones fused together to form a rigid structure which houses and protects organs such as the brain, auditory apparatus and eyes. The bones of the skull form the *face* and *cranium* (brain case) and consist of 6 single bones (*occipital, frontal, ethmoid, sphenoid, vomer* and *mandible*) and 8 paired bones (*parietal, temporal, maxillary, palatine, zygomatic, lacrimal, inferior concha* and *nasal*) The *lower jaw* or *mandible* is the only movable bone of the skull (head); it articulates with the temporal bones.

Other Parts: Other bones considered part of the axial skeleton are the *middle ear bones* (*ossicles*) and the small U-shaped *hyoid bone* that is suspended in a portion of the neck by 3uscles and ligaments.

Appendicular Skeleton

The appendicular skeleton forms the major internal support of the appendages—the *upper* and *lower extremities* (limbs).

Pectoral Girdle and Upper Extremities: The arms are attached to and suspended from the axial skeleton via the *shoulder* (*pectoral*) girdle. The latter is composed of two *clavicles* (*collarbones*) and two *scapulae* (*shoulder blades*). The clavicles articulate with the sternum; the two *sternoclavicular joints* are the only sites of articulation between the trunk and upper extremity.

Each upper limb from distal to proximal (closest to the body) consists of hand, wrist, forearm and arm (upper arm). The *hand* consists of 5 *digits* (fingers) and 5 *metacarpal* bones. Each digit is comprised of three bones known as *phalanges,* except the thumb which has only two bones. The *wrist* consists of eight *carpal* bones which articulate with metacarpals. The *forearm* consists of two bones, the *ulna* on the side of the fifth digit (little finger) and the *radius* on the thumb side. The articulation between radius and ulna at the wrist permits rotation of the radius over the ulna during pronation (palm facing backward) and supination (palm turned forward). The ulna articulates at the elbow joint with the *humerus* creating a hinge joint and movement of the arm. The humerus, in turn, is connected to the shoulder girdle at the *glenoid cavity* of the scapula.

Pelvic Girdle and Lower Extremities: The lower *extremities,* or legs, are attached to the axial skeleton via the *pelvic* or *hip girdle.* Each of the two coxal, or *hip, bones* comprising the pelvic girdle is formed by the fusion of three bones—*ilium, pubis* and *ischium.* The coxal bones attach the lower limbs to the trunk by articulating with the sacrum.

From distal to proximal the lower limb consists of foot, ankle, shank and thigh. The *foot* consists of 5 digits *(toes)* and 5 *metatarsals.* The digits contain 3 *phalanges* each, except for the big toe, which has two. The *ankle* is formed by 7 *tarsal* bones. The shank region is supported by two bones, the *tibia* and *fibula.* The tibia is larger, is located medially, forms the shin, and articulates at the knee joint with the *femur (thigh bone).* The knee joint is protected anteriorly by the kneecap, or *patella.* The femur articulates with the *acetabular fossa* of the coxal bone.

THE HUMAN SKELETAL SYSTEM

Part of the Skeleton	Number of Bones
Axial Skeleton	**80**
Skull	22
Ossicles (malleus, incus and stapes)	6
Vertebral column	26
Ribs	24
Sternum	1
Hyoid	1
Appendicular Skeleton	**126**
Upper extremities	64
Lower extremities	62

Characteristics of Bone

Bone is a specialized type of connective tissue consisting of cells *(osteocytes)* embedded in a calcified matrix which gives bone its characteristic hard and rigid nature. Bones are encased by a *periosteum,* a connective tissue sheath. All bone has a central marrow cavity. *Bone marrow* fills the marrow cavity or smaller marrow spaces, depending on the type of bone.

Types of Bone: There are two types of bone in the skeleton: *compact bone* and *spongy* (cancellous) bone.

Compact Bone. Compact bone lies within the periosteum, forms the outer region of bones, and appears dense due to its compact organization. The living osteocytes and calcified matrix are arranged in layers, or *lamellae.* Lamellae may be circularly arranged surrounding a central canal, the *Haversian canal,* which contains small blood vessels. This unit of a Haversian canal circumscribed by Haversian lamellae is known as an *Haversian system,* or *osteon.* Osteons are oriented along the longitudinal axis of the bone and communicate with each other, the periosteum, and the marrow cavity via oblique or transverse canals known as *Volkmann's canals.* Blood vessels enter and leave and are distributed throughout bone via the Haversian and Volkmann's canals. Irregular lamellae structures, the *interstitial lamellae,* are present between the Haversian systems. They are remnants of resorbed lamellar systems resulting from the remodelling of bone. The inner (next to marrow cavity) and outer (next to periosteum) limits of compact bone are formed by lamellar structures, the *inner (endosteal)* and *outer (periosteal) circumferential lamellae,* respectively. The Haversian systems are the major component of compact bone and lie between these two circumferential lamellae. The marrow cavity and Haversian canals are lined by *endosteum,* a thin layer of connective tissue. Both the endosteum and periosteum contain *osteogenic cells,* which can transform into bone-forming cells, or *osteoblasts.*

Spongy bone. Spongy bone consists of *bars, spicules* or *trabeculae,* which form a lattice meshwork. Spongy bone is found at the ends of long bones and the inner layer of flat, irregular and short bones. The trabeculae consist of osteocytes embedded in calcified matrix, which in definitive bone has a lamellar nature. The spaces between the trabeculae contain bone marrow.

Bone Cells: The cells of bone are osteocytes, osteoblasts, and osteoclasts. *Osteocytes* are found singly in *lacunae* (spaces) within the calcified matrix and communicate with each other via small canals in the bone known as *canaliculi.* The latter contain osteocyte cell processes. The osteocytes in compact and spongy bone are similar in structure and function.

Osteoblasts are cells which form bone matrix, surrounding themselves with it, and thus are transformed into osteocytes. They arise from undifferentiated cells, such as mesenchymal cells. They are cuboidal cells which line the trabeculae of immature or developing spongy bone.

Osteoclasts are found during bone development and remodelling. They are multinucleated cells lying in cavities, *Howship's lacunae,* on the surface of the bone tissue being resorbed. Osteoclasts remove the existing calcified matrix releasing the inorganic or organic components.

Bone Matrix: *Matrix* of compact and spongy bone consists of collagenous fibers and ground substance which constitute the organic component of bone. Matrix also consists of inorganic material which is about 65% of the dry weight of bone. Approximately 85% of the inorganic component consists of calcium phosphate in a crystalline form (hydroxyapatite crystals.) Glycoproteins are the main components of the ground substance.

MAJOR TYPES OF HUMAN BONES

Type of Bone	Characteristics	Examples
Long bones	Width less than length.	Humerus, radius, ulna, femur, tibia.
Short bones	Length and width close to equal in size.	Carpal and tarsal bones.
Flat bones	Thin flat shape.	Scapulae, ribs, sternum, bones of cranium (occipital, frontal, parietal).
Irregular bones	Multifaceted shape.	Vertebrae, sphenoid, ethmoid.
Sesamoid	Small bones located in tendons of muscles.	Patella (kneecap) in quadraceps femoris tendon.

Joints

The bones of the skeleton articulate with each other at *joints,* which are variable in structure and function. Some joints are immovable, such as the *sutures* between the bones of the cranium. Others are *slightly movable joints;* examples are the *intervertebral joints* and the *pubic symphysis* (joint between the two pubic bones of the coxal bones). These contain fibrocartilage plates separating the articulating bones and have a slight gliding motion. The most common joints are *freely movable joints.* They are also referred to as *synovial joints* since their joint capsules are lined by a serous *synovial membrane* which produces a lubricating fluid—*synovial fluid*—between the articulating bones. The *capsule* is a fibrous connective tissue sheath which encases the joint. Another feature of synovial joints is that a thin layer of *hyaline cartilage* lines the articular surfaces of the abutting bones. The synovial joints can be classified according to the type of motion permitted by the structure of the joint.

TYPES OF JOINTS

Joint Type	Characteristic	Example
Ball and socket	Permits all types of movement (abduction, adduction, flexion, extension, circumduction); it is considered a universal joint.	Hip and shoulder joints.
Hinge (ginglymus)	Permits motion in one plane only.	Elbow and knee, interphalangeal joints.
Rotating or pivot	Rotation is only motion permitted.	Radius and ulna, atlas and axis (first and second cervical vertebrae).
Plane or gliding	Permits sliding motion.	Between tarsal bones and carpal bones.
Condylar (condyloid)	Permits motion in two planes which are at right angles to each other (rotation is not possible).	Metacaro-phalangeal joints, temporomandibular.

Adjacent bones at a joint are connected by fibrous connective tissue bands known as *ligaments*. They are strong bands which support the joint and may also act to limit the degree of motion occurring at a joint.

Muscular System

Classification

A muscle cell not only has the ability to propagate an action potential along its cell membrane, as does a nerve cell, but also has the internal machinery to give it the unique ability to contract.

Most muscles in the body can be classified as striated muscles in reference to the fact that when observed under a light microscope the muscular tissue has light and dark bands or striations running across it. Although both skeletal and cardiac muscles are striated and therefore have similar structural organizations, they do possess some characteristic functional differences. Skeletal muscle contraction, for example, is made up of the contraction of many motor units. A motor unit consists of a single motor neuron coming from the spinal cord of the central nervous system and all the muscle fibers which it innervates (a few to 2000).

In contrast to skeletal muscle, cardiac muscle is a functional syncytium. This means that although anatomically it consists of individual cells the entire mass normally responds as a unit and all of the cells contract together. In addition, cardiac muscle has the property of automaticity which means that the heart initiates its own contraction without the need for motor nerves. Motor nerves may alter this inherent rhythm but the resource for initiating the contraction lies within the special cardiac cells called pacemaker cells. Here an action potential is initiated and spreads to the other cardiac cells.

Non-striated muscle consists of multi-unit and unitary (visceral) smooth muscle. Visceral smooth muscle has many of the properties of cardiac muscle. To some extent it acts as a functional syncytium e.g., areas of intestinal smooth muscle will contract as a unit. Smooth muscle is part of the urinary bladder, uterus, spleen, gallbladder, and numerous other internal organs. It is also the muscle of blood vessels, respiratory tracts, and the iris of the eye.

The basic contractile mechanism is probably the same in all muscle types although the structural organization of smooth muscle is very different from that of striated muscle. We will concentrate on skeletal muscle, knowing that what we discuss can be applied to cardiac muscle and to some extent to smooth muscle.

Skeletal Muscles

In order for the human being to carry out the many intricate movements that must be performed, approximately 650 skeletal muscles of various lengths, shapes, and strength play a part. Each muscle consists of many muscle cells or fibers held together and surrounded by connective tissue that gives functional integrity to the system. Three definite units are commonly referred to:

(1) endomysium—connective tissue layer enveloping a single fiber;
(2) perimysium—connective tissue layer enveloping a bundle of fibers;
(3) epimysium—connective tissue layer enveloping the entire muscle.

Muscle Attachment and Function

For coordinated movement to take place, the muscle must attach to either bone or cartilage or, as in the case of the muscles of facial expression, to skin. The portion of a muscle attaching to bone is the tendon. A muscle has two extremities, its origin and its insertion; the origin is the relatively fixed attachment site, while the insertion is the end attached to a structure that will be moved when the muscle contracts. A pair of muscles usually control the movement of a joint; they are opposing or antagonistic muscles. For example, a flexor muscle is opposed by an extensor.

Terms to Describe Movement

Flexion is bending, most often ventrally to decrease the angle between two parts of the body; it is usually an action at an articulation or joint.

Extension is straightening, or increasing the angle between two parts of the body; a stretching out or making the flexed part straight.

Abduction is a movement away from the midsagittal plane (midline); to abduct is to move laterally.

Adduction is a movement toward the midsagittal plane (midline); to adduct is to move medially and bring a part back to the mid-axis.

Circumduction is a circular movement at a ball and socket (shoulder or hip) joint, utilizing the movements of flexion, extension, abduction, and adduction.

Rotation is a movement of a part of the body around its long axis.

Examples: a. The atlas (1st cervical vertebra) rotates on the axis (2nd cervical vertebra).
b. The thigh may be rotated medially or internally; it may also be rotated laterally or externally.

Supination refers only to the movement of the radius around the ulna. In supination the palm of the hand is oriented anteriorly; turning the palm dorsally puts it into pronation. The body on its back is in the supine position.

Pronation refers to the palm of the hand being oriented posteriorly. The body on its belly is the prone position.

Inversion refers only to the lower extremity, specifically the ankle joint. When the foot (plantar surface) is turned inward, so that the sole is pointing and directed toward the midline of the body and is parallel with the median plane, we speak of inversion. Its opposite is eversion.

Eversion refers to the foot (plantar surface) being turned outward so that the sole is pointing laterally.

Opposition is one of the most critical movements in humans; it allows us to have pulp-to-pulp opposition, which gives us the great dexterity of our hands. In this movement the thumb pad is brought to a finger pad. A median nerve injury negates this action.

Muscle Names

The names of some muscles may appear strange; the naming, however, is based essentially on anatomical position, function, shape, or other feature. Here are some examples:

1. **Position and Location:**

   a. Pectoralis major and minor — pectoral region of thorax; the major is larger

   b. Temporalis — temporal region of head

   c. Infra- and supraspinatus — below and above spine of scapula

   d. External and internal intercostals — refers to their location in the intercostal spaces

2. **Principal Action:**

   a. pronators (e.g., pronator quadratus) and supinators — pronators refers to palm down and supinator to palm up; quadratus refers to the shape

   b. Flexors and extensors (e.g., flexor and extensor digitorum) — flexors and extensors of digits

   c. Levator scapulae — elevator of the scapula (shoulder)

3. **Shape:**

   a. Trapezius — trapezoid in shape

   b. Rhomboid major and minor — rhomboid in shape

4. **Number of Divisions (Heads) and Position:**

   a. Biceps brachii — two-headed muscle in anterior brachium (arm)

   b. Triceps brachii — three-headed muscle in posterior brachium (arm)

5. **Size, Length, and Shape:**

   a. Flexor pollicis longus and brevis — long and short flexors of the thumb

   b. Rhomboid major and minor — major is larger in size; rhomboid in shape.

6. Attachment Sites:

a. Sternocleidomastoid — extends from sternum and clavicle (cleido) to mastoid process

b. Sternohyoid — extends from sternum to hyoid bone

Structural Organization of a Muscle Fiber

A muscle fiber is a single muscle cell. If we look at a section of a fiber we see that it is complete with a cell membrane called the sarcolemma and has several nuclei located just under the sarcolemma—it is multinucleated. Each fiber is composed of numerous cylindrical fibrils running the entire length of the fiber.

The fibril exhibits light and dark bands—the "I" and "A" bands respectively. The "I" band is bisected by the "Z" line and the "A" band by the "M" line. There is a somewhat lighter band within the "A" band that is called the "H" band. An even lighter area in the middle of the "H" zone on either side of the "M" line is called the "pseudo-H" band.

These striations are produced by the arrangement within the fibril of myofilaments which make up the contractile machinery. A sarcomere, the area between two "Z" bands, is the functional unit of muscle; it is the region between two "Z" lines and consists of an "A" band and half of two abutting "I" bands. Refer to the illustration of the relaxed myofibril (page 35) for the positions of these lines and bands.

Myofilaments

1. The thick and thin myofilaments form the contractile machinery of muscle and are made up of proteins. Approximately 54% of all the contractile proteins (by weight) is myosin. The thick myofilament is composed of many myosin molecules oriented tail-end to tail-end at the center with myosin molecules staggered from the center to the myofilament tip.

2. The second major contractile protein is actin. Actin is a globular protein. The thin myofilament contains two chains of F-actin arranged in a twisted fashion. This configuration gives the thin myofilament a certain periodicity. Associated with the thin myofilament along its entire length is the globular protein troponin. The pressure of troponin along with tropomyosin-B inhibits myosin-actin interaction—it represses actomyosin formation. Calcium ions released following an action potential in the fiber membrane and T-tubules bind with troponin. Calcium-troponin binding removes the inhibition of actomyosin formation.

Sarcoplasm

The sarcoplasm (cytoplasm of the muscle cell) contains Golgi complexes near the nuclei. Mitochondria are found between the myofibrils and just below the sarcolemma. The myofibrils are surrounded by smooth endoplasmic reticulum (*sarcoplasmic reticulum*) composed of a longitudinally arranged tubular network (*sarcotubules*). This network is continuous with dilated sacs, *terminal cisternae*, which lie transversely across the fiber near the center of the "I" band. Near this same point the sarcolemma invaginates into the sarcoplasm, forming a tubular channel called the T *(transverse) tubule*, which branches and extends among the myofibrils. A branch of the T system is interposed between the two terminal cisternae at the junction between any two sarcomeres (directly over the "Z" line).

The complex (terminal cistern–T tubule–terminal cistern) formed at this position is known as a *triad*. The T tubules function to bring a wave of depolarization of the sarcolemma into the fiber and thus into intimate relationship with the terminal cisternae. The sarcoplasmic reticulum concentrates calcium ions (CA^{2+}) within its lumen, but depolarization of the T-tubule membrane induces the nearby terminal cisternae of the sarcoplasmic reticulum to release this Ca^{2+} into the sarcoplasma among the myofilaments. The Ca^{2+} becomes associated with the troponin of the thin myofilament, bringing about contraction as discussed below.

Excitation

Contraction in a skeletal muscle is triggered by the generation of an action potential in the muscle membrane. Each motor neuron upon entering a skeletal muscle loses its myelin sheath and divides into branches with each branch innervating a single muscle fiber, forming a *neuromuscular junction*. Each fiber normally has one neuromuscular junction which is located near the center of the fiber. A *motor unit* consists of a single motor neuron and all the muscle fibers innervated by it. The *motor end plate* is the specialized part of the muscle fiber's membrane lying under the neuron.

The impulse arriving at the end of the motor neuron causes liberation of *acetylcholine* from vesicles in the neuron terminal. The acetylcholine acts at specific sites normally found only on the motor end plate section of the fiber membrane and increases the permeability of the motor end plate. The resulting Na^+ influx produces a depolarizing potential called the end-plate potential. This in turn depolarizes adjacent areas of the fiber membrane, triggering an action potential which is propagated in both directions from the central neuromuscular junction toward the fiber ends. Normally the magnitude of the end-plate potential is sufficient to discharge the muscle membrane, so that each impulse in the nerve ending produces a response in the muscle. The acetylcholine is rapidly destroyed by the enzyme *acetylcholinesterase* which is found in high concentrations at the neuromuscular junction.

Contraction

According to the sliding filament theory (Huxley) the sarcomere response to excitation involves the sliding of thin and thick myofilaments past one another making and breaking chemical bonds with each other as they go. Neither the thick nor thin myofilaments change in length. If we could imagine observing this contraction under a light microscope we would see the narrowing of the "H" and "I" bands during contraction while the width of the "A" band would remain constant.

The word *contraction* refers to those processes which are manifested externally by either a *shortening* of a muscle or by *tension development* in a muscle. If the muscle length is held constant, the contraction is referred to as an *isometric contraction*. In an isometric contraction the passive tension remains constant with the *active tension* being added to it to produce the *total tension* of the muscle.

If the muscle shortens during contraction, it is called an *isotonic contraction* and the total tension remains constant.

Muscle Twitch

A muscle's response to a single maximal stimulus is a *muscle twitch*. The beginning of muscular activity is signalled by the record of the *electrical activity* in the sarcolemma. The *latent period* is the delay between imposition of the stimulus and the development of tension.

Tetanus

When a volley of stimuli is applied to a muscle, each succeeding stimulus may arrive before the muscle can completely relax from the contraction caused by the preceding stimulus. The result is *summation*, an increased strength of contraction. If the frequency of stimulation is very fast, individual contractions fuse and the muscle smoothly and fully contracts. This is a *tetanus*.

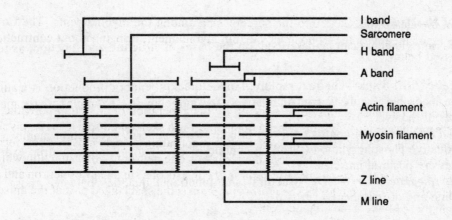

Relaxed Myofibril

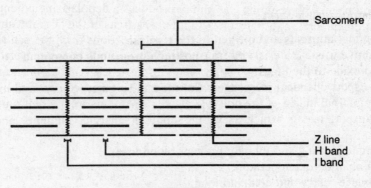

Contracted Myofibril

SCHEMATIC OF SKELETAL (STRIATED) MUSCLE

Energy Sources

In any phenomenon including muscular contraction the energy input to the system and the energy output from the system are equal. Let us consider first the energy sources for muscular contraction. The immediate energy source for contraction is ATP which can be hydrolyzed by actomyosin to give ADP, P_i, and the energy which is in some way associated with cross-bridge motion.

The ultimate source of this ATP is the ATP produced by the intermediary metabolism of carbohydrates and lipids. Skeletal muscle has the biochemical machinery to utilize both. With mild exercise oxygen availability after an initial period of adjustment is sufficient so that the aerobic pathways for ATP production can keep pace with the ATP utilization during the exercise—a new equilibrium is reached. During short-term, violent exertion, however, aerobic energy production cannot keep pace with energy utilization and even during the onset of mild exercise aerobic energy production initially lags behind energy utilization. Yet the ATP concentration remains constant. The reason is that there are stores of CP (creatine phosphate) in muscles and ATP levels can be maintained at the expense of CP levels. In these cases of insufficient oxygen availability ("oxygen debt") anaerobic pathways can produce enough additional ATP to permit those short-term bursts of exercise but lactic acid is generated. This incomplete oxidation produces substantially less energy than the complete aerobic oxidation to carbon dioxide and water.

Type of Muscle Fibers

Skeletal muscle fibers can be described, on the bases of structure and function, as follows:

1. *White (fast) fibers*—contract rapidly; fatigue quickly; energy production is mainly via anaerobic glycolysis; contain relatively few mitochondria; examples are the muscles of the eye.
2. *Red (slow) fibers*—contract slowly; fatigue slowly; energy production mainly via oxidative phosphorylation (aerobic); contain relatively many mitochondria; examples are postural muscles.
3. *Intermediate fibers*—have structural and functional qualities between those of white and of red fibers.

Circulatory System

Functions

The circulatory system serves:

(1) to conduct nutrients and oxygen to the tissues;

(2) to remove waste materials by transporting nitrogenous compounds to the kidneys and carbon dioxide to the lungs;

(3) to transport chemical messengers (hormones) to target organs and modulate and integrate the internal milieu of the body;

(4) to transport agents which serve the body in allergic, immune, and infectious responses;

(5) to initiate clotting and thereby prevent blood loss;

(6) to maintain body temperature;

(7) to produce, carry and contain blood;

(8) to transfer body reserves, specifically mineral salts, to areas of need.

General Components and Structure

The circulatory system consists of the heart, blood vessels, blood and lymphatics. It is a network of tubular structures through which blood travels to and from all the parts of the body. In vertebrates this is a completely closed circuit system, as William Harvey (1628) demonstrated. The heart is a modified, specialized, powerful pumping blood vessel. Arteries, eventually becoming arterioles, conduct blood to capillaries (essentially endothelial tubes), and venules, eventually becoming veins, return blood from the capillary bed to the heart. (Malpighi [1661] demonstrated the capillary system.) The system is lined entirely by endothelium. Fluids (mostly water) which leave capillaries return as lymph to the blood stream via lymphatic channels. The spleen, liver, and bone marrow function in the formation, destruction and replacement of blood cells.

Systemic arteries orginating from the left side of the heart (via the aorta) distribute oxygenated and nutrient-rich blood to the body. The systemic venous system returns deoxygenated blood to the heart. The pulmonary arterial circuit delivers this blood from the right side of the heart to the lungs and the pulmonary venous component returns oxygenated blood to the left side of the heart. Arteries travel away from the heart; veins come to it.

Course of Circulation

Systemic Route:

a. *Arterial system*. Blood is delivered by the pulmonary veins (two from each lung) to the left atrium, passes through the bicuspid (mitral) valve into the left ventricle and then is pumped into the ascending aorta; backflow here is prevented by the aortic semilunar valves. The aortic arch toward the right side gives rise to the brachiocephalic (innominate) artery which divides into the right subclavian and right common carotid arteries. Next arising from the arch is the common carotid artery, then the left subclavian artery; these two arise independently from the arch. In general the carotids split into external and internal carotids which supply the head and neck and brain. The subclavians supply the upper limbs. As the subclavian arteries pass the first rib they are renamed axillary arteries. When the axillary arteries leave the axilla (armpit) and enter the arm (brachium) they are called brachial arteries. Below the elbow these main trunk lines divide into ulnar and radial arteries, which supply the forearm and eventually form a set of arterial arches in the hand which give rise to common and proper digital arteries. The descending (dorsal) aorta continues along the posterior aspect of the thorax giving rise to the segmental intercostal arteries. After passage "through" (behind) the diaphragm it is called the abdominal aorta. Branches are:

inferior phrenic arteries to the diaphragm and adrenal gland,
middle suprarenal (adrenal) artery to the adrenal,
celiac artery to the stomach, part of duodenum, liver, and spleen,
superior mesenteric artery to the small intestines, the cecum, ascending, and transverse colon
renal arteries to the kidneys and adrenals,
ovarian and testicular arteries to the respective gonads,
inferior mesenteric artery to the descending and sigmoid colon, and to the superior portion of the rectum,
lumbar segmental arteries to the abdominal wall.

At the pelvic rim the abdominal aorta divides into the right and left common iliac arteries. These divide into the internal iliacs, which supply the pelvic organs, and the external iliacs, which supply the lower limb.

As the external iliac artery passes below the inguinal ligament into the thigh, its name changes to femoral artery. In the region posterior to the knee joint the artery is known as the popliteal artery; it divides into an anterior tibial artery to the anterior leg, a posterior tibial artery to the posterior leg, and a peroneal artery to the lateral aspects of the leg. The anterior and posterior tibial arteries eventually give rise to metatarsal and digital arteries for the supply of the dorsal and plantar aspects, respectively, of the foot.

b. *Venous system*. Veins are frequently multiple and variations are common. They return blood originating in the capillaries of peripheral and distal body parts to the heart. Tributaries converge and eventually all the blood of the body except that from the lungs and heart itself reaches the right atrium via the superior and inferior venae cavae.

The superior vena cava is formed in the following manner. The internal jugular veins, from the brain and deep face and neck, and the external jugular veins, from the superficial face and neck, join the subclavian veins, which receive the drainage of the upper limb and form right and left brachiocephalic (innominate) veins. The two brachiocephalic veins join to form the superior vena cava. Also joining the superior vena cava is the azygous system of veins, which drains the chest wall.

The inferior vena cava has the following origin. Femoral veins, from the lower limb, become in the abdominal cavity the external iliac veins, which receive the internal iliac veins from the pelvis and form the common iliac veins. The common iliac veins join to form the inferior vena cava. The inferior vena cava receives the renal veins, veins from the body wall, the right gonadal vein and the hepatic veins, from the liver, before passing through the diaphragm into the thorax to enter the right atrium of the heart.

Hepatic Portal System: Blood draining the alimentary tract (intestines), pancreas, spleen and gall bladder does not return directly to the systemic circulation, but is relayed by the hepatic portal system of veins to and through the liver. In the liver, absorbed foodstuffs and wastes are processed. After processing, the liver returns the blood via hepatic veins to the inferior vena cava and from there to the heart.

Pulmonary Circuit: Blood is oxygenated and depleted of metabolic products such as carbon dioxide in the lungs. The pathway is as follows:

(1) Deoxygenated blood arrives in the right atrium and passes through the tricuspid valve into the right ventricle.

(2) It leaves the right ventricle via the pulmonary (trunk) artery and passes to the lungs; backflow is prevented by the pulmonary semilunar valves.

(3) In the capillary network of the lung, blood is oxygenated. It then leaves the lung via two pulmonary veins each from the right and left lung and passes to the left atrium.

(4) Blood passes through the bicuspid valve into the left ventricle and from there is expelled to the rest of the body via the ascending aorta; backflow is prevented by the aortic semilunar valves.

Lymphatic Drainage: A network of lymphatic capillaries permeates the body tissues. Lymph is a fluid similar in composition to blood plasma, and tissue fluids not reabsorbed into blood capillaries are transported via the lymphatic system eventually to join the venous system at the junction of the left internal jugular and subclavian veins. Like veins, lymphatics possess valves. Interposed along the course of some lymph vessels are lymph nodes. These nodes filter lymph and add lymphocytes to the circulation. Lymph nodes possess an outer cortex and an inner medulla. Lymphoid follicles are present in the cortex; irregular cords of lymphocytes make up the medulla.

The Heart

The heart is a highly specialized blood vessel which pumps 72 times per minute and propels about 4,000 gallons (about 15,000 liters) of blood daily to the tissues. It is composed of:

endocardium (lining coat; epithelium)

myocardium (middle coat; cardiac muscle)

epicardium (external coat or visceral layer of pericardium; epithelium and mostly connective tissue)

impulse conducting system

Mammals possess modified cardiac muscle fibers specialized for conduction (Purkinje system). The heart has an automatic rythmic beat. Cardiac (autonomic) nerves exert an influence on heartbeat but serve only to change the force and frequency of the contractions in accordance with the physiologic needs of the organism.

Cardiac Nerves: Modification of the intrinsic rhythmicity of the heart muscle is produced by cardiac nerves of the sympathetic and parasympathetic nervous system. Stimulation of the sympathetic system increases the rate and force of the heartbeat and dilates the coronary arteries. Stimulation of the parasympathetic (vagus nerve) reduces the rate and force of the heartbeat and constricts the coronary circulation. Visceral afferent (sensory) fibers from the heart end almost wholly in the first four segments of the thoracic spinal cord.

Cardiac Cycle: Alternating contraction and relaxation is repeated about 75 times per minute; the duration of one cycle is about 0.8 second. Three phases succeed one another during the cycle:

(a) atrial systole: 0.1 second,

(b) ventricular systole; 0.3 second

(c) diastole: 0.4 second

The actual period of rest for each chamber is 0.7 second for the atria and 0.5 second for the ventricles, so, in spite of its activity, the heart is at rest longer than at work.

Blood

Blood is composed of cells (corpuscles) and a liquid intercellular ground substance called plasma. The average blood volume is 5 to 6 liters (7% of body weight). Plasma constitutes about 55% of blood volume, cellular elements about 45%.

Plasma: Over 90% of plasma is water; the balance is made up of plasma proteins and dissolved electrolytes, hormones, antibodies, nutrients, and waste products. Plasma is isotonic (0.85% sodium chloride). Plasma plays a vital role in respiration, circulation, coagulation, temperature regulation, buffer activities and overall fluid balance. The plasma proteins (albumin, globulin and fibrinogen) are responsible for the viscosity of blood, carry immune material and control osmotic pressure. Fibrinogen, in bleeding, is transformed into fibrin and helps form a clot. Plasma defibrinated by clotting is known as *blood serum.*

Blood Cells: There are two types of blood cells: red blood cells (RBC), or erythrocytes, and white blood cells (WBC), or leukocytes. Cell fragments called blood platelets are also present in mammalian blood.

a. *Erythrocytes—RBC.* These cells are biconcave discs about 7.7 microns in diameter. Mature cells lack a nucleus. The normal RBC hematocrit is about 36–45. The normal RBC counts are $5.2 \times 10^6/mm^3$ in males and $4.5 \times 10^6/mm^3$ in females. *Hemoglobin,* a complex molecule of iron and protein, is present in the cell. Red blood cells carry oxygen (in the form of oxyhemoglobin) from the lungs to the tissues and transport carbon dioxide from the tissues to the lungs. The membranes of the RBC carry Rh antigen and blood group antigens. Red blood cells have a life span of about 3 months. They are removed from the circulation by the spleen and replaced by new red blood cells formed in bone marrow. In the breakdown of hemoglobin, bilirubin is excreted and iron is retained.

b. *Leukocytes—WBC.* These cells differ from red blood cells by having nuclei and by exhibiting ameboid movement. A normal count of WBC in circulating blood is about $5–9 \times 10^3/mm^3$. WBC contain phosphatases, liberate proteolytic enzymes, and function mainly in phagocytosis, proteolysis and antibody formation. An increase in the number of leukocytes is called *leukocytosis,* a decrease *leukopenia.*

There are two main types of leukocytes: nongranular and granular.

Non- or Agranular Leukocytes

1. *Lymphocytes* make up between 20 and 25% of total leukocytes and are seldom phagocytic. They originate from lymphoid tissue and bone marrow, function in immunologic responses and the detoxification of noxious substances; and are prevalent at sites of chronic inflammation. Some live several years.

2. *Monocytes* make up between 3 and 8% of total WBC. They are sometimes phagocytic and help in debridement.

Granular (possess abundant, specific granules) Leukocytes

1. *Neutrophils* make up about 65–75% of leukocytes. They are twice as large as a RBC and have a lobulated nucleus. They are the most active and phagocytic, providing the first line of defense against invading organisms. Dead neutrophils become *pus.*

2. *Eosinophils* make up about 2–5% WBC. They possess large red acidophilic granules and a bilobed nucleus. Large numbers are found at sites of parasitic infections and allergic reactions (specifically, in the respiratory and digestive tracts). Eosinophils function in the destruction of antigen-antibody complexes.

3. *Basophils* make up 0.5% or less of the total white blood cell count. They are rarely phagocytic. Basophils contain large quantities of basophilic granules. They are involved in immune phenomena, and produce heparin, which prevents the clotting of blood.

c. *Blood platelets.* These cytoplasmic structures are not true cells but are cell fragments characteristic of mammalian blood. (In lower vertebrates, cells called thrombocytes have a function similar to platelets.) Blood platelets average about three microns in diameter. About $250–350,000/mm^3$ are normally present. These structures arise by the fragmentation of cytoplasmic processes of giant bone marrow cells. Platelets agglutinate and adhere to regions of injured vessels; they plug wounds of blood vessels. They help physically in clotting and form thromboplastin (thrombokinase), an integral chemical component of clot formation.

Blood Clotting: Platelets contribute thromboplastin (thrombokinase), an enzymatically active substance. Thromboplastin interacts with calcium ions and prothrombin (a plasma protein). Prothrombin is an inactive precursor of the catalyst thrombin. In the presence of these components prothrombin is converted to thrombin. Subsequently thrombin reacts with the plasma protein fibrinogen, forming fibrin. Fibrin is an insoluble, coagulated protein which clots. A clot also contains blood cells. Diagrammatically we can represent clotting reactions as follows:

$$\text{platelets} \longrightarrow \text{thromboplastin}$$
$$\downarrow$$
$$\text{prothrombin} + Ca^{2+} \longrightarrow \text{thrombin}$$
$$\downarrow$$
$$\text{fibrinogen} \longrightarrow \text{fibrin.}$$

Anticoagulants. An anticoagulant is a substance that prevents or retards coagulation of blood. Examples are: *heparin,* an acid mucopolysaccharide which occurs most abundantly in the liver; *aspirin* (acetylsalicylic acid), which also acts as an analgesic, antipyretic, antirheumatic compound; and the drug *Dicumarol,* a tradename for bihydroxycoumarin.

Blood Pressure: Blood pressure is usually measured by placing a sphygmomanometer cuff around the arm compressing the brachial artery and vein. Maximum blood pressure is obtained during ventricular contraction (systole) and minimum blood pressure indicates ventricular rest (diastole). The normal blood pressure listed for a young adult is 120 systolic and 80 diastolic (mm Hg).

Respiratory System

The respiratory system is composed of a conduit for air and an air-blood interface for gaseous exchange in the alveoli of the lungs. The function of the lung is to facilitate movement of oxygen from the air into the pulmonary circulation and the movement of carbon dioxide from the body out. This is accomplished by simple diffusion from an area of high concentration to one of a low partial pressure.

The conducting passages of the respiratory system can be listed as:

1) external (anterior) nares
2) nasal cavity with conchae, meatuses and sinuses
3) internal (posterior) nares
4) nasopharynx
5) oropharynx (communicates with oral cavity and mouth anteriorly)
6) laryngeal pharynx
7) larynx (possesses false and true vocal cords)
8) trachea
9) primary (left and right) bronchi
10) secondary (three named ones per lung—one per lobe) bronchi
11) tertiary bronchi
12) respiratory bronchioles
13) alveolar ducts
14) alveolar sacs
15) alveoli

The tracheobronchial tree (anatomic dead space) consists of about 16 generations of branches, while the respiratory unit is made up of an additional seven generations of respiratory bronchioles, alveolar ducts, and alveolar sacs for a total of 23 generations. The last seven are functional in gas exchange. (The upper parts of the respiratory system function in the removal of inhaled particles.)

Removal of Inhaled Particles

Large particles are filtered by hairs and mucous material in the nose and respiratory tract. Air is also warmed and humidified. Mucus is continually moved by cilia towards the throat and expelled by swallowing, expectoration or through the nose. No cilia are present in alveoli; macrophages and leukocytes debride this area. Material so gathered is removed via the lymphatic system.

Pulmonary Ventilation

Respiration refers to the gaseous exchanges which occur between the body as a whole and the environment. It entails:

1) ventilation of the lungs
2) gas exchange between lungs and blood
3) transport of gases in the blood
4) gas exchange between blood and interstitial fluids of the body

Ventilation must be adequate in environments ranging from sea level to high altitude and under degrees of physical activities ranging from sleep to exertion.

Respiratory minute ventilation is the amount of air which one inspires or expires each minute. It is equal to the amount of air inspired with each breath (the *tidal volume*) times the frequency (the number of breaths per minute). Normally with each breath we inspire about 500 ml and breathe at a rate of 12 breaths per minute. The resting respiratory minute ventilation under these conditions is 6 1/min. During severe exercise, the respiratory minute ventilation may reach 80 to 100 1/min; this is an indication of the practical upper limit of our respiratory system. Thus a 15-fold increase in ventilation is possible, indicating that the respiratory system has considerable reserve.

Inspiration and Expiration

During inspiration the thoracic cavity expands, its volume increases and air rushes into the respiratory tract due to the creation of negative pressure; the musculature involved is the diaphragm (innervated by the phrenic nerve) and the external intercostal muscles (innervated by intercostal nerves). During its contraction the diaphragm descends as much as 7 cm; the external intercostal muscles raise the rib cage. Relaxation of these muscles, the stabilization of the thoracic cage by the internal intercostals, contraction of the abdominal musculature, plus the elasticity of the lung, return the organ to the pre-inspiratory resting phase. A normal breath involves a volume of about 500 ml. Normal expiration is passive and involves no great muscular contraction. When ventilation exceeds about 40 1/min, expiratory (abdominal) muscles come into play to speed up expiration. By contracting, they push on contents of the abdominal cavity which then push the diaphragm upward, forcing air out of the lungs.

Positive and Negative Pressure Breathing

Gases flow from regions of higher pressure to those of lower pressure. Thus, when the gas pressure in the alveoli is equal to that of the surrounding atmosphere, no movement of gas occurs. For inspiration to occur, the alveolar gas pressure must be less than the atmospheric pressure. There are two ways in which this pressure difference can be produced. The first is by positive pressure breathing as is the case when using a resuscitator. Here the pressure at the nose and mouth (the atmospheric pressure) is made greater than the alveolar gas pressure. The second method is by negative pressure breathing as is the case when using the iron lung. Here the alveolar gas pressure is lowered below atmospheric pressure.

Normal breathing is a form of negative pressure breathing. If we plot intra-alveolar pressure (intrapulmonary pressure) during inspiration and expiration, we see that enlarging the thorax and lungs enables the alveolar gas to expand until its pressure drops below that of the surrounding atmosphere and the inflow of gas then occurs. For expiration to occur, the alveolar gas pressure must be made greater than the atmospheric pressure. This is produced by the natural recoil of the lungs, during which time the alveolar gas is compressed until its pressure is above atmospheric pressure. Gas then flows out of the lungs. Resistance to respiration arises due to the elastic fibers of the lung itself and the surface tension phenomena (forces) present at any liquid-air interface.

Since the inner surface of the lung is lined with a fluid (surfactant, which has a low surface tension), surface tension forces play a role. As a result of this surface tension the alveolus will tend to collapse unless opposed by the inflating pressure. The amount of pressure needed to oppose surface tension and maintain inflation is determined by the Law of Laplace:

$$p = \frac{2T}{\text{radius}}$$

where p = the inflation pressure, T = surface tension forces, and radius means the radius of the alveoli.

With a plasmalike liquid lining the lungs (constant surface tension), as the radius decreases (deflation) the distending pressure increases. Also, smaller alveoli would require a greater distending force than the larger alveoli.

The density of the surfactant molecules at the liquid-air interface is such that at high lung-volumes there are few surfactant molecules per unit of area and the surface tension is relatively high (like plasma). As deflation occurs, the surfactant molecules become more concentrated at the liquid air interface, and surface tension becomes relatively low (like surfactant). Thus, during deflation, the alveolar radius is decreasing tending to increase the needed distending pressure, but the surface tension is becoming less, which tends to decrease the required distending pressure. The lung, therefore, has alveoli which will not collapse until very low pressures are reached (because the surface tension is low), and can have small and large alveoli existing side by side (because the surface tension is area dependent).

Absence of the ability to produce surfactant is a key element in hyaline membrane disease. Infants afflicted die of respiratory distress because their lungs collapse with each breath due to the high surface tension. Extreme muscular efforts are required for reinflation and respiration is very labored in these cases.

Neuronal Control and Integration of Breathing

Normal spontaneous breathing is under control of motor neurons (primarily the phrenic nerves) which innervate the respiratory muscles. Brain impulses regulate and modulate the process. Voluntary activity originates in the cerebral cortex, automatic (autonomic) control rests in the pons and medulla of the brain.

The respiratory center, located in the medulla, has an inspiratory and an expiratory portion. The ventral portion produces forced and deep inspiration; the dorsal portion produces expiration.

Rhythmicity is spontaneous (12–15 times/minute) but is modulated by centers in the pons and medulla and by input from afferent vagal (stretch) receptors located in the lung. Stretching of the lung during inspiration reflexly limits the inspiratory drive.

Smooth muscle in the walls of the airways is innervated by parasympathetic and sympathetic nerves. Parasympathetic stimulation causes bronchoconstriction and an increase in airway resistance. Sympathetic stimulation produces relaxation. (Therefore, during an asthmatic attack it is helpful to inhale an aerosol containing a sympathomimetic drug, a drug that mimics the action of stimulating the sympathetic nervous system.)

Gas Exchange in the Alveoli

Abutting the alveoli (about 150 million/lung) is a large capillary bed providing an enormous diffusion area (about 90 m^2) with an extremely thin barrier (about 5000 Å) for gaseous exchange. Gas exchange takes place only in the alveoli and not in the tracheobronchial tree; the nonfunctional space (anatomic dead space) volume comprises about 150 ml. The alveolar portion, known as the respiratory zone, has a volume of about 2,000 ml. The diffusion pathway for alveolar gas may be listed as:

1) surfactant (lowers surface tension)
2) alveolar epithelium
3) interstitium (fused basement membranes)
4) capillary endothelium (epithelium)
5) plasma
6) red blood cell

Oxygen Transport

Oxygen is transported mainly in the form of oxyhemoglobin. Normal hemoglobin (Hb) values are, respectively, 14 g/100 ml for women and 16 g/100 ml for men. Blood then contains an average of 15 g hemoglobin/100 ml blood; each gram of hemoglobin can combine with 1.39 ml of oxygen. Fully oxygenated blood can be calculated thus:

$$(15 \text{ g Hb}/100 \text{ ml blood}) \times (1.39 \text{ ml O}_2/\text{g Hb})$$

to contain 21 ml O_2/ml blood. This is known as the *oxygen capacity* of blood.

If the concentration of oxygen against the PO_2 is plotted, a sigmoid shaped curve, also called the *oxygen dissociation curve*, is obtained.

Four factors affect the affinity of hemoglobin for oxygen:

1) pH
2) temperature
3) concentration of 2,3-diphosphoglycerate (DPG)
4) carbon dioxide

A decrease in pH, an increase in temperature or an increase in DPG will facilitate the release of oxygen in the tissue capillaries.

Actively metabolizing tissues have a higher temperature and produce metabolic acids (e.g., lactic acid) and carbonic acid via the reaction of released carbon dioxide and water. An increase in CO_2 and a decrease in affinity of hemoglobin for oxygen with a decrease in pH and an increase in carbamino Hb is called the *Bohr effect*. Most of the oxygen released is due to the decrease in PO_2 in the interstitial fluid but an extra amount is released due to these factors. Chronic hypoxia increases the amount of DPG and thus facilitates oxygen release by this mechanism.

Carbon Dioxide Transport

While some carbon dioxide remains in plasma, most diffuses into red blood cells. Here, it can be (1) transported in physical solution, (2) bound to the amino groups of hemoglobin as carbamino hemoglobin, or, most importantly, (3) converted to bicarbonate ions via its interaction with water to form carbonic acid, which almost completely dissociates into bicarbonate and hydrogen ions. This reaction occurs rapidly in red blood cells because the cells contain the enzyme carbonic anhydrase, which catalyzes the reaction.

The carbon dioxide in plasma can also be transported (1) in physical solution, (2) bound to the amino groups of plasma proteins (although the amount carried as carbamino compounds in plasma is small compared to the amount carried in red blood cells as carbamino hemoglobin), or (3) as bicarbonate ions. Few bicarbonate ions are produced in the plasma, however, since there is no carbonic anhydrase in plasma.

Bicarbonate ions produced in the red blood cells diffuse into the plasma because of the concentration gradient. However, the red blood cell membrane is not very permeable to cations so no positively charged ion can accompany the bicarbonate ions into the plasma. The result is that the inside of the red blood cell is slightly positive and so attracts negatively charged chloride ions from the plasma. This exchange of chloride for bicarbonate is referred to as the *chloride shift*. Thus, although bicarbonate is produced in red blood cells it is transported in plasma.

The hydrogen ions produced are buffered to a great extent by hemoglobin. The fact that reduced hemoglobin holds hydrogen ions more strongly than oxyhemoglobin means that as oxygen is released to tissues hydrogen ions generated by the addition of carbon dioxide can be taken up by the deoxygenated (reduced) hemoglobin. Slightly more hydrogen ions are produced than can be handled by the reduced hemoglobin produced. Thus, the pH of venous blood is slightly lower than that of arterial blood.

Since deoxygenated hemoglobin forms carbamino compounds much more readily than oxygenated hemoglobin does, venous blood can handle more CO_2 than can arterial blood.

The changes in the quantity of oxygen and carbon dioxide in the lungs are as indicated:

	Inspired Air, %	Expired Air, %	Change, %
Oxygen	20.96	16.02	4.94 loss
Carbon dioxide	0.04	4.48	4.44 gain

The carbon dioxide resulting from cellular metabolic activity diffuses into the blood since it is less concentrated there; here it then either combines with hemoglobin or is converted into carbonic acid:

$$CO_2 + H_2O \longrightarrow H_2CO_3$$

The carbonic acid reacts with sodium in the plasma to form sodium bicarbonate:

$$H_2CO_3 + Na^+ \longrightarrow NaHCO_3 + H^+$$

or it can react with potassium in the hemoglobin to form potassium bicarbonate:

$$H_2CO_3 + K^+ \longrightarrow KHCO_3 + H^+$$

In the lungs the carbon dioxide is dissociated from the bicarbonate and hemoglobin and diffuses into alveolar space air for exchange.

Chemical Regulation of Respiration

Chemical stimulants of physiological importance that affect respiration are:

1) increased arterial PCO_2 (hypercapnia),
2) decreased arterial PO_2 (hypoxia),
3) an increased arterial hydrogen-ion concentration (acidosis).

Arterial $[H^+]$ and PO_2 are monitored by carotid and aortic bodies which contain nerve endings that are sensitive to arterial pH and PO_2. The carotid bodies lie near the carotid sinus at the bifurcation of the common carotid arteries and send impulses through fibers of the glossopharyngeal nerves. The aortic bodies lie near the arch of the aorta; their neural fibers are part of the vagus nerves.

Increases in arterial PCO_2 are also sensed to some extent by these peripheral chemoreceptors (carotid and aortic bodies) but, more importantly, by a central chemosensitive area on the surface of the medulla overlying the medullary respiratory center. This central chemosensitive area, bathed in cerebrospinal fluid (CSF), is sensitive to changes in $[H^+]$ in the CSF. Although hydrogen ions poorly penetrate the blood-brain barrier which separates arterial blood and CSF, carbon dioxide can rapidly diffuse between the two fluids. Thus, arterial PCO_2 and CSF PCO_2 equilibrate. Once in the CSF, carbon dioxide reacts with water to form carbonic acid, which dissociates into bicarbonate and hydrogen ions. The central chemosensitive area is sensitive to the pH changes thus produced. In a similar manner (but of less importance) arterial PCO_2 alters arterial pH, which is best detected by the carotid and aortic bodies.

Oxygen lack stimulates ventilation solely by its effect on the peripheral chemoreceptors, but alveolar PO_2 must fall to low levels (50–60 mm Hg) before ventilation begins to increase. However, some chemoreceptor discharge is present at normal oxygen tensions. Hypercapnia, which often accompanies hypoxia, will potentiate sensitivity of peripheral chemoreceptors to hypoxia. Hypoxia is the stimulus for increased ventilation observed at high altitudes.

Acidosis stimulates ventilation mainly via peripheral chemoreceptors. Arterial $[H^+]$ may also effect the central chemosensitive area but its influence there is slow in onset and much less pronounced. Hyperventilation driven by acidosis will "blow off" CO_2 and generate alkalosis in the CSF, which tends to depress ventilation. The results of these opposing forces is a lesser increase in ventilation than would occur with a constant arterial PCO_2. The effects of acidosis and either hypoxia or hypercapnia are additive with no complicated potentiation occurring.

Ventilation is much more sensitive to hypercapnia than to either hypoxia or acidosis. Changes in ventilation produced by hypercapnia are only slightly altered when the peripheral chemoreceptors are denervated, indicating the importance of the central chemosensitive area in monitoring CO_2. Hypoxia potentiates this CO_2 sensitivity.

Urinary System

The urinary system helps maintain homeostasis of the body by excreting wastes and regulating the content of the blood. It consists of two kidneys, two ureters, a urinary bladder and a urethra. Kidneys produce the excretory product; three tubular structures serve as a passageway for the excretory material (urine) to reach the outside of the body.

Structure of the Kidney

The kidney is a bean-shaped organ encased by a fibrous capsule and embedded within a fatty connective tissue and perirenal fascia. The kidney lies deep to the *peritoneum* (i.e., retroperitoneal) which lines the abdomino-pelvic cavity. It is approximately 10 centimeters long, 5 centimeters wide and 3 centimeters thick. Its medial aspect, which is indented or concave, is known as the *renal hilus (hilum)*; it is the location for the renal arteries and veins as well as for the renal pelvis. The hilus leads into a cavity, the *renal sinus*, within the kidney which contains fat, blood vessels, nerves, calyces and renal pelvis.

The internal aspect of the kidney when bissected in a medial to lateral plane presents two zones, an outer *cortex* and an inner *medulla*. The medulla is adjacent to the renal sinus. The cortex is redder in appearance and has fine striations known as *medullary rays*. These striations are due to medullary structures (collecting tubules) extending into the cortex. The medulla consists of triangular (pyramidal) structures, *the renal pyramids*, separated by columns of cortical material known as *renal columns*. The bases of the renal pyramids face the cortex while the apices or *papillae* extend into the *minor calyces*.

The kidney is divided into functional *lobes*, each defined as one renal pyramid, its abutting cortex and part of the two adjacent renal columns. There are about 6 to 18 lobes. A *lobule* of a kidney is considered to be a medullary ray and the adjacent nephrons draining into the collecting ducts forming the ray.

The functional unit of the kidney is the *uriniferous tubule*, which consists of a *nephron* and a *collecting tubule* (duct) within the kidney. There are 1 to 3 million per kidney. The individual nephron is considered by many as the functional unit and the collecting tubule as a separate entity being part of the internal excretory pathway for urine.

Nephron: The nephron is a tubular structure about 30 to 40 millimeters long and lined by epithelium. It functions in producing an ultrafiltrate and then reabsorbing material from and excreting substances into the filtrate resulting in an excretory product. It consists of several morphologically and physiologically different sections forming a continuous tubular unit. The regions of a nephron sequentially are: Bowman's capsule, proximal convoluted tubule, loop of Henle, and distal convoluted tubule. The latter is continuous with the collecting tubule (excretory duct) draining it. The loop of Henle extends into the medullary pyramid while the other three regions are found entirely in the cortex.

Nephrons vary in their level or position in the cortex with some, the *cortical nephrons,* being at the periphery of the cortex, and others, the *juxtamedullary nephrons,* abutting the medulla. These vary in that the size of the renal corpuscle and the length of the loop of Henle are larger in the juxtamedullary nephrons.

Bowman's capsule is an invaginated blind sac lined by a simple squamous epithelium. The latter forms two layers, the *visceral* and *parietal layers,* continuous with each other at the capsule's vascular pole, as well as separated by a cavity, *Bowman's space.* The visceral layer of Bowman's capsule is intimately related with the capillary network, known as the *glomerulus,* located between an *afferent and an efferent arteriole.* The Bowman's capsule forms a unit with the glomerulus referred to as the *renal corpuscle* (*corpuscle of Malpighi*). The proximal and distal convoluted tubules are located adjacent to their renal corpuscle. The region of the capsule where the arterioles enter and exit is the *vascular pole,* while the *urinary pole* is located where Bowman's space is continuous with the proximal convoluted tubule. The visceral layer consists of specialized star-shaped epithelial cells, the *podocytes,* abutting the endothelium of the tuft of capillaries.

The lumen of the capillary and Bowman's space are separated by the *filtration membrane or barrier,* which consists of fenestrated endothelium; *basement membrane,* between endothelium and podocyte; and *filtration-slit membranes,* between the podocyte processes known as *pedicels* (end feet) abutting the basement membrane. The ultrafiltrate formed enters the capsular space and then passes into the proximal convoluted tubule which is lined by a low columnar or cuboidal epithelium.

The loop of Henle consists of the following three sequential regions:

(1)   descending thick limb (straight portion of proximal tubule)
(2)   thin limb, forming a loop which connects descending and ascending thin limbs; lined by simple squamous epithelium
(3)   ascending thick limb (straight portion of distal tubule).

Collecting Tubules: The route for the filtrate and excretory product is from Bowman's space through the proximal convoluted tubule, descending thick and thin limbs of the loop of Henle, ascending thin and thick limbs, distal convoluted tubule and then into the collecting tubule. The latter unite and form 10–25 larger collecting ducts (papillary ducts of Bellini) which extend into the renal pyramids and terminate at the papillae.

The urine passes from the ends of these large collecting ducts into funnel-shaped collecting vessels, the *minor calyces,* into which the papillae extend. The 7 to 18 minor calyces empty into 2 to 3 *major calyces,* which are larger funnels that terminate in the *renal pelvis.* The renal pelvis is the terminal collecting site for urine in the kidney and is continuous with the ureter at the hilum of the kidney.

Tubular Passageways

The *ureter* is a long muscular tube which connects the renal pelvis to the urinary bladder. It passes inferiorly on the posterior abdominal wall, enters the pelvis by crossing the pelvic inlet, and then pierces the wall of the urinary bladder at its posterior-lateral aspect. The smooth muscles which are part of the bladder and surround the oblique path of the ureter through the wall act as a sphincter of the ureter.

The *urinary bladder* is located in the pelvis superior and posterior to the pubic bone, anterior to the uterus in the female, anterior to the rectum in the male. The bladder consists of a thick wall composed of three intermeshing smooth muscle layers known as *detrusor muscles.* The bladder functions to store urine as well as to expel it. The excretory pathways and the bladder are lined by the urinary type of the epithelium known as transitional epithelium.

The *urethra* is a fibromuscular tube that transmits urine to the outside of the body. It is continuous inferiorly with the urinary bladder. It traverses the prostate gland and then exits the pelvic cavity by passing through the pelvic floor (urogenital diaphragm) and terminates at the external urethral orifice of the penis or in the vestibule of the female.

The male urethra (20 centimeters in length) is longer than the female urethra (2–6 centimeters) and consists of three parts: the *prostatic, membranous* and *spongy urethrae*. The spongy urethra is within the corpus spongiosum of the penis which forms the glans penis.

Functions of the Kidney and Uriniferous Tubules

The kidney, during production of urine,

a) excretes the waste products of metabolism;
b) maintains the fluid volume of the extracellular regions of the body;
c) excretes foreign materials from the body;
d) regulates the type and concentration of salts retained in the body (maintain electrolyte balance);
e) regulates the total body water;
f) regulates the acid-base balance of the body.

The physiological processes occurring during the production of urine are

a) *filtration*—the production of an ultrafiltrate of plasma within Bowman's space;
b) *reabsorption*—the selective removal of material from the ultrafiltrate as it passes through the tubular nephron and the return of these substances into peritubular capillaries;
c) *secretion*—the cells forming the nephron actively secrete material into the filtrate;
d) *passive diffusion*—diffusion of fluids along the osmotic gradient.

Filtration: Filtration occurs at the renal corpuscles through the filtration barrier, which permits the passage of water and various solutes from the capillary lumen into Bowman's space but retains cells and large proteins. The ultrafiltrate produced (125 ml/min) enters the capsular space to be transported through and modified by the remaining portions of the nephron. Approximately 170–180 liters of ultrafiltrate are produced in 24 hours; this results in about 1 to 2 liters of urine per day. The production of the ultrafiltrate results from:

a) the filtration pressure (about 25 mm Hg), which is the differential between hydrostatic pressure within the glomerular capillaries (about 75 mm Hg) and total pressure resulting from osmotic pressure (30 mm Hg) and the intratubular pressure in Bowman's space and nephron (20 mm Hg). The resulting filtration pressure forces substances from the blood through the filtration barrier and into the nephron;

b) blockage of proteins larger than 70,000 molecular weight by the filtration membrane.

The ultrafiltrate is similar to plasma and isotonic to blood. It is composed of amino acids, urea, uric acid, salts, creatinine, glucose and small amounts of albumin.

Reabsorption: The isotonic ultrafiltrate enters the proximal convoluted tubules which are lined by cuboidal or low columnar epithelium with numerous apical microvilli (brush border). Filtrate volume is decreased by approximately 80% as it passes through the proximal convoluted tubule (PCT) through reabsorption of substances from the tubule lumen into interstitial spaces and then peritubular capillaries. Major resorption of substances from the ultrafiltrate occurs, therefore, in the PCT and results in:

a) the active reabsorption of all the glucose;
b) the active reabsorption of 85% of the sodium chloride;

c) the passive diffusion, due to the osmotic gradient, of 85% of the water from the filtrate;

d) the active transport of all amino acids, ascorbic acid and proteins. (Protein is broken down to amino acids in phagolysosomes following pinocytosis at the apical microvillar border.)

Secretion: The cells of the proximal convoluted tubule also secrete creatinine into the tubular lumen, as well as materials foreign to the body, such as phenol red, antibiotics and various radiopaque dyes. The amount of a substance reabsorbed is controlled; what is not resorbed from the tubule lumen is excreted. (In diabetes, glucose concentration in the blood and thus the ultrafiltrate is high; not all glucose is resorbed, and the remainder or excess is excreted in the urine.)

Passive Diffusion: The loop of Henle functions by setting up the mechanism (counter-current multiplier system) in the renal medulla for the production of *hypertonic urine*. The descending limb of the loop is permeable to water, Na^+ and Cl^-. These materials pass through the walls according to osmotic gradients. Water diffuses out of the tubule lumen into the more concentrated (hypertonic) interstitial tissue of the renal pyramids; Na^+ and Cl^- diffuse passively into the tubule.

The ascending limb of the loop differs in that its wall is impermeable to water. Therefore, water remains in the tubule. Also, chloride ions are actively reabsorbed and pumped into the interstitium surrounding the loop of Henle, as well as into the collecting ducts passing through the medullary pyramid. Sodium ions are thought to diffuse passively out of the tubules in conjunction with the Cl^-. This decrease in sodium chloride concentration of the filtrate results in a hypotonic filtrate at the distal end of the loop of Henle as it enters the distal convoluted tubule. The flow of the sodium chloride out of the tubule also increases its concentration in the surrounding interstitial tissue, which thus becomes hypertonic. This hypertonic interstitium is essential for production of hypertonic urine as the filtrate passes through the collecting ducts of the renal pyramid.

Hormonal Control of More Secretion and Resorption

The simple cuboidal epithelium lining the distal convoluted tubule may also increase the Na^+ concentration in the interstitium by reabsorbing Na^+. At the same time potassium ions (K^+) are excreted into the tubular lumen. The latter processes are regulated by *aldosterone*, a hormone produced by the adrenal cortex. The distal convoluted tubules also participate in maintaining the acid-base balance of the blood by adding hydrogen and ammonium ions into the filtrate.

The permeability of water through the walls of the distal convoluted tubules and collecting tubules is regulated by the *antidiuretic hormone* (ADH) secreted by the posterior lobe of the pituitary gland (neurohypophysis). The presence of this hormone makes these tubules more permeable to water. Since the interstitium of the renal pyramids is more highly concentrated (hypertonic) than the filtrate, water exits the collecting tubules and passes into the interstitium. This process continues along the length of the collecting ducts and results in concentrating the urine which therefore is *hypertonic*. The amount of water resorbed is regulated by ADH production. For example, an increase in ADH increases resorption of water resulting in a more hypertonic urine, while a decrease in ADH decreases resorption resulting in the excretion of more water and therefore, a diluted or hypotonic urine. Diuretic drugs counteract the action of ADH, causing less water resorption and increased urine volume. The osmotic gradient in the renal pyramids is also maintained by the *vasa recta* adjacent to the collecting tubules due to flow of water and Na^+ into and out of the vessel lumen. This establishes a countercurrent exchange system between the arterioles and venulae rectae.

Integumentary (Skin) System

The skin and the specialized organs derived from the skin (hairs, nails and glands) form the integumentary system.

Skin

The skin lines the external surface of the body. It is continuous with the mucous membranes of (1) the respiratory pathways via the nose; (2) the digestive tract via the mouth and anus; (3) the genitourinary system via urethra and/or vagina.

Functions: The skin functions by surfacing the body and thus protecting it from dehydration as well as from damage by the elements in the external environment. The skin also helps maintain normal body activities. The skin

(1) Protects the body against dehydration. The skin is impermeable to water which, therefore, prevents loss of body fluids. This property permits humans, as well as other animals, to live in a non-fluid environment such as land.

(2) Protects the body against abrasive forces. The ability to withstand frictional forces also allows humans to walk and perform manipulatory skills with the hands.

(3) Protects the body against damage from toxic chemicals and extreme heat.

(4) Protects the body from the harmful effects of ultraviolet rays. This is primarily the function of the melanin pigment secreted by the melanocytes in the epidermis.

(5) Acts as a barrier to infectious organisms invading the body.

(6) Takes part in regulating the temperature of the body. The degree of heat loss or retention is regulated by neurovascular processes. The body is cooled by the evaporation of water (sweat) from its surface.

(7) Functions to excrete body wastes and fluids via the production of sweat by the sweat glands.

(8) Acts as a primary sense organ of the body for general somatic sensations, such as touch, pressure, heat, cold and pain.

(9) Plays a role in the production of vitamin D through the action of ultraviolet light. The latter transforms vitamin D precursors (7-dehydrocholesterol) found in the skin into vitamin D.

Structure: Skin consists of the *epidermis* and *dermis (corium)*. Deep to the dermis and therefore, the skin, is the *hypodermis,* which is also known as the *subcutaneous* or superficial connective tissue of the body. The latter comprises loose connective tissue with various amounts of adipose cells (tissue).

Epidermis: The epidermis is derived from the ectoderm and is composed of a keratinized stratified squamous epithelium. The epidermis varies in thickness depending on the function of the specific region of the body. Its thickness is used to differentiate two types of skin—thick and thin.

Thick skin denotes skin with a thicker epidermis which contains more cell layers when compared to *thin skin.* The epidermis ranges in thickness from 0.07 millimeter to 1.4 millimeters. Skin itself (both epidermis and dermis) ranges from 0.5 millimeter to greater than 4 millimeters. The epidermis, similar to other epithelial layers, is avascular and lies on a basal lamina (basement membrane). The latter separates it from the underlying dermis to which the basal layer of epidermal cells is anchored.

The epidermis consists of specific cell layers which differ in their morphology and function. The layers of the epidermis of thick skin (sole of foot and palm) from the basal lamina (dermis) to the free surface are:

1. stratum basale or germinativum
2. stratum spinosum
3. stratum granulosum
4. stratum lucidum
5. stratum corneum

The combined layers of the strata basale and spinosum are also referred to as the *stratum malpighi* or *malpighian layer.*

In thin skin the stratum lucidum is absent and the stratum granulosum often appears as a discontinuous layer. The strata spinosum and corneum are always present as distinct layers but are thinner than in thick skin.

The layers of skin represent the different stages through which the epidermal cells (keratinocytes) pass as they undergo the process of keratinization from their origin in the stratum basale to their sloughing off as dead keratinized cells at the free surface.

The five layers of thick skin are characterized as follows:

1. Stratum basale
   a) Simple cuboidal to columnar epithelial cell layer resting on the basal lamina.
   b) Cells with the ability to divide (mitosis) and thus give rise to cells which migrate into the overlying stratum spinosum. This continuous process replenishes the keratinized epithelial cells which are shed from the surface.
   c) *Melanocytes,* which synthesize the brown pigment, *melanin,* in the form of pigment granules *(melanosomes).* Melanocytes have long cell processes which extend among the cells of the strata basale and spinosum. Via these processes they release and transfer melanosomes to the cells of the stratum malpighi. Increased exposure to UV light stimulates an increase in the secretion and release of melanosomes by the melanocytes, which results in the darkening of the skin (tanning). Dark color skin results from melanin, from carotene, a yellowish pigment, and from the degree of vascularity of the area, which adds a reddish-blue tint.

2. Stratum spinosum—consists of several layers of polygonal (polyhedral) cells which adhere to each other via desmosomes.

3. Stratum granulosum
   a) Consists of 3 to 5 layers of flat epithelial cells with pycnotic nuclei.
   b) Has a granular appearance due to the accumulation of irregular granules, the *keratohyalin granules,* within the cytoplasm. The granules are basophilic and are not encased by a membrane. The keratohyalin granules are associated with the numerous tonofilaments; both are involved in the production of keratin.
   c) The cells also contain *membrane-coating granules* (lamellated granules) composed of mucopolysaccharides and phospholipids. The latter are secreted into the intercellular regions surrounding the cells of the stratum granulosum. This intercellular matrix appears to block the passage of substances through the epidermis.
   d) The keratinocytes die in this stratum.

4. Stratum lucidum
   a) It is a homogeneous translucent layer separating the strata granulosum and corneum in thick skin.
   b) Consists of 3 to 5 layers of flat, elongated cells whose organelles and nuclei are indistinct or absent.

5. Stratum corneum
   a) Composed of layers of compressed, flat, cornified (keratinized) cells which lack nuclei and organelles. These scalelike cells are often referred to as *horny cells.*
   b) The most superficial horny cells slough off or desquamate constantly.

Dermis: The *corium,* or dermis, is the connective tissue layer between the epidermis and hypodermis. Depending on the region, its thickness may range between 0.5 millimeter to 4 millimeters. The border between these two strata is irregular in contour. This is caused by the irregular pattern of the surface of the dermis, to which the epidermis conforms. In a section perpendicular to the skin's surface, the dermis is seen to project into folds of the epidermis. These connective tissue projections are known as *dermal ridges (or papillae);* the epidermal regions between these ridges are the *epidermal or interpapillary pegs (ridges).* The dermal ridges are more numerous in thick skin (palm and soles), where greater abrasive forces occur. Since the epidermis follows the contours of the skin, the irregular contour of the dermis is projected onto the surface of the skin as ridges and grooves. The orientation and patterns of these surface grooves differ according to the skin region. They are very evident in the palm and fingers. The pattern is also extremely specific for each individual as is illustrated by the use of fingerprints to identify a person. These fingerprints, therefore, are actually the impressions of the grooves on the surface of the skin which represent the contour of the dermo-epidermal junction.

The dermis consists of two strata, the *papillary* and *reticular* layers.

Papillary layer. The *papillary layer* abuts the epidermis and forms the dermal ridges (papillae). It is thinner than the reticular layer and is composed of loose connective tissue. It consists of fine collagen, reticular, and elastic fibers associated with typical connective tissue cells (mainly fibroblasts and macrophages). The region abutting the basal cell layer is organized into a basement membrane. The processes of the basal cells anchor in the fibers of the membrane. The dermal ridges have extensive capillary networks. The epidermis is nourished by the diffusion of nutrients from this vascular bed. The papillary layer also contains encapsulated sensory receptors.

Reticular layer. The *reticular layer* is thicker and is composed of dense irregular connective tissue. The collagen and elastic fibers are thicker and coarser and form an interlacing network. Most fibers are primarily oriented parallel to the surface forming lines of skin tension called *Langer's lines,* which are important for surgical incisions. Capillaries are sparse. A rich nerve supply as well as encapsulated receptors are present in this layer. The reticular layer is the location of epidermal derivatives such as sweat and sebaceous glands and hair follicles. It also contains smooth muscles (arrector pili) associated with hair follicles and skeletal muscles in the head and neck (muscles of facial expression).

Glands

Glands are specialized organs derived from skin. There are two basic types: sebaceous and sweat.

Sebaceous Glands: Sebaceous glands are *simple branched alveolar (acinar) glands* with a *holocrine* mode of secretion. They are found in all areas of the body except the palms and soles. The excretory ducts of several glands open into the necks of a hair follicle.

The cells of the gland differentiate and become progressively larger as they accumulate lipid droplets in their cytoplasm. The cells eventually rupture releasing their lipid content and cell remnants into the lumen. The latter comprise the oily secretion of the sebaceous glands called *sebum,* which helps protect the skin from becoming extremely dry.

Sweat Glands: Sweat is a watery fluid containing ammonia, urea, uric acid and sodium chloride. The production of sweat is important for the excretion of some body wastes and the regulation of body temperature and is under nervous system control.

There are two types of sweat glands: eccrine and apocrine.

Eccrine Sweat Glands: The *eccrine sweat glands* are simple, coiled tubular glands with a merocrine mode of secretion. These glands are the ones that are typically considered when discussing sweat glands. Up to three million are found distributed all over the body in humans, except at the margin of the lip, glans penis, and ear drums. The largest number occur in the thick skin of the palms and soles. The *secretory tubular* unit is very coiled and is located in the reticular layer of the dermis near the hypodermis.

Apocrine Sweat Glands: The *apocrine sweat glands* are very large glands which are thought to have a merocrine mode of secretion. They occur mainly in the hypodermis of the axilla, areola of breast, labia majora and scrotum. They are branched tubular glands whose secretory tubule is very dilated. Their secretory product is more viscous. The excretory ducts open into the hair follicles above the openings of this sweat gland.

The *ceruminous glands* of the external auditory canals, which secrete wax, and the *glands of Moll,* in the eyelid margin, are also considered to be apocrine sweat glands.

Hair

Hairs are long, filamentous keratinized structures derived from the epidermis of skin. The process of keratinization is similar to that in skin since cells divide, differentiate, and move toward the surface and become keratinized. Hairs are found covering the whole body except palms, soles, sides of fingers and toes, glans and prepuce of penis, clitoris and labia minora.

Structure: A hair consists of a *shaft,* which extends above the skin surface, and a *root,* which lies within the skin. The root is encased by a tubular *hair follicle* composed of epidermal and dermal cell layers. At its deeper end, the follicle dilates and forms an invaginated *hair bulb* which is continuous with the root. The invaginated portion of the hair bulb contains a connective tissue papilla, the *dermal papilla,* which has a rich blood supply.

Hairs consist of three concentrically oriented epidermal layers, the *medulla, cortex* and *cuticle.* The *medulla* forms the center of the hair and consists of two or three layers of cuboidal cells found only in coarse hair; these cornified cells contain soft keratin. The medulla is encased by the *cortex,* which constitutes the largest part of the hair. It consists of several layers of keratinized cells which contain numerous filaments embedded in an amorphous matrix. The latter form the *hard keratin* found in these compactly arranged spindle-shaped cells. Melanin granules are found in the cells of the cortex giving hair its coloration. Air in the intercellular region of these cells also affects the pigmentation of hairs. The *cuticle* surrounds the cortex and consists of a single layer of transparent, enucleated cells which form keratinized scales.

Hair Follicle: The *hair follicle* consists of two sheaths, the *epithelial root sheath* and the *connective tissue root sheath.* The epidermally derived epithelial root sheath abuts the cuticle and is subdivided into the *inner epithelial root sheath* and the *outer (external) epithelial root sheath.* The *inner epithelial root sheath* extends from hair bulb to the level of the excretory duct of the sebaceous glands. It comprises three layers: (1) the *cuticle root sheath,* abutting the cuticle; (2) *Huxley's layer;* and (3) *Henle's layer,* adjacent to the outer epithelial root sheath. These layers are composed of keratinized cells containing soft keratin. The cells of the inner epithelial root sheath arise from the *hair matrix* in the hair bulb and migrate upward from it.

The *outer epithelial root sheath* is continuous with the epidermis of the skin. Close to the hair bulb the outer epithelial root sheath consists of a simple cuboidal layer similar to the stratum germinativum.

The *connective tissue root sheath (or dermal root sheath)* is derived from the dermis and consists of three layers: (1) the *glassy membrane,* the innermost layer which is a noncellular translucent membrane that corresponds to the basal lamina deep to the epidermis; (2) the *middle layer,* similar to the papillary layer of the dermis, and consisting of fine connective tissue fibers arranged in a circular pattern; and (3) the *outer layer,* similar to the reticular layer and consisting of longitudinally arranged coarse collagen fibers.

Hair Growth: Growth of a hair depends on the viability of the epidermal cells of the hair matrix which lie adjacent to the dermal papilla in the hair bulb. The matrix cells abutting the dermal papilla proliferate and give rise to cells which move upward to become part of the specific layers of the hair root and the inner epithelial root sheath. The hair matrix, therefore, functions similarly to the malpighian layer of the epidermis since it gives rise to cells which become cornified as they move toward the surface. Due to this upward movement of the cells arising from the hair matrix, the hair (root and shaft) grows outward. Hairs do not grow continuously but have specific growth and rest periods which vary according to the area of the body. Hair growth is influenced by growth hormone and the sex hormones.

Hair Musculature: Hairs are oriented at a slight angle to the skin surface and are associated with *arrector pili muscles.* These smooth muscle bundles extend from the dermal root sheath to a dermal papilla. Contraction results in the standing up of the hairs and raising of the skin surrounding the hair. This produces what is referred to as *gooseflesh* or *goose pimples.*

Nails

Nails are translucent plates of keratinized epithelial cells on the dorsal surface of distal phalanges of fingers and toes. The nail plate consists of a *body* and *root,* formed by compact layers of cornified epithelial cells similar to the stratum corneum. The *nail body* is the main portion of the plate lying on the *nail bed,* which is an epidermal layer consisting primarily of the malpighian cell layer. The proximal end of the body is continuous with the *nail root* at the *lunula.* The lunula is the crescentric whitish region at the proximal part of the nail.

Deep to the root and continuous with the proximal end of the nail bed is the *nail matrix.* The latter is a thickened stratum malpighi which gives rise to new cells that migrate upward and become keratinized. The matrix, therefore, functions in producing cornified cells composed of hard keratin which are added to the proximal end of the nail plate (root). This process increases the length of the nail. Nails increase in length about 0.5 millimeters per week.

The *cuticle*, or *eponychium*, is a fold of the stratum corneum which extends over the surface of the nail body in the area of the lunula.

A similar fold, the *hyponychium*, occurs deep to the distal free margin of the nail plate. The hyponychium is actully a thickening of the stratum corneum of the skin where the nail bed and epidermis of the skin are continuous.

Digestive System and Nutrition

Nutrition

The environment must supply its organisms with adequate nutrients via the food supply. Organisms require the basic elements making up protoplasm, the enzymes that catalyze and control the metabolic activity, and vitamins and hormones that have profound effects on the overall function of the system. Elements that are needed in very small quantities are called trace elements. No organism is independent of the environment, but on nutritional self-sufficiency we can classify organisms into autotrophs and heterotrophs. Heterotrophs include all animals; autotrophs include all those that carry out photosynthesis and can manufacture organic constituents from inorganic material. Although all organisms require intake of nutrients, we shall confine this discussion to nutrition and digestion in higher animals (particularly humans).

Unit for Measuring Value of Foods: The kilocalorie (kcal) is the unit of heat used in measuring the value of foods for producing heat and energy in the human body. It is equivalent to the amount of heat that is required to raise the temperature of one kilogram of water one degree Celsius. The kilocalorie is $1000 \times$ calorie, the amount of heat required to raise the temperature of one gram of water 1°C.

Proteins: Few free amino acids are available in the diet. Amino acid intake is primarily in the form of proteins (high molecular weight heteropolymers of amino acids). Amino acids are necessary for the production and maintenance of protoplasm. Certain amino acids are denoted as essential in all higher animals; these are: L-leucine; L-methionine; L-phenylalanine; L-valine; L-lysine; L-isoleucine; L-threonine and L-tryptophan. In the rat, however, all of the above eight plus histidine and arginine are essential. Among the nonessential amino acids (synthesized by the organism) are glycine, alanine, serine, cystine, tyrosine, and proline. Not all proteins have a complete complement of all amino acids; therefore, dietary intake must be adjusted to meet the needs of the organism.

Carbohydrates: Of primary importance in human nutrition are the monosaccharides, disaccharides, and polysaccharides. Monosaccharides ordinarily are simple 5- or 6-carbon sugars; they cannot be broken down into smaller units. Common examples are glucose and fructose.

Disaccharides are formed by the union of two 6-carbon monosaccharides and thus contain 12 carbons; they can be broken down by hydrolysis into their component hexose sugars. Common examples are sucrose (containing glucose and fructose) and lactose (containing glucose and galactose). Polysaccharides are large molecules formed by the union of many monosaccharides; they can be broken down into their respective monosaccharides. Common examples are glucose polymers, starch, and glycogen.

Fats: Fats may be grouped into simple lipids, compound lipids, and lipids derived from simple and compound lipids by hydrolysis. Fat is composed of three fatty acid molecules joined to a molecule of glycerol. Simple lipids are esters of fatty acids with various alcohols. Waxes possess alcohols other than glycerol. Cholesterol esters are a combination of fatty acids and sterol alcohols such as cholesterol. Compound lipids are composed of esters of fatty acids and glycerol; they also incorporate other chemical groups. Derived lipids are obtained by hydrolysis of simple and compound lipids and can be grouped into free fatty acids, alcohols, and sterol alcohols. Fatty acids may be either saturated or unsaturated. The unsaturated fatty acids may contain cis or trans double bonds, but cis double bonds are more common.

Vitamins: Vitamins are organic substances which are needed in minute quantities; vitamins often play a role as part of an enzyme system. Vitamins are used up in the metabolic activities and must be constantly replaced; the organism, however, is not capable of synthesizing a vitamin (at least in sufficient quantities) and must obtain it from the outside. Autotrophs have no requirement like heterotrophs for vitamins. Deficiency of a vitamin reduces the metabolic efficiency of the process which depends on it and symptoms arise for the deficiency diseases. Most deficiency diseases in the young will lead to stunting. Vitamins can be grouped into fat-soluble and water-soluble substances.

Fat-soluble Vitamins:

1. *Vitamin A.* This vitamin is formed from the carotenoid provitamins (yellow pigments of most vegetables and fruits). Deficiency in man causes poor dark vision adaptation, conjunctivitis and keratinization of the cornea.

2. *Vitamin D.* This vitamin does not occur naturally and is manufactured in the animal body by the utilization of ultraviolet light. Deficiency in humans mainly affects calcification of bones and teeth; in the child, rickets and in the adult, osteomalacia are consequences. The vitamin enhances the absorption of calcium and phosphorus from the intestinal tract.

3. *Vitamin E.* This vitamin is essential for normal reproduction in a variety of animals. Deficiency causes non-motility of sperm (sterility) and general loss of sexual instincts in the male. In the female, while conception and early embryological development are not impaired, about halfway through the pregnancy the fetus will abort. In the human the need for this vitamin is unclear.

4. *Vitamin K.* This vitamin is necessary for the production of prothrombin and thus for normal blood clotting to occur. Deficiency causes abnormally long clotting times and hemorrhage.

Water-soluble Vitamins:

1. *Thiamine (Vitamin B_1).* This vitamin is essential for the proper functioning of the nervous system; it is an antagonist to acetylcholine. Deficiency will result in beriberi in humans and polyneuritis in birds.

2. *Riboflavin (Vitamin B_2).* Riboflavin functions in the conversion of tryptophan to nicotinic acid. No recognized disease is associated with a deficiency. General problems with vision, skin, coordination and growth do occur.

3. *Niacin (Nicotinic acid).* Niacin is the functional group of the coenzymes NAD and NADP. Deficiency results in blacktongue in canines and pellagra in humans. Dermatitis and neurological lesions are manifestations of pellagra. As noted above, tryptophan may be converted to nicotinic acid.

Minerals: Minerals are also utilized by the tissues of the body. Among the most common ones found on the label of a bottle of vitamin and mineral supplements are calcium, phosphorus, potassium, sodium, magnesium chlorine, manganese, iodine, iron, zinc, copper, cobalt, bromine and fluorine. Except in unusual circumstances, of course, these will be in the normal diet and need not be taken in pills.

The Digestive System

Regionalization of the Embryonic Gut:

1) Foregut (supplied mainly by celiac artery): pharynx, esophagus, stomach, and cranial portion of duodenum from which the primordia of the liver, gall bladder and pancreas arise.

2) Midgut (supplied by superior mesenteric artery): caudal duodenum, jejunum, ileum, and ascending colon and 2/3 of transverse colon including the appendages cecum and vermiform appendix.

3) Hindgut (supplied by inferior mesenteric artery): distal third of transverse colon, descending colon, sigmoid colon, and rectum.

Parts of the Adult Digestive Tract: The parts of the human intestinal tract may be listed in the following order: oral cavity (receives salivary gland secretions); oral and laryngeal pharynx; esophagus; cardiac sphincter; stomach; pyloric sphincter; duodenum (receives bile and pancreatic secretions); jejunum (absorption of nutrients); ileum (absorption of nutrients); cecum, ascending colon (water absorption); transverse colon; descending colon; sigmoid colon; rectum; and anal sphincter.

The Oral Cavity. The oral cavity is divided into:

a) Vestibule: the area between cheek and teeth.
b) The Lip: composed of a core of skeletal muscle and covered externally by skin.
c) The Cheek: structure similar to the lip.
d) Oral Cavity Proper: area from teeth to fauces.
e) The Tongue: composed primarily of a core of skeletal muscle and glands and covered by a mucous membrane. The anterior 2/3 of the upper (oral) portion is separated from the posterior 1/3 (pharyngeal) portion by the sulcus terminalis.

Three types of lingual papillae appear as surface projections:

a) Circumvallate papillae, located along the sulcus terminalis and possessing taste buds;
b) Filiform papillae, the most numerous;
c) Fungiform papillae, relatively few but possessing taste buds.

f) The Teeth: two sets occurring during lifetime. In childhood, there are 20 temporary primary (deciduous) teeth present; this dentition lacks premolars (bicuspids) and has only two instead of three pairs of molars (tricuspids) in each jaw. After about the age of six, the primary dentition is replaced by a set of 32 symmetrically arranged permanent (succedaneous) teeth. Each jaw contains beginning at the front: 2 central incisors, 2 lateral incisors, 2 cuspids, 4 premolars (bicuspids), and 6 molars (tricuspids).

The basic parts of a tooth are:

a) crown—above gum margin;
b) root—1 to 3 cm below gum margin;
c) alveolus—root socket in jaw bone;
d) neck—junction of root and crown;
e) periodontal membrane—attaches the root to the alveolar wall;
f) pulp chamber—extends from crown into root canals;
g) apical foramen—canal opening at the tip of root;

h) dental pulp—soft core of loosely arranged connective tissue occupying the chamber and containing blood vessels and nerves to teeth;

i) tooth wall with dentin, which borders pulp; enamel, which covers the crown and thins at the neck; and cementum, which encrusts the root and thins at the neck.

g) Salivary Glands: There are 3 pairs of major salivary glands.

1) Parotid (largest gland)—located in relation to the mandibular ramus below and anterior to the ear. It is a compound tubulo-alveolar, serous gland of the merocrine type. Connective tissue divides the gland into lobes and lobules. The major duct (Stenson's) opens into the vestibule of the oral cavity opposite the second upper (maxillary) molar.

2) Submandibular (intermediate in size)—located in relationship to the mylohyoid muscle, medial and inferior to the mandible. It is a tubulo-alveolar, merocrine gland (mixed-mucus and serous). The major duct (Wharton's) opens on the anterolateral margin of the frenulum of the tongue.

3) Sublingual (smallest gland)—a collection of glands located under the mucous membrane of the floor of the mouth. It is a tubulo-alveolar merocrine gland with mostly mucous acini. The major duct (Bartholin's) empties on the side of the frenulum of the tongue, having joined the submandibular duct.

Tubular Digestive Tract. The adult tubular digestive tract has a general structural plan of mucosa, submucosa, muscular tunic and adventitia.

1) Mucosa
   a) moist surface epithelium
   b) connective tissue (lamina propria)
   c) thin muscular layer (muscularis mucosae)
   d) villi (evaginations of the mucosa)
2) Submucosa
   a) connective tissue
   b) plexi of nerves and ganglion cells termed Meissner's plexus
   c) some areas may contain glands
   d) rich in blood vessels
3) Muscular tunic
   a) inner circular smooth muscle layer
   b) outer longitudinal smooth muscle layer
   c) Auerbach's myenteric plexus—between the two muscle layers is located a parasympathetic plexus of nerves associated with numerous ganglion cells
4) Adventitia
   a) connective tissue containing blood vessels, nerves and lymphatics
   b) peritoneal covering (mesothelium) known as a serosa, located in some regions

Esophagus (about 10–12 inches). The upper ⅓ of the esophagus features skeletal muscle (voluntary), the middle ⅓ both skeletal and smooth (involuntary) muscle, the lower ⅓ as the rest of the digestive tract only smooth muscle.

The Stomach. The stomach is highly vascular, contains gastric glands, and has smooth muscle fibers extending around the glands. There are two types of gastric glands: cardiac and fundic.

1) Cardiac glands secrete mucus
2) Fundic glands:
   a) mucous and epithelial cells—secrete mucus; this mucus protects against autodigestion and neutralizes acid to a small degree.
   b) parietal or oxyntic cells—secrete hydrochloric acid (HCl). Acid (pH below 5.5) is necessary to convert pepsinogen into pepsin; at pH 2, this reaction is almost instantaneous. Parietal cells secrete acid under the influence of the hormone gastrin (probably of greatest importance); parasympathetic mediation via acetylcholine; histamine; and the presence of foodstuffs, such as peptides and amino acids.

c) chief (zymogenic) cells—secret pepsinogen, the precursor of pepsin (proteolytic enzyme). These cells also secrete and release the hormone gastrin, and some are also implicated in the production of rennin and gastric intrinsic (anti-pernicious anemia) factor.

d) argentaffin cells—thought to secrete serotonin, a vasoconstrictor substance.

Small Intestine. The small intestine has 3 major regions:

1) Duodenum (10 inches)
2) Jejunum (8.5 feet)
3) Ileum (12.5 feet)

The small intestine has mucosal surface modifications:

a) Villi (projections of mucosa)—covered by simple columnar epithelium and having a core of connective tissue; they are broad in the duodenum, fingerlike in the ileum. In the core of the villus (in the connective tissue layer called the lamina propria) are found lymphocytes, eosinophils, plasma cells, macrophages, capillaries and *lacteals* (lymphatic capillaries).

b) Microvilli—present on columnar absorptive cells covering villi and lining crypts; we speak in terms of a striated border.

Large Intestine (cecum, ascending, transverse and descending colon)

Colon and Rectum

The Major Digestive Glands

Pancreas: The pancreas has both an exocrine and endocrine secretory function. Two excretory ducts are usually present and enter the second part of the duodenum. Exocrine glandular elements are arranged in acini. Acinar cells have a basal zone which is basophilic and an apical zone with zymogen granules which are the precursors of the enzymes in pancreatic juice—namely trypsin, chymotrypsin, amylase, and lipase. Acinar cells secrete:
(1) trypsinogen, which will be converted into trypsin.
(2) chymotrypsinogen, which will be converted into chymotrypsin.
(3) procarboxypeptidase, which will be converted into carboxypeptidase.

The above reactions are autocatalyzed (trypsinogen-trypsin). Trypsin, chymotrypsin and carboxypeptidase attack proteins and polypeptides and eventually render amino acids which can be absorbed.

Pancreatic lipase, amylase and proteases are controlled by the presence of foodstuffs and hormones. As acid chyme enters the duodenum from the stomach, secretin is released and fluid and bicarbonate are secreted.

Pancreatic juice:

1) neutralizes the acid chyme in the duodenum
2) provides enzymes for the digestion of proteins, carbohydrates and fats.

Islets of Langerhans are the endocrine portion of the pancreas. The endocrine cell aggregations are interspersed irregularly among the acini. Three cell types can be identified:

1) A, or alpha, cells, which are presumed to form glucagon.
2) B, or beta, cells which are more numerous than A cells and produce insulin.
3) D, or delta, cells; their significance is uncertain but they might represent multipotent resting cells.

Liver: The liver has the following functions:

a) Removal of bile pigments from blood which are excreted in bile.
b) Storage of glycogen.
c) Conversion of fats, and perhaps proteins, to carbohydrates (*gluconeogenesis*).

d) Maintenance of the constancy of blood glucose level.
e) Deamination of animo acid with urea as a by-product.
f) Metabolism of fat and storage in the liver.
g) Synthesis of plasma proteins such as fibrinogen, prothrombin, and albumin.
h) Storage of essential vitamins (A, D, B_2, B_3, B_4, B_{12}, and K).
i) Embryonic hemopoietic (blood cell forming) organ.

Gallbladder: *Bile,* which is secreted continuously by the hepatocytes, is collected and transported via the hepatic ducts and cystic duct into the gallbladder, where it is stored and concentrated. When demand exists bile is released and flows into the cystic duct which connects with the common bile duct (formed by union of common hepatic and cystic ducts), which empties into the second part of the duodenum.

General Functional Schema of the Digestive Tube (ingestion, digestion, egestion)

Oral Cavity:

a) Receives food and perceives taste, odor, texture and temperature.
b) Grinds foodstuffs to facilitate the action of enzymes.
c) Adds enzymes, mucus and moisture and shapes the bolus for the process of swallowing.

Pharynx and Esophagus: The oral and laryngeal pharynx, and the esophagus are essentially conduits for food to reach the stomach.

Stomach: Food is received, stored and churned; digestive juices are added; and the digestive process started in the mouth is continued. Intrinsic factor (anti-pernicious anemia factor) is secreted.

Small Intestines: Digestion is completed and most absorption takes place in jejunum and ileum.

Large Intestines:

a) Water and electrolytes are reabsorbed to preserve that delicate balance in the body.
b) Food is propelled along for elimination (egestion).

Intestinal Motility

Intestinal motility facilitates:

1) the mixing of food with secretions and enzymes
2) the contact of foodstuffs with the intestinal mucosa
3) propulsion along the tube (peristalsis).

This process is controlled by the nervous system, hormonal secretions, and intestinal distension and similar phenomena.
Epinephrine (from the adrenal) inhibits contraction; serotonin (from the small intestines) stimulates contractions.

Innervation of the Intestinal Tract

The nerves supplying the intestinal tract affect smooth muscle, glands, endocrine tissue and control motility and secretion. Motility or *peristalsis* is a wave of compression (contraction) that is followed by a regional relaxation. The gut musculature (smooth) is controlled by the autonomic nervous system.

Sympathetic Innervation: Effects of sympathetic innervation are:

a) some excitation of salivary secretion
b) a decrease of motility and secretion in the stomach and small intestines due mainly to the vasoconstrictive action

c) an inhibition of muscular contraction and intrinsic ganglion cell activity due to the release of the neurotransmitters epinephrine and norepinephrine

Parasympathetic Innervation: Effects of the parasympathetic innervation are:

a) stimulation of motility and secretion via its supply of the intrinsic plexi and the release of the neurotransmitter acetylcholine
b) release of gastrin

Summary of Digestive Juices

Saliva: Saliva is protective and digestive. In this manner, it

a) dissolves food and passes it over the taste buds
b) lubricates food
c) starts starch digestion (contains amylase which breaks down 1,4-glycosidic bonds of glucose molecules as in starch)
d) contains antibacterial enzymes (lysozymes)

Saliva is composed of

a) water
b) electrolytes
c) enzymes (chiefly ptyalin, or salivary amylase)
d) mucin
e) glycoproteins
f) blood group proteins
g) gamma globulins

Ptyalin. Ptyalin (salivary amylase), produced chiefly by the parotid, submandibular, and sublingual salivary glands, functions in the breakdown of starch into molecules of the disaccharide maltose.

Gastric Juices: Gastric juice is composed of

a) water
b) hydrochloric acid (HCl)
c) inorganic salts
d) mucus
e) enzymes (pepsin, rennin, and lipase)

About 2 to 3 liters of gastric juices are secreted within a 24-hour period. Food usually remains in the stomach for 3 or 4 hours. The pH of gastric juice usually varies from about 0.9 to 1.5. This acidity allows pepsin to act and inhibits ptyalin (salivary amylase).

Pepsin, a proteinase of gastric juice, is derived from its precursor pepsinogen, which is secreted by the chief cells of the gastric mucosa. Pepsin acts upon protein substrates, breaking them down to amino acids, proteoses, and peptones.

Rennin. Rennin is secreted by the stomach. This enzyme splits some peptide bonds in casein to produce a calcium-precipitable paracasein.

Mucus. Mucus is composed of proteins, glycoproteins, polysaccharides, intrinsic factor, plasma proteins, and blood group substances.

Intrinsic factor. Intrinsic factor, produced by the parietal cells of the stomach, is a mucoprotein. It binds to vitamin B_{12} and "protects" it until it is absorbed in the ileum and then transported actively into the circulation.

Pancreatic Juice: Pancreatic juice contains proteolytic, lipolytic, and amylolytic enzymes.

Pancreatic amylase. Pancreatic amylase is an enzyme which hydrolyzes starch to maltose.

Steapsin. Steapsin, or pancreatic lipase, facilitates the digestion of fats.

Trypsinogen. Trypsinogen is secreted by the pancreas and converted by enterokinase to the active enzyme *trypsin*. Trypsin's substrates are proteins but specifically it further disintegrates proteoses and peptones.

Chymotrypsinogen. Chymotrypsinogen is the precursor in pancreatic juice of the enzyme *chymotrypsin*. Trypsin is active in this conversion. Chymotrypsin acts with trypsin to hydrolyze proteins and protein products to polypeptides and amino acids.

Bile: Bile is secreted by the liver, stored and concentrated in the gall bladder, and poured into the duodenum. It primarily contains bile salts (such as cholic acid, chenodeoxycholic acid, deoxycholic acid and lithocholic acid), cholesterol phospholipids (lecithins), pigments (bilirubin), mucin and sodium, potassium, calcium and other elements. It aids in the emulsification, digestion, and absorption of fat. It also contributes to the alkalinization of the intestinal contents.

Lacteals are found in the villi of the small intestines; they are part of the lymphatic system and function to take up chyle containing fat in lipoproteins.

Hormones of the Digestive Tract

Endocrine cells of the gut originate from the neural crest. Hormones of the gastrointestinal tract are produced by the mucosa of the stomach (gastrin) and by the small intestines (secretin and cholecystokinin). These gastrointestinal hormones are polypeptides which affect:

1) water balance;
2) electrolyte balance;
3) enzyme secretions;
4) motility;
5) digestion;
6) absorption;
7) growth; and
8) hormonal release.

The general stimuli for their release are:

1) nervous activity;
2) physical extension;
3) chemical stimuli.

Specific stimuli for three key hormones are:

1) Gastrin—distension, vagal stimulation, and presence of proteins and amino acids.
2) Secretin—acid chyme (hydrogen ion) released when the pH falls below 4.5.
3) Cholecystokinin—presence of proteins and amino acids and of monoglycerides, fatty acids.

Primary actions are as follows:

1) Gastrin
   a) stimulates gastric acid and pepsinogen secretion.
   b) increases the distension of the stomach and gastric motility.
2) Secretin
   a) stimulates the pancreas to secrete pancreatic fluid and bicarbonate
   b) stimulates biliary fluid secretion and bicarbonate
   c) potentiates the enzymatic response to cholecystokinin
   d) slows gastric motility and emptying
   e) stimulates pepsinogen secretion and
   f) inhibits gastrin release.

3) Cholecystokinin
   a) stimulates pancreatic enzyme secretion
   b) increases the pancreatic bicarbonate response to secretin
   c) increases the distensibility of the stomach and inhibits gastric emptying
   d) induces gallbladder contractions and emptying.

General Digestion of the Major Food Groups

Carbohydrates: Starch digestion begins in the oral cavity under the influence of α-amylase and ends in the small intestines after exposure to pancreatic amylase. Products resulting from the above processes are further hydrolyzed by enzymes associated with the microvilli of the intestinal cells. For example: (1) maltase acts on maltose and maltotriose to yield glucose units; (2) sucrase acts on sucrose to produce glucose and fructose; (3) lactase breaks down lactose to yield monosaccharide subunits.

Proteins: Digestion begins in the stomach by the action of pepsin, which has a specificity for peptide bonds; it is inactivated by pancreatic juice. When products are transferred from the stomach to the duodenum, this stimulus results in the release of cholecystokinin (CCK) which is responsible for the release of pancreatic proteolytic enzymes such as: (1) endo- and exopeptidases, (2) trypsin, (3) chymotrypsin, (4) elastase.

Fats: In the stomach fat products are acted upon by pepsin; when the products are released into the duodenum, cholecystokinin stimulates the pancreas to secrete lipases and the gallbladder to release its contents, which emulsify fat droplets resulting in the formation of micelles. The absorption is completed in the jejunum.

Nervous System

The nervous system is usually divided into: a) central nervous system (brain and spinal cord) and b) peripheral nervous system (peripheral nerves and ganglia). The peripheral nervous system is divided into a somatic system and visceral (autonomic) system.

Nervous Tissue

Nervous tissue consists of neurons (nerve cells and their processes) and supportive elements. Neuroglia in the central nervous system and Schwann cells in the peripheral nervous system are the supportive elements.

The Neuron

The neuron is a cellular element and, as a highly specialized cell, it carries out the function of nervous transmission. The neuron is like many other cells within the body in that it consists of a nucleus with an associated nucleolus and a cytoplasm which is rich in organelles, the most prominent of which are the rough-surfaced endoplasmic reticulum (Nissl substance), mitochondria, and the Golgi apparatus. In addition to the above characteristics, it should be noted that neurons possess numerous cytoplasmic processes or appendages. In almost all of the many varieties of neurons, there are two kinds of processes: the *dendrites* and the *axon*.

The Dendrites:
1. are direct extensions of the cytoplasm.
2. are generally multiple.
3. provide an increased surface area, the dendritic zone, to allow for synaptic interaction.

The Axon:
1. There is only one per neuron.
2. This process arises from a conical elevation of cytoplasm which is devoid of rough-surfaced endoplasmic reticulum (Nissl) and this area is called the *axon hillock*.

3. It is usually thinner and longer than the dendrites of the same neuron.

4. It may be surrounded by a *myelin sheath* which is produced by the *oligodendrocytes* in the CNS and by the *Schwann cells* in the PNS. Discontinuities in this myelin sheath occur at intervals known as the *nodes of Ranvier*. Though many axons are myelinated and are referred to as myelinated nerve fibers, numerous others possess no myelin ensheathment and thus are referred to as unmyelinated nerve fibers.

5. At its ending, the axon transmits impulses: a. to other neurons—the site of this impulse transmission being called a *synapse;* and, b. to effector cells such as muscle fibers or gland cells. This junction with skeletal muscle fibers constitutes a *motor end plate*.

The Action Potential: An impulse traveling along a neuron is an electrical phenomenon initiated by a temporary change in the permeability of the neuron's cell membrane. To understand this change, one must first examine the condition of a resting, or unstimulated, neuron. The membrane possesses specific sites for the active transport of sodium ions (Na^+) and potassium ions (K^+). At these sites, sodium is transported out of the cell, and potassium is transported inward. Both ions tend to return to their original positions through pores, but Na^+ ions are less successful than are K^+ ions. Thus, the unstimulated neuron accumulates a larger concentration of positive ions (both Na^+ and K^+) outside its membrane than in its cytoplasm. A voltmeter would measure this difference as about 70 millivolts, with the inside of the neuron being negative; this is called the *resting potential* or *membrane potential*.

A sufficient stimulus—whether it be mechanical, chemical, or electrical—causes a radical but temporary change in the permeability of the affected membrane region. The membrane possesses specific channels that can allow sodium to pass, and others for potassium; in a resting membrane both are closed. A stimulus causes the sodium channel to open, and accumulated sodium ions outside the membrane rush into the interior by diffusion. Their number is sufficient to reverse the interior charge, making it about 40 millivolts positive. This change, in turn, causes the potassium channels to open, allowing a loss of potassium ions from the cytoplasm. Thus, the initial gain of interior positive ions (Na^+) is countered by a loss of positive ions (K^+), and the cytoplasm once again is negatively charged. The charge reversal, from negative to positive to negative, occurs within only a few milliseconds. The phenomenon is termed an *action potential*.

Immediately after an action potential, the sodium and potassium channels close again, and the two types of ions are pumped back to their original sites. During this refractory period of several milliseconds, an additional stimulus will not lead to another action potential.

Initiation of the action potential at any point of a neuron's membrane acts as a stimulus to the adjacent membrane material; therefore, the effect is of an action potential flowing along the membrane. The result is the "message" that moves quickly over the length of a motor neuron's axon. It is also the message that flows along and into a muscle fiber that has been stimulated by events at a motor end plate, because the membrane of a muscle fiber can act like that of a neuron.

The Synapse: The synapse is the site of contact between two neurons; it may be, and most commonly is, between an axon and a dendrite; however, contacts between an axon and the cell body and between axons and axons have also been observed. A typical synapse seen between an axon and dendrite (axodendritic synapse) has the following properties:

1. As the axon terminal reaches the synaptic site, it forms a bulbous head called a *bouton*. This bouton, which constitutes the presynaptic element of the synapse, contains numerous mitochondria and specialized vesicles, the synaptic vesicles, which contain the various neurotransmitters (acetylcholine is the primary one).

2. The dendrite, which constitutes the postsynaptic element of the synapse, is separated from the bouton by a cleft which varies in width from 150 to 200 Å.

3. This axo-dendritic synapse is *not* a site where cytoplasmic continuity is established between the axon and the dendrite, as both the pre- and postsynaptic elements are separated by a cleft. However, via the process of synaptic vesicle release, this axodendritic synapse establishes a functional (chemical) continuity across the expanse of the cleft.

Classification of Neurons

Multipolar Neurons: Most abundant; somatic and visceral motor, and associational.

Unipolar Neurons: Somatic and visceral *sensory* neurons; cell bodies are located in cranial sensory and dorsal root ganglia; peripheral process goes out to receptor and central process travels into the central nervous system.

Bipolar Neurons: Special *sensory* neurons; cell bodies are located in special sense organs; i.e., eye (retina), ear (spiral and vestibular ganglia), and nose (olfactory epithelium).

Groups of Neurons

Nucleus: cluster of nerve cell bodies *within* the central nervous system.

Ganglion: cluster of nerve cells bodies *outside* the central nervous system.

Cortex: layered arrangement of nerve cells bodies on the surface of the cerebrum and cerebellum (gray matter).

Supportive Elements

Neuroglia—Supportive Elements of the Central Nervous System: Neuroglia, the supportive elements of the central nervous system, are of several types.

1. Astrocytes. Astrocytes are fibrous and protoplasmic; their perivascular feet end on capillaries. They are located between capillary (or pia matter) and neurons and are implicated in the blood-brain barrier. Eighty percent of brain capillary surfaces are covered by perivascular end feet of astrocytes.
2. Oligodendrocytes. Oligodendrocytes function in the myelinization of central nervous system axons.
3. Microglia. Microglia are of questionable origin and role; they may be macrophages of the central nervous system.

Supportive Elements of the Peripheral Nervous System:

1. Schwann (neurolemmal) Cells. These are involved in the myelinization of peripheral nervous system axons.
2. Satellite Cells. These cells surround nerve cell bodies in the ganglia (e.g., dorsal root ganglia) of the peripheral nervous system.

The Central Nervous System

The central nervous system is made up of the brain and the spinal cord.

Spinal Cord: Before one can appreciate the organization of the cerebral mass and brain stem, it is necessary to understand the basic structural organization found throughout the extent of the spinal cord.

Cross Section View. If one were to examine a cross section through any level of the spinal cord, the following would be seen:

1. A centrally located H-shaped mass which contains the cell bodies of neurons. This H-shaped mass is divided into dorsal and ventral columns, or *horns*. Cell bodies responsible for sensory phenomena are located in the dorsal horns, cell bodies for motor phenomena in the ventral horns. This H-shaped mass is collectively referred to as the *gray matter*.

2. Peripheral to this H-shaped mass, *white matter,* made up primarily of myelinated nerve fibers.

3. Entering the spinal cord at the apex of the dorsal horn, or column, is the dorsal root of the spinal nerve. The cell bodies of these fibers are unipolar and are located in the dorsal root ganglion. The ventral root exits from the ventral horn of the gray matter. The cell bodies of these fibers are multipolar and located in the ventral horn.

4. White matter is divided into three masses of fibers known as *funiculi.* These three funiculi are:

    a) the dorsal funiculus, located between the dorsal midline and the dorsal root,

    b) the lateral funiculus, located between the dorsal and ventral roots,

    c) the ventral funiculus, located between the ventral root and the ventral midline.

Within each funiculus are found bundles of fibers (axons) called *tracts.* The fibers within a specific tract have a common origin, termination, and function and either descend or ascend in the cord.

5. An orderly arrangement of gray and white matter that remains constant throughout the spinal cord, varying only in relative mass.

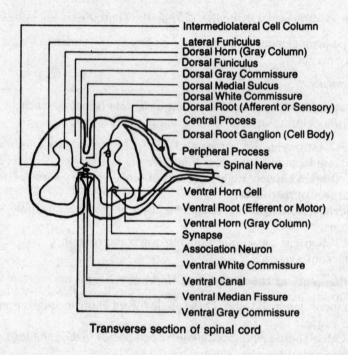

Intermediolateral Cell Column
Lateral Funiculus
Dorsal Horn (Gray Column)
Dorsal Funiculus
Dorsal Gray Commissure
Dorsal Medial Sulcus
Dorsal White Commissure
Dorsal Root (Afferent or Sensory)
Central Process
Dorsal Root Ganglion (Cell Body)
Peripheral Process
Spinal Nerve
Ventral Horn Cell
Ventral Root (Efferent or Motor)
Ventral Horn (Gray Column)
Synapse
Association Neuron
Ventral White Commissure
Ventral Canal
Ventral Median Fissure
Ventral Gray Commissure

Transverse section of spinal cord

Gross Anatomy and Relationships. The spinal cord viewed as a whole also has the following characteristics:

1. It is cylindrical, about ½ inch in diameter and 18 inches in length, and has *cervical* and *lumbar enlargements* due to the involvement of these cord levels with the innervation of the upper and lower limbs, respectively.

2. It runs within the bony *vertebral canal* but is shorter than the canal since vertebral column growth exceeds cord growth. The spinal cord ends at vertebral level L_1–L_2 (Lumbar 1–2).

3. It is protected not only by the bony vertebral column but also by three connective tissue sheaths known collectively as the *meninges* (dura mater, arachnoid membrane and pia mater). *Cerebrospinal fluid* is in the subarachnoid space (between arachnoid and pia) and bathes the cord and cushions it from shock.

4.   There are 31 pairs of *spinal nerves* that are connected to the cord by *dorsal* and *ventral roots:* 8 *cervical,* 12 *thoracic,* 5 *lumbar,* 5 *sacral* and 1 *coccygeal.*

5.   The spinal nerves exit from the vertebral canal through *intervertebral foramina.*

6.   It is because the cord ends at vertebral level L_2 that *lumbar punctures* (spinal taps) can be done safely below that level. (Nerve roots arise from the cord and extend below this level to exit at the specific vertebral level. These roots are collectively called *cauda equina* and are deflected away from the needle and therefore are not damaged.)

The Brain: The brain is divided into three parts: the cerebrum (two cerebral hemispheres), the brain stem, and the cerebellum. The brain stem is, in turn, divided into the medulla, pons, midbrain, and diencephalon. Important facts about the structure and functions of each of the parts is given below.

Cerebrum. The cerebrum consists of two hemispheres that are joined by a broad band of commissural fibers, the *corpus callosum.* Eminences on the surface are known as *gyri* and the furrows as *sulci* or *fissures.*

Each cerebral hemisphere is divided into five lobes:
1.   *frontal*—contains the major motor areas (motor speech area).
2.   *parietal*—is concerned with sensory impressions such as touch, pressure, and pain.
3.   *occipital*—is concerned with vision.
4.   *temporal*—is concerned with hearing.
5.   *insula*—is found deep within the Sylvian fissure.

The cerebrum is the seat of intelligence, consciousness and rational behavior and possesses areas for speech and writing.

Medulla Oblongata. The medulla oblongata is structurally derived from the myelencephalon and is continuous with the spinal cord at the *foramen magnum* and extends to the caudal portion of the pons. The medulla controls movement of eyelids (in blinking), sneezing, coughing, chewing, swallowing, and vomiting, and contains centers for the autonomic control of respiration (breathing), heartbeat (rate and force), contractility of blood vessels, visceral movement (gastric juice production and peristalsis), and glandular secretion (salivation).

Pons. The pons is essentially a crossing and relay station for nerve tracts. It is a conduit through which the cerebral cortex communicates with the cerebellum. It contains the motor nuclei that exert control over facial expression and mastication, and it possesses cell bodies that control lacrimation and salivation, and it serves as a relay station of tactile sensation for the facial system.

Midbrain. The midbrain serves as a relay center for auditory and optic phenomena. It houses the oculomotor nucleus, which controls extraocular movements, and exerts autonomic control over pupillary constriction and the process of accommodation.

Diencephalon. The diencephalon is itself divided into the thalamus and the hypothalamus.

Thalamus.
1.   Maintains the internal environment of the organism.
2.   Processes all sensory input except olfactation.
3.   Maintains a subconscious sense of comfort.
4.   Serves as the main relay station between the cerebrum and the rest of the nervous system.
5.   Serves in the integration of motor activities via its relay activity between the basal ganglia, the cerebellum and the cerebral cortex.

Hypothalamus. The hypothalamus regulates body temperature, osmotic balance, blood pressure, and sleep.

Cerebellum. The cerebellum is derived from the metencephalon. It integrates unconscious proprioceptive impulses, integrates and modulates vestibular functions and body equilibrium. The cerebellum is also responsible for muscular synergy of the body; it coordinates the smooth, accurate and orderly sequences of muscular contraction and movement. Without cerebellar influence muscle activity is disorganized and crude. There is, however, no conscious perception.

The Peripheral Nervous System

The peripheral nervous system is made up of a somatic portion and an autonomic portion.

Somatic Peripheral Nervous System: The somatic portion of the peripheral nervous system is made up of cranial nerves and spinal nerves.

Cranial Nerves. The cranial nerves are those peripheral nerves which leave the brain. It is customary to subdivide the cranial nerves into twelve pairs and to number and name these pairs as follows:

I. Olfactory nerve	VII. Facial nerve
II. Optic nerve	VIII. Vestibulocochlear (auditory) nerve
III. Oculomotor nerve	
IV. Trochlear nerve	IX. Glossopharyngeal nerve
V. Trigeminal nerve	X. Vagus nerve
VI. Abducens nerve	XI. Spinal accessory nerve
	XII. Hypoglossal nerve

No.	Nerve	General Components	Peripheral Termination and Modality Supplied	Damage to Nerve Results in
I	Olfactory	Sensory	Nasal mucosa—olfaction	Anosmia; Parosmia
II	Optic	Sensory	Rods and cones of retina—vision	Visual field defects
III	Oculomotor	Motor	Superior, inferior and medial rectus muscles and inferior oblique muscle—rotate eyeball	Strabismus or squint—deviation of the eyeball; Diplopia—double vision
		Motor	To a muscle which constricts pupil	Dilated pupil; Loss of light reflexes
			To ciliary muscle whose contraction thickens lens	Loss of accommodation
IV	Trochlear	Motor	Superior oblique muscle—rotates eyeball	Strabismus and diplopia
V	Trigeminal	Motor	Muscles of mastication—mastication	Paralysis of the muscles of mastication
		Sensory	Skin of face and mucosa of mouth and nose—supplies sensation	Loss of sensation over the distribution of V; Loss of reflex; Tic douloureux—pain over the distribution of V

No.	Nerve	General Components	Peripheral Termination and Modality Supplied	Damage to Nerve Results in
VI	Abducens	Motor	Lateral rectus muscle—moves eyeball laterally	Loss of the ability to abduct eyeball
VII	Facial	Motor	Muscles of facial expression	Facial paralysis (Bell's palsy); Expressionless face with a drooping mouth
		Sensory	Taste buds on the anterior ⅔ of the tongue	Loss of taste on the anterior ⅔ of the tongue
VIII	Vestibu-locochlear	Sensory (Vestibular portion)	Cristae of semicircular canals—provide for equilibrium	Vertigo, nystagmus and nausea
		Sensory (Cochlear portion	Hair cells in the organ of Corti—provide for hearing	Deafness
IX	Glosso-pharyngeal	Motor	Parotid gland—provides for glandular secretion	Loss of secretion
		Sensory	Taste buds in the posterior ⅓ of the tongue	Loss of taste in the posterior ⅓ of the tongue
		Sensory	Epiglottis, root of tongue, soft palate	Loss of gag reflex
X	Vagus	Motor	Palate and pharyngeal constrictors and intrinsic muscles of larynx	Aphonia and dysphonia
		Motor	Via the cardiac and pulmonary ganglia to the cardiac muscle and to the smooth muscle and the glands of the pulmonary and gastrointestinal systems—provides for autonomic regulation of the above named organs	Autonomic disturbances
XI	Spinal Accessory	Motor	Trapezius and sternomastoid muscles	Difficulty in rotating head or raising shoulder
XII	Hypoglossal	Motor	Muscles of the tongue	Paralysis of tongue

Spinal Nerves. Thirty-one pairs of spinal nerves are connected to the spinal cord. Like any nerve, a spinal nerve is composed of nerve fibers (axons and their sheaths) coursing together outside the central nervous system. Spinal nerves are surrounded by well-organized, protective connective tissue sheaths, i.e., endoneurium, perineurium and epineurium.

Spinal nerves contain both sensory and motor fibers.

a) Sensory:
   1) from recpetors in skin and skeletal muscle (G.S.A.—general somatic afferent)
   2) from receptors in smooth muscle in walls of organs and blood vessels (G.V.A.—general visceral afferent).

b) Motor:
    1) to skeletal muscle (G.S.E.—general somatic efferent)
    2) autonomic fibers to smooth muscle, cardiac muscle, and glands (G.V.E.—general visceral efferent).

Sensory Pathway. A typical sensory pathway contains three neurons in a chain from the receptor on the surface of the body to consciousness in the cerebral cortex (Primary: 1°, Secondary: 2°, and Tertiary: 3° neurons).

1° neuron: has its unipolar cell body in the dorsal root ganglion; its peripheral process goes out to the receptor through the spinal nerve; its central process follows the dorsal root and synapses in the C.N.S. with a second order (2°) neuron.

2° neuron: has its cell body in the central nervous system; those cell bodies concerned with pain and temperature are found within the spinal cord; those concerned with touch and pressure are localized in the medulla of the brain. The axon of this 2° neuron then crosses the midline and ascends to the thalamus, where it synapses with a third order (3°) neuron.

3° neuron: has its cell body in the thalamus; its axon ascends to the cerebral cortex.

Voluntary Motor Pathway. A typical voluntary motor pathway contains two neurons from the cerebral cortex to the effector organ in skeletal muscle.

Neuron 1: (upper motor neuron) has its cell body in the cerebral cortex; its axon descends, crosses in the medulla and terminates in relation to lower motor neurons found in the ventral horn.

Neuron 2: (lower motor neuron) has its cell body in the ventral horn of the spinal cord; its axon (efferent fiber) leaves the spinal cord through the ventral root and follows the spinal nerve to the skeletal muscle, where it terminates as a motor end plate.

Autonomic Nervous System: The autonomic nervous system innervates all smooth muscle, cardiac muscle, and glands. The autonomic nervous system is divided into a sympathetic (flight and fight) component and parasympathetic (maintains homeostasis) component. The autonomic nervous system exerts important influences on the intrinsic eye musculature, skin glands, the cardiovascular, gastrointestinal, respiratory, endocrine, and reproductive systems.

Fear, rage, pain, and the like evoke sympathetic activity that mobilizes the resources of the body. Gastrointestinal activity is curtailed; heart rate and blood pressure increase and coronary arteries and bronchioles dilate.

Reflex Arc

The typical pathway of a reflex may be outlined as follows: sensory receptor on dendrite of dorsal root ganglion cell ⟶ ganglion cell ⟶ axon of cell ⟶ dorsal root ⟶ dorsal horn of spinal cord ⟶ either directly to motor cell in ventral horn or via internuncial (association) neuron to ventral horn motor cell ⟶ axon via ventral root ⟶ spinal nerve ⟶ effector organ (e.g., muscle).

Organs of Special Sense

The Eye

The visual system is made up of the eye and complex nerve pathways for interpretation by the cerebral cortex and subcortical centers for the purpose of:

1) Refraction of light rays and the focusing thereof on the retina for the production of an image;
2) Conversion of light rays into a nervous impulse;
3) Transmission to visual centers of the brain for interpretation.

The visual system is composed of the following structures: eyelids, tearing apparatus (lacrimal gland), extrinsic muscles, and the eyeball and optic nerve. We will concentrate on the eyeball and optic nerve.

Eyeball and Optic Nerve: The eye is nearly spherical and about 2.5 cm in diameter. The eyeball is composed of three coats—namely, an outer fibrous layer, a middle vascular and pigmented layer, and an inner or retinal layer—and the refractive elements—the cornea, the aqueous humor, the lens and the vitreous humor.

Two clinical problems concerned with the size of the eyeball must be identified:

1) *myopia* (near-sightedness)—In this condition the eyeball is longer than normal and light rays come to focus in front of the retina.

b) *hyperopia* (far-sightedness)—In this condition the eyeball is shorter than normal and light rays come to focus in back of the retina.

Outer Layer. The outer fibrous tunic is the opaque *sclera* (white of the eye), which anteriorly becomes the transparent, non-vascular *cornea*. The sclera maintains the shape of the eye and gives attachment to the external ("extrinsic") ocular muscles. The cornea is composed of five layers and is one of the refractive elements.

Middle Layer. The middle vascular and pigmented tunic is the *choroid*, which anteriorly becomes the *ciliary body* and the *contractile iris*. The ciliary body, attached to the *lens* via the suspensory ligaments, aids in focusing light rays on the retina. Contraction of the ciliary muscles mediated by the parasympathetic portion (Edinger-Westphal nucleus) of the oculomotor nerve decreases the tension on the suspensory ligaments, allowing the lens to increase in thickness. The *pupil* is the central opening of the iris; its size is regulated by the amount of light present. Two smooth muscles regulate the opening; the constrictor, or sphincter pupillae, is innervated by the parasympathetic system (oculomotor nerve) and reduces the size of the pupil, while the dilator, or dilator pupillae, receives its innervation from the sympathetic system and enlarges the diameter of the pupil.

Inner Layer. The innermost tunic, the retinal layer, consists of ten layers of cells and fibers. Three layers are of neuronal importance:

a) rod and cone layer; here light energy is transformed into chemical and electrical energy;
b) bipolar cells, which allow for internal nerve impulse transmission;
c) ganglion cells which give rise to the *optic nerve.*

There are about 120 million rods and 6 million cones present per eye. The rods contain rhodopsin, or visual purple, which converts photons (basic unit of light) into chemical and then into electrical energy. Rhodopsin is formed from vitamin A; a deficiency of vitamin A may result in night blindness. Rods are very sensitive and function in dim light but yield no color discrimination. Cones contain iodopsin: they are concerned with bright light vision, visual acuity (scotopic vision) and color perception.

Bipolar cells make contact with many rods and cones to receive their impulses which they in turn transmit to the ganglion cells whose axons give rise to the optic nerve. It is estimated that the one million ganglion cells receive information from approximately 130 million rod and cone receptors.

The area at which optic nerve fibers exit is called the *optic disc* or *blind spot*. No photoreception takes place there but the central artery and vein of the retina may be observed there.

Directly in line (visual axis) with the center of the cornea is the *macula lutea*. This area exhibits a high concentration of cones; the center, known as the *fovea centralis,* is the area of most acute vision. The image formed on the retina is inverted; this is inverted again—corrected—by the brain.

The Ear

The ear, which is located in the temporal bone, essentially seves in a dual capacity. It is an auditory organ for the sense of hearing (40–20,000 cycles/second) and a vestibular organ monitoring the effects of gravity and position of the head. Hearing utilizes the cochlear mechanism; vestibular functions are modulated by the utricle, saccule and the three semicircular canals.

Irritative lesions to the vestibular system may result in nystagmus, vertigo, nausea, incoordination or any other disorders of equilibrium or posture.

The auditory functions of the ear are:

1) reception and conduction of sound waves,
2) amplification of the waves,
3) transduction of the waves into nerve impulses,
4) transmission of the impulse to conscious centers.

The vestibular functions of the ear are:

1) reception of stimuli and response to movements of the head and gravitational influences on the head,
2) nerve transmission to higher centers for reflex and postural adjustments to maintain equilibrium.

The ear is commonly divided into the external ear, the middle ear, and the inner ear.

The External Ear: The auricle, or pinna, is composed of skin molded on a complex elastic cartilage; it serves to gather and funnel sound waves into the external auditory meatus (canal), which terminates at the tympanic membrane, or eardrum. In the skin of the meatus are located fine hairs and large sebaceous glands. Coiled, tubular ceruminous glands are also present; they discharge a brownish secretion which in conjunction with the sebaceous products and desquamated cells produce a waxy product known as cerumen.

The Middle Ear: The middle ear is a cavity continuous superiorly with the mastoid air cells and inferiorly, via the auditory (Eustachian) tube, with the nasopharynx. The auditory tube is ordinarily closed and serves to equalize the internal and external pressures on the eardrum. Within the cavity are located three ossicles. From external (eardrum) to internal (oval window), they are respectively the malleus (hammer), the incus (anvil), and the stapes (stirrup). These small bones function in transduction: they translate the displacement of the tympanic membrane, produced by sound waves, into mechanical energy.

On the medial wall of the middle ear are the vestibular window (oval) and the cochlear window (round). The vestibular window houses the base of the stapes; the cochlear window is closed by a membrane. Movement of the eardrum sets up vibrations of the stapes in the oval window; these are transmitted to perilymph in the scala vestibuli (bony labyrinth). The movement is transferred to the endolymph in the cochlear duct (membranous labyrinth) and from there to perilymph in the scala tympani and then is dissipated through the movement of the membrane in the round window. Sound vibrations may be transmitted by surrounding bone in case of middle ear disease (deafness); therefore, the outer and middle ear are not absolutely essential for hearing.

The Inner Ear: The internal ear, located in the petrous portion of the temporal bone, consists of a complex series of fluid (endolymph)-filled sacs, the membranous labyrinth, housed within bony cavities (bony labyrinth), which are filled by perilymph. The interconnecting membranous channels serve static and kinetic senses (vestibular) as well as hearing (auditory).

The vestibular apparatus comprises: three semicircular canals, utricle, and saccule.

The auditory mechanism is housed in the cochlear duct. Both senses are transmitted by the stato-acoustic nerve (cranial nerve VIII) to the brain. This nerve is also named "vestibulocochlear nerve"; in the past it had been called the "auditory nerve."

The Cochlea. The cochlear duct is a helical tube of about 2½ turns housed in its bony labyrinth. The duct separates the bony tube into two channels, the scala tympani and scala vestibuli. At the apex the scala tympani and scala vestibuli communicate; this point is termed the helicotrema. The scala vestibuli begins at the oval window and the scala tympani terminates at the round window.

Pulsations are set up in the perilymph of the scala vestibuli by movements of the stapes at the oval window. They are propagated either via the helicotrema directly to the scala tympani or may pass through the vestibular membrane, activate movement in the endo-lymph of the cochlear duct, and then pass via the basilar membrane into the perilymph of the scala tympani. The pulsations stimulate the receptor (hair) cells located on the basilar membrane and elicit the phenomenon of hearing. Movements of the endolymph, varying with the volume and pitch of the sound waves are registered in specific regions of the organ of Corti. The cochlear division of the stato-acoustic nerve transmits the information to the medulla, then to the midbrain, the thalamus, and, finally, interpretation takes place in the cerebrum.

The Vestibular Apparatus. Head movements are perceived by the three semicircular canals, attached at right angles to the utricle. Displacement of the head causes endolymph to elicit a response in the sensory hair cells of the crista. Position with respect to gravity is monitored by movement of otoliths (calcium carbonate crystals) on the sensory hair cells, in the macula of the utricle and sacculus. The vestibular division of the stato-acoustic nerve (CN VIII) relays the information to the medulla, then to the cerebellum, where muscle coordination is elicited.

Semicircular Canals. There are three canals. Each possesses an ampulla with a modified, sensory epithelium (crista ampullaris) which is associated with neuronal reception. Each crista is stimulated by movements occurring in the plane of its specific canal. Rotational movement leads to a compensatory response of the eyes, head and limbs.

Utricle. The sensory epithelium is located in a region known as the macula. Gelatinous material in which are embedded crystals (otoliths) cover the hair cells. Any change in position of the head in space and any linear acceleration will result in pressure from the crystals on the hair cells and a compensatory reaction such as righting of the body and eye coordination.

Saccule. The morphology of the saccule is similar to that of the utricle. The saccule responds to vibrational stimuli.

The Olfactory System

The olfactory system may be visualized as a highly specialized mucous membrane located in the roof of each nasal cavity. Four primary odors—fragrant, acid, burnt and rancid—are perceived. Olfactory stimulation is caused by gaseous and odiferous substances in solution. Olfactory sero-mucous glands secrete a watery fluid continuously. This allows for reception of dissolved substances and also lessens retention and lingering of stimulation. The receptive cells, bipolar ganglion cells, end in bulbous knobs that possess about 10 olfactory hairs; these serve as the sensory receptors. The sense of smell is subject to fatigue; no structural differences are correlated with discrimination of different kinds of odors. Reception follows this route:

Bipolar cells of olfactory epithelium → Olfactory bulb → Olfactory tract (cranial nerve I) → Olfactory stria → Olfactory cortex.

The Gustatory System

In higher vertebrates the sense of taste is generally restricted to the oral cavity (tongue and epiglottic region). Taste buds are located in vallate, foliate and fungiform papillae. The receptors in the taste bud are neuroepithelial cells. Substances must be in solution and the four modalities of taste—sweet, sour, salt and bitter are specific and regionalized. Sweetness is localized mainly on the tip of the tongue, sour and salt mainly on the central areas and bitter on the back of the tongue.

Endocrine System

Two systems modulate, integrate, and control the activities of the body; they are the nervous and endocrine systems. The response in nervous control is rapid while control via the endocrine system is fairly slow and longer lasting. The endocrine glands are ductless and secrete their products, called hormones, into the capillaries (bloodstream). Hormones are substances that are secreted into the bloodstream and travel to their target organs to elicit their effects. The product of the target organ may also feed back upon the organ that stimulated its activity and production and thus manipulate its cycle of function. It may shut off the supply of stimulating hormone; this activity is called a negative feedback. The controlling mechanism can be thought of as a neuro-endocrine-somatic tissue relationship, or the brain affecting the pituitary gland, which in turn affects the target organs, which then elicit their effect upon the body tissues and cells. Hormones cannot be classified into one chemical class; they are, however, all organic substances and may be proteins, peptides, amino acids (or amino acid derivatives), and steroids, or prostaglandins (derivatives of essential fatty acids). Generally the glands which produce protein hormones embryologically origninate from the alimentary tract; they are the anterior pituitary, thyroid, parathyroids, and pancreas. Glands which produce steroid products are derived from the celomic mesothelium and are the testes, ovaries, and adrenal cortex. Glands whose products are small molecular weight amines arise from cells of nervous tissue derivation and are the neurohypophysis and the adrenal medulla.

It is the purpose of this chapter to give the student a brief description of each endocrine organ, its products, and the results of hypo- and hypersecretion.

The Pituitary Gland (Hypophysis)

The pituitary gland is commonly divided into an anterior and a posterior lobe according to origin. The anterior lobe (adenohypophysis) originates from the oral epithelium of the roof of the mouth in the embryo (Rathke's pouch) while the posterior lobe (neurohypophysis) is a downgrowth of the floor of the brain (in relation to the third ventricle and the hypothalamic areas).

Three cell types are found in the anterior lobe: chromophobes 50%; acidophils 40%; basophils 10%. Chromophobes are considered to be resting cells.

Hormones Secreted by Acidophils (Alpha Cells):
1. *Somatotropic hormone (STH)*
   a. Stimulates general body growth
   b. Hypersecretion—before ossification is complete, giantism
                     —after ossification is complete, acromegaly
   c. Hyposecretion—dwarfism
2. *Lactogenic hormone* or luteotrophic hormone (LTH) or prolactin
   a. Promotes growth of breast which was already stimulated by estrogen and progesterone, especially during the last trimester of pregnancy
   b. Promotes and maintains lactation
   c. Helps in the maintenance of the corpus luteum
   d. Promotes maternal instinct

Hormones Secreted by Basophils (Beta and Delta Cells):
1. *Beta cells*
   a. Thyroid stimulating hormone (TSH)
      (1.) Stimulates the thyroid gland to produce its hormones T_3 (triiodothyronine) and T_4 (tetraiodothyronine or thyroxin)

        (2.) Modulates the iodide trapping mechanisms

        (3.) Hypersecretion—goiter, exophthalmos

        (4.) Hyposecretion—diminished thyroid function and lethargy

   b. Adrenocorticotropic hormone (ACTH)

        (1.) Stimulates the adrenal cortex to produce glucocorticoids (cortisol, etc.)

        (2.) Does *not* stimulate mineralocorticoid activity (aldosterone production)

        (3.) Affects production of adrenal androgens

   c. Melanocyte stimulating hormone (MSH) or intermedin

        (1.) Function poorly understood in humans

        (2.) This hormone causes the dispersion of pigment in the chromatophores of the skin of cold-blooded vertebrates and a darkening of the skin results; the action of MSH allows for quick changes in the skin color in response to changes in the external environment.

  2. *Delta cells*

   a. Luteinizing hormone (LH) in female

      Interstitial cell stimulating hormone (ICSH) in male

        (1.) In the female this hormone is necessary for preovulatory development of the ovarian follicle, ovulation, and formation of the corpus luteum.

        (2.) In the female it modulates the production of estrogen and progesterone.

        (3.) In the male this hormone stimulates the interstitial cells of the testes, which results in a secretion of testicular androgens.

   b. Follicle stimulating hormone (FSH)

        (1.) In the female this hormone stimulates the growth of the ovarian follicle.

        (2.) In the male FSH stimulates the testes to produce sperm (spermatogenesis).

Hormones of the Neurohypophysis:

The posterior lobe or neurohypophysis develops from the floor of the third ventricle of the brain. The function of this portion of the pituitary gland is to store and release the hormones oxytocin (produced by the paraventricular nucleus of the hypothalamus) and vasopressin or antidiuretic hormone (ADH, produced by the supraoptic nucleus of the hypothalamus).

  1. *Oxytocin*

   a. Stimulates the contraction of the smooth muscle of the uterus and may play some role in the initiation of labor

   b. Stimulates the ejection of milk by affecting the myoepithelial cells of the breast tissue (mammary gland)

  2. *Vasopressin; antidiuretic hormone (ADH)*

   a. Acts upon the renal tubules to aid water resorption and thereby restricts diuresis; a lack of hormone results in the condition known as diabetes insipidus (the production of large volumes of dilute urine).

The Pituitary Portal System: In humans the pituitary gland receives its blood supply via the right and left superior and the right and left inferior pituitary arteries from the internal carotid artery system. These vessels supply the hypothalamic areas, the pituitary stalk, and the posterior lobe. The anterior lobe, however, receives no arterial blood supply. The entire blood supply to the anterior lobe is derived from the pituitary portal veins. These veins arise from the capillary network of the median eminence and the infundibular stem. The vascular tufts of the primary capillary system are in close relationship with the nerve endings of the hypothalamo-hypophyseal tract. It is hypothesized that upon excitation these nerve fibers liberate their secretory products into this system, which then, via the portal veins, transports these neurosecretory products to the sinusoids of the anterior lobe. It is in this manner that the activity of the anterior lobe is governed by the hypothalamic areas.

The Thyroid Gland

The thyroid gland is derived from the pharynx (the foramen cecum of the tongue). Its structural unit is the follicle; the follicle is composed of a unit of epithelial cells that surround a colloid space. Colloid is located extracellularly and contains thyroglobulin. The function of the thyroid gland is to produce colloidal material which contains the thyroid hormones (T_3—triiodothyronine and T_4—thyroxin) which affect the rate of metabolism of all the tissues of the body.

The iodides consumed in our food and water are absorbed and carried to the iodide pool in the extracellular fluid via the circulatory system. Five basic events can be identified in thyroid hormone production: a. trapping iodide; b. oxidation of iodide to organic iodine; c. synthesis of hormone; d. storage of hormone as the thyroglobulin moiety in the follicle; and e. release of the hormone into the circulation. TSH from the anterior pituitary influences greatly the trapping mechanism; thiocyanates block this mechanism while thiouracil blocks the oxidation and synthetic steps. These compounds are classified as antithyroid agents.

The production of the hormone thyrocalcitonin has been implicated with the parafollicular cells of the thyroid gland. This hormone is an antagonist of parathyroid hormone and its functions are to lower the serum calcium level and to enhance the deposition of calcium in bone.

Action of Thyroid Hormone:

1. *Controls the rate of metabolism.*
2. *Controls the growth, maturation, and differentiation of the organism.*
3. *Influences nervous system activity.*

Problems Associated with Thyroid Function:

1. *Cretinism.* Congenital failure of proper development of the thyroid gland. The cretin is a dwarf physically and mentally.

2. *Myxedema.* Acquired thyroid deficiency in the adult. This deficiency can be of two types:

    a. Thyroid deficiency due to thyroidectomy, neoplasms, thyroiditis, and so forth.

    b. A pituitary deficiency in the secretion of TSH.

The thyroid in these cases appears atrophic, hard, and fibrous. The clinical picture is the presentation of a patient who is fairly heavy, phlegmatic, and devoid of expression; his skin is rough and dry and sensitive to cold. The patient is sluggish mentally and physically. Laboratory tests would show a low basal metabolic rate, low protein bound iodine, and a high serum cholesterol level.

3. *Goiter.* Any enlargement of the gland not due to neoplasm or inflammatory disease. Endemic goiters are due to lack of intake of iodine caused by deficiency in the soil and water. This results in increased TSH production, thyroid compensatory hypertrophy, and eventual exhaustion of the gland.

4. *Hyperthyroidism.* Increased activity by the organ. The patient exhibits loss of weight, nervousness, irritability, increased metabolic rate, rapid heart rate, sweating, and so forth. Exophthalmos, a protrusion of the eyeballs, is exhibited and thought to be due to an increased production of TSH. Hyperthyroidism may be an adjunct to the development of a goiter or may arise *de novo*.

The Parathyroid Glands

There are usually four parathyroid glands which are embedded in the thyroid gland. The parathyroid glands produce parathyroid hormone, which governs the metabolism of calcium and phosphorus. The parathyroids are essential to life; their removal results in cramps, convulsions, tremors, and eventually death due to tetany. The condition is due to the increased irritability of the muscular and nervous system caused by the decrease of calcium levels in the blood and body fluids. The activity of the parathyroids depends on the level of ionized calcium in the serum.

Problems Associated with Parathyroid Function:

1. *Hypoparathyroidism.* This condition results in a decrease of urinary excretion of phosphorus and its concomitant rise in the serum; this results in a shift in the calcium-phosphorus serum levels and a decline in calcium resorption from bone. The fall in serum calcium will produce tetany. Low serum levels of calcium may also be influenced by deficient intake of calcium, deficiency of vitamin D in the diet, problems with intestinal absorption or increased demand for calcium during pregnancy.

2. *Hyperparathyroidism.* Tumor is the most frequent cause of this condition. In this condition urinary phosphorus excretion is elevated and serum levels are decreased. Calcium resorption from bone is increased and serum levels rise. The glomerular filtrate is saturated and stones may form. Secondary renal disease may occur.

The Pancreas

The pancreas is both an endocrine and exocrine gland. The endocrine portion to be discussed is located in the islets of Langerhans. The function of the islets of Langerhans is to produce insulin by the beta cells and glucagon by the alpha cells. A deficiency of insulin production results in the disease known as diabetes mellitus (elevated blood sugar level). The beta cells do not seem to depend upon any outside trophic influences and the primary physiologic stimulus for insulin production seems to be the level of the blood sugar.

Insulin promotes the removal of glucose from the blood and also the conversion of glucose to glycogen in muscle and liver. It increases the rate of oxidation of glucose in the tissues, the conversion of carbohydrates into fats, the mobilization of fatty acids from adipose tissue, and the rate of protein synthesis.

Glucagon is the glycogenolytic hormone produced by the alpha cells of the pancreas; its principal action is to stimulate the conversion of glycogen to glucose by the liver. Glucagon also increases the peripheral utilization of glucose; therefore, it should not be referred to as simply the antagonist of insulin. Its secretion is controlled by the concentration of blood glucose and blood insulin levels. If insulin levels rise and blood glucose levels drop, glucagon secretion increases.

The Adrenal Glands

The adrenal is composed of a cortex and a medulla. The cortex is derived from mesoderm of the Wolffian ridge in conjunction with the sex glands, while the medulla is of ectodermal, neural crest origin in conjunction with the anlage of the sympathetic nerve cells. In fetal life the adrenal is composed almost completely of cortex, but after birth the entire fetal cortex rapidly degenerates and is replaced by the adult cortex and medulla. The cortex, which produces the mineralocorticoids and glucocorticoids, is divided into three zones: a. the most peripheral zona glomerulosa; b. the intermediate zona fasciculata; and c. the zona reticularis bordering the medulla. The function of the adrenal cortex is to produce the sex hormones: androgens, estrogens, and progesterone, and the corticosteroids: glucocorticoids and mineralocorticoids.

The zona glomerulosa is rich in lipids, especially cholesterol, from which the mineralocorticoids are formed. Aldosterone is the most powerful mineralocorticoid. Mineralocorticoids function in the retention of water, sodium, and chloride, and increase urinary loss of potassium and phosphorus by action on the renal tubules. This regulation of the electrolytes is essential to life. No pituitary control is present.

The zona fasciculata and reticularis are the sources of the glucocorticoids; i.e., 17-hydroxycorticosteroids. Corticosterone (hydroxycorticosterone), cortisone (compound E), and hydrocortisone (cortisol or compound F) are the most widely known compounds.

The levels of these hormones are increased by ACTH; they are gluconeogenic in nature. They convert amino acids into sugar instead of protein and in this way increase blood sugar and liver glycogen levels. Cortisone—in addition to influencing protein, carbohydrate, and fat metabolism—a. affects the permeability of cell membranes; b. interferes with the antigen-antibody response by inhibiting antibody formation; and c. suppresses the inflammatory response. Cortisone, however, only relieves the symptoms of disease without influencing the cause.

The zona reticularis is responsible for the production of the sex hormones or 17-ketosteroids. The action of these hormones is no different from the action of the estrogens, androgens, and progesterone (the regular sex hormones produced by the testes and ovaries); i.e., they masculinize the body and increase the synthesis of amino acids and protein from nitrogen; they favor the retention of nitrogen, phosphorus, potassium, sodium, and chloride. ACTH has some control of these hormones.

Problems Associated with Adrenal Cortex Function:

1. Hypofunction *or chronic adrenal insufficiency*. Addison's disease. This condition is due to inadequate amounts of steroid hormones. Deficiency of glucocorticoids makes the patient easily susceptible to stress; deficiency of mineralocorticoids leads to a fall in serum sodium and rise in serum potassium. These patients lack proper resistance to infection and are easily dehydrated. Patients exhibit general languor and debility, a very weak heart, irritability of the stomach, and a peculiar change in skin color due to the deposition of melanin; this feature is highly characteristic.
2. Hyperadrenalism
   a. Overfunction of zona glomerulosa—aldosteronism (Conn's syndrome).
   b. Overfunction of zona fasciculata—(Cushing's syndrome).
   c. Overfunction of zona reticularis—adrenal virilism (Adreno-genital syndrome).

Primary Aldosteronism—Conn's Syndrome:

Characterized by:
1. Periodic severe muscular weakness or paralysis.
2. Intermittent tetany and paresthesia.
3. Hypertension.
4. Renal disfunction.

Cushing's Syndrome:

Characterized by:
1. Painful adiposity of face, neck, and trunk (full moon face).
2. Excess hair growth in the female and preadolescent males.
3. Peculiar body striations.
4. Sexual dystrophy.
5. Muscular weakness and atrophy.
6. Hypertension.

Adrenal Virilism—Adrenogenital Syndrome:

1. Excess hair growth.
2. Virilism.
3. Excessive muscularity.

The adrenal medulla is intimately connected with the nervous system and develops from the neural crest. The cells of the adrenal medulla are modified ganglion cells and receive stimulation from the preganglionic fibers whose cell bodies are located in the intermediolateral cell columns of the spinal cord in the thoraco-lumbar segments dealing with the sympathetic outflow of the autonomic nervous system. Sectioning of the splanchnic nerves to the adrenal medulla will result in cessation of secretion, while stimulation of these nerves enhances secretion markedly. The function of the adrenal medulla is to secrete adrenalin (epinephrine) and nor-adrenalin (nor-epinephrine).

In general these hormones help the body in frightful and stressful situations. They affect the vascular system, the heart, respiration, carbohydrate metabolism, the pupillary dilators, the intestines, and uterine musculature.

A clinical picture of nor-adrenalism during which these pressor amines are produced in excess will show: a. hypertension; b. headache; c. palpitation; d. dyspnea; e. weakness; and f. chest and/or abdominal pain, etc.

The Testes

The testes function in the production of sperm and also contain interstitial cells, which produce the male sex hormone testosterone. Testosterone promotes and maintains the development of the male accessory genital organs (prostate and seminal vesicles) and secondary sex characteristics, i.e., beard growth, hair growth (pubic, axilla, trunk and limbs), and scrotal growth. It maintains spermatogenesis, is responsible for the deepening of the voice, the greater muscular development of men, sex urge, and acne at puberty. It also exerts an influence upon nitrogen, electrolyte and water balance within the system. Both males and females produce estrogens and androgens; it is the ratio of the two which determines male and female characteristics.

General Functional Schema of Both Sexes

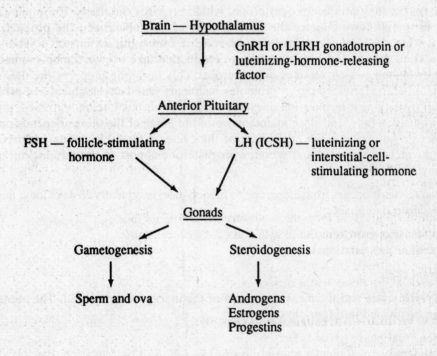

Steroidogenesis is similar in the ovary and the testis; the difference is in the predominance and quantity of the secretions. The androgen testosterone is the predominant secretion of the testis, while in the ovary the estrogen estradiol and the progestin progesterone predominate.

Actions of LH and FSH in the Male: These hormones act on the testis to promote:

1) androgen secretion,
2) spermatogenesis.

Hormonal Control of Spermatogenesis:

1. Pituitary secretions regulate spermatogenic activities.
2. Interstitial-cell-stimulating hormone (ICSH) affects seminiferous tubules via androgen secretion.
3. FSH affects maturation of spermatids.
4. FSH and GH maintain spermatogenesis.

Androgenic and Anabolic Actions of Testosterone:

1. Maintenance of spermatogenesis.
2. Maintenance of structure and function of the accessory sex organs.
3. Promotion of secondary sex characteristics (size of genitalia, voice, glandular secretions, muscle development, and hair distribution),
4. Normal development and body growth.
5. Psychological balance.
6. Suppression of LH via feedback mechanism.

The Ovaries

Like the testes, the ovaries are endocrine glands; they have three functions: a. they produce the female gamete (ovum); b. they produce estrogens, which function in the preparation for fertilization of the egg and in the production of secondary female sex characteristics; and c. they produce progesterone, which prepares the uterus for implantation. FSH from the pituitary initiates the development of the follicle and the production of estrogen; when the level of estrogen rises above a certain point, it shuts off FSH production, ovulation occurs, and LH and prolactin production take over in the development of the corpus luteum, which secretes progesterone. This hormone prepares the uterus for implantation of the fertilized egg; it promotes mammary gland development and prohibits additional ovulation. If fertilization does not occur, the corpus luteum regresses, progesterone production falls, and since maintenance of the lining of the uterus depends on progesterone, menstruation is the next phase of the cycle. If fertilization has occurred, the corpus luteum is maintained and secretes progesterone almost to the termination of the pregnancy.

Ovarian Cycle: It occurs from menarche to menopause, is typically 28 days long, and can be divided into two phases:

1) follicular or estrogenic,
2) luteal or progestational.

Menstrual Cycle

The ovarian cycle and the menstrual cycle of the uterus are integrated. The menstrual cycle can be divided into four phases:

1) menstrual phase (days 1–5);
2) proliferative or follicular phase (days 6–13), followed by ovulation (day 14);
3) secretory or luteal phase (days 15–25);
4) ischemic phase (days 26–28).

Uterine Changes during the Menstrual Cycle: Menses (days 1–5) involves the sloughing off of necrotic endometrium, blood, and uterine fluid, which is discharged as menstrual flow. During the proliferative phase (days 6–13) the primary hormonal stimulus is estrogen from the follicle, which promotes proliferation of uterine epithelium and glandular tissue. Ovulation generally occurs on day 14 of the cycle. During the postovulatory phase (days 15–25) the uterus is under the combined effects of estrogen and progesterone from the corpus luteum. This hormonal milieu promotes increased vascularity, further development of glands, their increased secretory activity (including glycogen accumulation), hypertrophy, and fluid accumulation. These changes prepare the uterus for implantation of a fertilized ovum, should fertilization occur. If fertilization does not occur, the corpus luteum begins to regress after day 25, leading ultimately to the onset of menses.

Hormonal Control of the Menstrual Cycle: The suppressed (and even declining) plasma gonadotropin (FSH and LH) levels during the follicular phase are due to the negative-feedback inhibitory effects of estrogen being secreted from developing follicles. The small, abrupt rise in plasma estrogen is believed to trigger the ovulatory LH surge (by suspension of negative feedback or by positive feedback). During the luteal phase negative-feedback suppression is reestablished, but in this period feedback is due to the combined effects of estrogen and progesterone. Luteal failure occurs at about 26 days. It results in an abrupt withdrawal of estrogen and progesterone and hence in a release of feedback inhibition, which accounts for the rise in FSH and LH at the beginning of a new cycle.

Female Contraception

Female oral contraceptives represent combinations of synthetic progestational compounds (19-nortestosterone derivatives such as norgestrol and norethindrone) with synthetic estrogen. The original rationale behind the pill was that the synthetic progestin in the presence of estrogen would block the ovulatory LH surge. The progestins are effective because they also cause the cervical mucus to produce an environment (like that in the luteal phase) hostile to sperm.

The Placenta

While the placenta is mainly concerned with support and nourishment of the developing embryo, it secretes estrogens, progesterone, and chorionic gonadotropin. Excess chorionic gonadotropin (similar to luteinizing hormone) is excreted in the urine and is the basis of most pregnancy tests. The estrogen production by the placenta inhibits FSH production and in this manner inhibits follicle development during pregnancy.

The Pineal

The pineal organ is a diencephalic outgrowth. It has been linked to photoperiodism and seasonal breeding; experimental evidence now suggests that it produces an antigonadotropic substance. How the pineal influences the reproductive organs remains to be established.

The Prostaglandins

Prostaglandins (PGs) are hormonelike substances; they play a role in cellular metabolism. Their function, unlike that of hormones, is limited to immediate areas; in this respect they may be labeled as tissue hormones. These substances, which are derivatives of prostanoic acid, are C_{20} fatty acids containing a five-membered ring; they are found in almost every type of human and animal tissue and elicit a multitude of effects. Prostaglandins exert control over processes such as reproduction, inflammation, nerve impulse transmission, blood pressure and blood clotting, smooth muscle activity, and hormone secretion.

Major Actions of the Prostaglandins:

1. Lower blood pressure.
2. Modulate smooth muscle activity.
3. Inhibit the release of glycerol and fatty acid from adipose tissue.
4. Decrease nervous system excitability.
5. Modulate uterine smooth muscle.
6. Induce labor.
7. Modulate the bronchial tree.
8. Suppress gastric secretions.
9. Amplify pain response.

10. Stimulate renin secretion.
11. Modulate platelet aggregation.
12. Shrink swollen nasal passages.
13. Increase intraocular pressure.
14. Mediate inflammation.
15. Stimulate steroid production.
16. Promote sodium excretion.
17. Potentiate the pain-producing action of bradykinin.
18. Modulate norepinephrine release.

The Small Intestine

Food materials stimulate the secretion of certain hormones by the gastrointestinal mucosa and they may be summarized as follows:

1. Secretin: from duodenal mucosa—stimulates pancreatic juice secretion which is low in enzymatic content.

2. Pancreozymin: from duodenal mucosa—stimulates pancreatic juice secretion rich in enzymes.

3. Cholecystokinin: from duodenal mucosa—stimulates the contraction and emptying of the gall bladder.

4. Enterogastrone: from duodenal mucosa—inhibits motility and depresses the acid secretion by the stomach.

5. Gastrin: from pyloric region of stomach—enhances acid secretion by the stomach.

Reproductive System

Reproductive Organs

Male: Seminiferous tubules of the testis, epididymis, vas deferens, seminal vesicles, prostate, prostatic urethra, membranous urethra, penile urethra, glans penis.

Female: Ovaries, oviduct, uterus, vagina; the breasts (accessory organs).

Hormonal Control

For a detailed discussion of the hormonal interactions concerning the reproductive system, the reader is referred to the section dealing with the endocrine system. However, the cyclic activity of the female organism is briefly summarized since it is of the utmost importance and quite difficult.

The reproductive cycle is under hormonal regulation; gonadotropic hormones of the pituitary (anterior lobe) stimulate the ovaries to produce a mature egg. The pituitary and ovaries have a reciprocal effect upon each other. FSH (follicle stimulating hormone) from the pituitary elicits estrogen production from the developing follicle. When estrogen concentration reaches a certain blood level, it inhibits FSH production. At that time the egg is discharged and the cells lining the follicle come under the influence of another gonadotropin, LH (luteinizing hormone), which influences the development of the corpus luteum. The corpus luteum produces the hormone progesterone, which influences the wall of the uterus in preparation for implantation. As the concentration of progesterone rises, LH production is checked. If fertilization has occurred, the production of FSH is curtailed throughout the period of gestation through the production of estrogen by the placenta and ovary. If fertilization does not occur, the cycle begins anew.

Gametogenesis and Meiosis

The production of gametes, or sex cells—egg and sperm, is known as gametogenesis. Since an individual possesses an equal amount of genetic material from both parents and the same number of chromosomes as either parent, a reduction to one half that number must be accomplished in the development of the egg and sperm. Eggs and sperms are haploid; and a fertilized egg (zygote) possesses the diploid number of the parent again. The reduction occurs during meiosis.

The process of meiosis is best demonstrated in the following manner:

Haploid gametes; either sperm (spermatids) or egg (ova).

$$\underline{1,2} + \underline{1a, 2a}$$

The above unite in fertilization (form zygote) and the diploid adult somatic and primary germ cells are formed.

$$\downarrow$$
$$\underline{1, 1a, 2, 2a}$$

Primary germ cell in the adult undergoes spermatogenesis (male) or oogenesis (female); the result eventually will be haploid cells.

Tetrad formation

$$\downarrow$$
$$\underline{1, 1, 1a, 1a, 2, 2, 2a, 2a}$$

The first meiotic or reduction division occurs next, and results in the following:

$$\downarrow$$
$$\underline{1, 1a, 2, 2a} \quad + \quad \underline{1, 1a, 2, 2a}$$

Meiosis II occurs now and four haploid cells are produced.

$$\downarrow$$
$$\underline{1, 2} \quad \underline{1a, 2a} \quad \quad \underline{1, 2} \quad \underline{1a, 2a}$$

Even though we have not indicated it, random assortment does take place during the process and chromosome combinations other than those illustrated are possible. In the human male four functional cells (sperms) are produced while in the human female one functional cell (egg) and three polar bodies are produced. This is the general gamut of the process of meiosis.

Mature Gametes

Types of Eggs: Isolecithal eggs are primitive and have a small amount of yolk that is distributed equally; examples are sea urchin eggs and amphioxus eggs. Telolecithal eggs have a large amount of yolk concentrated at one pole (lower or vegetal pole); examples are fish, amphibia, reptile, and bird eggs. Centrolecithal eggs show a concentration of yolk in their center; insect eggs are the prime example.

Semen: Semen is a fluid secreted by the male accessory sex glands, namely the prostate, seminal vesicles, and bulbo-urethral glands. Fructose is added by the prostate, as are acid phosphatase, citric acid, calcium, and fibrinolysin. The seminal vesicles add phosphorylcholine. The vas deferens is just a tube through which sperm are transported from the testes to the urethra. Between 3 and 4 ml of semen comprise one ejaculation, which contains between 300 and 400 million sperm cells.

Chromosomes: Forty-four autosomal chromosomes are present in every diploid cell of the human body. Mature gametes, however, are haploid. The total chromosome number of the human being is 46 (male 44 plus X and Y; female 44 plus X and X).

Other Modes of Reproduction

Budding, as in hydra, involves the multiplication of cells in one region of the organism and the organization of these cells into a new individual.

Binary fission or mitosis is a division of a cell into two equal parts and in this respect two new organisms (cells).

Parthenogenesis involves a mechanism in which a single cell is set apart for the purpose of reproduction. This cell has the capability to develop into a new organism.

A hermaphrodite possesses both male and female reproductive tissue.

Development

Fertilization

The development of a new organism starts with fertilization, the process during which the male and female gametes unite in the *ampulla* of the oviduct (Fallopian tube). The *diploid* (2N) number of chromosomes is achieved in this fusion. The egg (oocyte) is transported from the ovary down the oviduct by the *ciliary* movement and *peristaltic* action of the tube. Sperm pass quite rapidly from the vagina into the uterus, and then into the oviduct; they are propelled by the contractions of the musculature of the uterus and the oviduct and by the tail motion of the sperm itself.

Before fertilization can occur the spermatozoa must undergo *capacitation,* a process during which some of the protective coating of the head is removed. An *acrosome reaction* also occurs; during this process enzymes which are necessary to penetrate the protective barrier of the oocyte are released.

Of the approximately 350 million sperm deposited in a single ejaculation only about 350 reach the egg. Only one is necessary for fertilization but the others, it is thought, help in the dispersal of *corona radiata* cells (a circle, or "crown," of ovarian nurse cells that accompany the egg to this point) by release of enzymes such as hyaluronidase.

After passing through the corona radiata, the fertilizing sperm touches the *zona pellucida,* a protective membrane surrounding the oocyte. The zona reaction then takes place; this prevents multiple sperm penetration. The sperm next touches the inner oocyte cell membrane and fusion of both membranes occurs. Upon entrance of the sperm, the secondary oocyte completes its second maturation division. The nucleus of the now mature ovum is known as the *female pronucleus.* When the male and female pronuclei come in contact, their nuclear membranes vanish, and the chromosomes intermingle. Fertilization is now complete, and the fertilized egg is known as a *zygote.*

Fertilization therefore consists of:

a) penetration of the corona radiata barrier,
b) penetration of the zona pellucida,
c) penetration of the oocyte membrane.

Fertilization results in:

a) restoration of diploid number of chromosomes and variation of species,
b) determination of sex,
c) initiation of cleavage.

Cleavage

About 30 hours after fertilization, the zygote reaches the two-cell stage. Mitotic divisions rapidly increase the number of cells at this time; these small cells are termed *blastomeres* and the developing organism (now a solid ball) is called the *morula.* At approximately the 16-cell stage the zygote consists of centrally located cells, the *inner cell mass,* and a covering layer, the *outer cell mass.* The inner cell mass gives rise to the embryo proper, while the outer cell mass forms the *trophoblast,* which becomes the fetal component of the placenta. (In some species, cleavage of an ovum may occur without fertilization; the process is referred to as *parthenogenesis.*)

Blastocyst Formation

As the morula reaches the uterine cavity, fluid starts to accumulate internally between the inner cell mass and the outer cell mass and eventually forms a single cavity, the *blastocele.* The zygote is then referred to as the *blastocyst.* The inner cell mass (at this point located at one pole) now assumes the name *embryoblast,* and the outer cell mass, or *trophoblast,* at this time forms the epithelial wall of the *blastocyst.* By two weeks of gestation, the developing zygote has passed through the morula and blastocyst stages and has begun the implantation process by which it invades the uterine tissue to establish contact with the maternal circulation.

Implantation in the Uterus

Endometrium (uterine mucosa, an epithelium) lines the uterus; *myometrium* forms the thick, middle muscular layer; and *perimetrium* covers the outside of the organ. When the blastocyst arrives the *uterine mucosa* is in the *secretory* or *progestational* phase. Uterine arteries are dilated, glands are enlarged, mucin and glycogen are being produced and the tissue resembles a sponge. Implantation usually occurs either along the anterior or posterior wall of the uterus.

Second Week (Bilaminar Germ Disc Formation)

As the blastocyst embeds the trophoblast differentiates into an inner *cytotrophoblast* and an outer *syncytiotrophoblast* layer. Syncytiotrophoblastic processes invade the endometrial epithelium and stroma. *Lacunae* (spaces) soon appear in the syncytiotrophoblast and fill with maternal blood and secretions; this nutritive material, called *embryotroph,* reaches the embryoblast by diffusion (a primitive uteroplacental circulation). The embryoblast differentiates into *endoderm* and *ectoderm* (two of the three primary germ layers) which form a flat disc known as the *bilaminar germ disc.* Between the cytotrophoblast and ectoderm layer the *amniotic cavity* develops, while beneath the ectoderm, the single layer of endoderm proliferates to form the definitive *yolk sac.* As development proceeds, the extraembryonic coelom, the cavity between the embryoblast and the trophoblast, expands and the large *chorionic cavity* is formed. Within the chorionic sac, the embryo and its amnion and yolk sac are suspended. Extraembryonic mesoderm lines this cavity and covers the embryoblast, thus connecting it to the trophoblast. As soon as blood vessels develop this connecting stalk will become the *umbilical cord.*

Highlighting this period is the development of the *primitive streak* on the surface of the ectoderm facing the amniotic cavity. The primitive streak functions as the *blastopore* during gastrulation. The cephalic end of this streak is known as the *primitive node.* During gastrulation, mesoderm cells segregate from the ectoderm layer and migrate between the ectoderm and endoderm by way of the primitive streak. In this manner the third primary germ layer, the *mesoderm* is formed between the ectoderm and endoderm except at the prochordal plate (buccopharyngeal membrane) and cloacal membrane.

The *allantois* appears as an outpocketing in the caudal end of the primitive gut around day 16. It stores excretory products in lower forms; it remains rudimentary in humans but plays a vital role as a source of vascular stem cells. During this period, formation of the *somites* from *mesoderm* and formation of the *central nervous system* from *ectoderm* begins. Mesoderm also gives rise to the blood vessels which eventually connect the placenta and the embryo.

Second Month (Germ Layer Differentiation)

During this period the main organ systems become established and external body features such as limb buds, face, ear, nose and eyes become apparent.

Ectodermal Derivatives:

1. The *central and peripheral nervous system,* which develops in conjunction with the notochord. The notochord develops from the notochordal process and establishes a primitive axis for the embryo. (The nucleus pulposus of the intervertebral disc in the adult is the remnant of the notochord.) The established *neural plate* (composed of neuroectoderm above the notochord) forms a neural groove by differential growth and eventually becomes a *neural tube* giving rise to *brain vesicles* and the central canal of the *spinal cord. Neural crest cells,* intermediate in position between the neural tube and surface ectoderm, develop into *dorsal root* and *cranial sensory* ganglia and their associated neurons.

2. *Placodes.* Many complex sensory structures begin their development as placodes, which are simple, localized ectodermal thickenings which invaginate into the underlying tissues and there differentiate into their definitive structures.

   a) An *otic placode* forms the *otic pit* and the *otic vesicle* giving rise eventually to organs of hearing and equilibrium.

   b) A *lens placode* under induction of the *optic vesicle* gives rise to the lens of the eye.

   c) A *nasal placode* gives rise to the *olfactory epithelium* of the nose.

3. The *epidermis,* including hair and nails, and subcutaneous connective tissue.

4. *Mammary glands,* the *pituitary gland* and the *enamel of the teeth.*

Mesodermal Derivatives: The sheet of mesoderm first gives rise to *paraxial mesoderm* (it will become the future paired *somites*), second to the *intermediate mesoderm* (it will become the future excretory units) and third to the *lateral plate* mesoderm (it will split into *somatic* and *splanchnic* (visceral) layers) which will line the intraembryonic *coelomic cavity.*

a. *Somite Differentiation.* Somites are individual blocks of paraxial mesoderm arranged as paired chains along the length of the notochord and neural tube. Each somite will form bone, muscle, and dermis for a specific body segment. At the beginning 4 occipital, 8 cervical, 12 thoracic, 5 lumbar, 5 sacral and 8–10 coccygeal pairs of somites are present; the first occipital and the last 5–7 coccygeal disappear at a later stage. Each somite is organized into a sclerotome, a myotome, and a dermatome.

1. *Sclerotome.* This is formed by *mesenchyme,* or primitive connective tissue, which is multipotent and differentiates into:

   a) *fibroblasts,* which give rise to reticular, collagenous and elastic fibers of connective tissue;

   b) *chondroblasts,* which give rise to cartilage;

   c) *osteoblasts,* which give rise to bone of the vertebral column.

2. *Myotome.* Each myotome gives rise to the skeletal musculature of its segment.

3. *Dermatome.* Cells of this nature give rise to the dermis (skin) and subcutaneous tissue under the skin.

b. *Intermediate Mesoderm Differentiation.* Cells in the cervical and thoracic region will give rise to *nephrotomes;* more caudally located cells form the *nephrogenic cord.* These will become the excretory units of the urinary system.

c. *Lateral Plate Mesoderm*

1. *Somatic.* These cells form the lining of the intraembryonic coelomic cavity and give rise to the non-segmental skeletal muscle of both wall and serous membranes which will eventually line the pericardial, pleural and peritoneal cavities of the adult.

2. *Splanchnic.* These cells differentiate into *angioblasts,* which will give rise to blood cells and the cardiovascular and lymphatic systems. True blood formation starts in the second month and occurs in the liver, spleen, bone marrow and lymph nodes.

Other Mesoderm Derivatives. Besides the structures described, mesoderm also gives rise to the gonads and their ducts, the cortex of the adrenal glands, and the spleen. It is also the source of the smooth muscle of the viscera.

Endodermal Derivatives: This germ layer provides:

1) the epithelial lining of the gastrointestinal system
2) the epithelial lining of the respiratory system
3) the parenchyma of the tonsil, thymus, thyroid, parathyroid, liver and pancreas
4) the epithelial lining of the urinary bladder and urinary tract
5) the epithelial lining of the auditory (Eustachian) tube and the tympanic cavity (middle ear).

At eight weeks the fetus stage has been reached and the dramatic changes leading to organ formation have taken place. The embryonic period now enters a phase of remarkable growth until the *conceptus* is ready for delivery.

Fetal Membranes and Placenta

The fetal membranes are the: amnion, yolk sac, allantois, and chorion. While these membranes originate from the zygote only the *yolk sac* and *allantois* contribute to embryonic structures.

The Amnion: The amniotic cavity is filled with fluid derived from the maternal circulation and from excretory products of the fetus. Amniotic fluid is swallowed by the fetus and taken up by the gastrointestinal system. The embryo, suspended by the umbilical cord, floats in the amniotic fluid. Amniotic fluid:

1) serves as a cushion and absorbs jolts,
2) allows the fetus to move,
3) helps in temperature regulation,
4) separates the amnion from the embryo,
5) provides a hydrostatic wedge during birth.

The Yolk Sac: The yolk sac is formed in the chorionic cavity and is connected to the umbilical cord. No yolk storage takes place in the human. However, the yolk sac plays a role in:

1) nutrient transfer before placental circulation is established,
2) blood development,
3) formation (endodermal component) of the gut,
4) formation (epithelial component) of the respiratory system,
5) formation of the germ cells (spermatogonia and oogonia).

The Allantois: This structure serves in the following manner:

1) it contributes to blood formation,
2) the allantoic blood vessels become the umbilical arteries and vein,
3) via the urachus the bladder is connected to the umbilicus.

The Placenta:

Structure. The placenta is composed of two parts:

1) the maternal part, derived from the endometrial decidua basalis,
2) the fetal part, derived from the chorionic villi.

Decidua. The decidua is the functional layer of the endometrium during pregnancy. Three zones are differentiated:

1) decidua basalis—this is the part deep to the conceptus, which forms the maternal placenta,
2) decidua capsularis—this is the part superficial to the conceptus and closest to the uterine cavity,
3) decidua parietalis—this is the term applied to the remaining portion of the uterine mucosa.

Chorionic Component. Originally the entire chorionic sac is covered by villi; however, around week eight, the villi not associated with the decidua basalis start to degenerate. The villi in relation to the decidua basalis increase in number and size and become the functional fetal portion of the placenta. The maternal and fetal components form an intimate anatomical and functional unit.

Function. Deoxygenated blood is carried from the fetus via the umbilical arteries to the placenta (villi). No mixing of maternal and fetal blood occurs. Exchange takes place over the endothelial barrier of the fetal vessels. Oxygenated blood passes into fetal placental veins, which form the umbilical vein, which supplies the fetus.

The main functions of the placenta are:

1) exchange of metabolic and gaseous products,
2) synthesis of glycogen, cholesterol and fatty acids,
3) synthesis of hormones,
4) transmission of antibodies

Fetal and Neonatal Circulation

The cardiovascular system is designed to meet the needs of the fetus and at birth quickly to adapt to the demands of a new circuit and environment.

Fetal Circulation: Placenta → umbilical vein → ductus venosus of liver (half of the blood bypasses in this manner the hepatic circulation) → inferior vena cava → right atrium → foramen ovale, between right and left atria (blood bypasses the pulmonary circuit) → left atrium → left ventricle → ascending aorta → descending aorta → two umbilical arteries → placenta.

Blood that enters the right ventricle from the right atrium leaves via the pulmonary artery but bypasses the pulmonary circuit by passing through the ductus arteriosus, which connects the pulmonary artery to the aortic arch. In this manner blood reaches the aorta.

Changes at Birth: Due to a cessation of placental blood flow and the activation of the respiratory system because of pressure on the thoracic cavity and the replacement of amniotic fluid by air in the bronchial tree, certain changes are necessary:

1) ductus arteriosus closes due to muscular constriction of its wall,
2) blood flow through the lungs increases and results in a rise of pressure in the left atrium,
3) right atrial pressure drops due to cessation of placental circulation,
4) the above pressure differentials result in the closing of the foramen ovale and complete pulmonary circulation is established,
5) the umbilical arteries close
6) the umbilical vein and ductus venosus close.

Adult Derivatives

	Fetal structure	Adult structure
1)	umbilical vein	→ ligamentum teres
2)	ductus venosus	→ ligamentum venosuum
3)	umbilical arteries	→ a) superior vesicle arteries
		b) medial umbilical ligaments
4)	foramen ovale	→ fossa ovalis
5)	ductus arteriosus	→ ligamentum arteriosum

Multiple Pregnancy

Twinning: Twinning occurs in about 1% of normal births; about ⅔ are of the *dizygotic* (fraternal) twin type. The frequency of dizygotic twins increases with the age of the mother and is influenced by heredity. (No age correlation exists as far as *monozygotic* [identical] twins are concerned.) If a first pregnancy results in twins, subsequent twinning is about 3 to 5 times greater than in the normal population. The *genotype* of the mother seems to be the key determining factor in the frequency of twin births.

Monozygotic Twins (Identical Twins). A single ovum and sperm are involved. The zygote usually splits by the blastocyst stage of development. These embryos have a common placenta and chorionic cavity but possess separate amniotic cavities. These individuals have the same sex and blood groups, and a strong resemblance in external features. (Their phenotypes and genotypes are identical.)

Dizygotic Twins (Fraternal Twins). Two separate oocytes and two separate sperms are involved. Both zygotes are totally different genetically. They may or may not be of the same sex. These zygotes implant independently and develop their own placenta and membranes. (Fraternal twins are not identical in phenotype or genotype. They are no more similar than any other non-twin siblings.)

Triplets: Triplets occur once in about 8,000 pregnancies. They may result from:

1)   one zygote and therefore be identical,
2)   two zygotes, and therefore give rise to one set of identical twins and one independent infant,
3)   three zygotes and result in three independent individuals.

Types of multiple births higher than triplets are rare but similar combinations do occur.

Genetics

Chromosomes within the nucleus of the cells are the source of DNA (deoxyribonucleic acid), the inheritable material; chromosomes contain specific units called genes which are arranged in linear order on the chromosomes. Genes are paired elements, held together in a specific linkage arrangement. One member of each pair of genes separates during germ cell production; therefore, each germ cell contains only one set. An allele is one of a pair of genes that occupies the same locus on homologous chromosomes. Genotype refers to the genetic make-up of the organism. The genotype is expressed via phenotypic characteristics that are visible and observable under normal circumstances.

Mendel is responsible for the discovery of several intriguing phenomena:

1. He showed that each member of a pair of genes will be found in a different gamete; they were contributed to that individual by his parents and underwent no change such as blending while they were associated. This is Mendel's first law (law of segregation) which affirms that *allelomorphs segregate.*

2. Mendel also documented that the distribution of members of one pair has absolutely no bearing on the distribution of another pair. For example, if an individual possesses one pair of alleles Y and y, and another pair Z and z, the individual will produce approximately equal numbers of gametes of the four possible chance combinations of one member from each pair (YZ; Yz; yZ; yz). This law is known as independent assortment; the law does not apply to linked genes but only to genes located on different chromosomes. Independent behavior of chromosomes during meiosis is essential.

Mendel also showed that certain characteristics mask other traits; this phenomenon is known as dominance.

Genetic phenomena are best explained and demonstrated by problem solving, and it will be attempted in this manner.

Mendelian Characteristics

Dominance: Dominance is expressed in terms of a pair of alleles. A gene which produces and expresses the same characteristic whether it is present alone (in the heterozygous state matched to a gene not possessing the same trait) or with a gene possessing the same trait (in the homozygous state) is said to be dominant to the allele with which it is paired. The allele which is ineffective in the expression of its trait in the heterozygote is said to be recessive to the dominant. Let us illustrate with the following example.

The trait of green eyes did not occur in the F_1 (offspring from parents) but made its appearance in the F_2 (offspring of F_1 or offspring of offspring from the parents) generation. We are dealing with a recessive trait that is being masked by a dominant one. AA (brown eyes) bred with aa (green eyes) results in all F_1, Aa (genotypically heterozygous but phenotypically A; all brown eyes). Breeding of the offspring Aa with Aa results in 1 AA 2 Aa 1 aa genotype and 3:1 phenotype. The above demonstrates a one factor cross.

Let us now demonstrate several typical two-factor crosses:

1. Crossing of two types of organisms yields the classical 9:3:3:1 ratio. The cross would be considered an expression of phenotypic ratio.

The example calls for a cross between individuals possessing a genetic makeup of RrSs × RrSs. Construct the Punnett square below and see the results in a 9:3:3:1 phenotypic ratio.

	RS	Rs	rS	rs
RS	RRSS	RRSs	RrSS	RrSs
Rs	RRSs	RRss	RrSs	Rrss
rS	RrSS	RrSs	rrSS	rrSs
rs	RrSs	Rrss	rrSs	rrss

R__S__ or RS = 9
R__ss or Rss = 3
rrS__ or rrS = 3
rrSS or rrss = 1

2. In rabbits, rough coat is dominant over smooth coat. Brown is dominant over grey fur color. A rough, brown male is mated to a couple of smooth, grey females. The offspring are counted as: 18 rough, brown; 21 rough, grey; 16 smooth, brown; 24 smooth, grey. If this male had been mated to a female of his own genotype, what proportion of the offspring would have exhibited rough, grey coats? The answer is 3 out of 16 and is obtained in the following manner.

Basic genetic knowledge is applied.

rough   = (dominant)
smooth = (recessive)
brown = (dominant)
grey = (recessive)

The male is crossed to several smooth grey females; they had to be homozygous recessive genotype. Since all four combinations appeared, we can assume that the male was genotypically heterozygous even though he appeared phenotypically dominant. If first we crossed this heterozygous male RrBb × rrbb, the result would be RrBb; Rrbb; rrBb; rrbb; in other words the four combinations given. Now let us cross the RrBb male × RrBb female; the following combinations would have to be considered in both male and female: RB; Rb; rB; rb. If these are crossed, we find 3 out of 16 possess rough grey coats (namely RRbb; Rrbb and Rrbb).

Incomplete Dominance: Seeds from a self-pollinated gold flowering plant produce 56 charcoal, 130 gold and 61 beige flowering plants. The plant is heterozygous with incomplete dominance of its traits.

The phenomenon illustrated here is incomplete dominance (blending of two traits). Let us assume:

	charcoal	C
	beige	B
	gold	BC
Cross: →	BC × BC	
Result:	1 BB (beige)	
	2 BC (gold)	
	1 CC (charcoal)	

Backcross: A backcross consists of crossing a dominant phenotype with a pure homozygous recessive. In this manner a breeder can determine if the phenotype is heterozygous or homozygous. The backcross is used, therefore, to determine if a line is genotypically pure.

Probability Ratios: Genetic ratios are probability ratios. If, for example, we mate (B = black dominant; b = grey recessive) two heterozygous black squirrels (Bb) and 4 offspring are produced, the ratio of 3 black and 1 grey should be probable. However, what are the chances of all black and all grey litters?

Many crosses of heterozygous (Bb) animals will result in a fairly close 3:1 ratio. We, therefore, can see that we have 3 chances out of 4 to produce an individual exhibiting the dominant trait, and 1 chance out of 4 to show the recessive trait.

Therefore, to produce black squirrels (BB or Bb, 3 out of 4) we multiply $\frac{3}{4} \times \frac{3}{4} \times \frac{3}{4} \times \frac{3}{4} = 81/256$; to produce grey squirrels (bb, 1 out of 4) we multiply $\frac{1}{4} \times \frac{1}{4} \times \frac{1}{4} \times \frac{1}{4} = 1/256$.

Polygenic Traits

In morning glories, genes C and P are necessary for pink flowers. In the absence of either (ccP__ or C__pp) or both (ccpp) of these genes, the flowers are blue. What will be the result of the following crosses as far as flower color of the offspring and proportion of the offspring are concerned? Cross a. Ccpp × ccPp = 1 pink : 3 blue; b. ccpp × CcPp = 1 pink : 3 blue.

In essence the expression of pink requires C__ P__, and all others will be blue. The offspring may be Cc or cc with equal probability (i.e., 50%); the same is true for Pp and pp (50%). If the chance of C__ is 0.5 and the chance of P__ is 0.5, then the chance of C__ P__ is $0.5 \times 0.5 = 0.25$. Thus, 1/4 will be pink and 3/4 will be blue.

Sex Determination: A male carries an XY and a female an XX complement of chromosomes. If a male embryo were to result, the sperm that fertilizes an egg would have to possess a Y chromosome.

Sex-Linked Traits: Both sexes carry a complete complement of sex-linked genes. A female, however, with the XX arrangement will only exhibit a recessive gene if it has received it from both parents (a rare event if we are dealing with an uncommon gene of the population) while in the male with the XY arrangement the recessive gene cannot be masked since there is no partner X chromosome and, therefore, a larger number of recessive genes are expressed (examples are hemophilia and color blindness). A man receives his X chromosome from his mother and passes it on to his daughters not his sons. His daughters in this respect are the carriers of his sex-linked traits and their sons will be the affected ones. Let us illustrate with an example. The normal czarinas of Russia produced sons suffering from hemophilia, a disease that is caused by a sex-linked recessive gene, h. The more dominant gene, H, produces normal blood clotting. Genotypically, these women must have carried Hh (X_H and X_h). A daughter, depending on the father ($X_H Y$ or $X_h Y$), could have carried $X_H X_h$ or $X_H X_H$ while a son could have been born with either an $X_H Y$ or an $X_h Y$ (hemophilic) chromosomal complement.

Another way of expressing a sex-linked or, strictly speaking, sex-limited phenomenon is shown in the example below.

A cattle breeder has in his herd a y-linked trait which produces white stockings. A calf sired by a white-stockinged bull is born. The breeder determines that the chances of white stockings by this inhertance are 50%. If the calf born had been a female, the chances of exhibiting the trait (or serving as a carrier) were zero. The explanation is that the male may contribute gametes containing either X or Y chromosomes, but the female can contribute only gametes containing X chromosomes. If the X chromosome is contributed by the male, an unaffected female offspring will result; if the Y chromosome is contributed by the male, an affected male offspring will result. These two possibilities are of equal probability (i.e., 50%). If the sex of the offspring is known, there is no doubt about whether it has the trait. All males (100%) and no females (0%) would have the trait. Females could not even be carriers for a Y-linked trait.

Mutation: A mutation may be thought of as a sudden change in the genetic makeup of the organism. It may be beneficial or harmful. It may occur spontaneously or may be experimentally produced with chemicals, X-rays, cosmic rays, and so forth. It may or may not be passed on to the next generation because, for example, it may be lethal or otherwise preclude reproduction.

Blood Types: The ABO blood grouping system is explained on the basis of a single triallelic system with genes A, B, and O operating at a single genetic locus. Phenotypic and genotypic characteristics may be expressed as follows:

Phenotype	Genotype
A	A/A; A/O
B	B/B; B/O
O	O/O
AB	A/B

The A and B genes appear to be codominant; they are dominant over O, which is recessive.

As can be seen from the above table, there are four major blood types and the explanation as to universal donor and recipient is based on the following:

Type	Agglutinogens on Cells	Agglutinins in Serum and Plasma
AB—can receive A, B, AB or O (universal recipient)	A, B	none
A—can receive A, O	A	anti b
B—can receive B, O	B	anti a
O—can receive only O, but can give to all; therefore, O is the universal donor	O	anti ab

Rh Factor: Rhesus (Rh) agglutinogen is present in humans and is represented by a dominant gene R. The agglutinogen of an Rh positive fetus passes across the placenta, enters the maternal blood stream, and elicits the production of an agglutinin (antibody) by the mother. The agglutinin passes into the circulation of the fetus and if present in sufficient concentration can produce agglutination, at times fatal to the developing fetus.

Mode of Inheritance of Some Common Human Traits: Among the human traits inherited as single-gene dominants are:

a) brachydactyly (short digits),
b) white forelock in the hair,
c) blue sclera (white of the eye),
d) Rh-positive blood.

Among the traits inherited as recessives:

a) albinism (lack of skin pigment),
b) alkaptonuria (urine turns black).

Sex-linked traits:

a) hemophilia,
b) colorblindness.

Crossing-Over: During the process of meiosis a recombination of genetic material is possible. One way this is effected is through crossing over. In crossing-over, comparable portions of chromatids are exchanged. Since crossing-over is more the rule than the exception, we shall illustrate it with two diagrams. These portions may differ in alleles but they do carry the same gene sites (loci) and control the same specific trait, as, for example, eye color.

Let us start with one pair of homologous chromosomes:

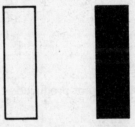

As illustrated, replication results during the first part of meiosis in four chromatids:

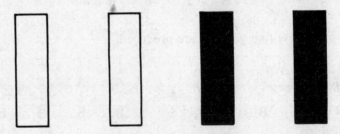

Of the four chromatids, two may exchange materials in a process known as crossing-over:

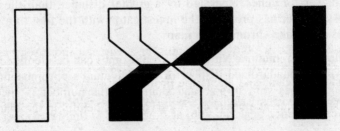

The configuration shown by the central two chromosomes is termed a chiasma, the region where crossing-over occurs. After separation in the second reduction division of meiosis, the resulting chromatids include two recombinants, having new combinations of genetic material.

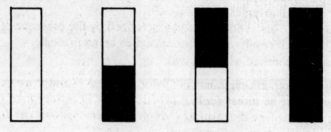

We shall next illustrate crossover using two specific genes.

Two gametes unite and form a new hybrid individual (F_1).

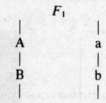

Without crossover these four gametes are produced:

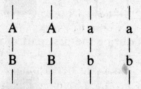

With crossing-over these four gametes are produced,

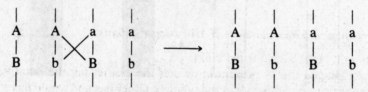

and the result is two new types of gametes with new combinations of genes.

Crossing-over may occur anywhere along the chromosome; however, the recombination frequency is higher for genes separated by a greater distance than those that are close together. Crossing-over has provided the investigator with the tool to measure distances between genes and make chromosome maps.

Abnormalities in Chromosome Number: Chromosomes can be identified in somatic cells and a *karyotype*, a standardized display of an individual's chromosomes, can be constructed. Chromosomes vary in size and shape but the number is species specific. In humans the chromosome number is 46. A karyotype is helpful in the diagnosis of genetic abnormalities.

In humans some abnormalities of chromosome number are:

Down's syndrome (formerly called mongolism) This phenomenon is most often character-ized by three, instead of two, chromosomes 21 in group G; a total number of 47 chro-mosomes are present in these individuals.

Turner's syndrome Females possess only one X chromosome (not the normal female XX). Total number of chromosomes present is 45.

Klinefelter's syndrome This syndrome is characterized by the presence of two X chromo-somes and a Y, which results in 47 chromosomes being present.

Epistasis (or Gene Interaction): In morning glories, genes *C* and *P* are necessary for pink flowers. In the absence of either (*ccP__* or *C__ pp*) or both (*ccpp*) of these genes, the flowers are blue. What will be the result of the following crosses as far as flower color of the offspring and proportion of the offspring are concerned?

$$Ccpp \times ccPp = 1 \text{ pink:3 blue;}$$

$$ccpp \times CcPp = 1 \text{ pink:3 blue}$$

In essence the expression of pink requires *C__ P__*, and all others will be blue. In this example, the epistasis is of the complementary interaction type. The offspring may be *Cc* or *cc* with equal probability (i.e., 50%); the same is true for *Pp* and *pp* (50%). If the chance of *C__* is 0.5 and the chance of *P__* is 0.5, then the chance of *C__ P__* is $0.5 \times 0.5 = 0.25$. Thus, 1/4 will be pink and 3/4 will be blue.

Polygenic Traits: Certain conditions are determined by genes at several loci. Each of the genes involved has a small effect which may be additive. Expression of this kind of trait is usually very sensitive to environmental influences.

Lethal Genes: Certain genes are lethal in the homozygous condition and cause the demise of the organism. An example is yellow coat in mice. If two hybrid yellow mice are mated the typical 1:2:1 genotypic ratio results—namely, 1/4 homozygous dominant (yellow dead embryos), 1/2 hybrid (yellow mice), and 1/4 homozygous recessive (wild type or agouti mice), but the phenotypic ratio among the live born mice is 2 yellow: 1 gray.

Modifying Genes: These genes affect the performance of other genes but apparently exhibit no trait of their own. If, for instance, in mice the gene for black hair is present, the gene for agouti color will elicit a yellow banding. When it is absent there is no effect.

Paternity Exclusion and Reassignment of Misassigned Infants

1) Paternity will be excluded if the child
   a) Has an antigen that is present in neither the mother nor the putative father;
   b) Does not have an antigen that the putative father has and would have had to give to his progeny (for example, a type O child and a type AB putative father).
2) Correct reassignment of infants misassigned to parents in a hospital is often achieved by looking for any of the following kinds of incompatibilities between the infants and the couples and then assigning each infant to the couple with which only compatibilities exist:
   a) The child has an antigen present in neither spouse;
   b) The child lacks one or more antigens that either or both spouses would have had to give him/her.
3) Increased probability of exclusion of a falsely accused male or of correct parental reassignment of misassigned infants results if several kinds of blood groups, HLA, and some of the following kinds of other genetically determined proteins are also included in the studies: hemoglobins, serum proteins, red cell enzymes, and several other enzymes.

The Animal Kingdom

Distribution of Living Organisms

Every living organism has a distinct yet interactive role, a place, and a mode of life, which are determined by that individual's structure and physiological makeup. The earth represents diverse *habitats* (places where one lives), which are characterized by conditions such as temperature, moisture, soil conditions, terrain, pressure, chemical cycles (gases and minerals), sunlight, seasonal variations, and others; organisms (species) must adapt and adjust their *life cycles* to the *climate* they live in. No species lives in a vacuum and is entirely independent; all are part of an integrated, systematically functioning, living (dynamic) *community* that includes many varieties of plants, animals, viruses, etc.

Although many populations of different species live together as a *community*, and although *turnover* is continuous, automatic, and self-adjusting, the result is an internally balanced community; there is a remarkable numerically steady state that is determined essentially by food supply, reproduction, and protection of the bonds of interdependency of community members.

Six factors are important to any habitat.

1. *Temperature* controls the speed of every reaction; raising the temperature by 10°C doubles the speed. While there exists a large range of temperature, most life exists in a narrow range; species have limits, and most are destroyed by excess at either end of the scale. Warm-blooded organisms (mammals and birds) possess internal regulation of body temperature, whereas cold-blooded animals (fishes, reptiles, amphibians, and invertebrates) do not and their function is directly related to their external environment. The oceans represent a fairly stable environment, and marine organisms are less prone to seasonal variations. Many land animals have adapted to seasonal changes by migration or hibernation.

2. *Moisture* (water) is critical to the existence of life since it is a solvent (minerals used by plants), a constituent of tissues, and the medium in which many species live and breed. The water cycle (evaporation, cloud formation, precipitation, drainage, and soil percolation) is dynamic and continuous (between sea, land, and air) and affects every particle of the universe. Also, water prevents rapid temperature fluctuations, a critical element in homeostasis.

3. *Soil conditions* are a crucial factor. The chemical makeup of the soil determines the presence or type of plants and, in some cases, the animals of the region. Texture and porosity play a role in moisture content, pH, and the presence or absence of burrowing animals. Slope affects drainage, while exposure to sunlight modulates absorption of heat.

4. *Pressure* varies with elevation (atmospheric pressure reflected in barometric reading) and with depth (water pressure: 15 pounds/10 meters equals one atmosphere of pressure). Availability of oxygen decreases with increasing altitude and depth. People living at high altitudes have higher red blood cell (erythrocyte) counts to compensate.

5. *Chemical interchange* occurs continuously in all habitats. Here are three good examples:

   a. Oxygen derived from air and water serves the oxidative machinery of life; after usage it returns to the life cycle in the form of carbon dioxide or, combined with hydrogen, as water. Carbon dioxide is used in the process of photosynthesis; some of the oxygen released is utilized by plants in respiration, but most is returned to the environment.

   b. Nitrogen is utilized directly by nitrogen-fixing bacteria to produce plant proteins; after utilization by animals these become animal proteins, and their eventual metabolic fate results in nitrogenous wastes. These wastes are converted by bacteria into nitrites and ammonia with release of nitrogen into the atmosphere; the nitrites are converted into nitrates, which again are utilized to make plant proteins.

c. Carbon is the backbone of protoplasm; it is derived from carbon dioxide (via photosynthesis) and synthesized into carbohydrates, which, together with proteins and fats, comprise the tissues of all plants and animals. Metabolism returns carbon for recycling as carbon dioxide.

6. *Sunlight* provides all the energy utilized by most living organisms. Energy is transformed from one type to another, but it is neither created nor destroyed. Lavoisier (1743–1794) showed that processes of organisms conform to the First Law of Thermodynamics—namely, the total amount of energy in a system is constant but is capable of transformation. Radiation from the sun includes heat, visible light, and ultraviolet radiation. Solar radiation, especially of the longer wavelengths, controls most climatic variations because of the effects of soil heating, water evaporation, and air expansion. Light controls the photoperiod responsible for the flowering of plants and the migration of animals.

Interrelationships of Animals

Competition for food, shelter, and mates is considerable; some organisms (termites, bees), however, have developed a cooperative society based on distinct roles (workers, protectors, reproducers, nurses, etc.). Plants (producers—autotrophs) commonly compete for sunlight (energy), minerals, and water. The passing of energy from one organism to another constitutes the *food chain* or pyramid; the small (more abundant) are eaten by the large (fewer in number). Plants are eaten by *herbivores* (primary consumers); these in turn are eaten by *carnivores* (secondary consumers); and as larger carnivores eat smaller ones the energy is passed along the chain. As the energy is transferred through the predator chain, the total declines progressively, and successive members are usually larger in size but fewer in number. Organisms eaten by a predator are called *prey*; an organism that consumes its own species is considered a *cannibal,* and one that devours dead material is a *scavenger*.

Factors such as disease control the number of organisms in the food chain; organisms such as viruses, rickettsias, bacteria, protozoans, parasitic worms, and arthropods which by themselves are populations also control the populations on/in which they live. The *parasite* obtains its food from its host, generally harming the host. *Ectoparasites* (lice) live *on* the host, while *endoparasites* (trichina worm) live *in* the host (gut or tissues). Some parasites such as the tick are intermediate hosts, as demonstrated in the transmission of Rocky Mountain spotted fever. Parasites that may destroy the host are called *pathogenic,* and are a considerable element in the regulation and control of the host population. All viruses are parasitic, and bacteria that lack photosynthetic abilities (are saprotrophic) are also parasitic.

The long-term relationship of two organisms of different species is commonly referred to as *symbiosis*. When one gains without harming the other, we speak of *commensalism* (barnacles on whales and epiphytes—plants—that grow on another host plant); in *mutualism* both parties are benefited (the flagellate in the termite digests the wood the termite eats, and the tick bird on the rhinoceros eats ticks, and cleans and warns the larger animal of danger).

Saprophytism is the obtaining of food from dead or decaying material (bacteria of decay and filamentous fungi are examples); the saprophytes essentially function to release chemicals back to the food chain. Without their role many essential elements would soon be unavailable, and the balance of energy transfer and transformation would be disturbed.

As previously emphasized, no organism can be successful in isolation since every specialized being depends on others for some product or process. The smallest congregation of like organisms is the *family*; a larger number comprises a *population*. The key element of a population is the fact that its members interbreed with one another; all populations are composed of *species*. Reproductive barriers exist between species. Speciation has many causes, such as separation by differences in climate, mountain ranges, rivers, or just distance. Only inheritable variations (e.g., skin color) controlled by genes are transmitted to new generations; acquired ones (e.g., muscle build) die with the individual. Individual variations of the members of a species are denoted as *polymorphism,* while the differences due only to sex are referred to as dimorphism.

All organisms live together in a dynamic state under the influence of environmental (chemical and physical) factors; not all are friendly since natural enemies exist for every species (they consume one another or compete for the same food source). Protective adaptation helps in survival. Many organisms blend well into their surroundings (polar bears are white), so that they are hard to see; some organisms such as the flounder can adapt readily to several backgournds, and others (insects are good examples) mimic their surroundings (butterflies look like flowers and leaves).

Population Dynamics

According to their mode of mobility, organisms are classified as *free-living* (the organism gets around by itself) or *sessile* (it is fixed to another structure). Among both groups there are *solitary* (independent) individuals and others that live in colonies (groups).

All organisms of one species that live in a definable area comprise a population that has distinct organizational features.

As part of the group dynamics of a population, certain factors must be considered:

1) *population density*—the number of organisms in a unit of area,
2) *birth rate*—the number of new organisms per unit of time,
3) *mortality rate*—the number of organisms dying per unit of time,
4) *reproductive or biotic potential*—the potential of a population to increase its numbers under optimal conditions.

Populations are usually considered in terms of the number per unit occupying a given area. As mentioned before, the number of larger organisms is considerably smaller. *Biotic potential* (maximum rate of increase) is continuously checked by *environmental resistance* (competition, disease, inclement climate, etc.). When a population settles in a new area, growth at first is slow (lack of mates), then increases rapidly (exponentially), and finally levels off as an equilibrium is reached because of limits of food supply, the settling of suitable habitats, and the increase of parasites and predators. Usually, as a population increases the environmental resistance, which initially was low, also increases as a result of population density.

A dynamic community of different plants and animals (interdependent) evolves to form an *ecosystem* with the physical environment. No situation is permanent; and while some changes occur rapidly, most are due to a sequential *succession* (lake–pond–swamp–grassland). No one species is present in every corner of the world; geography (geographical range) and environment (ecological range) are key elements. Physical (land and water), climatic (temperature and moisture), and biological (food and predators) barriers are limiting factors to the spread of populations.

Each species requires certain minimal elements for growth and reproduction; this fact led Liebig in 1840 to formulate the "law of the minimum," which states that the rate of growth of an organism is limited by the factor present in the scarcest amount. Too much of a certain factor, according to Shelford (1913), can be just as limiting since the well being of a species is determined by its *range of tolerance*. Organisms are usually more sensitive during development and early and late in life. The range varies greatly from factor to factor. *Stenothermic* organisms can tolerate only slight variations in temperature, while *eurythermic* organisms are able to survive a wide range.

Major Environments–Habitats

1. Water:

a. *Salt Water*. Over 70 percent of the earth is covered by salt water, and the environment, while varying widely overall, is quite stable in a specific region in regard to temperature (a range of 35°C), gas composition, and salinity (30–37 parts of salt per thousand). Ocean currents affect movements of marine organisms and the adjacent regional climate. Tidal fluctuations affect organisms in the shore region. Depth varies, pressure increases with depth, while light decreases with depth (about a 600-ft limit).

b. *Fresh Water*. Freshwater bodies are scattered in their distribution, have less volume and depth, and exhibit great variability in temperature, gas composition, mineral content, light penetration, and mobility. Organisms living in fresh water, because of its low salinity (low osmotic pressure), have had to develop organs for effectively regulating the osmotic pressure. Unlike oceans, freshwater bodies are subject to periodic drying, changing flow rates, and high turbidity.

2. Land or Terrestrial Habitat: The greatest variability is present on land, when one considers minerals, topography, temperature, water content, air movement, and light. Temperature and moisture vary tremendously with the seasons, altitude, latitude, and with topography. Soil and air temperatures vary as much as 120°C.

Learning, Conditioning, Rhythms

1. Learning: Many definitions of learning exist, but the process of learning, simply defined, is a change in the behavior of an organism based on some experience or practice. Many organisms have been very successful without much learning; their inborn patterns or instincts allow them to compete for food, find shelter, mate, and live out their life spans. Familiar examples of instinctive behavior are spiders spinning webs (specific patterns), birds building nests and migrating and returning, and fish returning to spawning grounds thousands of miles away. More complex, but still instinctive, are societies of bees and ants where a definite division of labor exists. Humans, on the other hand, while high in the evolutionary scale, must learn from their interaction with the environment and use that knowledge to succeed; for many years a human child is quite dependent, while most animals from day 1 are quite independent. Changes in behavior are often hard to assess but might include:

(a) a new pattern of the organism, and
(b) a change in the response to a stimulus not previously exhibited.

2. Conditioning: Many of our actions seem automatic, and in most instances we cannot attribute definite reasons for them. These behaviors (responses) may be learned even though we have no recollection of the learning process. On the other hand, many actions are unlearned reflexes. An example of the latter is the fact that the autonomic nervous system (sympathetic and parasympathetic) allows an organism to adapt to certain phenomena. When we walk into bright sunlight the sphincter pupillae contracts, but if we enter a dark area the dilator opens the pupillary opening; the sphincter is under parasympathetic, and the dilator under sympathetic, control. For close vision (reading) convergence and change in the shape of the lens allow the eye to accommodate. Salivary secretion (parotid, submandibular, and sublingual glands) and tearing by the lacrimal gland of the eye are other superb examples of these homeostatic reflexes. Fright produces an increase in heart rate, blood pressure, and metabolic states to prepare an organism to cope; all this takes place at the subconscious level.

Classical Conditioning. Some actions, however, can be learned by a process called *classical conditioning,* that is, learning to associate two previously linked phenomena.

First reported by Pavlov in 1927, it is exemplified by the responses of dogs to the introduction of food. When a dog sees or smells food, it is stimulated to begin a reflexive behavior—secretion of saliva. Pavlov restrained dogs in a harness and then simply used an auditory stimulus such as a bell. When the bell was rung, the dog did not secrete saliva. When food alone was provided, the expected salivary secretion occurred. If, thereafter, the two stimuli—bell and food—were presented for some time simultaneously, salivary secretion occurred. After many trials, the bell alone elicited the salivary response; the dog had learned to react to a different stimulus via conditioning. In 1920 Watson showed the same reaction in an 11-month-old baby, who was conditioned by a loud noise and the presentation of a furry object to eventually be frightened by fur alone. Many of the results of conditioning can be reversed through reconditioning the organism to a different association.

Pavlov identified five components of classical conditioning:

1) unconditioned stimulus—the food; it automatically stimulates salivation;
2) conditioned stimulus—the bell; it is neutral at the beginning but eventually effective and undistinguishable;
3) reinforcement—the pairing of two stimuli;
4) unconditioned response—salivation—the automatic response by the parasympathetic division of the autonomic nervous system;
5) conditioned response—the bell—the response as a result of learning by the central nervous system; the unconditioned and conditioned stimuli function as one.

Five other aspects of conditioning should be mentioned.

1. Extinction. The conditioned response can be reversed. Pavlov showed that, after an animal was conditioned, if for some time thereafter only the bell was rung without food being offered, the flow of saliva started to decrease and eventually stopped.
2. Spontaneous Recovery. In this set of experiments, Pavlov let a response achieve extinction and then gave the animal a long rest from the experimental protocol. After this rest the bell was rung and the response reappeared. This spontaneous recovery may explain phenomena we all experience, such as fears or preferences for certain things for which we have no conscious basis.
3. Stimulus Generalization. In these experiments, Pavlov was able to show that somewhat different but basically similar stimuli (e.g., different tones of music) may evoke the same response and effect. The more similar the new stimulus is to the familiar one, the stronger the response usually will be.
4. Stimulus Discrimination. In another set of experiments, food was offered to animals only at the sound of a specific bell, and salivation was elicited only when that particular bell was rung. The animal did not salivate at the ringing of a different bell; it had learned to discriminate between different stimuli.
5. Onset of Neurotic Behavior. In 1927 Pavlov also observed that, after an animal had learned stimulus discrimination and then the difference between the two stimuli was decreased to the point where the animal could not recognize it, the animal's behavior become unpredictable and aberrant.

In general, conditioning is best accomplished when a short interval between stimuli is used and when positive phenomena are elicited or are the end result. Conditioning is also enhanced when the stimulus is truly different (strong and novel) from many of the background stimuli.

Operant Conditioning. The results described above are due chiefly to the influence of the learning process on autonomic reflexes. However, other forms of behavior are also of consequence in reactions to stimuli. When, for instance, a cat is introduced into a new environment, the animal will react by exploring and marking its territory. In this case, the organism itself is acting on the environment, and the activity is referred to as *operant behavior.* Learning can modify these actions, as Skinner demonstrated in the 1930s with the help of a box and a food bar to reward the animal for a certain action.

In 1938 Skinner observed that a rat placed in a box explored actively and even pressed a bar that released a pellet of food. At first the animal did not make an association but soon learned to connect the pressing of the food lever with the dispensing of food and a reward for the action of pressing. The key element in this situation is that reinforced operant behavior is repeated (the lever is pressed frequently), while nonreinforced activities are quickly abandoned. Extinction, spontaneous recovery, and stimulus generalization and discrimination are also part of operant behavior.

Instrumental Conditioning (Operant) and the Law of Effect. In 1898 Thorndike addressed similar issues and found that, when cats were placed in a box and had to learn to open the door in order to obtain food, the reward enhanced their conditioning. The law of effect essentially states that, when a stimulus is followed by a reward, the response is strong, consistent, and likely to be repeated by the experimental subject.

Certain factors called *reinforcers* have been identified by psychological researchers:

1. Primary—in animals, food and water.
2. Secondary—love and affection, shown, for example, by petting.
3. Immediate—a reward given upon accomplishing a feat produces the most efficient learning.
4. Constant—repeated (short-interval) stimuli result in very efficient and rapid learning.
5. Partial—extinction is less apt to occur if there is at least partial reinforcement.

Operant Escape—Escape Learning. When an animal is exposed to an unpleasant stimulus (shock), it will quickly learn to leave the environment to avoid the experience.

Operant Avoidance—Active Avoidance Learning. If an animal is conditioned to a warning signal (bell) and knows that a shock will follow it will heed the warning and rapidly leave the hostile environment.

Aversive Conditioning. In this experimental setup the unconditioned stimulus is offensive and is of negative value to the organism. In this case the organism (e.g., after a shock is administered) not only exhibits a specific response such as muscular twitching but also develops a generalized "fear reaction," which results in modification of heart rate, respiratory activity, sweating, etc.

Primary Activities. Many activities occur as the organism goes through life, but some very organized ones are limited to early development. Human beings are fairly helpless, but other animals (e.g., rats) on day 1 can perform highly complex motor patterns independently. Two classical phenomena of rat behavior will serve as examples:

1. Suckling. Suckling involves some very complicated sensory input aspects, helps meet the nutritional needs of the organism, is an effective reinforcing activity leading to other skills, and provides thermal support and transport for the young. In order for suckling to occur, the mother's nipple must be coated by amniotic fluid, saliva, or both; the pup *in utero* swallows and excretes amniotic fluid during the last trimester and it is that familiarity with the substances that directs the pup's first act of suckling. Also, since the mother licks the pups and the nipples (milkline), saliva is a behavioral stimulus. The key factor in this primary activity is that it is the animal's previous exposure to the stimulus that leads it to react to it (it has had gustatory and olfactory clues). Thereafter, however, the pup's saliva becomes the stimulus. Ability of the pup to adapt to its new environment is categorized as developmental plasticity.

2. Huddling. This activity is undertaken by neonates and is beneficial in temperature regulation, which results in less energy expenditure by the young (a homeostatic response). Huddling is not a self-serving mechanism; it benefits the whole brood. An

animal starting at the periphery will eventually end up in the center, and so on; the shifting of places helps the group to survive and to adapt to and identify with litter-mates. Young animals that know their littermates will find their nest readily.

Conditioning and Biofeedback. Biofeedback manipulation is an attempt by the physician to let the individual know what his/her spontaneous functions—heart rate, blood pressure, respiratory activity, skin and internal body temperature, brain waves, peristaltic activity, muscular activity—are at a particular time and circumstance. Patients learn, for example, to recognize when their muscles are tense and may with conditioning be able to relax them to avoid spasms or relieve tension; in the same way vascular headaches may perhaps be avoided. In these procedures patients learn to manipulate and control nonconscious pro-cesses. Although results have been mixed, this arena has excited the imagination of researchers and is undergoing active analysis.

3. Rhythms—Biological Clocks: Interest has mainly focused on rhythms that appear in close approximation with natural periodicities such as day-night cycles; tidal rhythms; monthly, seasonal and annual phenomena; circadian rhythms (about 24 hours); and circa-tidal rhythms (12-hour cycles in marine organisms).

Rhythms are present from the cellular to the tissue–organ–system–organismal level, and from unicellular organisms to humans. Circadian rhythms persist even when the cues for the cycle are deleted. When cues are controlled, cycles are extremely constant and exact, but in the wild they tend to vary slightly. There is considerable evidence that endogenous and autonomic, genetically controlled mechanisms account for the persistence of rhythms.

Most living things, both animals and plants, show a circadian rhythm of activity and rest. It is well documented that humans perform differently on physiological and psychological tests at different periods of the day and night. Local time is not a critical factor, as has been well established by shift workers who work at night and sleep during the day; the shift worker's temperature is falling during the daytime, while in the rest of the population, which is working, temperatures are rising. The shift worker at the same time exhibits low levels of adrenal steroids, while in the rest of the population levels are high. These are relevant examples that the body's biological clock adjusts to the mechanical clock of soci-ety.

Characteristics of Rhythms. Rhythms are usually described in terms of four character-istics.

1) *Period*—the number of times required to complete the cycle; it is the time between peaks.
2) *Frequency*—the number of times that a peculiar event, such as sleeping occurs.
3) *Phase*—time location when a specific event occurs in a particular organism; the highs and lows of a substance are phase phenomena. Adrenal corticosteroid levels in day and night workers can be described as 180 degrees out of phase;
4) *Amplitude*—the extent (amount) of change that takes place (e.g., body temperature varies as much as 2° during one cycle).

Factors that Affect Rhythms. Among the commonly cited factors that influence rhythms are these six:

1) geomagnetic fields,
2) cosmic rays,
3) electric fields,
4) X-rays,
5) light and darkness,
6) atmospheric pressure.

Cycles can be disrupted by many factors; commonly cited ones are shift work, jet travel, and space flight.

Importance of Rhythms. As a consequence of our daily circadian rhythms we have a susceptibility or a resistance to drugs, stress, allergy, pain, infection, and many other factors. The responsiveness to different regimens, doses, and procedures have ramifications in therapeutic plans. The outcome of surgical procedures and the effect of anesthetic agents certainly are influenced by rhythms and the time they were performed and administered, respectively. Pain tolerance, for instance, shifts according to the time of day (more pain is experienced at night). What is just an annoyance at one time in the cycle is fatal at another point. Births and deaths mainly occur at night and in the early morning. Ulcers, allergies, and psychoses are more prevalent in the spring. Arctic hysteria is a winter phenomenon. In humans, deaths from arteriosclerotic disease peak in January and suicides in May.

To illustrate the importance of rhythms in every activity, here is a partial list of the factors they influence:

1. Body and skin temperature
2. Blood pressure
3. Pulse rate
4. Respiration
5. Blood sugar levels and glucose tolerance
6. Hemoglobin levels
7. Protein utilization and amino acid levels
8. Production and breakdown of ATP
9. Adrenal hormone levels
10. Urinary production, volume, and rate and urinary electrolytes
11. Mitosis
12. Enzyme activities
13. EEG rhythms
14. Stamina and physical vigor
15. Emotional state
16. Metabolic rate
17. Pancreatic enzymatic activity and insulin production

Evolution

The cornerstone of evolution is the fact that species arise from preexisting species.

Key People and Concepts

Aristotle (384–322 B.C.) philosophized that living organisms represent a succession and progression of more suitable forms, rather than random creations.

Redi (1626–1898) showed by experiment that organisms do not arise spontaneously from nonliving material; he demonstrated that maggots did not appear in meat unless the meat was exposed to flies, which laid their eggs on it.

Spallanzani (1729–1799) repeated Redi's work and showed that no life appeared in solutions first boiled and then protected from air.

Lamarck (1744–1829) believed that simple animals and plants are spontaneously generated but that lineage presents a series of evolutionary forms and that there can be independent branching and development. However, his incorrect ideas of inherited characteristics and of use and disuse of parts overshadowed his correct ideas that individual variations are retained because of adaptive value and that these variations lead to the emergence of different species suited for particular environments.

John Ray (1627–1705) was the first to attempt to define a species and to point out the difference between constant and incidental features of organisms.

Louis Pasteur (1822–1895) showed that life cannot arise in a medium from which all living things are excluded.

Charles Darwin (1809–1882) and *Alfred Russel Wallace* (1823–1913) documented the fact that natural processes can bring about a gradual development of new types.

Alfred Russel Wallace sent a manuscript to Darwin that dealt with the tendency of organisms to depart from the original type. Wallace had observed the same things as Darwin had on his voyage on the *Beagle*, and Darwin, being the scholar and gentleman he was, forwarded Wallace's article for publication and included a short article on his own observations. The failure of the articles to arouse much interest gave Darwin the impetus to proceed with his own work, and in 1859 he published his *Origin of Species by Natural Selection*. He argued two main premises:

1. No two members of a species are exactly alike even if they have the same parents.
2. Some variations are advantages, giving the organism the chance to branch out into new enviroments and to enlarge its numbers, while others are detrimental and diminish its chances of survival.

These premises lead to the conclusion that a population is likely to change in the relative frequency of its various characteristics (i.e., it *evolves*), because of the *natural selection* of some characteristics over others. The environment was cited as a major cause of natural selection, because it weeds out organisms with unfavorable characteristics and strengthens those with favorable variations.

As one can gather, the modern theory of evolution is not the work of a single individual, but it was Darwin, via his careful documentation and voluminous writings, who marshaled the evidence.

Process of Evolution

The basis of evolution is the inheritable genetic material; the forces (natural selection) can be demonstrated by the principles of Mendelian population genetics. Free reproduction within a population results in the shuffling and reshuffling of the genetic pool. As two populations (sister populations) interbreed, the total genetic material of a species continues to be shuffled, and one can readily see that inheritable features may arise by sexual recombination or by mutation. The individuals whose genes are passed on to the next generation with greater frequency will be those whose genes give them the ability to produce many viable offspring, because of their favorable ability to survive, to mate, to produce gametes, and to have the offspring survive to their own age of reproduction. It is via this mode that a genetically favorable trait is spread and a change that starts in one individual is distributed to the whole population. Generally, many such changes occur before a new species evolves; evolution is a very slow process. Thus, this basic process of evolution consists of:

1) The appearance of an inheritable trait by sexual recombination or mutation, and
2) the spreading of this trait via reproduction to successive generations.

In 1906 De Vries proposed that mutations (sudden changes in the genetic material) were largely responsible for many evolutionary features exhibited, since they are transmitted to future generations. Radiation (cosmic and other), mutagens (chemicals), and temperature probably cause most mutations. Most are unfavorable; advantageous ones, however, survive if occurring in gametes and are often utilized by humans (short-legged sheep that cannot jump fences readily and many varieties of flowers are good examples).

Adaptive Radiation

In speciation one ancestor species gives rise to several descendant species, and as the process continues the new type in turn becomes a potential ancestor for many lines; it can be likened to a tree trunk and its branches and branches of branches. This is not a ladder effect since many presently living species had a common ancestor and simply represent contemporary specimens of adaptive radiation.

Extinction

Obviously, not all the branches reach the top, and for many reasons not always clearly understood certain species became extinct. Lack of adaptation to the constantly changing environment and competition (basically for food) between two different species in the same location are the dominant factors controlling the fine balance between survival and extinction.

When a common ancestor gives rise to several descendent lines that, although closely related, have adapted in different ways and developed dissimilar characteristics in response to diverse states, one speaks of evolutionary *divergence*. On the other hand, when unrelated groups adapt to the same environment and a common set of features is developed, even though there is no common ancestry, the process is termed *convergence*. Even though similarities are developed, however, there is never identity.

Analogy and Homology

In unrelated organisms, structures performing similar functions have developed; if function is the only unifying element these structures are said to be *analogous* (examples are the wing of a bird and the wing of a bee).

If body parts exhibit similar structure but their functions are diverse, one suspects a common ancestry and speaks of *homology* (the wing of a bird and the upper extremity of a human have a common bone pattern). When a structure becomes nonfunctional, as the appendix has in humans, it is termed *vestigial*.

This association of structure and function led to the biogenetic law, which states, "Ontogeny repeats phylogeny"; in other words, as an individual develops it passes through the developmental stages of the larger group to which it belongs. For example, embryos of land vertebrates possess rudiments of gills at one state. However, the embryonic stages are far from perfect recapitulations of ancestors' evolutionary history.

CHEMISTRY

General Chemistry

The Atom

John Dalton's theories—still accepted

a. An element is composed of atoms. All atoms of an element possess the same chemical properties.

b. Atoms of different elements have different properties.

c. During a chemical reaction (nuclear reactions excepted, of course) atoms and elements are not created nor do they dissappear.

d. Atoms of more than one element may react to form compounds. In a pure compound the number of atoms of each element is constant.

Components of the Atom

1. Nucleus: The nucleus—found at the center of an atom—contains neutrons and protons.

a. Neutrons—no charge—mass of about 1 dalton

b. Protons—charge of +1—mass of about 1 dalton. Number of protons in an atom determines the atomic number and the identity of the element.

2. Electrons: Electrons—charge of −1—mass of about 0.0005 dalton. Number of electrons circling the nucleus is equal to the number of protons in the nucleus.

Placement of Electrons—Energy Levels

1. **Quantum numbers:**

    a. Principal quantum number, n, determines the shell. It may be 1, 2, 3, 4, etc., in increasing distance from the nucleus and increasing energy. The K shell has a principal quantum number of 1.

    b. Angular momentum quantum number, l, determines the subshell. $l = 0, 1, 2, \ldots, (n - 1)$.

    c. Magnetic quantum number, m_l, determines the orbital: $m_l = l, l - 1, \ldots, 0, \ldots, 1 - l, -l$. The energies are virtually identical.

    d. Spin quantum number, m_s, describes the spin of an electron. Allowed values are $+\frac{1}{2}$ and $-\frac{1}{2}$.

2. **Pauli exclusion principle:** No two electrons in an atom may have exactly the same quantum number (i.e., all four).

3. **Total number of electrons in a shell:** The total number of electrons in a shell is $2n^2$.

4. **Order of filling orbitals:** Orbitals are filled from lower to higher energy levels. They may be designated in shorthand form. For example, the following oxygen atom may be designated as $1s^2 2s^2 2p^4$. Within the $2p$ orbitals, it is possible for an electron to be in $2p_x$, $2p_y$, or $2p_z$. Hund's rule states that one electron of parallel spin will go into each of these until each has one electron; additional electrons of antiparallel spin will then be added as necessary until all are filled.

$$
\begin{array}{ccccc}
 & & & \overline{\hspace{2cm} 2p \hspace{2cm}} & \\
1s & 2s & 2p_x & 2p_y & 2p_z
\end{array}
$$

Oxygen $(\uparrow\downarrow)\,(\uparrow\downarrow)\,(\uparrow\downarrow)\,(\uparrow)\,(\uparrow)$

5. **The excited state:** The situation described above is that of the ground state. By input of energy it is possible to raise electrons to higher energy levels. When electrons drop back from these higher energy levels (excited state) to the levels required by the ground state, there is emission of radiation (emission spectrum).

Periodic Table

The Periodic Table arranges the elements from left to right in order of increasing atomic number. The Periodic Law states that: The properties of the elements are periodic functions of their atomic numbers.

1. **Groups:** Vertical columns are called groups. All elements in the same group have the same number of valence electrons and, therefore, related chemical properties. For example, Group IA elements have only one electron in their outermost principal energy level. They tend to lose this electron readily to form $+1$ ions. Group VIIA elements have seven valence electrons. They tend to gain one electron to form -1 ions. At the extreme right of the table is the group known as the noble gases. These elements have complete outer shells and are essentially non-reactive. Properties of elements in other groups are now known to be related to placement of their electrons.

2. **Periods:** Horizontal rows of the table are called periods. Elements in the same period have the same number of principal energy levels. From left to right across a period, many properties exhibit periodicity (change with changes in atomic structure). For example, from left to right, atomic radii and metallic characteristics decrease while ionization energy and electronegativity increase.

   Gases

1. **Ideal gas law:** Although early laws were formulated by Boyle, by Charles, and by Gay-Lussac to explain parts of the interrelationships between temperature, pressure, and

volume of a gas, one simple formula sums it up:

$$\frac{P_1 V_1}{T_1} = \frac{P_2 V_2}{T_2} = nR$$

where P = pressure in atmospheres or torr
V = volume
T = absolute temperature in convenient units
n = moles of the gas
R = universal gas constant in appropriate units

Real gas behavior deviates from the ideal gas law at low temperature and high pressure.

2. Partial pressures:

$$P_T = P_1 + P_2 + \cdots + P_n$$

(i.e., the total pressure of a mixture of gases is equal to the sum of the partial pressures)

3. Diffusion — Graham's Law: Rate of diffusion is inversely proportional to the square root of the molecular weight.

$$\frac{v_1}{v_2} = \sqrt{\frac{m_2}{m_1}}$$

where v = velocity
m = molecular weight

Thus, a gas of twice the molecular weight will diffuse 0.71 as fast.

Liquids and Solids

Ideal gases are assumed to have negligible intermolecular interactions. Within a homologous series of organic compounds, the boiling point increases with increasing molecular weight. The same relationship may be seen within the halogens.

There are, however, forces in some compounds that cause them to be liquids or even solids at temperatures at which their molecular weights would suggest that they should be gases.

1. Dipole forces: In certain asymmetrical molecules the electrons become unevenly distributed between regions, and there results a partial positive charge in one region (and a partial negative charge in another). Molecules become arranged so that there is electrostatic attraction between adjacent molecules.

2. Hydrogen bonds: Hydrogen in one molecule may bond to oxygen, nitrogen, or fluorine in another molecule. The energy required to break this bond is about 10 kcal.

3. London-van der Waals dispersion forces: These forces involve interaction between molecules on the basis of their polarizability. They may be important in nonpolar compounds.

4. Ionic forces: Oppositely charged ions exhibit coulombic attraction.

Phase Changes

1. Nature of the solid, liquid, and gaseous phases:

where A is melting or fusion
B is freezing
C is vaporization or boiling
D is condensation

$$\text{Solid} \underset{B}{\overset{A}{\rightleftharpoons}} \text{Liquid} \underset{D}{\overset{C}{\rightleftharpoons}} \text{Gas}$$

2. **Energy of phase transition:**

   a. The energy involved in conversion from the solid to the liquid phase is H_f.
   b. The energy involved in conversion from the liquid to the gaseous phase is H_v.
   c. All molecules in one phase do not have the same energy—there is a range. A liquid at a temperature below its boiling point is subject to some of its molecules being vaporized by virtue of the fact that some molecules are sufficiently energetic to be converted into the gaseous state. The temperature of the liquid, however, is a measure of the average kinetic energy.

   3. **Phase diagram:** The phase diagram allows the visualization of possible phases at particular temperatures and pressures.

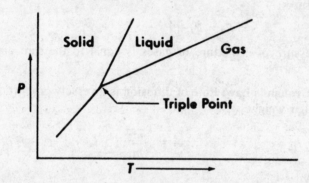

Note that the lines between phases in the phase diagram represent those conditions of pressure and temperature at which the phases indicated on the two sides of the lines may coexist. The point of intersection of the three lines is designated as *the triple point;* at this temperature and pressure all three phases may coexist.

Chemical Compounds

1. **Percent Weight and Empirical Formula:** Chemical compounds are pure substances that may be broken into two or more elements. A molecule is the smallest unit of a compound that still retains the properties of the compound; an atom is the smallest unit of an element.

A particular chemical compound will always have the same percentage composition by weight. Considering the compound iron (III) oxide, it is found to consist of:

$$Fe = 69.94\%$$

$$O = 30.06\%$$

Since it is agreed that a molecule of a compound is made up of whole atoms of elements, we will try to find the lowest multiple(s) of whole numbers. We may do this in two steps:

(1) Divide each percentage by the atomic weight of that element.

$$Fe = \frac{69.94}{55.85} = 1.252$$

$$O = \frac{30.06}{16.00} = 1.879$$

(2) Convert these numbers to the lowest whole multiple(s).

$$\frac{1.879}{1.252} = 1.501$$

This would indicate 1.5 atoms of oxygen for each atom of iron. Since it is agreed that whole atoms are involved, the simplest formula would be Fe_2O_3. This is known as the empirical formula.

2. Molecular Formula: In some cases, however, the molecular weight of a compound does not agree with its empirical formula. (This is often true of organic compounds and sometimes true of inorganic ones.) The organic compound glucose may be used as an example. Its elemental composition would give an empirical formula of CH_2O. From molecular weight determination, however, we can show that the molecular formula is $C_6H_{12}O_6$.

3. Mole and Avogadro's Number: If the molecular weight is known, we may weigh that many grams of the compound and we will have a mole. A mole of any compound contains 6.023×10^{23} molecules of that compound. This is known as Avogadro's number.

Balanced Chemical Equations

Chemical equations may be written in unbalanced or balanced form.

1. Inorganic Chemistry:

$$H_2 + O_2 \rightarrow H_2O$$

This equation tells us that diatomic molecules of hydrogen and oxygen react to form water. Inspection indicates, however, that there are 2 atoms of oxygen on the left side but there is only 1 atom of oxygen on the right side. This does not agree with what we know about conservation of matter.

We could increase the atoms of oxygen on the right side by placing the coefficient 2 before H_2O, thus indicating 2 molecules of H_2O. This unbalances the hydrogen, however, with 2 atoms of hydrogen on the left and 4 on the right. We can correct this by placing the coefficient 2 before the H_2:

$$2H_2 + O_2 \rightarrow 2H_2O$$

Inspection indicates that there are now 4 atoms of hydrogen on each side and 2 atoms of oxygen on each side.

This is now a balanced equation. The coefficients tell us that 2 diatomic molecules of hydrogen will react with 1 diatomic molecule of oxygen to form 2 molecules of water. Since the same number of molecules (i.e., Avogadro's number) are required for a mole of any material, we can also say that 2 moles of hydrogen react with 1 mole of oxygen to produce 2 moles of water.

2. Organic Chemistry: The equation

$$C_3H_8 + O_2 \rightarrow CO_2 + H_2O$$

is not balanced. Since there are 3 atoms of carbon on the left and 1 atom on the right, we need to multiply carbon dioxide by 3. Similarly, we need to multiply water by 4 to balance the hydrogen. Then, however, there will be too few oxygens on the left. We need to multiply O_2 by 5. Our balanced equation is then:

$$C_3H_8 + 5O_2 \rightarrow 3CO_2 + 4H_2O$$

Check to see that this equation is balanced. It tells us that 1 mole of propane reacts with 5 moles of oxygen to produce 3 moles of carbon dioxide and 4 moles of water.

Solutions

1. **Concentration units:**
   a. Molarity
      moles/liter = grams/molecular weight/liters of solution
   b. Molality = moles of solute/kilograms of solvent
   c. Normality = equivalents of solute/liters of solution
   d. Equivalents = grams/equivalent weight

2. **Colligative properties:** Based on the number of dissolved particles, without regard to their nature.
   a. Boiling point elevation
      Boiling point elevation = $K_b m$
         where K_b is a constant for the specific solvent and m = molality of solute.
Note, however, that a 1 molal solution of NaCl would have twice the calculated effect since it would be 1 molal each in Na^+ and Cl^- (i.e., 2 molal total).
   b. Freezing point depression
      Freezing point depression = $K_f m$
         where K_f is a constant for the specific solvent and m = molality of solute particles (see comment above regarding ionizable solutes).
   c. Osmotic pressure. When an aqueous solution is placed on one side of a semipermeable membrane and pure water on the other side, there is net movement of water across the membrane. The applied pressure required to produce a net movement of zero is called the osmotic pressure.

$$\pi V = nRT$$

where π = osmotic pressure
   V = volume
   n = moles of particles in solution
   R is the universal gas constant
   T is the temperature, kelvin units (K)

3. **Solubility:** A comparatively insoluble inorganic compound in water is in equilibrium with its soluble ions.

$$Al(OH)_3 \downarrow \rightleftharpoons Al^{3+} + 3OH^-$$

The solubility product constant is K_{sp}.

$$K_{sp} = 5 \times 10^{-33} = [Al^{3+}][OH^-]^3$$

Thus, in the specific case of $Al(OH)_3$, if the product of the molar concentration of OH^- raised to the third power and Al^{3+} exceeds 5×10^{-33}, precipitation will occur.

Acids and Bases, pH, and Buffers

1. **Acids:**
   a. Brönsted-Lowry acid—a material that donates a proton:

$$HCl + H_2O \longrightarrow H_3O^+ + Cl^-$$
   (acid)

   b. Lewis acid—a material that accepts an electron pair

2. **Base:**
   a. Brönsted-Lowry base—a material that accepts a proton:

$$H_3O^+ + NaOH \rightleftharpoons 2H_2O + Na^+$$
      (base)

   b. Lewis base—a material that donates an electron pair

3. **Strength of acids and bases:**
   a. Strong acids and bases. A strong acid or base is assumed to be completely ionized. Therefore the concentration of acid is equal to the concentration of hydrogen ions (or hydronium ions).

$$HCl + H_2O \longrightarrow H_3O^+ + Cl^- \quad or \quad HCl \longrightarrow H^+ + Cl^-$$

b. Weak acids and bases

(1) $HF \rightleftharpoons H^+ + F^-$

$$K_a = \frac{[H^+][F^-]}{[HF]} = 7 \times 10^{-4} \text{ (in this specific case)}$$

Consider a $1M$ solution of HF for example:

$[H^+] = [F^-]$

So, $K_a[HF] = [H^+][F^-] = [H^+]^2$

and $[H^+] = \sqrt{K_a[HF]} = \sqrt{7 \times 10^{-4}} = 2.6 \times 10^{-2}$

In this example HF is called a conjugate acid, capable of releasing a proton. F^- is called a conjugate base, capable of combining with a proton.

(2) Bases

$NH_3 + H_2O \rightleftharpoons NH_4^+ + OH^-$

$K_b[NH_3] = [NH_4^+][OH^-]$

$K_b = 1.8 \times 10^{-5}$ for this particular base.

Computation similar to that for acid would allow one to determine the $[OH^-]$ for a 1 molar NH_3 solution. H_2O is not included in the equilibrium expression.

4. **pH, pOH, and pK_w:**

a. $pH = -\log[H^+]$

The pH of pure water is 7.

b. $pOH = -\log[OH^-]$

The pOH of pure water is 7.

c. $pK_w = pH + pOH = 14$

d. Changes in pH and hydrogen ions. Remember that pH is a logarithmic scale. A decrease of one unit in pH (e.g., from 7 to 6) indicates an increase in hydrogen ions by a factor of 10.

5. **Solution of salts:**

a. A solution of the salt of a strong acid and a strong base is highly ionized and neutral.

b. A solution of the salt of a strong acid and a weak base is acidic.

c. A solution of the salt of a weak acid and a strong base is basic.

6. **Buffers:** A buffer is a solution containing a weak acid or a weak base *and* a salt of that weak acid or weak base.

a. The ionization of a weak acid, HA, may be shown as

$$HA \rightleftharpoons H^+ + A^-$$

b. The ionization constant is defined as

$$K_a = \frac{[H^+][A^-]}{[HA]}$$

c. The negative logarithm of K_a is defined as pK_a. It is then possible to define a useful relationship called the Henderson-Hasselbalch equation:

$$pH = pK_a + \log\frac{[\text{conjugate base}]}{[\text{conjugate acid}]}$$

In the example we have already considered, of course, A^- would be the conjugate base and HA would be the conjugate acid in the buffer pair.

Although the conjugate acid is weakly ionized, it is assumed that the salt that produces the conjugate base is strongly ionized. Thus, the mixture of 500 ml each of $0.1M$ acetic acid and 0.1M sodium acetate would produce 1 liter of a solution that contains 0.05M acetic acid and 0.05M acetate ion. The Henderson-Hasselbalch equation would provide us with

$$pH = pK_a + \log \frac{(0.05)}{(0.05)} = pK_a + \log 1 = pK_a$$

Thus, a mixture of equal concentrations of the conjugate base and the conjugate acid will produce a pH equal to the pK_a. From a practical standpoint it is usually considered that a buffer system is useful in the restraint of changes of pH only over the range of $pK_a \pm 1$ pH unit.

7. **Volumetric calculations with acids and bases:**
    a.   Molarity = grams acid or base/molecular weight/liters
    b.   Normality = grams acid or base/equivalent weight/liters
For a monoprotic acid such as HCl, the normality equals the molarity. For a diprotic acid such as H_2SO_4, the normality is twice the molarity.
    c.   Number of equivalents in neutralization:

$$L_{acid} \times N_{acid} = L_{base} \times N_{base} = \text{number of equivalents}$$

    d.   Neutralizations may be done using the experimental technique of titration.

Electrochemistry

The electrolytic cell uses the flow of electrical current to cause a chemical reaction to occur. This type of chemical reaction is an oxidation-reduction (otherwise known as redox). In the electrolysis of molten NaCl, there is production of both Na and Cl_2. The half reactions involved are:

$$Na^+ + e^- \rightarrow Na^0 \qquad \text{(reduction)}$$
$$2Cl^- \rightarrow Cl_2^0 + 2e^- \quad \text{(oxidation)}$$

In balancing these half reactions, we must first balance one half reaction against the other to obtain the same number of electrons in each:

$$2[Na^+ + e^- \rightarrow Na^0] = 2Na^+ + 2e^- \rightarrow 2Na^0$$
$$1[2Cl^- \rightarrow Cl_2^0 + 2e^-] = 2Cl^- \rightarrow Cl_2^0 + 2e^-$$

When these balanced half reactions are added together, the electrons drop out to give a balanced equation for the net reaction:

$$2Na^+ + 2Cl^- \rightarrow 2Na^0 + Cl_2^0$$

or

$$2NaCl \rightarrow 2Na^0 + Cl_2^0$$

Thermodynamics

1. **Laws:**
    a.   *First law.* Energy can neither be created nor destroyed.
    b.   *Second law.* The spontaneous flow of heat is always unidirectional from the higher to the lower temperature.
    c.   *Third law.* The entropy of all pure crystalline solids may be taken as zero at the absolute zero of temperature.

2. **Change in enthalpy:** The change in enthalpy is ΔH. A negative ΔH for a reaction indicates that the products have a lower heat content than the reactants; therefore, heat is evolved. Since enthalpy is independent of the route of a reaction, it is possible to algebraically add reactions.

$$Pb(s) + O_2(g) \longrightarrow PbO_2(s) \qquad \Delta H = -66.1$$
$$2H_2O(g) \longrightarrow 2H_2(g) + O_2(g) \qquad \Delta H = +115.6$$

Sum $\overline{Pb(s) + 2H_2O(g) \longrightarrow PbO_2(s) + 2H_2(g)} \qquad \Delta H = +49.5$

In this example the overall reaction would require input of heat.

3. Change in entropy: The change in entropy is ΔS. Entropy may be described as the degree of disorder of a system. It is also seen as unrecoverable energy. Without the addition of energy to a system, entropy increases to a maximum.

4. Changes in Gibbs free energy: Changes in Gibbs free energy are ΔG. Some of the energy of a reaction is unavailable for useful work. The term ΔG indicates the energy that is available for useful work.

$$\Delta G = \Delta H - T\,\Delta S$$

where T = absolute temperature, K°

A negative ΔG indicates a spontaneous reaction. A positive ΔG indicates a reaction that would be spontaneous in the reverse direction. When $\Delta G = 0$, the system is at equilibrium.

Rate Processes in Chemical Reactions

1. Rate-Controlling Step: Although we sometimes write an equation in a simple way such as

$$A + B \rightarrow X + Z$$

it is not always so simple. There may be many intermediates in the process. For example, a product C could be formed, and then converted to D, etc. Somewhere along such a series of steps there would be a slowest or rate-controlling step. In spite of the other series of reactions, as the name implies, this step would control or determine the rate of the overall reaction.

2. Activation Energy, Catalysts, Enzymes: Although a reaction is thermodynamically favorable, it will often require a certain activation energy.

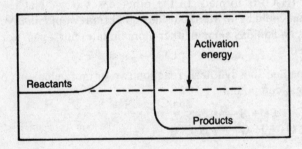

A catalyst or an enzyme (essentially a biological catalyst) may substantially increase the rate of a reaction by decreasing the activation energy that is required.

3. Equilibrium Constant: Consider a reversible reaction:

$$A + B \rightleftharpoons C + D$$

We may calculate an *equilibrium constant:*

$$K_{eq} = \frac{[C][D]}{[A][B]}$$

4. Le Chatelier's Principle: Le Chatelier's principle states that when a system is at equilibrium, it will shift to relieve any stress placed upon it. Thus, in the above example, addition of more C to the system would bring about the consumption of D and the production of more A and B (without changing the equilibrium constant).

General Principles

Characteristics of Mixtures and Compounds

Mixture	Compound
1. Physical union	Chemical union
2. No new substances are formed	New substances are formed
3. Can be separated by physical means	Can be separated by chemical means
4. Elements form no definite proportions	Elements form definite proportions

Reactions

1. Single Replacement Reaction: In a single replacement reaction a more active element reacts with a compound to replace a less active one. A new element and a new compound are the result.

Examples: $Fe + CuSO_4 \longrightarrow FeSO_4 + Cu$
$Zn + CuSO_4 \longrightarrow ZnSO_4 + Cu$

2. Double Replacement Reaction: Double replacement reactions involve a double exchange; compounds react chemically to form two new compounds.

Examples: $NaCl + AgNO_3 \longrightarrow NaNO_3 + AgCl$
$HCl + NaOH \longrightarrow NaCl + H_2O$

In the first example a precipitate ($AgCl$) is formed and in the second example a weakly ionized compound (H_2O) is formed. In the other cases (e.g., $NaCl + KNO_3$) a double replacement reaction could be written, but the equilibrium would involve all possible combinations of cations and anions since neither a precipitate, nor a gas, nor a weakly ionized compound is formed.

3. Synthesis Reaction: In a synthesis reaction two or more elements or compounds can unite to form a single compound.

Examples: $Fe + S \xrightarrow{\triangle} FeS$
$CO_2 + H_2O \longrightarrow H_2CO_3$

4. Decomposition Reaction: In a decomposition reaction a compound is broken down into simpler compounds or into its elements.

Examples $2KClO_3 \longrightarrow 2KCl + 3O_2$
$2HgO \longrightarrow 2Hg + O_2$

Role of Enzymes in a Reaction

Consider the following reaction:

$$A + B + C \xrightarrow{\text{E (enzyme)}} ABCE \longrightarrow D + F + E$$
$$1 \qquad\qquad 2 \qquad 3 \qquad 4 \quad 2$$

Substrate(s) or reactant(s) (1) react(s) with the enzyme (2) to form an enzyme-substrate complex (3). This complex breaks down into product(s) (4), and free enzyme (2) ready for the formation of a new enzyme-substrate complex is available again.

An enzyme speeds up the rate of the reaction but is not used up itself in the reaction.

Temperature Conversion Factors

On the Celsius scale (°C) the freezing point of water is 0°, and the boiling point is 100°. On the Fahrenheit scale (°F) they are respectively 32° and 212°.

The absolute Kelvin scale lists as absolute zero a temperature of −273°C, and therefore the Kelvin and Celsius scales differ only in the choice of point zero. Kelvin temperature is, therefore, 273 plus the Celsius temperature. Let us illustrate and work two examples:

1. 104°F is what temperature on the Kelvin scale? The answer is 313 K and is obtained in the following manner:

First we must convert Fahrenheit to Celsius by using the following formulas:

$$\text{Celsius equals } \frac{5}{9} \times (\text{Fahrenheit} - 32)$$

$$\text{Fahrenheit equals } \frac{9}{5} C + 32$$

$$\text{Celsius} = \frac{5}{9} \times (104 - 32)$$

$$C = \frac{5}{9} \times 72$$

$$C = 40°$$

Now we take 273°, add 40°, and obtain a Kelvin temperature of 313 K.

2. 45°C will equal how many degrees F?
We utilize the conversion factors:

$$F = \frac{9}{5} C + 32$$

or

$$C = \frac{5}{9} (F - 32)$$

$$F = \frac{9}{5} (45) + 32$$

$$F = 81 + 32$$

$$F = 113°$$

Formulas and Laws

1. **Specific Gravity:** Specific gravity is usually expressed as the weight of an object in air divided by the loss of weight when weighed in water.

Example: A ball of steel weighs 300 grams in air and 250 grams when submerged in water; its specific gravity is 6.

$$\text{Specific Gravity} = \frac{\text{Weight in Air}}{\text{Loss of Weight}}$$

$$\text{Specific Gravity} = \frac{300}{50} = 6$$

2. **Density:** Density is expressed as $\dfrac{M \text{ (mass)}}{V \text{ (volume)}}$

Example: A piece of iron 60 inches long, 12 inches wide and 2 inches high has a mass of 2000 lb. The density of this piece is 1.39 lb./in.^{3} and was obtained as follows:

$$D = \frac{M}{V} = \frac{2000 \text{ lb.}}{60 \text{ in.} \times 12 \text{ in.} \times 2 \text{ in.}}$$

$$D = \frac{2000 \text{ lb.}}{1440 \text{ in.}^3} = 1.39 \text{ lb./in.}^3$$

Organic Chemistry

It is not possible to present a course in organic chemistry in the limited space we have allotted. All we can hope to do is to help you review some of the high points.

General Considerations

1. **Definition:** Organic chemistry is the chemistry of compounds of carbon. Historically, it has been the study of chemical compounds from living or dead organisms. Until 1828, it was believed that these compounds could not be synthesized from "inorganic" compounds outside living organisms. This theory was first breached by Friedrich Wöhler in 1828; he was successful in synthesizing urea from the inorganic compound, ammonium cyanate.

2. **Bonds:** In general, the bonds in the stable organic compounds are covalent bonds, formed by the sharing of electrons between atoms. If the electrons are shared unequally between two atoms, the bond is said to be a polar bond (e.g., C—Br or C—O).

Such a polar bond is a dipole, and the molecule possesses a dipole moment. The dipole moment is calculated by multiplying the charge by the distance of separation. Thus methane (CH_4) has a dipole moment of zero. By comparison, CH_3Cl has a dipole moment of 1.87.

3. **Electronic Configuration of the Carbon Atom:** It is generally true that the orbital electrons in the outer unfilled shell are the most important in predicting the metal/non-metal character of the compound as well as the expected valence. The carbon atom has two electrons in the K shell and four in the L shell ($1s^2 2s^2 2p_x^1 2p_y^1$). It might be expected to lose four electrons to produce the electronic configuration of the noble element helium, or gain four electrons to produce the electronic configuration of the noble element neon. For the most part it shares electrons to complete the L shell. Thus it may be said to have a valence of 4 (see below).

4. **Bond Hybridization:** The orbital electrons of the carbon atom consist of two electrons in the $1s$ orbital, two electrons in the $2s$ orbital and one electron each in the $2p_x$ and $2p_y$ orbitals. (This may be written as $1s^2 2s^2 2p_x^1 2p_y^1$.) It exhibits a valence of 4. In simple compounds such as methane, four equivalent covalent bonds are formed. This may be considered to occur by raising one of the $2s$ orbital electrons to the $2p_z$ orbital and then forming four hybridized orbitals from the three $2p$ orbitals and the one remaining $2s$ orbital. These hybridized orbitals are sp^3 orbitals. The four covalent bonds in methane are the result of overlap of the one orbital electron of each of four hydrogen atoms with one sp^3 hybridized orbital electron of the carbon atom. These four bonds are called sigma bonds.

In a compound such as ethylene (ethene), however, there are pi as well as sigma bonds. Two of the three $2p$ orbital electrons are hybridized with the remaining $2s$ orbital electron. Thus there are three equivalent sp^2 hybridized orbital electrons for each carbon atom. These participate in the covalent sigma bond between the two carbon atoms and in the covalent sigma bonds between the carbon atom and the hydrogen atoms. The remaining $2p$ orbital electron in each carbon atom participates in the weaker second bond between the two carbon atoms (a pi bond).

Compounds such as acetylene (ethyne) have a triple bond, consisting of one sigma bond and two pi bonds. In each carbon atom participating in a triple bond, there is contribution of two hybridized *sp* orbital electrons to produce two pi bonds. The stronger sigma bond between the carbon atoms is produced by the contribution of one 2*p* electron from each carbon atom. In acetylene itself there is another sigma bond between the carbon atom and a hydrogen atom; this bond is produced by the overlap of a 2*p* orbital from the carbon atom and the sole electron from the hydrogen atom.

5. Stereochemistry: Chemical compounds with the same molecular formula but different structural formulas are termed *isomers*. Those having atoms joined in a different order are *structural isomers* (e.g., 2-propanol and 1-propanol). Those having their atoms joined in the same order are termed *stereoisomers*. Stereoisomers that are mirror images of each other are termed *enantiomers*. Stereoisomers that are not enantiomers are called *diastereomers*.

```
   H—C=O              H—C=O              H—C=O
     |                  |                  |
   H—C=OH             H—C—OH            HO—C—H
     |                  |                  |
  HO—C—H             HO—C—H             H—C—OH
     |                  |                  |
   H—C—OH             HO—C—H             H—C—OH
     |                  |                  |
   H—C—OH             H—C—OH            HO—C—H
     |                  |                  |
   CH₂OH              CH₂OH              CH₂OH

  D-glucose          D-galactose         L-galactose
```

D-Glucose and D-galactose are diastereomers. D-galactose and L-galactose are enantiomers.

To possess optical activity a compound must have a chiral center. A *chiral center* is a carbon atom that is attached to four different substituents. A compound possessing a chiral center may still not possess optical activity if there is a plane of symmetry in the molecule.

Light ordinarily oscillates in all planes. If it is passed through a polarizer, its oscillation is reduced to only one plane. If this plane-polarized light is allowed to pass through a solution of an optically active compound, the plane of the light will be rotated. If it is rotated to the right, the rotation is termed dextrorotatory or (+). If it is rotated to the left, the rotation is termed levorotatory or (−). The specific rotation [α] is characteristic of an optically active compound:

$$[\alpha] = \frac{\alpha}{(c)(l)}$$

where α = observed degrees of rotation

c = concentration, grams per milliliter

l = length of light path, decimeters

For comparison in the literature, the D line of sodium as the incident light and a temperature of 25°C have been agreed upon as standard.

A mixture of equal amounts of two enantiomers (called a *racemic* mixture) will have a rotation of zero. The rotations are opposite in sign and equal in numerical value, canceling each other.

The Alkanes

Alkanes are saturated noncyclic compounds of carbon and hydrogen. If carbon atoms are arranged in a straight chain sequence

$$C—C—C—C$$

and hydrogen atoms are added to account for each carbon atom's valence of four, we produce a compound like this:

$$
\begin{array}{cccc}
H & H & H & H \\
| & | & | & | \\
HC\!-\!\!&\!\!C\!-\!\!&\!\!C\!-\!\!&\!\!CH \\
| & | & | & | \\
H & H & H & H
\end{array}
$$

This compound is *n*-butane. The *n* designates the straight chain character. Another compound with the same numbers of carbon and hydrogen atoms is isobutane (or 2-methyl-propane).

$$
\begin{array}{ccc}
H_3C\!-\!\!&\!\!CH\!-\!\!&\!\!CH_3 \\
 & | & \\
 & CH_3 &
\end{array}
$$

It is useful to learn the names of many of the alkanes. With modification these names are an integral part of the names of the derivatives of alkanes.

Chain Length	Name	Chain Length	Name
1	Methane	11	Undecane
2	Ethane	12	Dodecane
3	Propane	13	Tridecane
4	Butane	14	Tetradecane
5	Pentane	15	Pentadecane
6	Hexane	16	Hexadecane
7	Heptane	17	Heptadecane
8	Octane	18	Octadecane
9	Nonane	19	Nonadecane
10	Decane	20	Eicosane

The IUPAC rules for nomenclature require that a compound that is not a straight chain be named on the basis of its longest chain. Thus, the following compound is 2-methyl-4-ethylheptane:

$$
\begin{array}{ccccccc}
H_3C\!-\!\!CH\!-\!\!CH_2\!-\!\!CH\!-\!\!CH_2\!-\!\!CH_2\!-\!\!CH_3 \\
\quad\quad | \quad\quad\quad\quad | \\
\quad\quad CH_3 \quad\quad\quad CH_2 \\
\quad\quad\quad\quad\quad\quad\quad | \\
\quad\quad\quad\quad\quad\quad\quad CH_3
\end{array}
$$

1. Synthesis — Wurtz Reaction:

$$2RBr + 2Na \longrightarrow RR + 2NaBr$$

(R will often be used to refer to an unspecified alkyl group.) More specifically:

$$2CH_3Br + 2Na \longrightarrow CH_3 - CH_3 + 2NaBr$$

If a mixture of two alkyl bromides is used, a mixture of three possible products is expected.

2. Reactions:
The alkanes are not very reactive, but they will undergo some reactions.

a. *Halogenation*

$$
Cl_2 +
\begin{array}{cc}
H & H \\
| & | \\
HC\!-\!\!&\!\!CH \\
| & | \\
H & H
\end{array}
\xrightarrow[\substack{u.v. \\ light}]{heat}
\begin{array}{cc}
H & H \\
| & | \\
HC\!-\!\!&\!\!C\!-\!Cl \\
| & | \\
H & H
\end{array}
+ HCl
$$

Reaction may continue and produce a more highly chlorinated product.

b. *Oxidation*

Alkanes may be oxidized to produce CO_2, water and energy.

The Cycloalkanes

The small ring cycloalkanes (cyclopropane and cyclobutane) are strained and are more reactive. Cyclopropane is planar, and the bond angles must be 60°. The normal bond angle is 109° 28'. Five- and six-membered rings are not appreciably strained. Larger rings were once thought to be unstable because of the strain (Baeyer), but puckering allows relative freedom from strain.

Example:

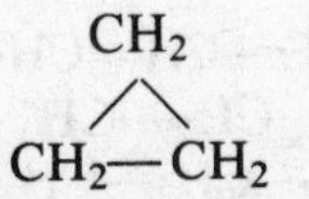

$$CH_2$$
$$\triangle$$
$$CH_2\text{—}CH_2 \qquad \text{cyclopropane}$$

The Alkenes

The alkenes may be considered as alkanes from which hydrogen has been removed, producing a carbon-to-carbon double bond. The simplest example of this series is ethene (ethylene).

$$H_2C{=}CH_2 \qquad \text{ethene}$$

$$H_2C{=}CH\text{—}CH_2\text{—}CH_3 \qquad \text{1-butene}$$

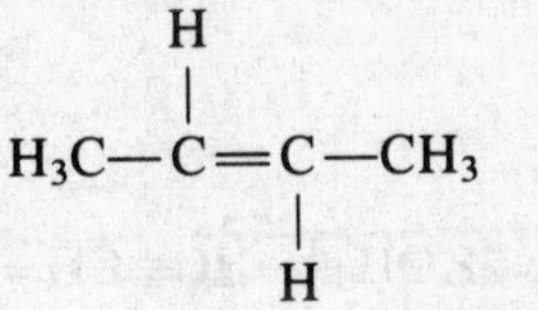

$$H_3C\text{—}\underset{\underset{H}{|}}{\overset{\overset{H}{|}}{C}}{=}C\text{—}CH_3 \qquad \textit{trans}\text{-2-butene}$$

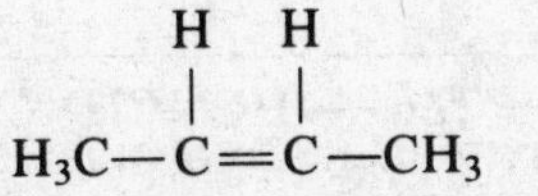

$$H_3C\text{—}\overset{\overset{H}{|}}{C}{=}\overset{\overset{H}{|}}{C}\text{—}CH_3 \qquad \textit{cis}\text{-2-butene}$$

1. Synthesis:

a. *Dehydrohalogenation*

$$H_3C\text{—}CH_2Br + \text{alcoholic KOH} \longrightarrow H_2C{=}CH_2 + H_2O + KBr$$

b. *Dehydration*

$$H_3C\text{—}CH_2OH \xrightarrow[H_2SO_4]{heat} H_2C{=}CH_2 + H_2O$$

c. *Dehalogenation*

$$Br\text{—}CH_2\text{—}CH_2\text{—}Br + Zn \longrightarrow H_2C{=}CH_2 + ZnBr_2$$

d. *Cracking* (relatively nonspecific denomposition reactions)

$$H_3C\text{—}(CH_2)_4\text{—}CH_3 \xrightarrow{\substack{heat \\ cracking}} H_2C{=}CH_2 + H_3C\text{—}CH_2CH_2\text{—}CH_3$$

2. Reactions:

a. *Addition of HX to the double bond*

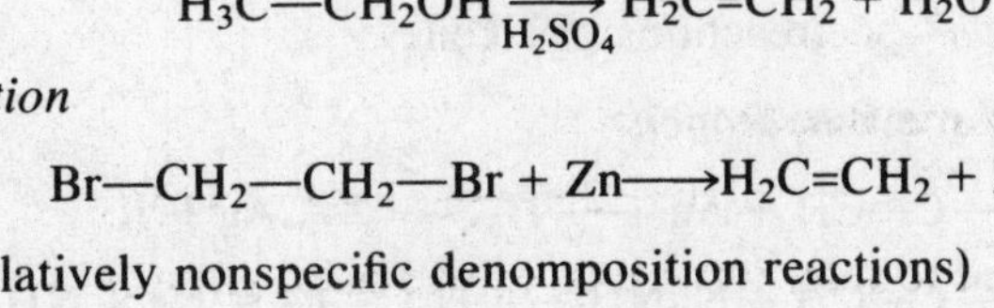

$$H_3C\text{—}CH{=}CH_2 + HBr \longrightarrow H_3C\text{—}\underset{\underset{Br}{|}}{\overset{\overset{H}{|}}{C}}\text{—}CH_3$$

The Markownikoff Rule says that in the addition of an acid across a double bond, the double-bonded carbon having the most hydrogen will receive the H of HX. The above is true for ionic addition, but in the presence of peroxides we see a free radical anti-Markownikoff addition:

$$H_3C—CH=CH_2 + HBr \xrightarrow{\text{peroxide}} H_3C—CH_2—CH_2Br$$

b. *Hydrogenation* (catalyst such as Pt, Pd, or Ni)

$$H_2C=CH_2 + H_2 \xrightarrow{\text{Pt}} H_3C—CH_3$$

$$3H_2C=CH—CH=CH_2 + 4H_2 \xrightarrow{\text{Pt}} H_3C—CH=CH—CH_3$$
$$+ H_2C=CH—CH_2—CH_3$$
$$+ H_3C—CH_2—CH_2—CH_3$$

c. $H_2C=CH_2 + Br_2 \longrightarrow BrCH_2—CH_2Br$

d. $H_2C=CH_2 \xrightarrow{\text{catalyst}} $ polymer (polyethylene in this case)

The Alkynes (derivatives of acetylene)

$HC\equiv CH$ acetylene or ethyne

1. Synthesis:
   a. $CaC_2 + H_2O \longrightarrow C_2H_2 + CaO$

   b. *Dehydrohalogenation*

   $$H_3C—CHBr_2 + \text{alcoholic } 2KOH \longrightarrow HC\equiv CH + 2H_2O + 2KBr$$

   c. *Dehalogenation*

   $$HCBr_2—CBr_2H + 2Zn \longrightarrow HC\equiv CH + 2ZnBr_2$$

2. Reactions:
   a. *Hydrogenation*

   $$HC\equiv CH + H_2 \xrightarrow{\text{Pt}} H_2C=CH_2 + H_2 \xrightarrow{\text{Pt}} CH_3—CH_3$$

   b. *Hydrohalogenation*—see reactions of alkenes

   c. *Halogenation*—see reactions of alkenes

   d. *Reaction of active hydrogen*

   $$H_3C—C\equiv CH + Ag^+ \longrightarrow H_3C—C\equiv CAg + H^+$$

   $$H_3C—C\equiv CH + NaNH_2 \longrightarrow H_3C—C\equiv CNa + NH_3$$

   $$H_3C—C\equiv CNa + CH_3Br \longrightarrow H_3C—C\equiv C—CH_3 + NaBr$$

Aromatic Compounds

Aromatic compounds consist of benzene and compounds whose chemical reactions are similar to those of benzene. Almost all aromatic compounds that you would be expected to recognize as such are derivatives of benzene; there are other unrelated aromatic compounds.

1. Nature of Benzene—Resonance: Although we may draw benzene as having three discrete double bonds and three discrete single bonds in conjugation, this does not adequately describe its structure. It may be shown as two structures in resonance:

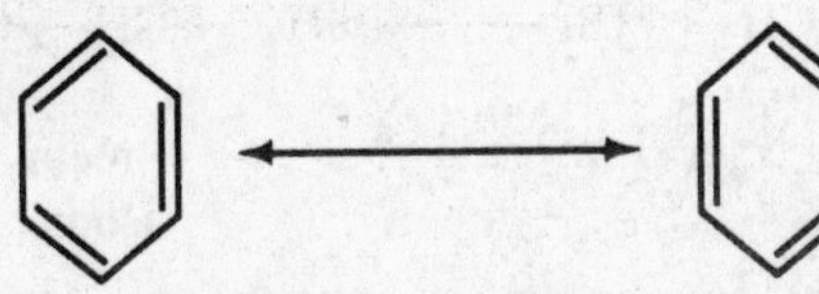

In reality, however, it appears that each carbon atom has three discrete covalent bonds, and the fourth bonding electron of each carbon atom is delocalized in electron clouds around the ring.

2. Synthesis of the Aromatic Ring: This is unusual; in general one will only be interested in reactions of compounds containing the benzene ring rather than in the synthesis of the aromatic ring.

3. Reactions: (ϕ is sometimes used as a shorthand designation for the phenyl group. Thus, benzene could be indicated as ϕ-H.)

a. *Monosubstitution*

$$\phi\text{-H} + HNO_3 \longrightarrow \phi—NO_2 + H_2O$$
$$\phi\text{-H} + H_2SO_4 \longrightarrow \phi—SO_3H + H_2O$$
$$\phi\text{-H} + Br_2 \xrightarrow{Fe} \phi—Br + HBr$$

b. *Friedel-Crafts reaction*

$$\phi\text{-H} + RCl \xrightarrow{AlCl_3} \phi—R + HCl$$

$$\phi\text{-H} + R—\overset{\overset{O}{\|}}{C}—Cl \xrightarrow{AlCl} \phi—\overset{\overset{O}{\|}}{C}—R + HCl$$

c. *Substitution in a benzene ring that already has one substituent*

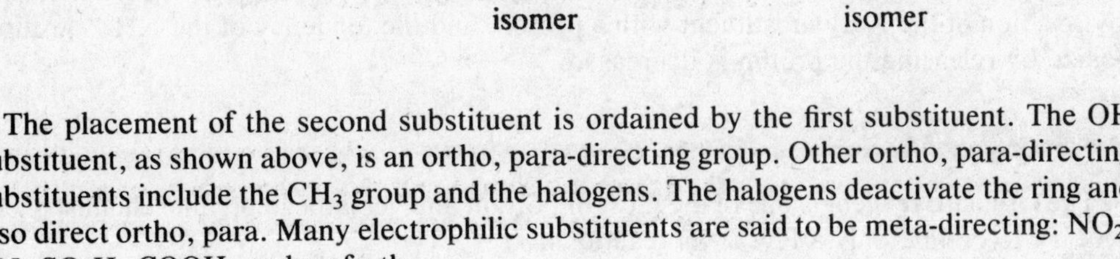

ortho isomer   para isomer

The placement of the second substituent is ordained by the first substituent. The OH substituent, as shown above, is an ortho, para-directing group. Other ortho, para-directing substituents include the CH_3 group and the halogens. The halogens deactivate the ring and also direct ortho, para. Many electrophilic substituents are said to be meta-directing: NO_2, CN, SO_3H, $COOH$, and so forth.

meta
isomer

The above meta-directing substituents also deactivate the ring.

Note that the reactions above *do* balance. In many cases below, we will write organic reactions that do not balance. This is done for the sake of simplicity and to emphasize the desired products.

d. *Diazotization of amines*

$$\phi-NH_2 + HNO_2 \longrightarrow \phi-N_2{}^+$$

e. *Reactions of diazonium salts* (see above)

$$\phi-N_2{}^+ + CuBr \longrightarrow \phi-Br$$
$$\phi-N_2{}^+ + CuCN \longrightarrow \phi-CN$$
$$\phi-N_2{}^+ + H_2O \xrightarrow{H^+} \phi-OH$$
$$\phi-N_2{}^+ + \phi-OH \longrightarrow \phi-N=N-\phi-OH \text{ (Coupling)}$$

$$\phi-N_2{}^+ + H_2 \xrightarrow{Pt} \phi\overset{\overset{\displaystyle H}{|}}{N}-NH_2$$

4. Acidity and Basicity:

A. *Acidity*. Phenol will ionize as an acid with a K_a of about 1×10^{-10}. A methyl substituent in the ortho position will lower the K_a (and the acidity) to about 6×10^{-11}. The electron-releasing methyl substituent contributes electrons to the ring and depresses release of H^+. A nitro substituent in the ortho position, conversely, increases the acidity (K_a about 7×10^{-8}) by withdrawing electrons from the ring.

b. *Basicity*. Aniline (aminobenzene or phenylamine) has a K_a of about 4×10^{-10}. The introduction of an electron-releasing methyl group in the para position (i.e., *p*-methylaniline) increases basicity (K_b about 1×10^{-9}). The introduction of the electron-withdrawing nitro group into the para position (i.e., *p*-nitroaniline) decreases basicity (K_b about 1×10^{-13}). The methyl substituent releases electrons into the ring, and the nitro substituent withdraws electrons from the ring. An electron-rich ring coincides with an electron-rich N in the NH_2 substituent. This will add stability to the $NH_3{}^+$ substituent which is formed by reaction of the NH_2 substituent with a proton, and the tendency of the $NH_3{}^+$ group to ionize by releasing the proton is decreased.

The Grignard Reagent

The Grignard reagent is one of the most important and versatile in organic chemistry. We will try to outline only a few of its reactions.

1. Synthesis: The Grignard reagent is synthesized by the reaction of an alkyl halide with elemental magnesium in the presence of anhydrous ether.

Example:

$$H_3C—CH_2Br + Mg \xrightarrow[\text{ether}]{\text{anhydrous}} H_3C—CH_2MgBr$$

or
$$RBr + Mg \xrightarrow[\text{ether}]{\text{anhydrous}} RMgBr$$

2. Reactions:

a. *Reaction with active hydrogen*. A Grignard reagent will react with any compound having active hydrogen (e.g., H_2O, an alcohol, an acid, or a 1-alkyne) to form a hydrocarbon.

$$RMgBr + H_2O \longrightarrow RH + MgBrOH$$

b. *Reaction with aldehydes and ketones*

$$RMgBr + HCHO \xrightarrow[\text{ether}]{\text{anhydrous}} R—CH_2OMgBr \xrightarrow{H^+} RCH_2OH \text{ (primary alcohol)}$$

$$RMgBr + R'CHO \xrightarrow[\text{ether}]{\text{anhydrous}} \underset{\underset{H}{|}}{RC}—OMgBr \xrightarrow{H^+} \underset{\underset{H}{|}}{\overset{\overset{R'}{|}}{RC}}—OH \text{ (secondary alcohol)}$$

$$RMgBr + R'—\underset{\underset{R''}{|}}{C}{=}O \xrightarrow[\text{ether}]{\text{anhydrous}} R'—\underset{\underset{R}{|}}{\overset{\overset{R''}{|}}{C}}—OMgBr \xrightarrow{H^+}$$

$$R'—\underset{\underset{R}{|}}{\overset{\overset{R''}{|}}{C}}—OH \text{ (tertiary alcohol)}$$

c. *Reaction with CO_2*

$$RMgBr + CO_2 \xrightarrow[\text{ether}]{\text{anhydrous}} R—\overset{\overset{O}{\|}}{C}—OMgBr \xrightarrow{H^+} RCOOH$$

d. *Reaction with an ester or an acyl halide*

$$RMgBr + R'COOR'' \xrightarrow[\text{ether}]{\text{anhydrous}} R'—\overset{\overset{O}{\|}}{C}—R$$

$$RMgBr + R'COBr \xrightarrow[\text{ether}]{\text{anhydrous}} R'—\overset{\overset{O}{\|}}{C}—R$$

Alcohols

Alcohols may be designated as ROH. The simplest alcohol is CH_3OH and is named methanol (i.e., methan-ol) as a derivative of the one-carbon hydrocarbon, methane. Other alcohols are similarly named as derivatives of hydrocarbons. The compound below is named 2-pentanol or 2-hydroxypentane.

$$H_3C—CH_2—CH_2—CH—CH_3$$
$$|$$
$$OH$$

The alcohols are very weak acids, even weaker than water. Polarity and hydrogen bonding cause short chain alcohols to be soluble in water.

1. **Synthesis:**
    a. *Hydration of alkenes*

$$H_2C{=}CH_2 + H_2O \overset{H^+}{\rightleftharpoons} H_3C—CH_2OH$$

    b. *Using Grignard reagents–discussed elsewhere*
    c. *Hydrolysis of alkyl halides*

$$R—I + H_2O \overset{KOH}{\rightleftharpoons} ROH + I^-$$

    d. *Reduction of aldehydes and ketones*

$$R—CHO + NaBH_4 \overset{H_2O}{\longrightarrow} R—CH_2OH$$

2. **Reactions:**

    a. *Oxidation to form aldehydes or ketones*

$$R—CH_2OH + K_2Cr_2O_7 \overset{H^+}{\longrightarrow} R—CHO$$

This is useful only if the aldehyde may be removed (sometimes by distillation) before further oxidation to the carboxylic acid. A ketone may not be easily oxidized further, but chain rupture is possible.

    b. *Dehydration to form alkenes–discussed elsewhere*
    c. *Formation of esters*

$$R—COOH + R—CH_2OH \overset{H^+}{\rightleftharpoons} R—COOCH_2—R$$

    d. *Conversion to halides*

$$ROH + HI \rightleftharpoons RI + H_2O$$

Amines

Amines have the structure $R—NH_2$. The simplest example is methylamine (or amino-methane):

$$H_3CNH_2$$

1. **Synthesis:**
    a. $RX + NH_3 \longrightarrow R—NH_2$
    b. $RCN + LiAlH_4 \longrightarrow R—CH_2—NH_2$
    c. *Hofmann degradation*

$$R—CONH_2 \overset{Br_2, NaOH}{\longrightarrow} RNH_2$$

2. Reactions:

$$R-NH_2 + HONO \xrightarrow{\quad H_2O \quad} ROH + N_2$$

a. (This is the reaction for a primary alkyl amine)

b. $\quad R-NH_2 + HONO \longrightarrow RN_2^+$

(This is the reaction for a primary aromatic amine. The diazonium salt is stable at the temperatures of ice water. It is capable of numerous further reactions under appropriate conditions.)

c. $\quad R-NH_2 + R'-COOH + \text{dicyclohexylcarbodiimide} \longrightarrow R-NH-COR'$

$$\text{(an amide)}$$

Amides

Amides have the structure R—NH—COR.
A simple example is acetanilide, ϕ—NH—CO—CH$_3$.

1. Synthesis:

a. $\quad R-NH_2 + R'-COCl \text{ (an acyl chloride)} \longrightarrow R-NH-\overset{\displaystyle O}{\overset{\|}{C}}-R'$

b. $\quad R-NH_2 + (R'-CO)_2O \text{ (an anhydride)} \longrightarrow R-NH-\overset{\displaystyle O}{\overset{\|}{C}}-R'$

c. $\quad R-NH_2 + R'-COOH + \text{dicyclohexylcarbodiimide} \longrightarrow R-NH-\overset{\displaystyle O}{\overset{\|}{C}}-R'$

(Primary amines are shown, but secondary amines may also be used.)

2. Reaction:

$$R-NH-COR' + H_2O \xrightarrow{\quad H^+ \quad} R-NH_3^+ + R'-COOH$$

(The reaction may also be accomplished in an aqueous base.)

Aldehydes and Ketones

1. Synthesis

a. *Reaction of a Grignard reagent with a carboxylic ester or an acyl halide to form a ketone* (outlined above under "Grignard Reagent"—Section 2;d)

b. *Mild oxidation of an alcohol* (often feasible in the synthesis of ketones and sometimes in the synthesis of aldehydes)

$$RCH_2OH \xrightarrow{\quad Cu, \triangle \quad} R-CHO \text{ (aldehyde)}$$

$$R-\overset{\displaystyle R'}{\underset{\displaystyle H}{\overset{\displaystyle |}{\underset{\displaystyle |}{C}}}}OH \xrightarrow{\quad Cu, \triangle \quad} R-\overset{\displaystyle R'}{\overset{\displaystyle |}{C}}=O \text{ (ketone)}$$

c. *Friedel-Crafts acylation to produce aromatic ketones* (see "Aromatic Compounds"—Section 3;b)

d. *Decarboxylation of acids to produce ketones*

$$2RCOOH \xrightarrow{\quad ThO_2, \triangle \quad} R-\overset{\displaystyle O}{\overset{\|}{C}}-R + CO_2$$

e. *Oxidation of diols to form aldehydes*

$$\underset{\substack{| \quad\; | \\ \text{OH}\;\;\text{OH}}}{R-CH-CH-R'} \xrightarrow{\text{HIO}_4 \text{ or Pb(OAc)}_4} R-CHO + R'-CHO$$

$$\underset{\substack{| \quad\; | \quad\; | \\ \text{OH}\;\text{OH}\;\text{OH}}}{R-CH-CH-CH-R'} \xrightarrow{\text{HIO}_4 \text{ or Pb(OAc)}_4} \begin{array}{l} R-CHO + R'-CHO \\ \quad + \text{HCOOH} \end{array}$$

$$\underset{\substack{| \qquad\qquad | \\ \text{OH}\qquad\quad\text{OH}}}{R-CH-CH_2-CH-R'} \xrightarrow{\text{HIO}_4 \text{ or Pb(OAc)}_4} \text{No reaction}$$

2. **Reactions:**

   a. *Reaction with Grignard reagents*

$$\underset{\substack{\| \\ \text{O}}}{R-C-R'} + R''MgBr \xrightarrow[\text{ether}]{\text{anhydrous}} \underset{\substack{| \\ R''}}{\overset{\overset{\text{OMgBr}}{|}}{R-C-R'}} \xrightarrow{\text{H}_2\text{O}} \underset{\substack{| \\ R''}}{\overset{\overset{\text{OH}}{|}}{R-C-R'}}$$

$$R-CHO + R'MgBr \xrightarrow[\text{ether}]{\text{anhydrous}} \underset{}{\overset{\overset{\text{OMgBr}}{|}}{R-CH-R'}} \xrightarrow{\text{H}_2\text{O}} \underset{}{\overset{\overset{\text{OH}}{|}}{R-CH-R'}}$$

$$HCHO + RMgBr \xrightarrow[\text{ether}]{\text{anhydrous}} R-CH_2-OMgBr \xrightarrow{\text{H}_2\text{O}} R-CH_2OH$$

   b. *Reaction of aldehydes or ketones with HCN*

$$R-CHO + HCN \longrightarrow \underset{\substack{| \\ H}}{\overset{\overset{\text{OH}}{|}}{R-C-CN}} \xrightarrow{\text{H}_2\text{O, H}^+} \underset{\substack{| \\ H}}{\overset{\overset{\text{OH}}{|}}{R-C-COOH}}$$

   c. *Reaction of aldehydes or methyl ketones with NaHSO₃*

$$R-CHO + NaHSO_3 \longrightarrow \underset{\substack{| \\ H}}{\overset{\overset{\text{OH}}{|}}{R-C-SO_3^-Na^+}}$$

   d. *Reaction with alcohols*

$$R-CHO + R'-OH \xrightarrow{\text{H}^+} \underset{\substack{| \\ H}}{\overset{\overset{\text{OH}}{|}}{R-C-OR'}} \xrightarrow{\text{R'OH, H}^+} \underset{\substack{| \\ H}}{\overset{\overset{\text{OR'}}{|}}{R-C-OR'}}$$

   (a hemiacetal)   (an acetal)

$$\underset{\substack{\| \\ \text{O}}}{R-C-R'} + R''OH \xrightarrow{\text{H}^+} \underset{\substack{| \\ \text{OR}''}}{\overset{\overset{\text{OH}}{|}}{R-C-R'}} \xrightarrow{\text{R''OH, H}^+} \underset{\substack{| \\ \text{OR}''}}{\overset{\overset{\text{OR}''}{|}}{R-C-R'}}$$

   (a hemiketal)   (a ketal)

e. *Reaction of ketones and aldehydes with hydroxylamine*

$$R-CHO + NH_2OH \xrightarrow{H^+} R-\overset{\overset{\displaystyle H}{|}}{C}=NOH$$

(an oxime)

f. *Reaction of ketones and aldehydes with hydrazine or hydrazine derivatives*

$$R-CHO + NH_2NH_2 \xrightarrow{H^+} R-\overset{\overset{\displaystyle H}{|}}{C}=N-NH_2$$

(a hydrazone)

g. *Oxidation of aldehydes*

$$R-CHO + Ag(NH_3)_2^+ \xrightarrow{OH^-} R-\overset{\overset{\displaystyle O}{\|}}{C}-O^- + Ag$$

(Tollens' reagent)   (silver mirror)

$$R-CHO + Cu^{++} \xrightarrow{OH^-,\ citrate} R-\overset{\overset{\displaystyle O}{\|}}{C}-O^- + Cu_2O$$

(Benedict's reagent)   (red ppt.)

h. *Haloform reaction with acetaldehyde or methyl ketones*

$$R-\overset{\overset{\displaystyle O}{\|}}{C}-CH_3 \xrightarrow{IO^-} RCO^- + CHI_3$$

i. *Aldol condensation* (requires alpha-hydrogen). Further reaction can also lead to polymers.

$$2CH_3-CHO \xrightarrow{OH^-} H_3C-\overset{\overset{\displaystyle OH}{|}}{\underset{\underset{\displaystyle H}{|}}{C}}-CH_2-CHO$$

j. *Cannizzaro reaction* (for aldehydes having no alpha-hydrogen)

$$2\ \phi-CHO \xrightarrow{OH^-} \phi-CH_2OH + \phi-\overset{\overset{\displaystyle O}{\|}}{C}-O^-$$

Carboxylic Acids

The carboxylic acids are organic compounds that ionize to produce free protons and

carboxylate anions. The simplest example is formic acid, $H-\overset{\overset{\displaystyle O}{\|}}{C}-OH$

1. Synthesis:

a. *Addition of carbon dioxide to a Grignard reagent*

$$R\ MgBr + CO_2 \rightarrow R-\overset{\overset{\displaystyle O}{\|}}{C}-OMgBr \xrightarrow{H^+} R-\overset{\overset{\displaystyle O}{\|}}{C}-OH$$

b. *Oxidation of alkene*

$$R-C=C-R' + KMnO_4 \rightarrow \underset{\substack{| \quad |\\ OH \quad OH}}{R-\underset{H}{\overset{H}{C}}-\underset{H}{\overset{H}{C}}-R'}$$

$$\underset{\substack{| \quad |\\ OH \quad OH}}{R-\underset{H}{\overset{H}{C}}-\underset{H}{\overset{H}{C}}-R'} + KMnO_4 \rightarrow RCOOH + R'COOH$$

c. *Oxidation of primary alcohol*

$$R-CH_2OH + KMnO_4 \rightarrow RCOOH$$

d. *Hydrolysis of nitrile*

$$RCN \xrightarrow{\text{H}_2\text{O, H}^+} RCOOH$$

e. *Hydrolysis of esters*

$$\overset{\overset{\textstyle O}{\|}}{R-C}-O-R' + H_2O \underset{}{\overset{\text{H}^+}{\rightleftharpoons}} R-COOH + R'OH$$

f. *Saponification of esters*

$$\overset{\overset{\textstyle O}{\|}}{R-C}-O-R' + NaOH \rightleftharpoons R'OH + \overset{\overset{\textstyle O}{\|}}{R-C}-ONa \xrightarrow{\text{H}^+} R-COOH$$

2. Reactions:

a. *Neutralization of base*

$$RCOOH + NaOH \rightarrow \overset{\overset{\textstyle O}{\|}}{RC}-O^- + Na^+ + H_2O$$

b. *Esterification*

$$RCOOH + R'OH \underset{}{\overset{\text{H}^+}{\rightleftharpoons}} \overset{\overset{\textstyle O}{\|}}{R-C}-OR' + H_2O$$

c. *Formation of acylhalide*

$$RCOOH \xrightarrow{\text{PBr}_3} \overset{\overset{\textstyle O}{\|}}{RC}-Br$$

d. *Formation of anhydride*

$$2RCOOH \longrightarrow \overset{\overset{\textstyle O \qquad\quad O}{\| \qquad\quad \|}}{R-C}-O-\overset{}{C}-R + H_2O$$

e. *High-temperature decomposition*

$$2RCOOH \xrightarrow{\text{ThO}_2,\ \Delta} \overset{\overset{\textstyle O}{\|}}{R-C}-R + CO_2 + H_2O$$

Esters

Esters may be formed from the reaction between an acid and an alcohol. Upon hydrolysis the products are an acid and an alcohol. We often think first of carboxylic acid esters, but they are not the only ones known. Phosphate esters are common in biochemistry.

The simplest carboxylic acid ester is methyl formate,

$$H-\overset{\overset{\displaystyle O}{\|}}{C}-O-CH_3$$

1. Synthesis:

a. $R-COCl + R'-OH \rightarrow R-\overset{\overset{\displaystyle O}{\|}}{C}-OR'$

b. $(R-\overset{\overset{\displaystyle O}{\|}}{C})_2O + R'-OH \rightarrow R-\overset{\overset{\displaystyle O}{\|}}{C}-OR'$

c. $R-COOH + R'-OH \overset{H^+}{\rightleftharpoons} R-\overset{\overset{\displaystyle O}{\|}}{C}-OR' + H_2O$

An equilibrium will be established. Removal of water by an appropriate method such as azeotropic separation will produce good yields. High yields based on one reactant can also be achieved by adding large quantities of the other reactant.

2. Reactions:

a. *Acid hydrolysis*

$$R-COOR' + H_2O \overset{H^+}{\longrightarrow} R-COOH + R'OH$$

b. *Saponification*

$$R-COOR' + H_2O \overset{OH^-}{\longrightarrow} R-COO^- + R'OH$$

Ethers

1. Synthesis:

a. *Dehydration. (Remember that the choice of conditions determines whether the ether or the unsaturated hydrocarbon, in this case ethylene, is the major product.)*

$$2CH_3-CH_2OH \overset{H_2SO_4,\Delta}{\longrightarrow} CH_3-CH_2-O-CH_2CH_3$$

b. *Williamson synthesis*. Much more useful than the dehydration method if an unsymmetrical ether is desired.

$$RONa + R'Br \longrightarrow ROR'$$

2. Reactions: Ethers are generally unreactive compounds. They are often useful as solvents in organic reactions because of their unreactive nature. They may be cleaved by heated halogen acids:

$$ROR + HI \overset{heat}{\longrightarrow} RI + ROH$$

The ROH which is formed may react with HI to form an additional RI.

Final Remarks

As stated earlier, you cannot learn organic chemistry from a brief presentation such as this. We recognize that we have been able to present only some of the more important points. It is our intent that you use this material (and the questions and answers in the practice tests) to review the organic chemistry you have learned in your coursework. If you find areas of weakness in your preparation, we would recommend that you study those areas in your organic chemistry textbook.

Biochemistry

Biochemistry or biological chemistry may be seen as an attempt to better understand life by studying the chemicals that are important in living cells and organisms. One must consider the amounts and identities of a variety of chemicals, as well as the ways in which they are transformed during different life processes. Perhaps it should not be surprising that biochemistry calls upon the background of other areas of chemistry, including organic chemistry, analytical chemistry, inorganic chemistry, and physical chemistry.

In these few pages we can only touch lightly on a few concepts in biochemistry. Those of you who continue in the life sciences, such as medicine, dentistry, or pharmacy, will be taught a great deal more about this fascinating area. Here we can only begin to delineate the forest, leaving you to study the trees at a later time. For those who have had little or no exposure to biochemistry, this brief introduction will help to prepare you for the Medical College Admission Test and will also lay the groundwork for your course in professional school. For those who have already taken a course in biochemistry, this material will assist in consolidating the information you already possess.

Areas of Biochemistry

Although there are a number of ways of subdividing biochemistry, there are substantial similarities among them. The subdivision is done according to similarities in the properties of the compounds within each subdivision. A biochemist usually specializes in the study of one of these subdivisions:

I. pH and Buffers
II. Amino Acids, Peptides, and Proteins
    A. Amino Acids
    B. Peptides and Proteins
III. Enzymes
    A. Nomenclature
    B. Cofactors
    C. Energy
    D. Velocity and Inhibition
IV. Carbohydrates
    A. Chemistry
    B. Functions
    C. Metabolism
        1. Glycolysis
        2. Krebs Cycle
        3. Hexose Monophosphate Shunt
V. Lipids
    A. Chemistry
    B. Metabolism
        1. Hydrolysis to Produce Fatty Acids
        2. Oxidation of Fatty Acids in the Mitochondria
        3. Synthesis of Fatty Acids
        4. Synthesis of Glycerides
VI. Nucleotides and Nucleic Acids; Biosynthesis of Nucleic Acids and Proteins
    A. Nucleotides
    B. Nucleic Acids
    C. Biosynthesis of Nucleic Acids and Proteins

pH and Buffers

The concepts of pH and buffers presented on page 109 under acids and bases are used also in biochemistry. The biochemist applies these principles in the context of the human body.

The human body (and other animal bodies) requires that the pH be maintained over a rather small range. The pH of human blood is ordinarily maintained from 7.36 to 7.42. Buffers prevent greater fluctuation, which could occur in response to loss or gain of acid or base.

The buffer pairs used in human blood include HCO_3^-/H_2CO_3; base/acid species of oxygenated hemoglobin; and base/acid species of deoxygenated hemoglobin. The phosphate pair $HPO_4^{2-}/H_2PO_4^-$ would offer a possible buffer, but little is present in the blood.

Amino Acids, Peptides, and Proteins

Amino Acids: The naturally occurring amino acids are primarily α-amino acids of the general structure

$$R-\underset{\underset{H}{|}}{\overset{\overset{NH_2}{|}}{C}}-COOH$$

If R does not represent H, then it will be noted that an asymmetric center exists, allowing for L and D isomers. The ones commonly found in nature, especially in higher animals, are usually of the L series. (The amino acid having no asymmetric center, and thus devoid of optical activity, is glycine.)

Although approximately 300 amino acids are found in nature, some are relatively rare. About 20 amino acids occur in all organisms. Amino acids can serve as biological active compounds in their own right (e.g., neurotransmitters), but we tend to think of them most often as the monomers of which the polymeric peptides and higher molecular weight proteins are composed.

Subdivisions of Amino Acids. It is possible to subdivide the amino acids based on their R groups. This is useful in predicting such things as the folding of a protein in a lipoprotein membrane; it is also helpful in remembering the different amino acids. Thus, they may be subdivided into aliphatic, hydroxy, sulfur, aromatic, dicarboxy (or dicarboxy with one carboxyl as an amide), diamino, and imino on the basis of the R groups.

They may also be subdivided into acidic, basic, and neutral. Those having a second amino function are basic (two basic functional groups and only one carboxyl). Those having a second proton-releasing functional group are acidic. (This second group could be a carboxyl. It could also be the more weakly ionized phenolic or sulfhydryl group.) The neutral amino acids contain only a single acidic and a single basic group, thus canceling each other.

Essential Amino Acids. Although many amino acids may be synthesized in the animal body, certain animals are unable to synthesize sufficient quantities of particular amino acids, called *essential amino acids.* (The term indicates no judgment of the importance of these amino acids compared to that of the other amino acids. It simply indicates that for optimal health these amino acids must be supplied in the diet.) In humans, ten amino acids are usually called essential: phenylalanine, valine, tryptophan, threonine, isoleucine, methionine, histidine, arginine, leucine, and lysine. Of these, histidine and arginine may be required in the diet only of infants or under special circumstances.

Forms of an Amino Acid. A simple amino acid such as glycine can exist in three forms. At a low pH such as 1, the amino group is protonated (and carrying a charge of +1); the carboxyl is not ionized or charged; and the net charge is +1. At an intermediate pH such as

7, the amino function and the carboxyl function carry equal and opposite charges of $+1$ and -1, and the net is a charge of zero. At a still higher pH such as 12, the carboxyl is ionized and the amino not ionized, resulting in a net of -1. The mean of the pK_a of these two ionizable groups is the pH at which the amino has no net charge and will not move in an electrical field. This pH is defined as the *isoionic point* and designated as pI.

Peptides and Proteins: Peptides are linear chains of amino acids with the carboxyl group of one amino acid attached in amide (specifically peptide) linkage to the amino group of the next amino acid.

$$H_3N^+\!-\!\underset{\underset{H}{|}}{\overset{\overset{R_3}{|}}{C}}\!-\!\overset{\overset{O}{\|}}{C}\!-\!\underset{\underset{H}{|}}{\overset{\overset{H}{|}}{N}}\!-\!\underset{\underset{H}{|}}{\overset{\overset{R_2}{|}}{C}}\!-\!\overset{\overset{O}{\|}}{C}\!-\!\underset{\underset{H}{|}}{\overset{\overset{H}{|}}{N}}\!-\!\underset{\underset{H}{|}}{\overset{\overset{R}{|}}{C}}\!-\!COO^-$$

Proteins are larger assemblies of amino acids. The linear sequence of amino acids in a chain is called the *primary structure*. The orientation of the peptide chain (e.g., the alpha helix) is called the *secondary structure*. The relationship of portions of the polypeptide chains to one another is called the *tertiary structure*. In some cases there are dimers, trimers, tetramers, etc., of the polypeptide chains. This is called the *quaternary structure*. Sometimes the units are identical, sometimes not. In the enzyme lactate dehydrogenase, two different monomers are assembled into an active tetramer. Five different active lactate dehydrogenase tetramers are possible and are separable by electrophoresis.

The primary structure of a peptide or protein may be determined by a combination of procedures. The carboxy terminal amino acid may be determined by its enzymatic release by carboxypeptidases. The rate of release allows determination of the sequence of a small number of amino acids at the carboxy terminal end. Another method, the Edman degradation, utilizes reaction of the amino terminus with phenylisothiocyanate, hydrolysis of the derivative of this amino acid from the peptide chain, and identification of the amino acid derivative. This Edman degradation allows determination of a number of amino acids in sequence at the amino terminal end.

Determination of a number of amino acids at each end of a peptide chain would not allow determination of the sequence of a long peptide chain. Fortunately there are also other enzymes (endopeptidases) that perform internal cleavage with a high degree of specificity. The smaller peptides thus formed may be separated and sequenced. By utilizing different endopeptidases, it is possible to prepare a series of overlapping peptides. When they are sequenced, it is possible to determine the sequence of the intact peptide.

By other methodology it is also possible to synthesize peptides. This procedure, referred to as the Merrifield synthesis, utilizes a solid material with a functional group to which the peptide chain is attached.

Enzymes

In 1926 Sumner isolated the enzyme urease from jack beans and claimed the enzyme to be a protein. Few believed this initially, and the claim was not accepted until about 1935.

Now, over 2600 enzymes have been isolated. Although biological in origin and protein in nature, enzymes are simply catalysts, serving to increase the rate of reactions in which they are involved.

Nomenclature: Some enzymes are given trivial names, such as the proteolytic enzymes trypsin or pepsin, names that provide no information unless one is familiar with these specific enzymes. Others have names that identify the substrate and type of reaction; examples are histidine decarboxylase (decarboxylating histidine to produce CO_2 and histamine), urease (breaking down urea to produce CO_2 and NH_3), and alcohol dehydrogenase (removing hydrogen and electrons from an alcohol to produce a reduced coenzyme and an aldehyde).

Since about 1965 (with a revision in 1972) there has been an attempt to confer more systematic nomenclature and classification on enzymes. An enzyme commission (EC) number is given as four numbers separated by periods. The first of these numbers indicates the main class.

1. Oxidoreductases—oxidation-reduction reactions
2. Transferases—transfer intact groups of atoms from donors to acceptors
3. Hydrolases—cleave by hydrolysis
4. Lyases—cleave C—C, C—O, C—N, and other bonds without hydrolysis or oxidation. (Hydration and dehydration reactions are included in this class.)
5. Isomerases—interconvert isomers, such as $cis \rightarrow trans$; D $\rightarrow$ L
6. Ligases—form bonds as a result of condensation of two different substances with energy provided by ATP.

An example of EC nomenclature and numbering is alcohol: NAD^+ oxidoreductase (EC1.1.1.1). The first number identifies it as an oxidoreductase; the second number identifies its subclass; the third number identifies its sub-subclass; and the final number is a serial listing within the sub-subclass. EC1.1.1.1 is more commonly known as alcohol dehydrogenase.

Cofactors: In addition to the protein portion, many enzymes need cofactors or coenzymes. The protein enzyme without cofactor is known as an *apoenzyme;* the complete enzyme with cofactor or coenzyme is called a *holoenzyme.* The term coenzyme is usually given to an organic cofactor. A cofactor may serve by altering the three-dimensional structure of the enzyme and/or the bound substrate, or it may participate effectively as a second substrate. Thus, the enzyme lactate dehydrogenase catalyzes the oxidation of lactate to pyruvate as the coenzyme NAD^+ is reduced to $NADH + H^+$.

Energy: Enzymes are often looked upon as defying or contradicting the laws of chemistry. This is not true, of course. The free energy of the substrate initially must be higher than the free energy of the products or the reaction will not occur (without net input of energy). In this case we say that the reaction is thermodynamically unfavorable. Indeed, in this case, the reverse reaction would be thermodynamically favorable.

In the case of a thermodynamically favorable reaction, however, input of energy may still be necessary. This energy input, called the *energy of activation,* will be released again as the energy of the system proceeds to the lower energy level of the final products. (This is sometimes compared to a large stone being rolled from one valley into a valley of lower elevation. The energy expended in rolling the stone to the crest of the intervening hill will be released as the stone proceeds downhill. In addition to the release of energy equal to the input of energy to reach the crest, there is also release of energy related to the difference in elevation of the starting and the ending positions.) The role of the enzyme or of other catalysts is seen as lowering the activation energy of the reaction, thus increasing the rate.

Velocity and Inhibition: In the study of enzymes several relationships must be considered: (1) the rate of the reaction will increase with temperature until there is partial denaturation of the enzyme; (2) rates of reactions of enzymes are affected by pH and will ordinarily exhibit a pH range over which maximal activity is seen; (3) reaction rates ordinarily increase linearly with substrate concentration up to the point of maximum velocity, where it is considered that all enzyme molecules have substrate bound at the same time; (4) reaction rates ordinarily increase linearly with enzyme concentration.

The determination of maximum velocity is somewhat difficult since a plot of velocity versus substrate *approaches* the maximum velocity with a reasonable substrate concentration. A more accurate method for determining maximum velocity involves a double reciprocal plot:

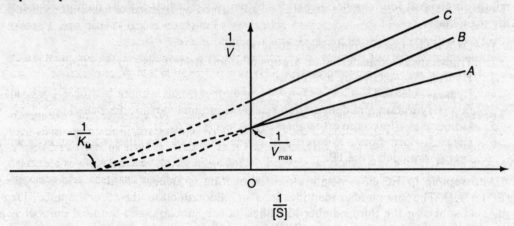

In this graph *A* is a plot of an uninhibited enzyme; *B* is a plot of the same enzyme in the presence of a competetive inhibitor; *C* is a plot of the enzyme in the presence of a noncompetetive inhibitor; *v* represents velocity and [S] represents substrate concentration. Note that the *y*-intercept is the reciprocal of maximal velocity, and the *x*-intercept is the negative of the reciprocal of the Michaelis constant, K_M, a characteristic of the individual enzyme. Note that the maximal velocity in the presence of a competetive inhibitor is the same as for the uninhibited enzyme. The maximal velocity in the presence of a noncompetetive inhibitor is lower (as noted by the fact that the reciprocal is higher).

Carbohydrates

Chemistry: Carbohydrates are a group of polyhydroxy aldehydes, polyhydroxy ketones, and closely related compounds. They may exist as monomers (monosaccharides), dimers (disaccharides), or polymers (polysaccharides).

D-glucose

α-D-glucopyranose

D-fructose

α-D-fructofuranose

D-Glucose and D-fructose are two of the most common monosaccharides found in the human body. They are shown above in straight-chain form and in ring form (as they are usually found in solution). Note that in the ring structure a hemiacetal or a hemiketal has been formed.

Disaccharides such as sucrose and lactose are formed by reaction of monosaccharides. Sucrose hydrolysis will produce equal quantities of D-glucose and D-fructose. Lactose hydrolysis will produce equal quantities of D-galactose and D-glucose.

Polysaccharides are polymers of ring-form monomers. Animal glycogen and plant starch are polymers of α-D-glucopyranose. Cellulose is a polymer of β-D-glucopyranose.

Functions: Carbohydrates play a number of roles in nature. For example, they are metabolized for energy (4 kcal/g), metabolized for production of other required compounds such as certain amino acids, serve as components of nucleic acids (ribose in RNA and deoxyribose in DNA), serve as a structural element (cellulose of plants and cell walls of bacteria), serve as components of lubricants of bone joints, serve as cellular antigens, and are components of heparin.

Metabolism: Many pathways of carbohydrate metabolism could be considered here. We will confine ourselves to comments about glycolysis, the Krebs cycle (also known as the citric acid cycle or the tricarboxylic acid cycle), and the hexose monophosphate shunt (also known as the pentose phosphate pathway).

The complete metabolism of a molecule of glucose proceeds in a series of linked reactions, as shown below. Energy associated with the bonds of glucose is eventually transferred to bonds of adenosine triphosphate (ATP) molecules, which are the molecules used most often to release this energy for work in the cell. Several of the steps shown in the diagram produce ATP directly; however, most ATPs made in the cell carry energy brought to them via "carrier" molecules, either NADH (reduced nicotinamide adenine dinucleotide) or $FADH_2$ (reduced flavin adenine dinucleotide), both of which are made in the reactions shown below. Glycolysis occurs in the cytoplasm; the Krebs cycle, in the mitochondria.

Glycolysis. Glycolysis, in a series of reactions, converts glucose to pyruvic acid (or to lactic acid under conditions of oxygen deficiency). Thus, there is a net formation of 2 moles of ATP from the anaerobic glycolysis of 1 mole of glucose.

Krebs Cycle. Pyruvic acid may be converted to acetyl coenzyme A, producing 3 moles of ATP for each mole of pyruvate. The Krebs cycle may then metabolize the acetyl CoA through a series of reactions to produce 12 moles of ATP for each mole of acetyl CoA. Since the Krebs cycle is often studied with carbohydrate metabolism, many people unconsciously associate them. It should be recognized, however, that acetyl CoA is produced in metabolism of fatty acids and amino acids as well. Acetyl CoA from these other sources is also metabolized in the Krebs cycle.

The Krebs cycle, unlike glycolysis, cannot operate under anaerobic conditions. Oxygen and a functioning electron transport system are required for regeneration of oxidized FAD and NAD^+ (from reduced $FADH_2$ and NADH), but they are also required to produce and capture most of the energy that is realized from the Krebs cycle.

Hexose Monophosphate Shunt. The hexose monophosphate shunt is a series of reactions that serve primarily to produce NADPH and the pentoses (D-ribose and D-deoxyribose). NADPH is important in numerous biosynthetic reactions, including those for biosynthesis of fatty acids and cholesterol. As noted earlier, the pentoses are required for biosynthesis of the nucleic acids (DNA and RNA).

Some Major Steps in Glycolysis and the Citric Acid Cycle*

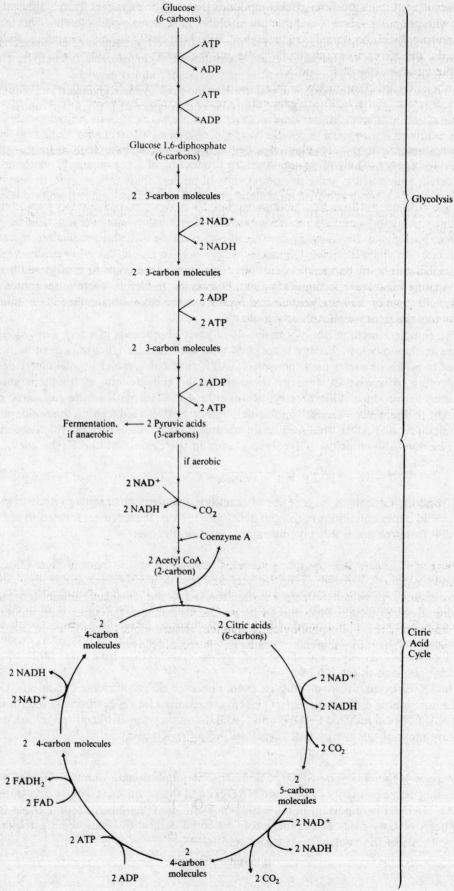

*Reprinted with permission from Barron's *How to Prepare for the Graduate Record Examination in Biology, Third Edition,* © 1989.

Lipids

Chemistry: Lipids are defined as compounds that may be extracted from biological materials with nonpolar solvents and that are insoluble in aqueous polar solvents. This includes the neutral glycerides (largely triglycerides), the phosphoglycerides, the sphingolipids, the steroids, the eicosanoids (particularly the prostaglandins), free fatty acids, and the lipid-soluble vitamins (A, D, E, and K).

Fatty acids are components of many lipids, thus suggesting the need for a discussion of their structure. Fatty acids are generally long, unbranched hydrocarbons with a carboxyl group at one terminus. In the simplest case there are no carbon-to-carbon double bonds, but unsaturation (presence of double bonds) is common. When double bonds are present, they are usually in a *cis*-configuration and in a methylene-interrupted sequence (if more than one double bond is present).

Neutral Glycerides. Neutral glycerides, or acylglycerols, are simply glycerol in ester linkage with one to three fatty acid molecules. Esterification with one fatty acid molecule produces a monoglyceride (monoacylglycerol); esterification with two fatty acid molecules produces a diglyceride (diacylglycerol); and esterification with three molecules of fatty acid produces a triglyceride (triacylglycerol). As previously stated, the triglycerides represent the principal form of storage of excess food. This appears to be a wise arrangement because triglyceride produces 9 kcal/g during metabolism, compared to 4 kcal/g for either carbohydrate or protein, and triglyceride is stored in a substantially water-free state, compared to the hydrated carbohydrates and proteins.

triglyceride   a fatty acid (linoleic acid)

Phosphoglycerides. The phosphoglycerides are similar to the neutral glycerides, but a phosphate group is substituted for the fatty acid that would be found in the 3-position in a triglyceride. Various substituents may be attached to the phosphate group, thus forming other phosphoglycerides. Attachment of choline, for example, produces phosphatidylcholine; ethanolamine → phosphatidylethanolamine; serine → phosphatidylserine; inositol → phosphatidylinositol; and glycerol produces phosphatidylglycerol.

phosphatidic acid

Sphingolipids. The sphingolipids are based on a long-chain amino alcohol, sphingosine, rather than on glycerol.

$$H_3C-(CH_2)_{12}-\overset{\displaystyle H}{\underset{\displaystyle H}{C}}=\overset{\displaystyle {}}{\underset{\displaystyle H}{C}}-\overset{\displaystyle OH}{\underset{\displaystyle H}{C}}-\overset{\displaystyle NH_2}{\underset{\displaystyle H}{C}}-CH_2OH$$

sphingosine

$$R-\overset{\displaystyle OH}{\underset{\displaystyle N}{C}}-\overset{\displaystyle H}{\underset{\displaystyle NH}{C}}-CH_2O-X$$

$$\underset{\displaystyle R'}{\overset{\displaystyle C=O}{|}}$$

a sphingolipid

In the preceding formula, R represents an unsaturated hydrocarbon chain, R' represents another hydrocarbon chain (from an R'—COOH that has reacted with the NH_2 to form an amide linkage). X can represent phosphorylcholine in phosphodiester linkage, giving us sphingomyelin. It can also represent a simple glucose (giving us a glucocerebroside), or it can represent a more complex carbohydrate containing sialic acid (giving us a ganglioside).

Steroids. The term steroid is understood by the layperson to designate a natural or synthetic hormone. As used by the biochemist and other professionals in this field, however, it refers to the structure only and does not signify hormonal activity. The structure of a steroid is based on the cyclopentanoperhydrophenanthrene nucleus or steroid nucleus:

An example of a steroid is the sterol cholesterol:

cholesterol

In addition to the sterols, the steroid group includes the bile acids, vitamin D, and the steroid hormones (estrogens, androgens, adrenal corticosteroids, and progesterone).

Eicosanoids. Some fatty acids, including linoleic acid, are very important to mammalian health, but cannot be synthesized in the body. These are therefore called *essential fatty acids.* Among the products of linoleic acid are the prostaglandins, 20-carbon fatty acids that include a 5-carbon ring. Prostaglandins are active in a variety of physiologically important ways and are sometimes used pharmacologically.

prostaglandin E₁
(PGE₁)

Free Fatty Acids. Free fatty acids may sometimes be found in small amounts in various tissues. Fatty acids are also found in unesterified form in blood plasma, but in this case they are ordinarily bound noncovalently to plasma proteins, particularly albumin.

Lipid-soluble Vitamins. The lipid-soluble vitamins A, D, E, and K may also be classified as lipids, based on their solubility. They are stored in the body, and, in contrast to water-soluble vitamins, *steady* dietary intake of these vitamins is not vitally important.

Metabolism:

Hydrolysis to Produce Fatty Acids. Neutral glycerides may be hydrolyzed by lipases such as pancreatic lipase or hormone-sensitive lipase, thus releasing free fatty acids. Fatty acids may also be released from phosphoglycerides by hydrolysis that is catalyzed by phospholipase A_1 and phsopholipase A_2.

Oxidation of Fatty Acids in the Mitochondria. Fatty acids may then be oxidized via β-oxidation to produce acetyl CoA + reduced flavin adenine dinucleotide ($FADH_2$) and reduced nicotinamide adenine dinucleotide ($NADH + H^+$). Thus a molecule of fatty acid 16:0 would produce 8 molecules of acetyl CoA, 7 moleucs of $FADH_2$, and 7 molecules of $NADH + H^+$. Each molecule of acetyl CoA can be metabolized in the Krebs cycle to produce 12 molecules of ATP. Each molecule of $FADH_2$ can produce 2 molecules of ATP when it is oxidized in the electron transport chain, and each molecule of $NADH + H^+$ can produce 3 molecules of ATP when oxidized in the electron transport chain.

Synthesis of Fatty Acids. Synthesis of fatty acids occurs in the nonparticulate cytoplasm. The pathway is not simply a reversal of β-oxidation; it requires biotin and carbon dioxide in addition to acetyl CoA. The carbon dioxide, however, is not incorporated into the fatty acid. Also the reducing equivalents required for the synthesis are derived from $NADPH + H^+$.

Synthesis of Glycerides. The neutral glycerides require L-3-glycerol phosphate in their biosynthesis. This glycerol phosphate may be formed by the enzymatic phosphorylation of glycerol or by the enzymatic reduction of dihydroxyacetone phosphate, which is produced in glycolysis.

Nucleotides and Nucleic Acids; Biosynthesis of Nucleic Acids and Proteins

Nucleotides: Both deoxyribonucleic acid (DNA) and ribonucleic acid (RNA) are polymers of nucleotides. A nucleotide consists of a nitrogen base (either a purine or a pyrimidine), a pentose (ribose or 2-deoxyribose), and a phosphate group. Deoxyribose is found in DNA; ribose, in RNA.

The nitrogen bases include the purines (adenine and guanine) in both DNA and RNA. The pyrimidines include cytosine and thymine in DNA; cytosine and uracil are present in RNA. Other nitrogen bases are found in small quantities. Some synthetic nitrogen bases are used in the treatment of cancer and certain viral infections.

Nucleic Acids: As mentioned above, DNA and RNA are polymers of appropriate nucleotides. The attachment between nucleotides is phosphate–pentose-phosphate-pentose–, etc. This leaves the nitrogen base as an appendage from the linear chain. In double-stranded DNA there are two strands that are paired and linked (noncovalently) through their nitrogen bases. Adenine pairs with thymine, and cytosine pairs with guanine. Methods are available to allow determination of the primary structures of both DNA and RNA.

Biosynthesis of Nucleic Acids and Proteins: It is recognized that DNA codes for its own duplication, as well as for RNA synthesis. Messenger RNA, in turn, codes for the biosynthesis of polypeptide chains. Since there is a triplet code without commas, there are $4 \times 4 \times 4 = 64$ possibilities and sequences for specification of a single amino acid. Only about 21 amino acids, however, are known to have codes. It turns out that some codes give other instructions (e.g., initiation or termination of a peptide chain biosynthesis) and some amino acids have more than one code for their placement. Arginine, for example, has six different codons that can specify its placement.

Mutations in the DNA chain can occur, of course, as a result of errors in duplication, spontaneous changes in DNA, or changes resulting from radiation or mutagenic chemicals. A point mutation results in the presence of a different nitrogen base. This may, in turn, cause problems, or it may be a silent mutation. It would be silent if the base change resulted in no difference in the amino acid or if it resulted in the substitution of a very similar amino acid.

A frame shift mutation is likely to be more serious. Consider that insertion or deletion of a nitrogen base will change the sequence of bases following it in the chain. (Remember that there are no commas.) This may be a lethal mutation.

Mutations can be repaired by a number of mechanisms. For example, sometimes an affected area is removed and replaced by a strand that is duplicated again from the complementary DNA strand. Specific cellular enzymes exist to aid in identifying and repairing mutations.

PHYSICS—FREQUENTLY ENCOUNTERED PHYSICS PROBLEMS AND THEIR ANSWERS

Accelerated Motion

Example: A boat accelerates uniformly from 15 mi/hr to 45 mi/hr in 10 sec.

1. Calculate acceleration.

$$a = \frac{v_2 - v_1}{t}$$

a = acceleration
v_1 = initial speed *or* velocity
v_2 = final speed *or* velocity
t = time

$$a = \frac{45 \text{ mi/hr} - 15 \text{ mi/hr}}{10 \text{ sec}} = \frac{30 \text{ mi/hr}}{10 \text{ sec}} = 3 \text{ mi/hr/sec, or } 3 \text{ mi/hr·sec}$$

2. Calculate average speed.

$$v = \frac{v_1 + v_2}{2} \qquad v = \text{average velocity}$$

$$v = \frac{15 \text{ mi/hr} + 45 \text{ mi/hr}}{2} = 30 \text{ mi/hr}$$

3. Distance covered?

$$s = \text{distance covered}$$

$$s = vt$$

Recall: There are 5280 ft/mi and 3600 sec/hr. In 30 mi, 158,400 ft are covered. So,

$$\frac{158,400}{3600 \text{ sec}} = 44 \text{ ft/sec}$$

Since the boat was in motion for 10 sec,

$$\text{distance covered} = 44 \text{ ft/sec} \times 10 \text{ sec} = 440 \text{ ft}$$

Example: An object is accelerated from rest to 600 mi/hr in 30 sec; the object has been subjected to an acceleration of 29 ft/sec^2

A convenient unit for acceleration is feet per second squared (ft/sec^2). First, convert the velocity units:

$$\frac{600 \text{ mi}}{\text{hr}} \times \frac{5280 \text{ ft}}{\text{mi}} \times \frac{\text{hr}}{3600 \text{ sec}} = 880 \text{ ft/sec}$$

Then

$$a = \frac{v}{t}$$

$$a = \frac{880 \text{ ft/sec}}{30 \text{ sec}} = 29 \text{ ft/sec}^2$$

Another way of expressing this type of phenomenon is to solve a problem as follows:

Example: A car is traveling at a speed of 31 mi/hr and accelerates for 8 sec to reach a speed of 55 mi/hr. Its rate of acceleration was 3 mi/hr/sec. Mathematically expressed:

$$a = \frac{\text{Final Velocity} - \text{Initial Velocity}}{\text{Time}}$$

$$a = \frac{55 \text{ mi/hr} - 31 \text{ mi/hr}}{8 \text{ sec}}$$

$$a = \frac{24 \text{ mi/hr}}{8 \text{ sec}} = 3 \text{ mi/hr/sec, or } 3 \text{ mi/hr·sec}$$

Falling Objects — Gravity Acceleration

Recall: $g = 32$ ft/sec^2 or 980 cm/s^2 or 9.8 m/s^2

Example: An object in free fall travels for 1 sec.

1. Calculate speed (velocity) obtained, when the body is released from rest.

$$v_2 = v_1 + at$$
$$v_2 = 0 + (32 \text{ ft/sec}^2)(1 \text{ sec})$$
$$v_2 = 32 \text{ ft/sec}$$

v_1 = initial speed = 0

v_2 = final speed

a = acceleration

t = time

2. The above body started from rest; the distance covered in the time was?

$$s = v_1 t + \frac{1}{2}at^2$$
$$s = 0 + \frac{1}{2}(32 \text{ ft/sec}^2)(1 \text{ sec})^2$$
$$s = 16 \text{ ft}$$

v_1 = initial speed = 0

t = time

s = distance traversed

a = acceleration

Example: A rocket traveling upward is going 400 ft/sec when its fuel is exhausted. Then:

1. The distance covered after 1 sec is?

$$s = v_1 t + \frac{1}{2}at^2 \qquad \begin{array}{l} v_1 = 400 \text{ ft/sec} \\ a = -32 \text{ ft/sec}^2 \\ t = 1 \text{ sec} \end{array}$$

$$s = (400 \text{ ft/sec})(1 \text{ sec}) + \frac{1}{2}(-32 \text{ ft/sec}^2)(1 \text{ sec})^2$$

$$s = 384 \text{ ft}$$

2. Calculate the speed obtained after 1 sec.

$$v_2 = v_1 + at$$
$$v_2 = 400 \text{ ft/sec} + (-32 \text{ ft/sec}^2)(1 \text{ sec})$$
$$v_2 = 368 \text{ ft/sec}$$

v_1 = initial velocity

v_2 = final velocity

a = acceleration

t = time

Example: a. At the end of 1 sec a falling object will attain a velocity of 32 ft/sec.

$$v_f = at = 32 \text{ ft/sec} \times 1 \text{ sec} = 32 \text{ ft/sec} \qquad v_f = \text{final velocity}$$

b. During this 1 sec of falling, however, an object previously at rest will have covered a distance of 16 ft.

$$s = v_0 t + \frac{at^2}{2}$$
$$s = (0 \text{ ft})(1 \text{ sec}).$$
$$+ \frac{(32 \text{ ft/sec}^2)(1 \text{ sec})^2}{2} = 16 \text{ ft}$$

s = distance traversed

v_0 = velocity at rest

= initial velocity = 0

t = time

Uniform Velocity

Example: a car travels with a constant velocity of 30 mi/hr for 40 mi. What time is needed to travel this distance?

$$t = \frac{s}{v}$$
$$t = \frac{40 \text{ mi}}{30 \text{ mi/hr}}$$
$$t = 1.33 \text{ hr}$$

v = velocity = 30 mi/hr

s = distance traversed = 40 mi

t = time

Nonuniform Motion

Example: A rocket with an initial velocity of 25 m/s is accelerated at 75 m/s^2 for 10 s.

1. The rocket covers a distance of how many meters during the period of acceleration?

$$s = v_0 t + \frac{1}{2} at^2 \hspace{3cm} s = \text{distance traversed}$$

$$s = (25 \text{ m/s})(10 \text{ s}) + \frac{1}{2} (75 \text{ m/s}^2)(10 \text{ s})^2$$

$$s = 250 \text{ m} + \frac{7500 \text{ m}}{2}$$

$$s = 250 \text{ m} + 3750 \text{ m}$$

$$s = 4000 \text{ m}$$

2. How far would the rocket travel if it started from rest?

$$x = \frac{1}{2} (75 \text{ m/s}^2)(10 \text{ s})^2$$

$$x = 3750 \text{ m}$$

Uniform Deceleration

Example: A train travels at 60 mi/hr (88 ft/sec); the brakes are applied for 2 sec, and it decelerates at a rate of 22 ft/sec^2. Calculate its final velocity.

$v = v_0 - at$

$v = 88 \text{ ft/sec} - (22 \text{ ft/sec}^2)(2 \text{ sec})$

$v = 44 \text{ ft/sec (or 30 mi/hr)}$

Free Fall

Example: A construction worker drops a brick while working at a height of 900 ft.

$$v_0 = 0$$

$$g = 32 \text{ ft/sec}^2$$

$$t = 3 \text{ sec}$$

$$y = \text{distance traversed}$$

1. What distance does the brick cover in 3 sec?

$$s = v_0 t + \frac{1}{2} gt^2$$

$$s = \frac{1}{2} gt^2$$

$$s = \frac{1}{2} (32 \text{ ft/sec}^2)(3 \text{ sec}^2)$$

$$s = 144 \text{ ft}$$

2. How long does it take for the brick to land on the ground?

$$s = \frac{1}{2}gt^2$$

$$t = \left(\frac{2s}{g}\right)^{1/2}$$

$$t = \left(\frac{(2)(900 \text{ ft})}{32 \text{ ft/sec}^2}\right)^{1/2}$$

$$t = (56/\text{sec}^2)^{1/2}$$

$$t = 7.5 \text{ sec}$$

3. What is the velocity of the brick at 2 sec of travel?

$$v = gt$$

$$v = (32 \text{ ft/sec}^2)(2 \text{ sec})$$

$$v = 64 \text{ ft/sec}$$

Forces and Motion

Forces and Acceleration

Newton's Second Law: Force = Mass × Acceleration or $f = ma$
Newton's Third Law: For every acting force there exists a reacting force of equal magnitude but in the opposite direction, that is, $F(\text{action}) = -F(\text{reaction})$.

$$f = \text{force}$$

$$m = \text{mass}$$

$$a = \text{acceleration}$$

Recall: A unit of force applied is the *dyne*; 1 dyne is the force that will impart to a 1-gram mass an acceleration of 1 cm/s², that is, 1 dyne $= 1 \frac{\text{g} \cdot \text{cm}}{\text{s}^2}$

Example: A force of 2000 dynes is applied to a mass of 250 g. Calculate the acceleration obtained.

$$a = \frac{f}{m}$$

$$a = \frac{2000 \text{ dynes}}{250 \text{ g}}$$

$$a = \frac{2000 \text{ g} \cdot \text{cm/s}^2}{250 \text{ g}}$$

$$a = 8 \text{ cm/s}^2$$

Example: What is the force exerted on the surface of an asteroid by a man of 70-kg mass if the acceleration due to gravity of the asteroid is 2.5 m/s²?

$$F = mg$$

$$F = 70 \text{ kg} \times 2.5 \text{ m/s}^2 = 175 \text{ N}$$

(A newton, abbreviated as N, is a unit of force expressed in kilograms × meter/second².)

Weight and Acceleration

$$F = \frac{w}{g} a \text{ OR } f = ma \qquad F \text{ or } f = \text{force}$$

$$w = mg$$

a = acceleration

w = weight

m = mass

g = acceleration due to gravity

Example: A force of 30 lb. is applied to a weight of 30 lb. Calculate the acceleration produced.

$$F = \frac{w}{g} a; \; a = \frac{Fg}{w}$$

$$a = \frac{30 \text{ lb} \times 32 \text{ ft/sec}^2}{30 \text{ lb}}$$

$$a = 32 \text{ ft/sec}^2$$

Example: A 180-lb. astronaut is accelerated upward by his rocket at 80 ft/sec². Calculate the force that the seat exerts on him.

$$F = \frac{w}{g} a$$

$$F = \frac{(180 \text{ lb})(80 \text{ ft/sec}^2)}{32 \text{ ft/sec}^2}$$

$$F = 450 \text{ lb}$$

This is the net accelerating force. The seat is also supporting his weight, so the total force is

$$F = 450 \text{ lb} + 180 \text{ lb} = 630 \text{ lb}$$

Example: A 20-kg mass located on a frictionless table is acted upon by a horizontal force of 240 N.

1. Calculate the acceleration of the object.

$$F = ma$$

$$a = \frac{F}{m}$$

$$a = \frac{240 \text{ N}}{20 \text{ kg}}$$

$$a = 12 \text{ m/s}^2$$

2. Calculate the distance the mass will travel in 10 sec.

$$s = v_0 t + \frac{1}{2} at^2$$

$$s = 0 + \frac{1}{2} (12 \text{ m/s}^2)(10 \text{ s})^2$$

$$s = \frac{1200 \text{ m}}{2}$$

$$s = 600 \text{ m}$$

Negative Acceleration

Example: A test vehicle weighing 3000 lb travels at 60 mi/hr (88 ft/sec.). Its stopping distance is 300 ft.

1. Calculate the negative acceleration.

$$v^2 = v_0^2 + 2ax$$

$$a = \frac{v^2 - v_0^2}{2x}$$

$$a = 0 - \frac{(88 \text{ ft/sec})^2}{2(300 \text{ ft})}$$

$$a = -12.9 \text{ ft/sec}^2$$

2. What is the mass?

$$m = \frac{w}{g}$$

$$m = \frac{3000 \text{ lb}}{32 \text{ ft/sec}^2}$$

$$m = 94 \text{ lb sec}^2/\text{ft or slugs}$$

3. What force is required to stop the vehicle?

$$F = ma$$

$$F = (93.75 \text{ slugs}) \times (-12.9 \text{ ft/sec}^2)$$

$$F = -1210 \text{ lb}$$

Example: A crane is lowering a 5000 kg air conditioning unit, and the tension in the cable is 40,000 N as the unit begins to go downward.

1. Net force on the unit?

The weight of the unit is

$$w = mg = (5000 \text{ kg}) \left(\frac{9.8 \text{ m}}{s^2} \right) = 49,000 \text{ N}$$

So the net downward force is

$$49,000 \text{ N} - 40,000 \text{ N} = 9000 \text{N}$$

2. Acceleration of unit?

$$a = \frac{F}{m} = \frac{9000 \text{N}}{5000 \text{ kg}} = 1.8 \text{ m/s}^2$$

3. How long will it take the unit to reach a speed of 4 m/s?

$$t = \frac{a}{v} = \frac{4 \text{ m/s}}{1.8 \text{ m/s}^2} = 2.2 \text{ s}$$

Resultant Forces

a. Forces Acting Upon Each Other at Right Angles.

Example: If a force of 3N and a force of 4N acted upon each other at right angles, the resultant would be 5N. The answer is obtained by utilizing the formula:

$$R = \sqrt{(\text{Force 1})^2 + (\text{Force 2})^2}$$

Thus,

$$R = \sqrt{(3N)^2 + (4N)^2}$$
$$R = \sqrt{25N^2}$$
$$R = \sqrt{5N}$$

b. Forces Acting in the Same Direction.

Example: The resultant of two forces of 3N and 10N acting in the same direction is 13N. Any combination of forces acting upon the same object in the same direction will result in an addition of the forces and the result will be equal to the sum of the forces.

Equilibrium States

An object is in equilibrium when all forces on it add to zero.

Example: An instrument weighing 35 N is placed in a stream, suspended by a rope that makes an angle of 40° with the vertical. A scale inserted in the rope reads 28 N. Find the force of buoyancy and the force exerted on the instrument by the current.

1. Determine the vertical and horizontal components of the tension in the rope.

$$T_{vert} = (28 \text{ N})(\cos 40°) = 21 \text{ N}$$

$$T_{hor} = (28 \text{ N})(\sin 40°) = 18 \text{ N}$$

2. Set all upward forces equal to all downward forces.

$$\text{Weight} = \text{Buoyancy } (B) + \text{Upward Component}$$

$$B = 35 \text{ N} - 21 \text{ N} = 14 \text{ N}$$

3. Set upstream forces equal to downstream forces.

$$\text{Horizontal Component} = \text{Current Force } (C)$$

$$C = 18 \text{ N}$$

Example: A 28-kg packing case is on a ramp inclined at 25° to the horizontal, and is pulled uphill at constant speed with a force of 160 N. Determine the coefficient of friction.

1. Determine the weight of the case.

$$w = mg = (28 \text{ kg})(9.8 \text{ m/s}^2) = 247N$$

2. Find the components of the weight parallel and perpendicular to the ramp.

$$W_{par} = (274 \text{ N})(\sin 25°) = 116 \text{ N}$$

$$W_{perp} = (274 \text{ N})(\cos 25°) = 248 \text{ N}$$

3. Find the friction by setting uphill forces equal to downhill forces.

$$160 \text{ N} = 116 \text{ N} + F$$

$$F = 44 \text{ N}$$

4. Find the coefficient of friction.

$$\mu = \frac{\text{friction}}{\text{normal force}} = \frac{44 \text{ N}}{248 \text{ N}} = 0.18$$

Projectile Motion

v = initial velocity

θ = angle with horizonal

v_h = horizontal component of path = $v \cos \theta$

v_v = vertical component of path = $v \sin \theta$

Example: A cannonball travels with a speed of 200 ft./sec. with a 30° horizontal projection.

1. Determine the height the ball reaches. Look up the sine and cosine in a standard table or use a scientific calculator.

$\sin 30° = 0.5$; $v_v = v \sin \theta = (200 \text{ ft/sec})(\sin 30°) = 100 \text{ ft/sec}$

$\cos 30° = 0.866$; $v_h = v \cos \theta = (200 \text{ ft/sec})(\cos 30°) = 173 \text{ ft/sec}$

Utilize the equation:

$$v_2{}^2 - v_1{}^2 = 2as \qquad v_1 = 100 \text{ ft/sec}$$

$$v_2 = 0$$

$$a = -32 \text{ ft/sec}^2$$

Thus we have:

$$0 - (100 \text{ ft/sec})^2 = 2(-32 \text{ ft/sec}^2)s$$

$$s = \frac{10,000 \text{ ft}^2/\text{sec}^2}{64 \text{ ft/sec}^2}$$

$$s = 156 \text{ ft}$$

2. Calculate the time necessary to reach maximum height.

$$v_2 - v_1 = at$$

$$0 - 100 \text{ ft/sec} = (-32 \text{ ft/sec}^2)t$$

$$t = \frac{100 \text{ ft/sec}}{32 \text{ ft/sec}^2}$$

$$t = 3.1 \text{ sec}$$

3. The ball will return to the earth in what time? If 3.12 sec are used for ascending, $2t$ should be required. The answer is 6.24 sec.

4. Determine the range (R) of the ball.

$$R = v_h t$$

$$R = (173 \text{ ft/sec})(6.24 \text{ sec})$$

$$R = 1080 \text{ ft}$$

Friction

$$\text{Formula } \mu = \frac{F}{N} \qquad \mu = \text{coefficient of friction}$$

$$F = \text{frictional force}$$

$$N = \text{normal or perpendicular force}$$

Example: a 2500-lb force draws a 30,000-lb railroad car at constant speed on level terrain.

1. Determine the coefficient of friction.

$$\mu = \frac{F}{N}$$

$$\mu = \frac{2500 \text{ lb}}{30,000 \text{ lb}} = 0.08$$

(The coefficient of friction is the ratio of the frictional force to the perpendicular force pressing the two surfaces together.)

2. The railroad car is pulled on a horizontal track at constant speed by a steel cable that makes a 30° angle above the horizontal. The tension in the cable is 300 lb. Determine the coefficient of friction.

$$F(\text{parallel frictional force}) = F = 300 \text{ lb} \times \cos 30°$$

$$= 300 \text{ lb} \times 0.866$$

$$= 259.8 \text{ lb}$$

The normal force N—which is the weight of the car—is 30,000 lb. However, the vertical component of tension must be subtracted from it.

$$N = 30,000 \text{ lb} - 300 \text{ lb} \times \sin 30°$$

$$= 30,000 \text{ lb} - 150 \text{ lb}$$

$$= 29,850 \text{ lb}$$

$$\mu = \frac{F}{N}$$

$$\mu = \frac{359.8 \text{ lb}}{29,850 \text{ lb}}$$

$$\mu = 0.009$$

Work and Power

Work (W) equals the force (F) times the displacement (d) in the direction of the force, that is, $W = Fd$.

Example: A machine is pushed 50 ft on a level floor. The frictional force is determined as 300 lb. Calculate the work performed.

$$W = Fd$$

$$W = (300 \text{ lb})(50 \text{ ft})$$

$$W = 15,000 \text{ ft-lb}$$

Example: Instead of being pushed, the above machine is dragged via a steel cable at an angle of 30° with the floor and a force on the cable of 300 lb. The work performed is?

$$W = (F \cos 30°)d$$

$$W = 300 \text{ lb.} \times 0.866 \times 50 \text{ ft}$$

$$W = 13,000 \text{ ft-lb}$$

Work and Energy

Example: A man pushes his snowblower with a constant force of 50 lb. The shaft makes an angle of 45° with the horizontal. The work done by the man in 150 ft is?

$$W = Fd \cos 45°$$

$$W = (50 \text{ lb})(150 \text{ ft})(0.707)$$

$$W = 5300 \text{ ft-lb}$$

Power and Power Units

$$\text{Power} = \frac{\text{Work}}{\text{Time}} \text{ or } P = \frac{W}{t}$$

Units: 1 watt = 10^7 ergs/sec = 1 joule/sec
1 horsepower (hp) = 550 ft-lb/sec = 746 watts
1 kilowatt = 1000 watts = 1.34 hp

Example: By means of its steel pulleys, a crane raises a machine weighing 500 lb to a height of 100 ft in 200 sec. The average horsepower necessary is?

$$P = \frac{W}{t}$$

$$P = \frac{\text{Force} \times \text{Distance}}{\text{Time}}$$

$$P = \frac{(500 \text{ lb})(100 \text{ ft})}{200 \text{ sec}}$$

$$P = 250 \text{ ft-lb/sec}$$

$$P = \frac{250 \text{ ft-lb/sec}}{550 \frac{\text{ft-lb/sec}}{1 \text{ hp}}}$$

$$P = 0.45 \text{ hp}$$

Example: A man weighing 180 lb is taking a stress test. The test equals the activity of climbing stairs a vertical distance of 30 ft in 5 sec. Calculate the horsepower he develops.

$$P = \frac{W}{t}$$

$$P = \frac{180 \text{ lb} \times 30 \text{ ft}}{5 \text{ sec}}$$

$$P = \frac{5400 \text{ ft-lb}}{5 \text{ sec}}$$

$$P = 1080 \text{ ft-lb/sec}$$

$$P = \frac{1080 \text{ ft-lb/sec}}{550 \dfrac{\text{ft-lb/sec}}{1 \text{ hp}}}$$

$$P = 1.96 \text{ hp}$$

Example: To take the MCAT examination you must climb stairs to a height of 60 ft, and you weigh 180 lb. The work you do against the force of gravity is 10,800 ft-lb.

$$W = F \times D$$

$$W = 180 \text{ lb} \times 60 \text{ ft} = 10,800 \text{ ft-lb}$$

Energy

Potential Energy

Potential energy (*PE*)—or energy of position—is the product of the weight (*w*) of an object and the height (*h*) to which the object is elevated, or the work done in elevating it: $PE = wh$.

Example: A machine weighing 5000 lb is raised onto the roof of a building 150 ft high. Calculate the increase in potential energy or the work done in lifting the machine.

$$PE = wh$$

$$PE = (5000 \text{ lb})(150 \text{ ft})$$

$$PE = 750,000 \text{ ft-lb}$$

Kinetic Energy

Kinetic energy = energy of motion.

Formulas: 1. $KE = \dfrac{1}{2}\dfrac{w}{g}v^2$ w = weight in lb.

2. $KE = \dfrac{1}{2}mv^2$ g = ft/sec^2

v = ft/sec

KE = ft-lb

Example: Determine the kinetic energy of a locomotive weighing 250,000 lb. and traveling at a speed of 30 mi/hr (44 ft/sec).

$$KE = \frac{1}{2}\frac{w}{g}v^2$$

$$KE = \frac{1}{2}\frac{(250,000 \text{ lb})(44 \text{ ft/sec})^2}{32 \text{ ft/sec}^2}$$

$$KE = 7,600,000 \text{ ft-lb}$$

Recall: The joule (J) is a unit of energy. It is a N · m, the work done by a force of 1 N through a distance of 1 m. It is the heat produced by an ampere flowing against an ohm for one second. One joule is equal to 10^7 ergs, and 4.185 J are equal to one calorie.

Example: A rocket with a mass of 2000 kg is fired vertically upward with an initial velocity of 100 m/s.
1. Calculate the change in kinetic energy at maximum height reached.

$$\Delta K = K - K_0$$

$$-K_0 = -\frac{1}{2} mv_0^2$$

$$-K_0 = -\frac{1}{2}(2000 \text{ kg})(100 \text{ m/s})^2$$

$$\Delta K = -K_0 = -10,000,000 \text{ J}$$

K = kinetic energy at maximum height = 0

K_0 = initial kinetic energy

V_0 = initial velocity

Answer: At maximum height reached, the rocket has lost 10,000,000 J of kinetic energy.
2. Calculate the potential energy at maximum height, and the change in kinetic energy upon return to lift-off point.

a.　$v^2 = v_0^2 - '2gy$

$$y = \frac{v_0^2}{2g}$$

$$y = \frac{(100 \text{ m/s})^2}{2(9.8 \text{ m/s}^2)}$$

$$y = \frac{10,000 \text{ m}^2/\text{s}^2}{19.6 \text{ m/s}^2}$$

$$y = 510 \text{ m}$$

v_0 = initial velocity

y = maximum height

g = gravitational acceleration

b. $PE = mgh$

$PE = (2000 \text{ kg})(9.8 \text{ m/s}^2)(510 \text{ m})$

$PE = 10,000,000 \text{ J}$

The increase in potential energy, then, is 10,000,000 J, and one can deduce that the rocket returns to its lift-off point with the same velocity it had at the beginning. The rocket had gained 10,000,000 J of kinetic energy on the original flight, but lost this amount in potential energy and, therefore, the total change in potential energy was zero. The *KE* and *PE* balance each other and are constant; the principle of conservation of energy is demonstrated.

Momentum

Momentum is the product of the mass and velocity of an object:

$$p = mv$$　p = momentum

$$m = \text{mass}$$

$$v = \text{velocity}$$

The change of momentum is equal to the force applied times time. You may use $\frac{w}{g}$ in place of m (mass), since $m = \frac{w}{g}$ (see p. 143).

Example: A 180-lb man is shot out of a cannon at the speed of 30 ft/sec. What is his momentum?

$$p = \frac{w}{g} v$$

$$p = \frac{180 \text{ lb}}{32 \text{ ft/sec}^2} (30 \text{ ft/sec})$$

$$p = 169 \text{ lb-sec}$$

Example: On landing, a plane is traveling at 60 mi/hr. Brakes are applied, and the plane comes to a stop in 10 sec. Assuming the average weight to be 160 lb, what is the force of the seat belts on each passenger? (60 mi/hr = 88 ft /sec)

Step 1   Calculate the change in momentum.

$$p = -mv_0 = -\frac{w}{g} v_0$$

$$p = -\left(\frac{160 \text{ lb}}{32 \text{ ft/sec}^2}\right) 88 \text{ ft/sec}$$

$$p = -440 \text{ lb-sec}$$

Step 2   Now calculate the force applied by the seat belt on a passenger.

$$F = \frac{p}{t}$$

$$F = \frac{-440 \text{ lb-sec}}{10 \text{ sec}}$$

$$F = -44 \text{ lb}$$

Uniform Circular Motion

Centripetal Acceleration

Example: A subway car traveling at a speed of 30 mi/hr (44 ft/sec) negotiates a curve whose radius is 600 ft. What is its acceleration?

$$a = \frac{v^2}{r} \qquad \begin{array}{l} a = \text{acceleration} \\ v = \text{velocity} \\ r = \text{radius} \end{array}$$

$$a = \frac{(44 \text{ ft/sec})^2}{600 \text{ ft}}$$

$$a = \frac{1936 \text{ ft}^2/\text{sec}^2}{600 \text{ ft}}$$

$$a = 3.22 \text{ ft/sec}^2$$

Circular Motion

Recall: $\dfrac{360°}{2\pi} = 1 \text{ rad} = 57.3°$

$360° = 2\pi \text{ rad}; \quad 180° = \pi \text{ rad}; \quad 90° = \dfrac{\pi}{2} \text{ rad}$

The radian is a unit of measurement equal to the angle obtained at the center of a circle making an arc equal to the length of the radius.

Example: An airplane has its automatic pilot fly a circular route at a constant speed of 60 mi/hr. The route has a diameter of 10,000 ft.

1. Calculate the plane's angular speed.

$\omega = \dfrac{v}{r}$ $\omega = $ angular speed

$v = $ velocity $= 60$ mi/hr $= 88$ ft/sec

$\omega = \dfrac{88 \text{ ft/sec}}{5000 \text{ ft}}$ $d = $ diameter $= 10{,}000$ ft

$\omega = 0.0176$ rad/sec $r = $ radius $= \dfrac{d}{2} = 5{,}000$ ft

2. Calculate the angular distance and the arc length flown in 45 sec.

Angular distance $\theta = \omega t$

$\theta = (0.0176 \text{ rad/sec})(45 \text{ sec})$

$\theta = 0.792$ rad

Arc length $s = r\theta$

$s = (5000 \text{ ft})(0.792 \text{ rad})$

$s = 3960$ ft

OR

$s = vt$

$s = (88 \text{ ft/sec})(45 \text{ sec})$

$s = 3960$ ft

Centripetal Force

Centripetal force may be expressed as mass times velocity squared divided by the radius, that is, $F_c = \dfrac{mv^2}{r}$ or $F_c = \dfrac{w}{g} \times \dfrac{v^2}{r}$.

Example: The previously cited subway car weighs 300,000 lb, travels at 30 mi/hr, and rounds the above radius of 600 ft. Its centripetal force is?

$F_c = \dfrac{w}{g} \times \dfrac{v^2}{r}$ $w = 300{,}000$ lb
$g = 32$ ft/sec^2
$v = 30$ mi/hr (44 ft/sec)
$r = 600$ ft

$F_c = \dfrac{300{,}000 \text{ lb}}{32 \text{ ft/sec}^2} \times \dfrac{(44 \text{ ft/sec})^2}{600 \text{ ft}}$

$F_c = 30{,}250$ lb

Example: A satellite is in circular orbit at an altitude of 5.0×10^2 km. One complete revolution takes 95 minutes.

1. Calculate the tangential velocity.

Radius of earth = 6400 km

Radius of orbit, r = 6400 km + 500 km = 6900 km, or 6.9×10^6 m

$$v = \frac{s}{t} = \frac{2\pi r}{t} = \frac{2\pi(6.9 \times 10^6 \text{ m})}{5700 \text{ s}} = 7600 \text{ m/s}$$

2. Calculate the angular speed

$$\omega = \frac{\theta}{t} = \frac{2\pi}{5700 \text{ s}} = 1.10 \times 10^{-3} \text{ rad/s}$$

To get the tangential speed from this:

$$v = r\omega = (6.9 \times 10^6 \text{ m})(1.10 \times 10^{-3} \text{ rad/s}) = 7600 \text{ m/s}$$

3. Calculate the centripetal acceleration, due to gravity:

$$a_c = \frac{v^2}{r} = \frac{(7600 \text{ m/s})^2)}{6.9 \times 10^6 \text{ m}} = 8.4 \text{ m/s}^2$$

Example: An astronaut weighing 160 lb is being spun in a centrifuge with a radius of 120 ft at a speed of 60 mi/hr. What is the centripetal force on the astronaut?

$$F_c = \frac{mv^2}{r} \qquad w = mg$$

$$m = \frac{160 \text{ lb}}{32 \text{ ft/sec}^2} = 5 \text{ slugs}$$

$$F = \frac{5 \text{ slugs } (88 \text{ ft/sec})^2}{120 \text{ ft}}$$

$$F = 320 \text{ lb}$$

Centrifugal Force

$$F_r = \frac{mv^2}{r} \text{ or } F_r = \frac{w}{g} \times \frac{v^2}{r}.$$

Example: A 0.5-kg object is traveling in a circular orbit 20 m in diameter at a speed of 2 m/s. The cord is subjected to a force of 0.2 N. What is the centrifugal force on the cord?

$$F_r = \frac{mv^2}{r} = \frac{(0.5 \text{ kg})(2 \text{ m/s})^2}{10 \text{ m}} = 0.2 \text{ N}$$

Since the mass is expressed in kilograms, velocity in meters per second, and distance in meters, the unit of force will be the newton. Note that the diameter of the circle was given, but the radius is required in the equation.

Fluids at Rest
Pressure

$$P = \frac{F}{A} \qquad P = \text{Pressure}$$

$$F = \text{Force}$$

$$A = \text{Area}$$

Example: The end of a pillar of a building has an area of 400 in². The air hammer applies a force of 600 lb as the pillar is driven into the ground. What is the pressure under the pillar?

$$P = \frac{F}{A}$$

$$P = \frac{600 \text{ lb}}{400 \text{ in}^2}$$

$$P = 1.5 \text{ lb/in}^2$$

Example: A man weighs 185 lb; his shoes have a surface area of 13 in², and therefore, the pressure exerted because of his weight is 14 lb/in². The formula to be employed is:

$$P = \frac{F}{A}$$

$$P = \frac{185 \text{ lb}}{13 \text{ in}^2} = 14 \text{ lb/in}^2$$

Density

Density is the mass per unit volume of a substance.

$P = hdg$ P = pressure

h = height

d = density

g = acceleration due to gravity

Example: A tank $10 \times 10 \times 10$ ft is filled with gasoline (weight-density 42 lb/ft³). Weight density $d_w = dg$.

1. Calculate the pressure at the bottom of the tank in lb/ft² and lb/in².

$$P = hd_w$$

$$P = 10 \text{ ft} \times 42 \text{ lb/ft}^3$$

$$P = 420 \text{ lb/ft}^3$$

$$P = \frac{420 \text{ lb/ft}^2}{144 \text{ in}^2/\text{ft}^2}$$

$$P = 2.92 \text{ lb/in}^2$$

2. Calculate the force at the bottom of the tank.

$$P = \frac{F}{A}$$

$$F = PA$$

$$F = (420 \text{ lb/ft}^2)(100 \text{ ft}^2)$$

$$F = 42,000 \text{ lb}$$

Example: Find the pressure due to a column of mercury 100 cm high.

$P = hdg$ h = 100 cm

$P = (100 \text{ cm})(13.6 \text{ g/cm}^3)(980 \text{ cm/s}^2)$ d = 13.6 g/cm³ (given)

$P = 1,330,000 \text{ dynes/cm}^2$ g = 980 cm/s²

Specific Gravity

$$\text{Specific Gravity} = \frac{d}{d_?}$$

d = density of a substance

$d_?$ = density of a standard substance, usually water (d_w)

Example: A metal bar is suspended from a spring scale that reads 300 oz in air and 200 oz when submerged in water.

1. Calculate the specific gravity.

$$\text{Specific Gravity} = \frac{\text{Weight in Air}}{\text{Weight Lost in Water}}$$

$$\text{Specific Gravity} = \frac{300 \text{ oz}}{100 \text{ oz}}$$

$$\text{Specific Gravity} = 3$$

2. Calculate the weight-density of the metal.

$$d_w = 62.4 \text{ lb/ft}^3$$

$$d = \text{Specific Gravity} \times d_w$$

$$d = (3)(62.4 \text{ lb/ft}^3)$$

$$d = 187.2 \text{ lb/ft}^3$$

Buoyancy

Example: A balloon on a transatlantic flight is operating where the weight-density of air is 0.050 lb/ft^3. It weighs 300 lb, has a volume of 8000 ft^3, and is filled with helium, with a d of 0.011 lb/ft^3. What load can it support?

Step 1. $w = Vd$ w = weight
V = volume
d = density
Weight of Air Displaced = 8000 ft^3 × 0.050 lb/ft^3 = 400 lb
Weight of Helium = 8000 ft × 0.011 lb/ft^3 = 88 lb
Weight of Balloon = 300 lb

Step 2. $L = w_a - w_h - w_b$ L = load balloon can support
$L = 400 \text{ lb} - 88 \text{ lb} - 300 \text{ lb}$ w_a = weight of air displaced
$L = 12 \text{ lb}$ w_h = weight of helium
w_b = weight of balloon

The load the balloon can support is 12 lb.

Gravity

All objects in the universe attract each other with a force equal to

$$F_{\text{grav}} = \frac{Gm_1m_2}{r^2}$$

where m_1 and m_2 are the two masses, r is the distance between them, and G is the universal constant of gravitation, equal to 6.67×10^{-11} N · m^2/kg^2.

Example: What is the force of attraction between a 10-metric-ton wrecking ball and a 50-kg man if they are 6 m apart?

$$F = \frac{(6.67 \times 10^{-11} \text{ N} \cdot \text{m}^2/\text{kg}^2)(10 \times 10^3 \text{ kg})(50 \text{ kg})}{(6 \text{ m})^2} = 9 \times 10^{-7} \text{ N}$$

Example: What is the mass of the earth? The force on 1 kg at the surface (6400 km from the center) is 9.8 N.

$$m_2 = \frac{Fr^2}{Gm_1} = \frac{(9.8 \text{ N})(6.4 \times 10^6 \text{ M})^2}{(6.67 \times 10^{-11} \text{ N} \cdot \text{m}^2/\text{kg}^2)(1 \text{ kg})} = 6.0 \times 10^{24} \text{ kg}$$

Temperature Calculations and Measurement

Recall:

	Freezing Point	Boiling Point of Water
Celsius	0°	100°
Fahrenheit	32°	212°
Kelvin	273	373

$$\text{Formulas:} \quad C = \frac{5}{9} \times (F - 32°)$$

$$F = \frac{9}{5}C + 32°$$

Example: A Celsius thermometer records a temperature of 37°C in a patient. What is the temperature on the Fahrenheit scale?

$$F = \frac{9}{5} \times 37° + 32°$$

$$F = 66.6° + 32°$$

$$F = 98.6°F$$

Example: An indoor arena is kept at a temperature of 72°F. What is the corresponding reading on the Celsius scale?

$$C = \frac{5}{9} \times (72° - 32°)$$

$$C = \frac{5}{9} \times 40°$$

$$C = 22°C$$

Absolute Scale: Absolute zero (0 on the Kelvin scale) is the theoretical temperature at which all molecular motion ceases. The Kelvin scale, therefore, has no negative degrees. Celsius temperatures can be expressed on the Kelvin scale ($K = 273 + C$).

Example: 40°C and −40°C can be expressed on the Kelvin scale as follows:

a. $K = 273 + 40$

$K = 313$ K

b. $K = 273 + (-40)$

$K = 233$ K

Heat

Heat is expressed in British thermal units or in calories. One British thermal unit (Btu) is the amount of heat required to raise the temperature of one pound of water one Fahrenheit degree, and one calorie (cal) is the amount of heat necessary to raise the temperature of one gram of water one Celsius degree. One British thermal unit equals about 250 calories.

Specific Heat

Example: How much heat is required to raise the temperature of 10 lb of ethylene glycol (0.528 cal/g · °C or Btu/lb · °F) from 70°F to 140°F?

$$H = (10 \text{ lb})(0.528 \text{ Btu/lb} \cdot °F)(140° - 70°F)$$

$$H = (10 \text{ lb})(0.528 \text{ Btu/lb} \cdot °F)(70°F)$$

$$H = 370 \text{ Btu}$$

Heat Lost = Heat Gained

Example: Five hundred lb of steel at 300°F are cooled in 700 lb of water at 100°F. The temperature obtained in the water is 125°F. Calculate the specific heat of the steel. Remember that the heat lost by the steel equals the heat gained by the water.

$$M_B = \text{weight of first object (steel)}$$

$$S_B = \text{specific heat of first object}$$

$$\Delta t_B = \text{initial temperature of first object}$$
$$- \text{final temperature of first object}$$

$$M_w = \text{weight of second object (water)}$$

$$S_w = \text{unit of heat (1 btu/lb} \cdot °F)$$

$$\Delta t_w = \text{final temperature of second object}$$
$$- \text{initial temperature of second object}$$

$$M_B S_B \ \Delta t_B = M_w S_w \ \Delta t_w$$

$$(500 \text{ lb}) S_B (300°F - 125°F) = (700 \text{ lb})(1.00 \text{ Btu/lb} \cdot °F)(125°F - 100°F)$$

$$S_B = \frac{(700 \text{ lb})(1.00 \text{ Btu/lb} \cdot °F)(25°F)}{(500 \text{ lb})(175°F)}$$

$$S_B = 0.20 \text{ Btu/lb} \cdot °F$$

Heat of Vaporization

Example: How much heat is necessary to change 100 lb of ice at 10°F to steam at 212°F? Ice, 0.51 Btu/lb · °F; heat of fusion of ice, 144 Btu/lb; water, 1.00 Btu/lb · °F; heat of vaporization of water, 970 Btu/lb.

Step 1.   Heat required to raise the temperature of ice to melting point

$$= M_i S_i (32°F - 10°F)$$

$$= (100 \text{ lb})(0.51 \text{ Btu/lb} \cdot °F)(22°F)$$

$$= 1122 \text{ Btu}$$

Step 2.   Heat required to melt ice

$$= (100 \text{ lb})(144 \text{ Btu/lb})$$

$$= 14,400 \text{ Btu}$$

Step 3.   Heat required to bring water to its boiling point

$$= (100 \text{ lb})(1 \text{ Btu/lb} \cdot {}°\text{F})(212° - 32°\text{F})$$

$$= 18,000 \text{ Btu}$$

Step 4.   Heat required to vaporize water

$$= (100 \text{ lb})(970 \text{ Btu/lb})$$

$$= 97,000 \text{ Btu}$$

Step 5.   Total heat required:

$$\begin{array}{r} 1,122 \text{ Btu} \\ 14,400 \text{ Btu} \\ 18,000 \text{ Btu} \\ \underline{97,000 \text{ Btu}} \\ 130,000 \text{ Btu} \end{array}$$

Thermodynamics

Work and Heat

The following conversion values of mechanical energy to heat should be utilized:

$$4.18 \times 10^7 \text{ ergs equals 1 cal}$$
$$4.18 \text{ J equals 1 cal}$$
$$1 \text{ J equals 0.239 cal}$$
$$778 \text{ ft-lb equals 1 Btu}$$
$$1055 \text{ J equals 1 Btu}$$

$$W = J \text{ (constant) } H \quad \begin{array}{l} W = \text{work} \\ J = \text{constant} \\ H = \text{heat} \end{array}$$

Example: Water drops 300 ft over the horseshoe falls at Niagara. Calculate the rise in temperature of the water if its potential energy were converted into heat.

Step 1.   Energy transformed per pound of water

$$= (1.00 \text{ lb})(300 \text{ ft})$$

$$= 300 \text{ ft-lb}$$

Step 2.   Heat produced

$$= \frac{300 \text{ ft-lb}}{778 \text{ ft-lb/Btu}}$$

$$= 0.39 \text{ Btu}$$

Step 3.   Rise in temperature:

Δt = rise (change) in temperature

H = heat change in material

M = mass (1 lb of water)

S = energy or units of work (Btu), or the specific heat of a substance (heat/unit mass-degree change in temperature)

$$\Delta t = \frac{H}{MS}$$

$$\Delta t = \frac{0.39 \text{ Btu}}{(100 \text{ lb})(1.00 \text{ Btu/lb} \cdot {}^{\circ}\text{F})}$$

$$\Delta t = 0.39{}^{\circ}\text{F}$$

Example: A compressed gas at a constant pressure of 75 lb/in^2 enters a cylinder 2 in diameter and pushes a piston 5 in. The work done by the gas is?

$W = P \, \Delta V$ $P = 75$ lb/in^2

$W = (75$ lb/in$^2)(5\pi$ in$^3)$ $\Delta V = \pi r^2 s$

$W = 1200$ in-lb $= \pi (1.0 \text{ in})^2 \times 5$ in

$W = 100$ ft-lb $= 5\pi$ in^3

Efficiency of a Boiler

Recall: The maximum efficiency of a heat engine supplied with heat at temperature T_1 and delivering heat to a reservoir at temperature T_2 can be calculated as follows:

$$E = \frac{T_1 - T_2}{T_1} = 1 - \frac{T_2}{T_1}$$

Example: An engine driven by a boiler receives steam at 300°C. Its exhaust temperature is 100°C. Its efficiency is?

$$E = \frac{T_1 - T_2}{T_1}$$

$$E = \frac{(300 + 273)\text{K} - (100 + 273)\text{K}}{(300 + 273)\text{K}}$$

$$E = \frac{573 \text{ K} - 373 \text{ K}}{573 \text{ K}}$$

$$E = 0.349$$

$$E = 34.9\%$$

Example: A heat engine removes 6000 J per cycle of heat energy from the heat chamber and exhausts 1000 J to a cold chamber.

1. What is the thermal efficiency of the engine?

$$E = 1 - \frac{T_{\text{cold}}}{T_{\text{hot}}} \text{ or } \frac{Q_{\text{cold}}}{Q_{\text{hot}}}$$

$$E = 1 - \frac{1000 \text{ J}}{6000 \text{ J}}$$

$$E = 1 - 0.17$$

$$E = 83\%$$

2. What is the work done by the engine?

$$W = Q_{\text{hot}} - Q_{\text{cold}}$$

$$W = 6000 \text{ J} - 1000 \text{ J}$$

$$W = 5000 \text{ J}$$

Electrostatics

The Electric Force

A positive and a negative charge attract each other; two similar charges repel each other. The force is given by Coulomb's Law:

$$F_{elec} = \frac{kq_1q_2}{r^2}$$

where q_1 and q_2 are electric charges in coulombs (C), r is the distance between them, and k is the electric constant of free space, equal to 9.0×10^9 N·m^2/C^2.

Example: What is the electric force between two plastic spheres, carrying charges of 20 nC and 12 nC, respectively, if they are 15 cm apart?

$$F = \frac{(9.0 \times 10^9 \text{ N} \cdot \text{m}^2/\text{C}^2)(20 \times 10^{-9}\text{C})(12 \times 10^{-9}\text{C})}{(0.15 \text{ m})^2} = 9.6 \times 10^{-5}\text{N}$$

Since the charges are alike, the force is a force of repulsion.

The Quantum of Charge

All electric charges are integral multiples of the charge on an electron, 1.60×10^{-19} C.

Example: How many electrons are there in a charge of 12 nC?

$$\frac{12 \times 10^{-9} \text{ C}}{1.60 \times 10^{-19} \text{ C}} = 7.5 \times 10^{10}$$

Electric Field

A positive charge in an electric field experiences a force in the direction of the field; a negative charge gets a force in the opposite direction. The magnitude of the force is

$$F_{elec} = \mathscr{E}q$$

where $\mathscr{E}$ is the electric field in newtons per coulomb.

Example: How strong an electric field will exert a force of 2.0×10^{-16} N on the electron?

$$\mathscr{E} = \frac{F_{elec}}{q} = \frac{2.0 \times 10^{-16}\text{N}}{1.60 \times 10^{-19}\text{C}} = 1250 \text{ N/C}$$

Example: How strong is the field at a distance of 30 cm from a point charge of 20 μC? The field is the force per coulomb of charge in the field. From Coulomb's law

$$\frac{F}{q} = \frac{kq_1}{r^2} = \frac{(9.0 \times 10^9 \text{ N} \cdot \text{m}^2/\text{C}^2)(20 \times 10^{-6}\text{C})}{(0.30 \text{ m})^2} = 2.0 \times 10^6\text{N/C}$$

which is the electric field strength.

Electric Potential Difference

The electric potential difference between two points in an electric field is the energy change in moving a unit charge from one point to the other. The unit is the joule per coulomb, called a volt (V).

$$V = \frac{E_{elec}}{q}$$

Example: The potential difference between the terminals of an automobile battery is 12 V. If the battery is charged using 1800 J of energy, how much charge is transferred from one terminal to the other?

$$q = \frac{E_{elec}}{V} = \frac{1800 \text{ J}}{12 \text{ V}} = 150 \text{ C}$$

Example: In a uniform electric field of 650 N/C, what is the potential difference between two points that are 20 cm apart in the direction of the field?

1. Determine the force on a coulomb in the field.

$$F = \mathscr{E}q = (650 \text{ N/C})(1 \text{ C}) = 650 \text{ N}$$

2. Determine the work done in moving the charge.

$$W = Fs = (650 \text{ N})(0.20 \text{ m}) = 130 \text{ J}$$

This is the electric energy difference between the points.

3. Determine the potential difference.

$$V = \frac{E_{elec}}{q} = \frac{130 \text{ J}}{1 \text{C}} = 130 \text{ V}$$

Electricity

Ohm's Law

In a metal conductor at constant temperature, the ratio of the voltage to the current is a constant, that is,

$$R \text{ (a constant)} = \frac{V}{I}$$

The constant is called resistance, measured in ohms = volts per ampere.

Example: The difference in potential between two terminals is 10 volts. A current of 5 A passes; calculate the resistance.

$$R = \frac{V}{I}$$

$$R = \frac{10 \text{ volts}}{5 \text{ A}}$$

$$R = 2 \text{ ohms}$$

Example: Increase the difference of the above potential to 20 volts. Calculate the current that passes. Remember that according to Ohm's law, the resistance (R) will remain the same when the voltage is increased—it is constant.

$$I = \frac{V}{R}$$

$$I = \frac{20 \text{ volts}}{2 \text{ ohms}}$$

$$I = 10 \text{ A}$$

Example: A motor needs a current of 8 A and has a resistance of 40 ohms. What voltage is necessary for the operation?

$$V = IR$$

$$V = 8 \text{ A} \times 40 \text{ ohms}$$

$$V = 320 \text{ volts}$$

Example: A 150-watt bulb operates on a potential difference of 110 volts.

1. Calculate the current drawn.

$$P = IV$$

$$I = \frac{P}{V}$$

$$I = \frac{150 \text{ watts}}{110 \text{ volts}}$$

$$I = 1.36 \text{ A}$$

2. Calculate the resistance.

$$V = IR$$

$$R = \frac{V}{I}$$

$$R = \frac{110 \text{ volts}}{1.36 \text{ A}}$$

$$R = 81. \text{ ohms}$$

Example: A current of 10 A flows through a wire for 45 min. The charge that passes through a cross section of the wire may be calculated as follows:

$$I = \frac{q}{t}$$

$$q = It$$

$$q = (10 \text{ A})(2700 \text{ sec})$$

$$q = 27,000 \text{ A} \cdot \text{sec or coulombs}$$

Electric Circuits

Electromotive Force (emf) and Internal Resistance

$$V = E - Ir \qquad$$ V = terminal potential difference
E = no-load potential difference or emf
r = internal resistance
I = current

Example: A battery powering a portable television has an emf of 10 volts and an internal resistance of 0.20 ohm. It supplies a current of 6 A. Calculate the terminal potential difference.

$$V = E - IR$$

$$V = 10 \text{ volts} - (6 \text{ A} \times 0.20 \text{ ohm})$$

$$V = 10 \text{ volts} - 1.2 \text{ volts}$$

$$V = 8.8 \text{ volts}$$

Resistors in Series

Example: A direct-current circuit is wired with resistances of 3 ohms, 6 ohms, and 2 ohms in series. These resistances could be replaced by one resistor of 11 ohms to produce equivalent resistance.

Example: Three lamps are connected in series and exhibit a resistance of 15, 10, and 5 ohms, respectively. How much current is produced by a potential difference of 100 volts across its terminals?

1. Determine the current in the lamp.

$$R = (15 + 10 + 5) \text{ ohms}$$
$$R = 30 \text{ ohms}$$
$$I = \frac{V}{R}$$
$$I = \frac{100 \text{ volts}}{30 \text{ ohms}}$$
$$I = 3.33 \text{ A}$$

2. Determine the voltage across each lamp; it is the product of its resistance and the current.

$$v_1 = (3.33 \text{ A})(15 \text{ ohms}) = 50 \text{ volts}$$
$$v_2 = (3.33 \text{ A})(10 \text{ ohms}) = 33 \text{ volts}$$
$$v_3 = (3.33 \text{ A})(5 \text{ ohms}) = 17 \text{ volts}$$

Resistors in Parallel

$$\frac{1}{R} = \frac{1}{R_1} + \frac{1}{R_2} + \frac{1}{R_3}$$

Recall that addition to a circuit of resistors in series increases the resistance while addition to a circuit of resistors in parallel decreases the resistance.

Example: Using the example of 3, 6, and 2 ohms, the equivalent resistance can be calculated as follows:

$$\frac{1}{R_{eq}} = \frac{1}{R_1} + \frac{1}{R_2} + \frac{1}{R_3}$$
$$\frac{1}{R_{eq}} = \frac{1}{3 \text{ ohms}} + \frac{1}{6 \text{ ohms}} + \frac{1}{2 \text{ ohms}}$$
$$= \frac{2}{6 \text{ ohms}} + \frac{1}{6 \text{ ohms}} + \frac{3}{6 \text{ ohms}} = \frac{6}{6 \text{ ohms}}$$
$$\frac{1}{R_{eq}} = 1 \text{ ohm, OR, } R_{eq} = 1 \text{ ohm}$$

Example: A circuit has resistances of 15, 10, and 5 ohms. If these are wired in parallel what is their combined resistance?

$$\frac{1}{R} = \frac{1}{R_1} + \frac{1}{R_2} + \frac{1}{R_3}$$

$$\frac{1}{R} = \frac{1}{15 \text{ ohms}} + \frac{1}{10 \text{ ohms}} + \frac{1}{5 \text{ ohms}}$$

$$\frac{1}{R} = (0.07 + 0.1 + 0.2) \text{ ohm}$$

$$\frac{1}{R} = 0.37 \text{ ohm}$$

$$R = \frac{1}{0.37} \text{ ohm}$$

$$R = 2.7 \text{ ohms}$$

Example: Find the current in a series circuit with two energy sources ($E_1 = 12$ volts, $E_2 = -4$ volt) and two resistors ($R_1 = 15$ ohms, $R_2 = 10$ ohms).

$$E_1 + E_2 = I_1(R_1 + R_2) \text{ or } V_1 + V_2 = I_1(R_1 + R_2)$$

$$I_1 = \frac{E_1 + E_2}{R_1 + R_2} \text{ or } \frac{V_1 + V_2}{R_1 + R_2}$$

$$I_1 \frac{(12 - 4) \text{ volts}}{(15 + 10) \text{ ohms}}$$

$$I_1 = \frac{8 \text{ volts}}{25 \text{ ohms}} = 0.32 \text{ A}$$

Example: A circuit has three resistors—of 2 ohms, 4 ohms, and 8 ohms.

1. What is the resistance of these three resistors when connected in series?

$$R_s = R_1 + R_2 + R_3$$

$$R_s = (2 + 4 + 8) \text{ ohms}$$

$$R_s = 14 \text{ ohms}$$

2. What is their resistance when connected in parallel?

$$\frac{1}{R_p} = \frac{1}{R_1} + \frac{1}{R_2} + \frac{1}{R_3}$$

$$\frac{1}{R_p} = \frac{1}{2 \text{ ohms}} + \frac{1}{4 \text{ ohms}} + \frac{1}{8 \text{ ohms}}$$

$$\frac{1}{R_p} = \frac{4}{8 \text{ ohms}} + \frac{2}{8 \text{ ohms}} + \frac{1}{8 \text{ ohms}}$$

$$\frac{1}{R_p} = \frac{7}{8 \text{ ohms}}$$

$$R_p = \frac{8}{7} \text{ ohms}$$

3. How much current would be drawn from a 12-volt battery?

SERIES

$$I = \frac{V}{R_s} = \frac{12 \text{ volts}}{14 \text{ ohms}} = 0.857 \text{ A}$$

Potential drop in each resistor:

$$V_1 = IR_1 = (0.857 \text{ A})(2 \text{ ohms})$$

$$= 1.7 \text{ volts}$$

$$V_2 = IR_2 = (0.857 \text{ A})(4 \text{ ohms})$$

$$= 3.4 \text{ volts}$$

$$V_3 = IR_3 = (0.857 \text{ A})(8 \text{ ohms})$$

$$= 6.9 \text{ volts}$$

The drop equals the voltage rise in the battery:

$$V_i = V_1 + V_2 + V_3$$

$$V_i = 12 \text{ volts}$$

PARALLEL

$$I = \frac{V}{R_p} = \frac{12 \text{ ohms}}{8/7 \text{ ohms}} = 10.5 \text{ A}$$

Current in each resistor:

$$I_1 = \frac{V}{R_1} = \frac{12 \text{ volts}}{2 \text{ ohms}} = 6 \text{ A}$$

$$I_2 = \frac{V}{R_2} = \frac{12 \text{ volts}}{4 \text{ ohms}} = 3 \text{ A}$$

$$I_3 = \frac{V}{R_3} = \frac{12 \text{ volts}}{8 \text{ ohms}} = 1.5 \text{ A}$$

$$I_i = I_1 + I_2 + I_3 = 10.5 \text{ A}$$

Cells in Series

Example: Three cells are connected in series; each has an emf of 10 volts and a resistance of 2 ohms. Calculate the current after the combination is connected to an external resistance of 20 ohms.

$$\text{Total emf} = 10 \text{ volts} + 10 \text{ volts} + 10 \text{ volts}$$

$$= 30 \text{ volts}$$

$$\text{Total Resistance } (R) = 2 \text{ ohms} + 2 \text{ ohms} + 2 \text{ ohms} + 20 \text{ ohms}$$

$$= 26 \text{ ohms}$$

$$\text{Total Current} = \frac{\text{Total emf}}{\text{Total Resistance}}$$

$$\text{Total Current} = \frac{30 \text{ volts}}{26 \text{ ohms}}$$

$$\text{Total Current} = 1.15 \text{ A}$$

Cells in Parallel

Example: Consider the following three arrangements:

    a. A single cell
    b. Two cells in series
    c. Two cells in parallel

Compare the currents maintained in a 5-ohm resistor under each condition. Each cell has an emf of 3 volts and negligible internal resistance. The emf of (a) is 3 volts, of (b) 6 volts, and of (c) 3 volts.

$$\text{(a):} \quad I_{total} = \frac{E_{total}}{R_{total}}$$

$$I_a = \frac{3 \text{ volts}}{5 \text{ ohms}}$$

$$I_a = 0.6 \text{ A}$$

$$\text{(b):} \quad I_b = \frac{6 \text{ volts}}{5 \text{ ohms}}$$

$$I_b = 1.2 \text{ A}$$

$$\text{(c):} \quad I_c = \frac{3 \text{ volts}}{5 \text{ ohms}}$$

$$I_c = 0.6 \text{ A}$$

In each cell, however, the current is 0.3 A.

Electric Energy

Joule's Law

$$\text{Voltage} = \frac{\text{Energy}}{\text{Charge}} \qquad V = \text{volts}$$

$$V = \frac{W}{Q} \qquad W = \text{usually in joules}$$

$$\text{OR } VIt = I^2Rt \qquad Q = \text{usually in coulombs}$$

Rewriting $W = VQ$, we can make the substitutions $Q = It$ and $V = IR$. Then, the basic equation for electric energy may be $W = VQ = VIt = I^2Rt$. This equation indicates that one joule must be expended in maintaining for one second a current of one ampere in a circuit of one-ohm resistance.

Example: A motor is used for 45 min to drive a conveyor belt. It uses 35 A at 110 volts. Calculate the electric energy used.

$$W = VIt$$
$$W = (110 \text{ volts})(35 \text{ A})(2700 \text{ sec})$$
$$W = 10,395,000 \text{ J}$$
$$W = 10.4 \times 10^6 \text{ J}$$

Example: How many calories are produced in a central electric resistance heating system in 5 min as it draws 30 A connected to a 220-volt line?

Recall: 1 cal = 4.18 J

$$H = \frac{VIt}{J} \text{ or } H = \frac{W}{J}$$

$$H = \frac{(220 \text{ volts})(30 \text{ A})(300 \text{ sec})}{4.18 \text{ J/cal}}$$

$$H = \frac{1,980,000}{4.18 \text{ J/cal}}$$

$$H = 470,000 \text{ cal}$$

Power and Resistance

Example: The above furnace operating at 220 volts requires 2 hp. What are the current and the resistance of the unit?

1. Current

$$P = 2 \text{ hp} \times 746 \frac{\text{watts}}{\text{hp}}$$

$$P = 1492 \text{ watts}$$

$$P = VI$$

$$1492 \text{ watts} = 220 \text{ volts} \times I$$

$$I = 6.78 \text{ A}$$

2. Resistance

$$R = \frac{V}{I}$$

$$R = \frac{220 \text{ volts}}{6.78 \text{ A}}$$

$$R = 32 \text{ ohms}$$

Alternating Current

Effective Values

In a sine-wave varying current, the average power is half the maximum power. The average power is $I_{rms}^2 R$, where I_{rms} is the root-mean-square, or effective, value of the current.

Example: A sine-wave alternating current with a peak current of 60 A is passing through a resistance of 2.0 Ω. Find the peak power, average power, effective current, and effective potential difference.

1. The peak power is $I_{max}^2 R$:

$$P_{max} = (60 \text{ A})^2 (2.0 \text{ Ω}) = 7200 \text{ W}$$

2. The average power is half the maximum, 3600 W.
3. The effective current produces the average power:

$$I_{rms}^2 R = 3600 \text{ W}$$

$$I_{rms} = \sqrt{\frac{3600 \text{ W}}{2.0 \text{ Ω}}} = 42 \text{ A}$$

4. Effective potential difference:

$$V_{rms} = I_{rms} R = (42 \text{ A})(2.0 \text{ Ω}) = 84 \text{ V}$$

Example: An effective potential difference of 120 V supplies a resistance of 40 Ω. Find the maximum potential difference and current.

1. Maximum is RMS value times the square root of 2:

$$V_{max} = (120 \text{ V})\sqrt{2} = 170 \text{ V}$$

2. Effective current is

$$I_{rms} = \frac{V_{rms}}{R} = \frac{120 \text{ V}}{40 \text{ }\Omega} = 3.0 \text{ A}$$

3. Maximum current is

$$(3.0 \text{ A})\sqrt{2} = 4.2 \text{ A}$$

Machines and Mechanical Advantage

Actual Mechanical Advantage (AMA) $= \dfrac{F_o}{F_i}$,

where F_o = output force and F_i = input force.

Theoretical Mechanical Advantage (TMA) $= \dfrac{d_i}{d_o}$

$$\text{Efficiency } (E) = \frac{F_o/F_i}{d_i/d_o} = \frac{\text{AMA}}{\text{TMA}} = \frac{\text{Output Work}}{\text{Input Work}}$$

Example: A man pushing down with a force of 50 lb lifts a 200-lb crate by utilizing a lever system. The lever arms are 6 and 1.2 ft, respectively.

1. Calculate the AMA.

$$\text{AMA} = \frac{F_o}{F_i}$$

$$\text{AMA} = \frac{200 \text{ lb}}{50 \text{ lb}}$$

$$\text{AMA} = 4$$

2. Calculate the TMA.

$$\text{TMA} = \frac{d_i}{d_o}$$

$$\text{TMA} = \frac{6 \text{ ft}}{1.2 \text{ ft}}$$

$$\text{TMA} = 5$$

3. What is the efficiency?

$$E = \frac{\text{AMA}}{\text{TMA}}$$

$$E = \frac{4}{5} (100\%)$$

$$E = 80\%$$

Example: A car weighing 1500 lb is pushed up a 50-ft ramp exhibiting an incline of 30°. A parallel force of 1000 lb is used to accomplish this task.

1. What is the AMA?

$$AMA = \frac{F_0}{F_i} = \frac{1500 \text{ lb}}{1000 \text{ lb}} = 1.5$$

2. What is the efficiency of the system?

$$TMA = \frac{50 \text{ ft}}{50 \text{ ft sin } 30°}$$

$$= \frac{1}{0.5} = 2$$

$$E = \frac{1.5}{2}$$

$$E = 75\%$$

Simple Harmonic Motion

Period and Frequency

The motion of an oscillating object is described by its:

displacement—distance from central position
amplitude—maximum displacement
period (T)—time for one full cycle
frequency (f)—cycles per unit time. One cycle per second is called a hertz (Hz)

Frequency is the reciprocal of period.

Example: What is the frequency of a vibrating rod that completes each cycle in 1/20 s?

$$f = \frac{1}{T} = \frac{1}{1/20\text{s}} = 20/\text{s} = 20 \text{ Hz}$$

Phase

Phase is the time difference, in fractions of a cycle, between two objects oscillating with the same frequency. One cycle is 360°.

Example: What is the phase difference between two identical pendulums with periods of 1.5 s if one reaches its maximum displacement 0.2 s before the other?

$$\text{Phase difference} = \left(\frac{0.2 \text{ s}}{1.5 \text{ s}}\right)(360°) = 48°$$

Waves

A wave is a system of oscillating particles or fields, in which each point transmits energy to the next point in turn. The next point follows with a slight time delay, so the phase varies continuously.

crest—a point of maximum displacement that appears to travel through the medium
trough—a traveling point of negative maximum displacement
wave velocity—speed of travel of crests and troughs
wavelength (λ, Greek lambda)—distance between successive points in phase.

Frequency, Wavelength and Phase

Wavelength depends on frequency and velocity:

$$v = \lambda f.$$

Example: If a wave in a rope travels at 4.6 m/s and the rope is shaken at one end with a frequency of 2.0 Hz, what is the wavelength of the wave in the rope?

$$\lambda = \frac{v}{f} = \frac{4.6 \text{ m/s}}{2.0/\text{s}} = 2.3 \text{ m}$$

Example: If a 120-Hz wave of vibration in a steel rail travels at 840 m/s, how far apart are two points that are 90° out of phase?

1. Find the wavelength.

$$\lambda = \frac{v}{f} = \frac{840 \text{ m/s}}{120/\text{s}} = 7.0 \text{ m}$$

2. Each phase cycle corresponds to a wavelength, so

$$\frac{90°}{360°} \times 7.0 \text{ m} = 1.75 \text{ m}$$

Interference

When two identical waves arrive simultaneously at a point, their displacements add. If they arrive out of phase, the interference is *destructive,* and a *node,* a point of no vibration, is formed. If they arrive in phase, the interference is *constructive,* and an *antinode,* a point of maximum vibration, develops.

Standing Waves

A standing wave in a string has alternate nodes and antinodes, spaced ¼ wavelength apart.

Example: In the fundamental mode, a string vibrates with a node at each end and an antinode in the middle. What is the frequency of vibration if the string is 25 cm long and the wave in it travels at 390 m/s?

1. Find the wavelength. Since there is a node at each end, the string is a half-wavelength long.

$$\lambda = 2 \times 25 \text{ cm} = 0.50 \text{ m}$$

2. Now find the frequency.

$$f = \frac{v}{\lambda} = \frac{390 \text{ m/s}}{0.50 \text{ m}} = 780 \text{ Hz}$$

Example: At a higher mode, there are 5 antinodes in the string of the preceding problem. What is the frequency at this mode?

1. Find the wavelength. Since there are 2 antinodes in each wavelength, there are 2½ wavelengths in the string.

$$\lambda = \frac{25 \text{ cm}}{2.5} = 10 \text{ cm}$$

2. Find the frequency.

$$f = \frac{v}{\lambda} = \frac{390 \text{ m/s}}{0.10 \text{ m}} = 3900 \text{ Hz}$$

Sound Waves

A vibrating object sets the adjacent air into vibration. This starts a longitudinal wave traveling through the air, a sound wave.

Pitch and Frequency

The *pitch* of the sound is its apparent tonal level, as defined by musical scales. An increase of 1 octave represents doubling the frequency.

Example: When the oboe sounds 440-A, what is the frequency of the tuba, sounding A two octaves lower? One octave lower is 220 Hz, the next octave below is 110 Hz.

In the equal-tempered chromatic scale, each increase of a half tone represents a frequency increase by a factor of $2^{1/12} = 1.05946$.

Example: What is the frequency of high C, which is 3 halftones above A?

$$\text{Frequency} = 440 \text{ Hz} \times 1.05946^3 = 523.2 \text{ Hz}$$

Intensity

The intensity, or loudness, of a sound in bels is the order of magnitude of its energy as compared with the softest audible sound. Thus, 3 bels (B), or 30 decibels (dB), has 10^3 times the zero level.

Example: If a rock band produces sound at 80 dB, how does the intensity of this sound compare with that of the softest audible sound?
The value of 80 dB is 8 B, so the loudest sound has 10^8 times the intensity of 0 B.

Speed of Sound

The speed of a sound wave depends on the nature of the medium in which it travels. It travels faster in liquids than in gases, and much faster in elastic solids. In air, the speed of sound depends on the temperature and can be calculated from the following formula:

$$v_{\text{air}} = 331\frac{m}{s} + 0.6\ T\frac{m}{s \cdot {}^\circ C}$$

Example: How far away is a wall if an echo is received from it 3.9 s after the sound is produced when the temperature is 26°C?

1. Find the speed of sound.

$$v_{\text{air}} = 331\ \frac{m}{s} + \left(0.6\ \frac{m}{s \cdot {}^\circ C}\right)(26{}^\circ C) = 346.6 \text{ m/s}$$

2. Calculate the distance the sound traveled:

$$s = vt = (346.6 \text{ m/s})(3.9 \text{ s}) = 1352 \text{ m}$$

3. Since the sound had to travel both ways, the distance of the wall is half this distance, or 676 m.

Beats

Two sound waves of different frequencies arriving at a point will interfere, alternating constructive and destructive interference. The beat frequency is the difference between the frequencies of the two sounds.

Example: As an orchestra tunes up, the oboe sounds 440-A. If the clarinetist hears 3 beats per second when he plays A, what is the frequency of the clarinet's A?
It could be either 443 Hz or 437 Hz.

Doppler Effect

If a sound source is moving away from an observer, the frequency heard is lower than the frequency emitted, and conversely.

$$f = f_s \frac{v}{v + v_s}$$

where f is the observed frequency, f_s is the frequency of the source, v is the speed of sound, and v_s is the speed of the source as it moves away from the observer.

Example: With the temperature at $-10°C$, a train moving toward the observer at 32 m/s sounds its horn at 380 Hz. What frequency does the observer hear?

1. Find the speed of sound.

$$v = 331 \frac{m}{s} + \left(0.6 \frac{m}{s \cdot °C}\right)(-10°C) = 325 \text{ m/s}$$

2. Apply the formula; v_s is negative because the source is moving toward the observer:

$$f = (380 \text{ Hz}) \frac{325 \text{ m/s}}{(325 - 32)\text{m/s}} = 421 \text{ Hz}$$

Light Rays

Light travels in straight lines (rays) unless deflected by reflection or refraction.

Reflection

In specular reflection, the angle of reflection is equal to the angle of incidence. Angles are measured with respect to the perpendicular to the surface (the normal).

Example: If a light ray strikes a mirror at an angle of incidence of 22°, what is the angle between the incident and reflected rays?

Since the angles are measured from the normal, there are 44° between the incident and reflected rays.

Refraction

When a light ray goes from one medium into another, it will bend. The speeds of light in the two media are proportional to the sines of the angles the rays make with the normal.

Example: A light ray in air enters a piece of glass, in which light travels at 2.20×10^6 m/s. If the angle of incidence is 25°, which is the angle of refraction?

$$\frac{\sin \theta_{glass}}{\sin 25°} = \frac{2.20 \times 10^8 \text{ m/s}}{3.00 \times 10^8 \text{ m/s}}$$

$$\theta_{glass} = 18°$$

Index of Refraction

The index of refraction (n) of a medium is the ratio between the speed of light in vacuum and the speed in the medium.

Example: What is the index of refraction of the glass in the preceding example?

$$n_{glass} = \frac{c}{v_{glass}} = \frac{3.00 \times 10^8 \text{ m/s}}{2.20 \times 10^8 \text{ m/s}} = 1.36$$

Refraction between Two Media

If light passes from medium A to B, or vice versa,

$$\frac{\sin \theta_A}{\sin \theta_B} = \frac{n_B}{n_A}$$

Example: A ray of light passes from crown glass ($n = 1.62$) into water ($n = 1.33$), making an angle of incidence of 40°. What is the angle of refraction?

$$\frac{\sin \theta_{\text{glass}}}{\sin \theta_{\text{water}}} = \frac{n_{\text{water}}}{n_{\text{glass}}}$$

$$\sin \theta_{\text{water}} = \sin 40° \left(\frac{1.62}{1.33}\right)$$

$$\theta_{\text{water}} = 52°$$

Total Internal Reflection

If a ray passes into a medium of higher index of refraction, the calculated angle of refraction may exceed 90°. Then the ray is totally reflected.

Example: What is the largest angle of incidence (the critical angle) at which a ray of light can pass from crown glass into water (constants given above)?

$$\frac{\sin i_c}{\sin 90°} = \frac{n_{\text{water}}}{n_{\text{glass}}} = \frac{1.33}{1.62}$$

$$i_c = 55°$$

Mirrors

Plane Mirrors

In a plane mirror, the image is virtual, erect, the same size as the object, and just as far behind the mirror as the object is in front of it.

Example: The image in a plane mirror of a book is 25 cm high when the book is 50 cm from the mirror. How high is the image if the book is moved to 150 cm?

The answer is 25 cm; the size of the image is always the same as the size of the object.

Convex mirrors

In a convex mirror, the focal length is half the radius of curvature and the image distance obeys the rule

$$\frac{1}{f} = \frac{1}{D_o} + \frac{1}{D_i}$$

where f is focal length, D_o is object distance, and D_i is image distance. The focal length is negative. The image is always erect, virtual, smaller than the object, and behind the mirror.

Example: A convex mirror has a radius of curvature of 60 cm. Where is the image of a lamp that is 180 cm from the mirror?

1. Find the focal length; it is half the radius of curvature, 30 cm.

2. Use the formula to find the image distance.

$$\frac{1}{-30 \text{ cm}} = \frac{1}{180 \text{ cm}} + \frac{1}{D_i}$$

$$\frac{1}{D_i} = \frac{-180 \text{ cm} - 30 \text{ cm}}{(180 \text{ cm})(30 \text{ cm})}$$

$$D_i = -26 \text{ cm}$$

A negative sign indicates that the image is behind the lens. The sizes of the object (S_o) and of the image (S_i) are in the same ratio as the respective distances.

Example: If the lamp in the preceding example is 40 cm tall, how tall is the image?

$$S_i = S_o\left(\frac{-D_i}{D_o}\right) = 40 \text{ cm}\left(\frac{+26 \text{ cm}}{180 \text{ cm}}\right) = +5.8 \text{ cm}$$

The image is virtual.

Concave Mirrors

Focal length is half the radius of curvature and positive. Image is either real, inverted, and in front of the lens, or virtual, erect, and behind the lens.

Example: (Object distance greater than focal length) A convex mirror has a radius of curvature of 80 cm. Find the size and location of the image of a lamp that is 60 cm high and 180 cm from the mirror.

1. Find the focal length; it is half the radius of curvature, −40 cm.
2. Apply the formula to find the image distance.

$$\frac{1}{D_i} = \frac{1}{f} - \frac{1}{D_o} = -\left(\frac{1}{40 \text{ cm}}\right) - \frac{1}{180 \text{ cm}}$$

$$-\left(\frac{(40 \text{ cm})(180 \text{ cm})}{180 \text{ cm} + 40 \text{ cm}}\right) = -33 \text{ cm}$$

3. Set the sizes proportional to the distances.

$$S_i = (60 \text{ cm})\left(\frac{33 \text{ cm}}{180 \text{ cm}}\right) = 11 \text{ cm}$$

Example: (Object distance less than focal length) A can 15 cm high is placed 25 cm in front of the same mirror as above. Find the size and location of the image.

1. Find the image distance.

$$\frac{1}{D_i} = \frac{1}{f} - \frac{1}{D_o} = -\left(\frac{1}{40 \text{ cm}}\right) - \frac{1}{25 \text{ cm}}$$

$$D_i = -\left(\frac{(25 \text{ cm})(40 \text{ cm})}{25 \text{ cm} + 40 \text{ cm}}\right) = -50.4 \text{ cm}$$

The image is behind the mirror.

2. Solve for the size.

$$S_i = (15 \text{ cm})\left(\frac{50.4 \text{ cm}}{25 \text{ cm}}\right) = 14 \text{ cm}$$

The image is virtual.

Lenses

Concave Lenses

Lenses that are thinner in the middle than at the edges form the same kinds of images as convex mirrors. They obey the same equations, and the focal length is negative.

Example: Find the size and location of the image formed in a lens of focal length -40 cm of a book 25 cm high placed 30 cm from the lens.

1. Find the image distance:

$$\frac{1}{D_i} = \frac{1}{f} - \frac{1}{D_o} = \frac{1}{-40 \text{ cm}} - \frac{1}{30 \text{ cm}}$$

$$D_i = \frac{(-40 \text{ cm})(30 \text{ cm})}{(30 \text{ cm}) - (-40 \text{ cm})} = -17 \text{ cm}$$

The negative sign shows that the image is behind the mirror.

2. Find the image size.

$$S_i = S_o\left(\frac{-D_i}{D_o}\right) = (25 \text{ cm})\left(\frac{17 \text{ cm}}{30 \text{ cm}}\right) = 14 \text{ cm}$$

The image is virtual.

Convex Lenses

Lenses that are thicker in the middle than at the edges form the same kinds of images as concave mirrors. They obey the same equations, and the focal length is positive.

Example: (Object distance less than focal length) Find the size and position of the image formed in a $+12.0$-cm lens of a postage stamp 2.4 cm high placed 10.0 cm from the lens.

1. Find the image position.

$$\frac{1}{D_i} = \frac{1}{f} - \frac{1}{D_o} = \frac{1}{12.0 \text{ cm}} - \frac{1}{10.0 \text{ cm}}$$

$$D_i = \frac{(10.0 \text{ cm})(12.0 \text{ cm})}{(10.0 \text{ cm}) - (12.0 \text{ cm})} = -60 \text{ cm}$$

The negative sign shows that the image is in front of the lens.

2. Find the image size.

$$S_i = S_o\left(\frac{-D_i}{D_o}\right) = 2.4 \text{ cm}\left(\frac{60 \text{ cm}}{10.0 \text{ cm}}\right) = 14 \text{ cm}$$

The image is enlarged and virtual.

Example: (Object distance greater than focal length) What focal-length lens is needed to form a real image 35 mm high of a man 2.0 m tall when the man is 1.7 m from the lens?

1. Find the image distance in centimeters.

$$D_i = D_o\left(\frac{S_i}{S_o}\right) = 170 \text{ cm}\left(\frac{3.5 \text{ cm}}{200 \text{ cm}}\right) = 3.0 \text{ cm}$$

The image is real.

2. Find the focal length.

$$\frac{1}{f} = \frac{1}{D_o} + \frac{1}{D_i} = \frac{1}{280 \text{ cm}} + \frac{1}{3.0 \text{ cm}}$$

$$f = \frac{(170 \text{ cm})(3.0 \text{ cm})}{170 \text{ cm} + 3.0 \text{ cm}} = 2.9 \text{ cm}$$

The image is real and small.

Combinations of Lenses

The power of a lens, in diopters, is the reciprocal of its focal length in meters. When lenses are combined, their powers add.

Example: What is the focal length of a combination of a +50-cm convex lens and a −20-cm concave lens?

1. Find the powers of the two lenses.

$$\frac{1}{+0.50 \text{ m}} = +2.0 \text{ diopters} \qquad \frac{1}{-0.20 \text{ m}} = -5.0 \text{ diopters}$$

2. Add the powers.

$$2.0 - 5.0 = -3.0 \text{ diopter}$$

3. Find the focal length.

$$\frac{1}{-3.0 \text{ diopter}} = -0.33 \text{ m, or } -33 \text{ cm}$$

Any number of lenses can be combined in this way.

Composition of the Atom

Subatomic Particles

Recall that the nucleus of an atom is composed of neutrons (no charge) and protons (positive electric charge). The total number of particles equals the mass number; the number of protons equals the atomic number. In an atom, the number of protons equals the number of electrons. The number of neutrons can be found by subtracting the atomic number from the mass number.

Example: How many particles of each type are there in an atom of $^{35}_{17}Cl$?
The atomic number is 17, so the element is chlorine (Cl). There are 17 protons in the nucleus and 17 electrons outside it. The number of neutrons in the nucleus is $(35 - 17) = 18$.

Isotopes

Isotopes of the same element have the same atomic number, but different mass numbers (because of different numbers of neutrons).

Example: Of the following, which are isotopes of the same element?

$$^{65}_{29}Cu \qquad ^{65}_{30}Zn \qquad ^{60}_{29}Cu \qquad ^{60}_{28}Ni$$

There are two isotopes of copper (Cu), both with atomic number 29.

Nuclear Reactions

In any nuclear reaction, the mass numbers and the electric charges must be the same on both sides of the equation.

Example: When aluminum atoms are bombarded with helium nuclei, which isotope is produced along with a neutron?

$$^{27}_{13}Al + ^{4}_{2}He \rightarrow ^{30}_{15}P + ^{1}_{0}n$$

An isotope of phosphorus is produced along with the neutron. The mass numbers are $27 + 4 = 30 + 1$. The electric charge (on the protons) is $13 + 2 = 15 + 0$.

Radioactivity

Large nuclei are unstable and break down, releasing particles and energy. There are two kinds of radioactivity in nature: alpha and beta.

Alpha Decay

In alpha decay, the nucleus releases an alpha particle, which is a nucleus of helium, $^{4}_{2}He$.

Example: What nucleus results from the alpha decay of a nucleus of radon-210?

$$^{210}_{86}Rn \rightarrow ^{4}_{2}He + ^{206}_{84}Po + \gamma$$

The γ (gamma ray) is a high-energy photon, which always accompanies alpha decay. The mass numbers agree: $210 = 4 + 206$. The electric charges agree: $86 = 2 + 84$.

Beta Decay

In beta decay, a neutron emits an electron, turning into a proton. It also produces a chargeless, massless particle called a neutrino.

Example: What is the result of the beta decay of radium-227?

$$^{227}_{88}Ra \rightarrow ^{227}_{89}Ac + ^{0}_{-1}e + \nu$$

Since the electron and the neutrino have negligible mass, there is no change in the mass number; $227 = 227 + 0$. The atomic number increases by 1, and the electric charge balance is $88 = 89 - 1$.

Half-life

The half-life of a nucleus is the time required for half of any given sample to undergo radioactive decay.

Example: The half-life of radon-214 is 2.5 seconds. If a sample of this gas contains 200 g, how much will be left at the end of 10 seconds?

Ten seconds is 4 half-lives, so the mass drops to half 4 times. The amount left will be

$$(200 \text{ g})(0.5)^4 = 13 \text{ g}$$

Example: What is the half-life of a radioactive nucleus if it takes 4 billion years for 40 g to decay down to 10 g?

The mass of the sample has dropped to half twice, so the half-life is 2 billion years.

Nuclear Energy

The mass of a nucleus is less than the sum of the masses of the protons and neutrons that compose it. The difference is called the mass defect of the nucleus, which corresponds to the binding energy ($E = mc^2$).

Units of Measure

The mass of nuclei is measured in atomic mass units, or daltons.

$$6.02 \times 10^{26} \text{ daltons (Dl)} = 1 \text{ kg}$$
$$6.25 \times 10^{18} \text{ electron-volts (eV)} = 1 \text{ J}$$
$$931 \text{ megaelectron volts (MeV)} = 1 \text{ Dl}$$

Example: If the mass defect of a nucleus is 0.0067 D1, how much energy will be needed to separate it into protons and neutrons?

$$0.0067 \text{ D1} \times \frac{931 \text{ Me V}}{\text{D1}} = 6.2 \text{ Me V}$$

Example: If a nuclear reaction yields 6.5×10^{12} J of energy, how much mass disappears?

$$m = \frac{E}{c^2} = \frac{6.5 \times 10^{12} \text{ J}}{(3.0 \times 10^8 \text{ m/s})^2} = 7.2 \times 10^{-5} \text{ kg, or 72 mg}$$

Fusion Reactions

When two small nuclei combine, their binding energy must be released.

Example: How much energy is released when lithium-6 combines with deuterium to form two helium nuclei (deuterium is hydrogen-2)?

1. Write the equation.

$$^6_3\text{Li} + ^2_1\text{H} \rightarrow 2^4_2\text{He}$$

The mass numbers are $6 + 2 = 2 \times 4$. The electric charge numbers are $3 + 1 = 2 \times 2$.
2. Add the nuclear masses on each side of the equation to find the mass deficit.

Li-6: 6.01512 D1
H-2: 2.0140 D1
        8.02912 D1
He-4: 2×4.00260 D1 = 8.00520 D1

The mass deficit is $8.0912 - 8.00520 = 0.0239$ D1.

3. Determine the energy equivalent of the mass deficit:

$$0.0239 \text{ D1}\left(\frac{930 \text{ MeV}}{\text{D1}}\right) = 22 \text{ MeV}$$

Nuclear Fission

When a very large nucleus splits into two medium-sized nuclei, the combined mass of the two fragments is less than the mass of the original nucleus. Thus, energy is released.

Example: When Uranium-235 is split by impact with a slow neutron, how many neutrons are produced?

$$^{235}_{92}\text{U} + ^1_0\text{n} \rightarrow ^{92}_{36}\text{Kr} + ^{141}_{56}\text{Ba} + ?^1_0\text{n}$$

Barium and krypton result. To balance the mass numbers, three neutrons must be produced. These neutrons can split additional uranium nuclei, producing a chain reaction.

Photons

Light has a dual nature; it can be described as a wave or a stream of particles (photons).

Wave Property of Light

As a wave, light obeys the equation

$$c = \lambda f$$

where c is the speed of the wave (3.00×10^8 m/s); λ (lambda) is the wavelength, and f (nu) is the frequency.

Example: What is the frequency of yellow light of wavelength 570 nm (nanometers)?

$$\nu = \frac{c}{\lambda} = \frac{3.00 \times 10^8 \text{ m/s}}{570 \times 10^{-9} \text{ m}} = 5.26 \times 10^{14}/\text{s} = 5.26 \times 10^{14} \text{ Hz}$$

Photon Energy

The energy of a photon obeys the equation

$$E = hf = \frac{hc}{\lambda}$$

where h is Planck's constant, 4.14×10^{-15} eV · s.

Example: What is the energy of a photon of red light with wavelength 730 nm?

$$E = \frac{hc}{\lambda} = \frac{(4.14 \times 10^{-15}\text{eV} \cdot \text{s})(3.00 \times 10^8 \text{ m/s})}{730 \times 10^{-9} \text{ m}} = 1.70 \text{ eV}$$

Photoelectric Effect

A photon may release an electron from a metal surface. The energy of the electron is equal to the energy of the photon minus the work function of the metal.

Example: What is the maximum energy of an electron emitted by a metal whose work function is 2.60 eV if the incident light is ultraviolet with a wavelength of 370 nm?

1. Find the energy of the photon.

$$E = hf = h\frac{c}{\lambda} = \frac{(4.14 \times 10^{-15} \text{ eV} \cdot \text{s})(3.00 \times 10^8 \text{ m/s})}{370 \times 10^{-9} \text{ m}} = 3.36 \text{ eV}$$

2. Subtract the work function of the metal.

$$3.36 \text{ eV} - 2.60 \text{ eV} = 0.76 \text{ eV}.$$

Example: What is the longest wavelength of light that will release an electron from a metal whose work function is 3.61 eV?

The minimum energy of the photon is the work function of the metal, so

$$\lambda = \frac{hc}{E} = \frac{(4.14 \times 10^{-15} \text{ eV} \cdot \text{s})(3.00 \times 10^8 \text{ m/s})}{3.61 \text{ eV}} = 3.4 \times 10^{-7} \text{ m}$$

or 340 nm, in the ultraviolet.

Atomic Energy Levels

The electrons in the outer shells of an atom can be raised from ground state to excited states in quantized steps.

Spectra

When an electron falls to a lower energy state, it loses a definite amount of energy by emitting a photon having that energy. The spectrum of the light emitted by a substance contains only photons of certain definite energies.

Example: What is the wavelength of the light emitted when an electron drops from a 4.70-eV excited state to a 3.22-eV state?

1. The energy of the photon is 4.70 eV − 3.22 eV = 1.48 eV.

2. The wavelength of the photon is

$$\lambda = \frac{hc}{E} = \frac{(4.14 \times 10^{-15} \text{ eV} \cdot \text{s})(3.00 \times 10^8 \text{ m/s})}{1.48 \text{ eV}} = 8.39 \times 10^{-7} \text{ m}$$

which is the wavelength of an infrared photon, at 839 nm.

Spectrum of Atomic Hydrogen

The single electron of a hydrogen atom occupies quantum states which can be represented by the expression $-13.6 \text{ eV}/n^2$, where n is any whole number.

Example: What is the wavelength of a photon that is emitted when a hydrogen electron drops from the fifth to the second state?

1. Find the energy levels of the two states.

$$\frac{-13.6 \text{ eV}}{2^2} = -3.40 \text{ eV} \qquad \frac{-13.6 \text{ eV}}{5^2} = -0.54 \text{ eV}$$

2. Subtract to get the energy of the photon.

$$-0.54 \text{ eV} - (-3.40 \text{ eV}) = 2.86 \text{ eV}$$

3. Find the wavelength of the photon:

$$\lambda = \frac{hc}{E} = \frac{(4.14 \times 10^{-15} \text{ eV} \cdot \text{s})(3 \times 10^8 \text{ m/s})}{2.86 \text{ eV}} = 4.34 \times 10^{-7} \text{ m}$$

Example: What is the wavelength of a photon that will ionize a hydrogen atom in its ground state?

1. The energy needed is enough to raise the total energy level to zero:

$$0 - \frac{(-13.6 \text{ eV})}{1^2} = 13.6 \text{ eV}$$

2. Calculate the wavelength of this photon:

$$\lambda = \frac{hc}{E} = \frac{(4.14 \times 10^{-15} \text{ eV} \cdot \text{s})(3.00 \times 10^8 \text{ m/s})}{13.6 \text{ eV}} = 9.1 \times 10^{-8} \text{ m or 91 nm}$$

Mathematics Review

An understanding of basic mathematical skills is essential for the science and quantitative skills test questions. This section reviews the most important mathematical concepts that may be present in these tests. This presentation does not attempt to cover all areas in great depth. Rather, it should be used in conjunction with texts so that the student will be prepared for mathematically oriented test questions.

Arithmetic

Operations on Numbers

Whole numbers are the counting numbers, 1, 2, 3, 4, 5, . . . *Integers* are the positive and negative whole numbers and zero: . . . , −3, −2, −1, 0, 1, 2, 3, . . . A *mixed number* consists of an integer combined with a fraction, for example, 3⅛. Many questions call for rounding off an answer "to the nearest integer." To round off a mixed number to the nearest integer, drop the fraction part of the number; if the fraction part is ½ or more than ½, increase the integer by 1; if the fraction part is less than ½, keep the original integer. For example, 4⅞ rounded off to the nearest integer is 5, but 3⅓ rounded off to the nearest integer is 3.

Questions often require that decimal answers be rounded off to some specified degree of precision, for example, to the nearest tenth, or to the nearest hundredth, or to the nearest thousandth. To answer such a question, drop all digits in the decimal which are to the right of the specified digit; if the first digit dropped is 5 or more, increase the last digit retained by 1; if the first digit dropped is less than 5, keep the last digit retained at its present value. As examples, 81.698 rounded to the nearest tenth is 81.7; 81.698 rounded to the nearest hundredth is 81.70 (note that the zero is retained to show a hundredths place); 45.639 rounded to the nearest tenth is 45.6.

The rules for rounding off decimals also apply to rounding off whole numbers to a specified degree of precision. For example, 102,681 rounded off to the nearest thousand is 103,000; 102,681 rounded off to the nearest hundred is 102,700; 49,294 rounded off to the nearest thousand is 49,000.

Precision and Significant Digits

All measurements are approximate. Consider a measurement said to be 43 grams to the nearest gram. The unit of measure is the smallest unit indicated by the number and is the unit which was applied in the measurement. In the illustration, the unit is the gram and the maximum possible error is one-half that unit. Thus 43 grams to the nearest gram means the true measure is between 43 ± 0.5 grams. A measure of 28½ feet means that the unit of measure is ½ foot and the maximum error is therefore ¼ foot. A measure of 28½ feet could represent a true measure of anywhere between 28¼ feet and 28¾ feet. A measurement of 2.05 inches means that the unit of measure is 0.01 inch (that is, ¹⁄₁₀₀ of an inch), and the 2.05 may represent a true measure anywhere between 2.045 and 2.055 inches.

If an approximate number is multiplied by some number greater than 1, the precision of the result is reduced since the maximum error is also multiplied by that number. If the approximate measure of 28½ feet, which has a maximum error of ¼ foot, is multiplied by 5, the result is 5 × 28½ or 142½ feet with a maximum error of 5 × ¼ or 1¼ feet. Thus, the 142½ foot approximation really represents a measure anywhere between 141¼ feet and 143¾ feet.

If an approximate number is represented as a decimal, every digit starting from the left-most non-zero digit and extending through the digit which represents the unit of measure is a *significant digit*. Thus, 2345 has 4 significant digits, 23.45 also has 4 significant digits, 0.00023 has 2 significant digits, and 2300 may have either 2, 3 or 4 significant digits depending on whether the two zeroes represent accurate measures in the tenths and units places or are merely used as "fillers" to locate the decimal point. Note that the position of the decimal point has nothing to do with the number of significant digits. The speed of light is 186,272 mi/sec; this figure has 6 significant digits; if we talk about the speed of light being 186,000 mi/sec., the figure has only 3 significant digits.

Performing mathematical operations on approximate numbers cannot increase the number of significant digits. If two approximate numbers are multiplied together or divided, you should carry out the multiplication or division and then round off your answer to the number of significant digits in the number with the *fewest* significant digits. Note that in the case of multiplication and division, the position of the decimal point has nothing to do with the number of significant digits in the answer. The situation in addition and subtraction is very different. If 231.2 is added to 15.623, the sum becomes 246.823, but digits beyond 246.8 are not significant since 231.2 was accurate to the nearest tenth only. Thus, in adding or subtracting approximate numbers, you should first carry out the operation and then round the answer to the first place where the *last* significant digit of any of the numbers is found. Note also that if 231.2 had been added to 15.673, the sum would first be 246.873, which would be rounded off to 246.9.

Percent and Percentage

Problems involving percent actually involve three quantities: the base, the percent (or rate), and the percentage. The *percent* (expressed as a decimal such as .20 or as a part of 100 such as 20%) is the ratio of one quantity (the percentage) to another (the base). The number of which the percent is taken is the *base*; the result after the percent of the base is taken is the *percentage*. For example, of we say that 40% of the 2000 bacteria in a certain culture are spirochetes, then there are 800 spirochetes present in the culture. 40% or .40 is the percent or rate, 2000 is the base, and 800 is the percentage. The best way to solve any problem involving percent or percentage is with an equation based on the formula $p = br$, that is, percentage equals base times rate. Thus, if asked to find what percent of the 2000 bacteria in a culture is represented by the 800 spirochetes, the equation $800 = 2000r$ is solved. If asked to find the number of bacteria in a culture in which 800 spirochetes are known to represent 40%, the equation $800 = b(.40)$ is solved. If asked to find how many spirochetes there are in a culture containing 2000 bacteria of which 40% are spirochetes, the equation $p = 2000(.40)$ is used.

Algebra

Ratio and Proportion

Ratio: A comparison of two values that are expressed in the same units. It may be expressed as an indicated division or as two numbers separated by a colon.

Example: A comparison of the length of two insects might be expressed as 2 cm:3 cm, that is, as 2:3 or as $\frac{2 \text{ cm}}{3 \text{ cm}}$, that is, as $\frac{2}{3}$. Note that in each case, the name of the units cancels and the ratio consists of two pure numbers, 2:3 or $\frac{2}{3}$. The units involved must be the same, however; the ratio of 3 inches to 2 yards is not 3:2, but 3 inches to 72 inches, that is 3:72 or $\frac{3}{72}$ or $\frac{1}{24}$.

Proportion: A statement that two ratios are equal. For example, 1:2 = 4:8 or $\frac{1}{2} = \frac{4}{8}$ represents a proportion.

The first and last terms of a proportion are called the *extremes* and the second and third terms of a proportion are called the *means*. In the proportion $\frac{1}{2} = \frac{4}{8}$, 1 and 8 are the extremes and 2 and 4 are the means. A most important relation used to solve problems involving proportions is this: In any proportion, the product of the means equals the product of the extremes.

Example: If two substances, A and B, are to be mixed in the ratio of 2 parts of A to 3 parts of B, how many milliliters of A must be mixed with 15 milliliters of B to make the proper mixture?

Let x = the number of milliliters of A.

Since the ratio of A to B equals the ratio $2:3$, a proportion is formed:

$$\frac{x}{15} = \frac{2}{3}$$

In a proportion, the product of the means equals the product of the extremes (cross multiply):

$$3x = 2(15)$$
$$3x = 30$$
$$x = 10$$

If the means in a proportion are equal, either of the means is called the *mean proportional* between the two extremes. Thus, in the proportion $\frac{1}{3} = \frac{3}{9}$, 3 is the mean proportional between 1 and 9.

Example: Find the mean proportional between 4 and 16.

If x is the mean proportional, then:

$$\frac{4}{x} = \frac{x}{16}$$

In a proportion, the product of the means equals the product of the extremes (cross multiply):

$$x^2 = 4(16)$$
$$x^2 = 64$$

Take the square root of both sides of the equation: $x = \pm 8$.

Note that every positive number has two square roots, one positive and one negative. In a practical problem, one of the roots (usually the negative one) may have to be rejected as meaningless (for example, if x represents a length).

Equations

Equations Containing Fractions: These are solved by multiplying all terms on both sides of the equation by the Least Common Denominator of all the fractions.

Example: Find a if $\frac{a}{4} - \frac{a}{6} = \frac{1}{2}$.

The least common denominator for 4, 6, and 2 is 12. Multiply all terms on both sides of the equation by 12:

$$12\left(\frac{a}{4}\right) - 12\left(\frac{a}{6}\right) = 12\left(\frac{1}{2}\right)$$
$$3a - 2a = 6$$
$$a = 6$$

Quadratic Equations: Second-degree equations may often be solved by factoring.

Example: Solve $2x^2 + 5x = 3$.

Rewrite the equation so that all terms are on one side in descending order of exponents, equal to 0:

$$2x^2 + 5x - 3 = 0$$

The quadratic trinomial on the left factors into two binomials. The factors of the first term, $2x^2$, become the first terms of the binomials:

$$(2x \quad)(x \quad) = 0$$

The factors of the last term, -3, become the second terms of the binomials, but they must be chosen in such a way that the product of the inner terms added to the product of the outer terms equals the middle term of the original trinomial, $+5x$. Try -1 and $+3$ as the factors of -3:

$$-x = \text{inner product}$$
$$(2x - 1)(x + 3) = 0$$
$$6x = \text{outer product}$$

Since $(-x) + (6x) = +5x$, these are the correct factors:

$$(2x - 1)(x + 3) = 0$$

Set each factor equal to zero:

$$2x - 1 = 0 \quad \text{OR} \quad x + 3 = 0$$
$$2x = 1 \qquad\qquad x = -3$$
$$x = \frac{1}{2}$$

The solution is $x = \frac{1}{2}$ or -3.

If a quadratic equation cannot be solved by factoring, the *quadratic formula* may be used: In a quadratic equation of the form $ax^2 + bx + c = 0$,

$$x = \frac{-b \pm \sqrt{b^2 - 4ac}}{2a}$$

Example: Solve $x^2 - 4x - 3 = 0$
Here $a = 1$, $b = -4$ and $c = -3$:

$$x = \frac{-(-4) \pm \sqrt{(-4)^2 - 4(1)(-3)}}{2(1)}$$

$$x = \frac{4 \pm \sqrt{16 + 12}}{2}$$

$$x = \frac{4 \pm \sqrt{28}}{2}$$

$$x = \frac{4 \pm \sqrt{(4)(7)}}{2}$$

$$x = \frac{4 \pm 2\sqrt{7}}{2}$$

$$x = 2 \pm \sqrt{7}$$

Radical Equations: Equations in which the variable appears under a radical sign. They may be solved by isolating the radical on one side of the equation and then squaring both sides.

Example: Solve $\sqrt{x^2 - 8} - x = 4$

Isolate the radical on one side of the equation:

$$\sqrt{x^2 - 8} = x + 4$$

Square both sides of the equation:

$$x^2 - 8 = (x + 4)^2$$
$$x^2 - 8 = x^2 + 8x + 16$$
$$-8 - 16 = 8x$$
$$-24 = 8x$$
$$-3 = x$$

The process of squaring may introduce an *extraneous root;* therefore, radical equations solved by squaring must always have the solution(s) checked to see if any are extraneous; checking must be done by substituting in the *original* equation:

$$\sqrt{(-3)^2 - 8} - (-3) \stackrel{?}{=} 4$$
$$\sqrt{9 - 8} + 3 \stackrel{?}{=} 4$$
$$1 + 3 \stackrel{?}{=} 4$$
$$4 \; ? \; 4 \surd$$

-3 is a true root.

Equations Containing Decimals: Such equations are best solved by removing all decimals by multiplying each term in the equation by the highest power of 10 that will remove all the decimals:

Example: Solve $153 + 0.085x = 0.85x$

Multiply each term by 1000:

$$153,000 + 85x = 850x$$
$$153,000 = 850x - 85x$$
$$153,000 = 765x$$
$$200 = x$$

Formulas

Questions may be asked requiring you to transform a given formula so that it is solved for a specified variable in terms of the others. This is accomplished in the same manner as the solution of a literal equation; the specified variable must be isolated on one side of the equation with all terms not containing this variable on the other side.

Example: The formula for obtaining the Fahrenheit temperature, F, when the Celsius temperature, C, is known is $F = \frac{9}{5}C + 32$. Find an expression for C in terms of F.

To solve for C, first multiply both sides by 5:

$$5F = 9C + 160$$

Isolate the term containing C on the right side:

$$5F - 160 = 9C$$

Divide both sides by 9:

$$\frac{5F - 160}{9} = C$$

Factor out a 5 in the numerator:

$$\frac{5(F - 32)}{9} = C$$

In another form:

$$C = \frac{5}{9}(F - 32)$$

Scientific Notation

Scientific notation is a method of writing a number as the product of a power of 10 and a decimal number whose whole number part is between 1 and 10. For example, 3.6903×10^4 is in scientific notation. Scientific notation is a convenient method for designating very large or very small numbers. It is particularly useful when only a small number of significant digits are used in the number. For example, the speed of light is said to be 186,000 mi/sec. The only significant digits are "186" since the three zeroes are merely used to indicate the placement of the decimal point. The speed of light is expressed more meaningfully in scientific notation as 1.86×10^5 mi/sec. Scientific notation makes the number easier to handle and also makes it clear that the zeros are not significant digits.

Questions may involve conversion from scientific notation to ordinary notation or vice versa. Since multiplication by 10 results in moving the decimal point one digit to the right, the number 1.25×10^4 becomes 12,500 in ordinary notation (the decimal point is moved 4 places to the right). Similarly, 10 raised to a negative exponent indicates division by 10 that many times. Division by 10 results in moving the decimal point to the left one place. Thus, 1.25×10^{-2} is equivalent to 0.0125 in ordinary notation. 81,250 in ordinary notation becomes 8.125×10^4 in scientific notation, and 0.002728 becomes 2.728×10^{-3}.

Exponents and Logarithms

Positive Exponents: A positive exponent is a number which indicates the number of times a quantity is to be used as a factor in a power. For example, 2^4 means (2)(2)(2)(2) or 16.

Zero Exponents: By definition $x^0 = 1$ for all values of x except $x = 0$, which is undefined. Thus, $5^0 = 1$ and $(-3)^0 = 1$.

Negative Exponents: By definition, $x^{-n} = \frac{1}{x^n}$ provided $x \neq 0$. Thus, $3^{-2} = \frac{1}{3^2} = \frac{1}{9}$.

Fractional Exponents: By definition $x^{m/n} = \sqrt[n]{x^m}$ or $(\sqrt[n]{x})^m$ provided $n \neq 0$. Thus, $x^{1/2} = \sqrt{x}$, and $8^{2/3} = (\sqrt[3]{8})^2 = 2^2 = 4$.

Law of Exponents:

For multiplication:	$(x^a)(x^b) = x^{a+b}$	Example: $y^3 \cdot y^4 = y^7$
For division:	$x^a \div x^b = x^{a-b}$	Example: $y^6 \div y^2 = y^4$
For powers:	$(x^a)^b = x^{ab}$	Example: $(y^2)^3 = y^6$
For roots:	$\sqrt[b]{x^a} = x^{a/b}$	Example: $\sqrt{y^6} = y^3$

Exponential Equations: An exponential equation is an equation in which the variable appears in an exponent. Simple exponential equations may be solved by expressing both sides of the equation as powers of the same base.

Example: Solve $3^{x-1} = 9$

Express both sides of the equation as powers of the same base, in this case, 3:

$$3^{x-1} = 3^2$$

Since the bases are the same, the exponents must be equal:

$$x - 1 = 2$$

$$x = 2 + 1$$

$$x = 3$$

If it is impossible to express both sides of the equation as powers of the same base, logarithms must be used to solve an exponential equation (see next section).

Logarithms: The logarithm of a number is the exponent to which a given base must be raised to produce the number. The given base for *common logarithms* is 10.

Thus, $\log_{10} 100 = 2$ since $10^2 = 100$

$\log_{10} 10{,}000 = 4$ since $10^4 = 10{,}000$

$\log_{10} 50 = 1.6990$ since $10^{1.6990} = 50$

$\log_{10} 10 = 1$ since $10^1 = 10$

In writing common logarithms, the base, 10, is generally omitted. Thus, we say $\log 100 = 2$, $\log 10{,}000 = 4$, $\log 50 = 1.6990$, and $\log 10 = 1$.

Of course, $\log 50 = 1.6990$ cannot be found readily. Like all common logarithms, it consists of two parts. The whole number part, or *characteristic,* is positive and is 1 less than the number of digits before the decimal point if the number is 1 or greater. Thus, the characteristic for $\log 839$ would be 2. If the number is a positive number less than 1, the characteristic is negative and its absolute value is 1 more than the number of zeroes between the decimal point and the first significant digit. Thus, the characteristic for $\log 0.0072$ would be -3.

The *mantissa,* or decimal part of the logarithm, is found in the Table of Common Logarithms. The mantissa is always positive and is the same for the same sequence of significant digits. Thus, the mantissas for 365, 36.5, and 0.0365 are the same. The mantissa for $\log 50$ is found by looking for the sequence of digits, 500; the table shows the mantissa for this sequence to be .6990. The characteristic for $\log 50$ is 1, so $\log 50 = 1.6990$. Since the mantissa is always positive and the characteristic may be negative, the log for a number such as 0.00372 must be written as $7.5705 - 10$.

Interpolation: If we have a Table of Common Logarithms that provides entries for numbers with a sequence of only 3 digits, we must interpolate to find a mantissa of a number having 4 significant digits. To find the mantissa for $\log 183.6$, we look for the mantissa for the sequence 183 (it is .2625) and for the mantissa for the sequence 184 (it is .2648). Since 1836 lies between 1830 and 1840, its mantissa will lie at a proportionate distance between their mantissas.

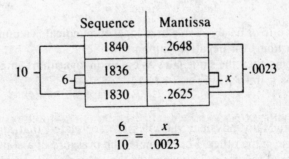

$$\frac{6}{10} = \frac{x}{.0023}$$

The product of the means equals the product of the extremes (cross multiply):

$$10x = 6(.0023)$$

$$10x = .0138$$

$$x = .00138 \text{ or } .0014$$

Mantissa for $\log 1836$ is $.2625 + .0014 = .2639$

Log 183.6 is 2.2639 since the characteristic for 183.6 is 2.

Laws of Logarithms: Since logarithms are exponents, they obey the the same laws of exponents:

For multiplication: $\log (ab) = \log a + \log b$
  Example: $\log 8 = \log (4 \cdot 2) = \log 4 + \log 2$

For division: $\log \left(\dfrac{a}{b}\right) = \log a - \log b$

  Example: $\log \left(\dfrac{12}{4}\right) = \log 12 - \log 4$

For powers: $\log a^n = n \log a$
  Example: $\log 2^3 = 3 \log 2$

For roots: $\log \sqrt[n]{a} = \dfrac{1}{n} \log a$

  Example: $\log \sqrt{5} = \dfrac{1}{2} \log 5$

Solving Exponential Equations by Logarithms:

Example: Solve for x: $3^x = 17$.
Since both sides cannot be written as powers of the same base, take logarithms of both sides of the equation:

$$x \log 3 = \log 17$$

$$x(0.4771) = 1.2304$$

$$x = \frac{1.2304}{0.4771}$$

The solution is completed by dividing 1.2304 by 0.4771.

Natural or Naperian Logarithms: Common logarithms use the base 10. In more advanced mathematics and in many scientific applications, it is more effective to use logarithms with a base called the natural number and represented by e; e is approximately 2.718. Logarithms using the base e are called natural or Naperian logarithms and are designated by ln. Thus, in $100 = 4.605$ since $e^{4.605} = 100$

$$\ln 10,000 = 9.210 \quad \text{since } e^{9.210} = 10,000$$

$$\ln e = 1.000 \quad \text{since } e^1 = e$$

$$\ln 1 = 0 \quad \text{since } e^0 = 1$$

Using either base 10 or base e, a negative logarithm indicates a number between 0 and 1. There are no logarithms for negative numbers.

Natural logarithms obey the same laws as common logarithms since both are exponents. For example, $\ln 65 = \ln (5 \cdot 13) = \ln 5 + \ln 13$.

Variation

Direct Variation: Many physical variables are so related that an increase in one will produce an increase in the other. For example, the pressure of a confined gas will increase as the temperature of the gas is increased. If the values of two variables bear a constant ratio to each other, they are said to be in direct variation; sometimes it is said that "y varies as x" or "y varies directly with x." Direct variation can be expressed in symbols as $\dfrac{y}{x} = k$ or $y = kx$, where k is called the constant of variation.

Example: If the work done, y, by a constant force varies directly as the distance, d, through which the force acts, and if $y = 16$ when $x = 3$, find y when $x = 9$.
Use the formula $y = kx$. Substitute 16 for y and 3 for x:

$$16 = 3k$$

Solve for k, the constant of variation:

$$\frac{16}{3} = k$$

Since k is a constant, substitute the new value of x in $y = \frac{16}{3}x$:

$$y = \frac{16}{3}(9)$$

$$y = 48$$

Inverse Variation: In many sciences, two variables are related so that their product is constant; when one gets larger, the other gets smaller. In an electrical circuit of constant voltage, for example, the product of the current and the resistance is constant. Current and resistance are said to vary inversely. Inverse variation involves a relationship of the form $xy = k$ or $y = \frac{k}{x}$, where k is the constant of variation.

Example: The volume, y, of a gas at a constant temperature is inversely proportional to the pressure, x. If $y = 30$ when $x = 2$, find y when $x = 12$.

Substitute in $xy = k$ to find the constant, k:

$$(2)(30) = k$$

$$60 = k$$

Since k is a constant and equal to 60, now substitute 12 for x in $xy = 60$:

$$12y = 60$$

$$y = 5$$

Joint Variation: Some physical phenomena involve the variation of more than two variables. If y varies directly with both x and z, then the basic relationship may be expressed as $y = kxz$. If y varies directly with x but inversely as the square of z, then the basic relationship may be expressed as $y = \frac{kx}{z^2}$.

Trigonometry and the Right Triangle

The Pythagorean Theorem

Many problems involving right triangles can be solved by use of the Pythagorean Theorem, which states that in any right triangle, the square of the length of the hypotenuse equals the sum of the squares of the lengths of the legs. In the diagram shown, where a and b are the lengths of the legs and c is the length of the hypotenuse, $a^2 + b^2 = c^2$. Thus, if the lengths of any two sides of a right triangle are known, the length of the third side can be found.

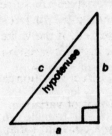

Example: If the hypotenuse of a right triangle is 7 feet, and the length of one leg is 4 feet, find the length of the other leg.

If b is the length of the other leg, apply the Pythagorean Theorem:

$$4^2 + b^2 = 7^2$$

$$16 + b^2 = 49$$

$$b^2 = 49 - 16$$

$$b^2 = 33$$

Take the square root of both sides of the equation:

$$b = \pm \sqrt{33}$$

Reject the negative value as meaningless for a length:

$$b = \sqrt{33}$$

Pythagorean Triples

Certain special cases result in right triangles in which the ratio of the lengths of the sides can be represented by integers. They are the 3-4-5, 5-12-13, and 8-15-17 right triangles. Note that in every case the largest number in the triple represents the hypotenuse; the other two represent the legs. These triples should be committed to memory as they make the solutions of many right triangles extremely easy.

Example: Find the remaining leg of a right triangle whose hypotenuse is 15 and one of whose legs is 12.

The hypotenuse, 15, is equal to 3 times 5 and the leg, 12, is equal to three times 4. Hence the triangle is a 3-4-5 right triangle with all the values multiplied by 3. The remaining leg is three times 3 or 9.

45°-45°-90° and 30°-60°-90° Triangles

The MCAT includes questions that may require knowledge of the relationships among the sides of two special right triangles, the 45°-45°-90° triangle and the 30°-60°-90° triangle. The relationships can all be determined by use of the Pythagorean Theorem and certain facts from plane geometry, but it is recommended that the student commit to memory the two diagrams below and use the values shown as formulas to apply in solving either of these special triangles.

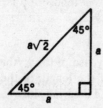 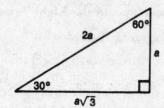

Example: Find the leg of an isosceles right triangle whose hypotenuse is $5\sqrt{2}$.

An isosceles right triangle is a 45°-45°-90° triangle. Applying the formulas from the diagram above, the hypotenuse is $a\sqrt{2}$:

$$a\sqrt{2} = 5\sqrt{2}$$

$$a = 5$$

From the diagram above, the length of a leg is a:

$$\text{leg} = 5$$

Example: If the hypotenuse of a 30°-60°-90° triangle is 6, find the length of the leg opposite the 30° angle and the length of the leg opposite the 60° angle.

The formula for the hypotenuse of a 30°-60°-90° triangle is $2a$:

$$2a = 6$$

$$a = 3$$

The formula for the leg opposite 30° is a:

$$a = 3$$

The formula for the leg opposite 60° is $a\sqrt{3}$:

$$a\sqrt{3} = 3\sqrt{3}$$

Trigonometric Functions

The three basic trigonometric functions are defined for acute angles from ratios in a right triangle:

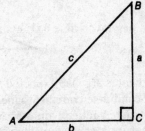

$$\sin A = \frac{\text{opposite side}}{\text{hypotenuse}} = \frac{a}{c}$$

$$\cos A = \frac{\text{adjacent side}}{\text{hypotenuse}} = \frac{b}{c}$$

$$\tan A = \frac{\text{opposite side}}{\text{adjacent side}} = \frac{a}{b}$$

A convenient way to remember these definitions is by memorizing the mnemonic *soh-cahtoa*. Split into three parts, *soh,cah,toa,* where "*s*" stands for sine, "*o*" for opposite, "*h*" for hypotenuse, etc., the mnemonic gives all three definitions. Note that sin is an abbreviation for sine, cos for cosine, and tan for tangent. When any 2 parts from among the two acute angles and the three sides of a right triangle are known, any of the other parts can be found.

Example: In the right triangle shown, find the length of side $\overline{EG}$.

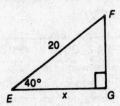

$\overline{EG}$ is the side adjacent to the 40° angle and 20 is the hypotenuse. Hence the cosine is used:

$$\cos 40° = \frac{\text{adjacent leg}}{\text{hypotenuse}}$$

From the Table of the Values of Trigonometric Functions, $\cos 40° = 0.7660$:

$$0.7660 = \frac{x}{20}$$

Multiply both sides of the equation by 20:

$$20(0.7660) = x$$

$$15.32 = x$$

A student taking the MCAT will be expected to know the sines and cosines of 0°, 90°, and 180°. These are shown in tabular form below:

	0°	90°	180°
sin	0	1	0
cos	1	0	−1
tan	0	∞	0

The sines, cosines, and tangents of 0° and 90° are deduced from consideration of what happens as angle A in the diagram of $\triangle ABC$ collapses toward 0°. BC will approach 0, and thus the sin 0° and the tan 0° will both be 0. As angle A collapses, the hypotenuse $\overline{AB}$ will approach $\overline{AC}$, and hence $\dfrac{AB}{AC}$ will equal 1 at 0°, or cos 0° = 1. The values for 90° are deduced in a similar manner; those for 180° are the result of an extension of the definitions of the trigonometric functions to values beyond the acute angles found in a right triangle.

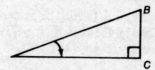

MCAT candidates are also expected to know the sines, cosines, and tangents of 30°, 45°, and 60°. If the candidate commits to memory the formulas for the sides as recommended in the section of this book on the 45°-45°-90° triangle and the 30°-60°-90° triangle, these values need not be memorized since they can be obtained by applying the definition of the sine, cosine, or tangent to the expressions in the formulas. For example, sin 45° = $\dfrac{\text{opposite side}}{\text{hypotenuse}} = \dfrac{a}{a\sqrt{2}} = \dfrac{1}{\sqrt{2}}$. The value $\dfrac{1}{\sqrt{2}}$ can be used for sin 45° or it can be changed to $\dfrac{1}{2}\sqrt{2}$, obtained by multiplying numerator and denominator by $\sqrt{2}$. As another example, cos 60° = $\dfrac{a}{2a} = \dfrac{1}{2}$. For the convenience of those candidates who would prefer to memorize the values of the sine, cosine, and tangent of 30°, 45°, and 60°, a table of these values is also given here:

	30°	45°	60°
sin	$\dfrac{1}{2}$	$\dfrac{1}{2}\sqrt{2}$	$\dfrac{1}{2}\sqrt{3}$
cos	$\dfrac{1}{2}\sqrt{3}$	$\dfrac{1}{2}\sqrt{2}$	$\dfrac{1}{2}$
tan	$\dfrac{1}{3}\sqrt{3}$	1	$\sqrt{3}$

Systems of Measurement

The MCAT candidate will be expected to understand and operate in either the metric system of measurement or in the system of common British units. It may be required to perform conversions from one system to the other, but in all such cases, the conversion factor will be supplied with the question.

The Common British System

The following equivalences and abbreviations should be known:

1 yard (yd) = 3 feet (ft) = 36 inches (in)
1 foot = 12 inches
1 mile (mi) = 5280 feet = 1760 yards
1 pound (lb) = 16 ounces (oz)
1 ton (T) = 2000 pounds
1 gallon (gal) = 4 quarts (qt) = 8 pints (pt)
1 quart = 2 pints
1 pint = 16 fluid ounces (oz)

This table of equivalences permits conversions within the British system.

Example: How many ounces are there in 3 tons?

$$3 \cancel{\text{tons}} \times \frac{2000 \cancel{\text{lbs}}}{\cancel{\text{ton}}} \times \frac{16 \text{ oz}}{\cancel{\text{lb}}}$$

$$3 \times 2000 \times 16 \text{ oz} = 96{,}000 \text{ oz}$$

Note that names of units which appear once in a numerator and a denominator are cancelled. For example, tons ÷ tons = 1 and lbs ÷ lbs = 1. This leaves only the name of the units in which the answer is denoted.

Balancing Equations Containing Physical Units: The preceding comment on cancelling the names of units in an equation points up the importance of balancing the names of units on both sides of an equation that deals with physical units.

Example: Given that the distance, d, that a body falls if dropped from rest is $\frac{1}{2}$ the acceleration due to gravity, a, times the time, squared, t^2, find the distance in meters that a body will drop in 3 minutes.

The given equation is:

$$d = \frac{1}{2} at^2$$

We cannot substitute 16 ft/sec^2 for a, or 3 min for t and expect to get a distance in meters because the units involved will not balance:

$$d(\text{meters}) \neq \frac{1}{2} \cdot \frac{16 \text{ ft}}{\text{sec}^2} (60 \text{ min})^2$$

Since 1 min = 60 sec, we can replace (60 min)^2 by $(60)^2$(sec)^2, and since 1 ft = 0.3 meter, we can replace 16 ft by 16(0.3 meter):

$$d(\text{meters}) = \frac{1}{2} \cdot \frac{16(0.3 \text{ meter})}{\text{sec}^2} (60)^2(\text{sec})^2$$

Cancelling names of units wherever possible shows that both sides of the equation are in meters only:

$$d(\text{meters}) = \frac{1}{2} \cdot \frac{16(0.3 \text{ meter})}{\cancel{\text{sec}^2}} (60)^2\cancel{(\text{sec})^2}$$

If the units in an equation cannot be balanced in this way, it is an indication that there is an error somewhere in the equation.

The Metric System

The basic units for the metric system are:

For length: meters (abbreviated m)
For volume: liters (abbreviated l or L)
For mass: grams (abbreviated g)

The following prefixes are attached to the names of the basic units to denote other units whose size equals the basic unit multiplied or divided by a power of 10:

pico (p) = 10^{-12}
nano (n) = 10^{-9}
micro (μ) = 10^{-6}
milli (m) = 10^{-3}
centi (c) = 10^{-2}
deci (d) = 10^{-1}

$$\text{deka (da)} = 10$$
$$\text{hecto (h)} = 10^2$$
$$\text{kilo (k)} = 10^3$$
$$\text{mega (M)} = 10^6$$

Thus, a kilometer (km) is 10^3 or 1000 times as large as a meter. A centimeter (cm) is 10^{-2} times a meter or $\frac{1}{100}$ the size of a meter. A milligram (mg) is 10^{-3} times the size of a gram or $\frac{1}{1000}$ the size of a gram.

Conversions may be made within the metric system simply by moving the decimal point. Thus, 53 cm = 0.53 m (since a meter is 10^2 centimeters). Similarly, 8.3 kg = 8300 g (since a kilogram is 10^3 grams).

Elementary Probability

The probability of an event occurring $= \dfrac{\text{the number of favorable cases}}{\text{the total possible number of cases}}.$

For example, the chance of a tossed coin landing heads up is $\frac{1}{2}$ or 0.5, since there is 1 favorable case, heads, out of a total possible number of 2 cases, either heads or tails. The probability of drawing a king on a single draw from a pack of 52 cards is $\frac{1}{13}$. The number of favorable cases is 4 (there are 4 kings) and the total possible number of cases is 52; $\frac{4}{52} = \frac{1}{13}$.

The probability of two or more independent events occurring is the product of their separate probabilities. Thus, the probability of tossing 3 coins and having them all land heads up is $\left(\frac{1}{2}\right)\left(\frac{1}{2}\right)\left(\frac{1}{2}\right) = \left(\frac{1}{2}\right)^3 = \frac{1}{8}$ or 0.125.

If a coin has been tossed 3 times and has landed heads up each time, what is the probability that a fourth toss will result in a head? The answer is still $\frac{1}{2}$ since the fourth result is not affected by the three previous cases (it is said that "coins and cards have no memory"). The probability that all of four tossed coins will land heads up is $\left(\frac{1}{2}\right)\left(\frac{1}{2}\right)\left(\frac{1}{2}\right)\left(\frac{1}{2}\right) = \left(\frac{1}{2}\right)^4 = \frac{1}{1} = 0.0625.$

In a medical situation, suppose that a patient requires ear surgery for which the success rate is 90%. Note that this is equivalent to saying that the probability of success is $\frac{9}{10}$ or 0.9. If the patient requires surgery on both ears, what is the probability of a successful outcome for both?

$$(0.9)(0.9) = 0.81 = 81\%$$

Note that in these calculations, the assumption has been made that the events are independent, that is, that one event does not influence another. Thus, it is assumed that the surgical patient is a normal patient and that success of surgery on one ear does not make success on the other ear more or less probable.

In a compound probability situation, be sure to examine the number of favorable cases and the total possible number of cases for each of the separate situations.

Example: What is the probability of drawing 2 blue marbles from a bag containing 4 red and 6 blue marbles if the first marble is not replaced before the second one is drawn?

The probability of drawing a blue marble on the first draw is $\frac{6}{10}$. But since this first blue marble is not replaced, there are now only 5 blue marbles in the bag out of a total of only 9 marbles. Therefore, the probability of drawing a blue marble on the second draw is

$\frac{5}{9}$. The probability of the two events occurring one after the other is $\frac{6}{10} \times \frac{5}{9}$ or $\frac{30}{90}$ or $\frac{1}{3}$.

Statistics

Some Measures of Central Tendency

Suppose you are asked to examine the fasting blood glucose concentrations of several patients in a hospital and obtain the results in mg/dl as 100, 80, 100, 90, 100, 120, and 125.

The *range* (the distance between the extreme values) is from 80 to 125, or 45.

The *mode* (the most common value in the series) is 100.

The *arithmetic mean* or *average* is the sum of all the values divided by the number of values:

$$\frac{100 + 80 + 100 + 90 + 100 + 120 + 125}{7} = 102.1$$

The *median* (the middle value when they are arranged in order of size) is 100 since arrangement in order of size gives 80, 90, 100, 100, 100, 120, 125, and the middle number is 100. If there were an even number of items in the series, there would be no single middle number; in such a case, the median is taken as the value half way between the two middle values.

The Standard Deviation

The standard deviation is a statistical measure that indicates the dispersion or spread of the values in a set of data. You will not be expected to calculate it on the MCAT, but you must be able to interpret it. In the previous illustration, the standard deviation is 15.8. You should know that in a normal distribution, 68% of the values will fall within the arithmetic mean ± 1 standard deviation, and 96% of the values will fall within the arithmetic mean ± 2 standard deviations. Thus, in the example shown, 68% of the values would be expected to lie between 102.1 − 15.8 or 86.3, and 102.1 + 15.8 or 117.9. The fact that only 4 out of the 7 values fall in this range $\left(\frac{4}{7} = 57.1\%\right)$ is due to the sample being so small. 96% of the values would be expected to fall between 102.1 − 31.6 or 70.5, and 102.1 + 31.6 or 133.7. Actually, all 7, that is 100% of them, do so.

Correlation

Suppose two variables change at random. The *coefficient of correlation* is a statistical measure of the degree to which the variation in one imitates the variation in the other. On the MCAT, you will not be expected to calculate a coefficient of correlation, but you will be expected to understand the nature of this measure.

The coefficient of correlation may have values between −1 and +1 inclusive; for example, values of +.86 or −.23 are typical. A correlation of +1 is a perfect positive correlation; the two variables involved move up and down together although they may be measured in different units and the moves may be of different magnitudes. A correlation of −1 is a perfect negative correlation; the variables involved move at the same times and to the same degree but in opposite directions (one decreases when the other increases). A correlation of 0 means that there is no relation between the variations in the two.

The output of a factory and its direct costs would tend to move together to some degree; hence the correlation between these two could be expected to be positive although not nearly as great as +1. It is usally true that the higher the price, the lower the sales; if there is a price increase, sales tend to drop; hence price and sales can be expected to be negatively correlated.

The three graphs below represent "scatter diagrams" obtained by plotting random readings of two variables, *x* and *y*. Graph *A* shows no association between *x* and *y* and hence the correlation would probably be close to 0. Graph *B* shows a generally negative correlation (*y* decreases when *x* increases), and Graph *C* shows a positive correlation.

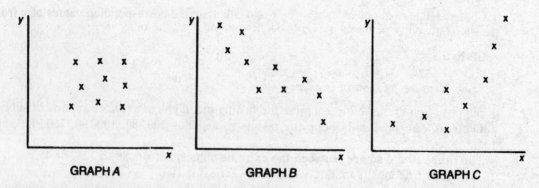

GRAPH A   GRAPH B   GRAPH C

Graphic Representation of Data and Functions

Medical and other scientific publications use graphic representation of data and of algebraic functions to make relationships clear and also to deduce other information from such a representation.

The Rectangular or Cartesian Coordinate System

This system permits the location of any point on a plane with reference to two perpendicular axes whose point of intersection is called the *origin*. The horizontal axis is the x-axis, and the vertical axis is the y-axis. The position of a point is specified by an ordered pair of numbers in parentheses, for example, (4,3), which are called the *coordinates* of the point. The x-coordinate, also called the *abscissa*, is always written first, and the y-coordinate, also called the *ordinate*, is second. The abscissa is the distance measured horizontally from the y-axis and the ordinate is the distance measured vertically from the x-axis to the point. In the diagram, P is the point (4,3), Q is the point (−2,5), and R is the point (−3,−6).

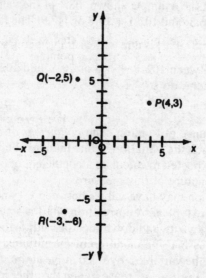

A first degree equation in two variables has an infinite number of pairs of values of x and y which satisfy it. These points may be plotted on a graph to represent the equation. A first degree equation always has a graph which is a straight line.

Example: Draw the graph of $x + 4y = 8$.

Solve the equation for y in terms of x:

$$4y = -x + 8$$

$$y = -\frac{1}{4}x + 2$$

Choose some convenient values for x and calculate the corresponding values of y from the equation:

x	-4	0	8
y	3	2	0

Plot the points $(-4,3)$, $(0,2)$, and $(8,0)$ and draw a straight line through them. This line is the graph of $x + 4y = 8$.

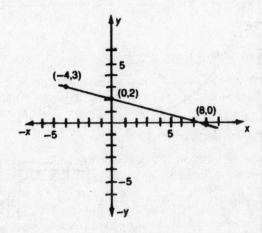

Slope of a Line: If Δy represents the change in the y-values from one point to another and Δx represents the change in the x-values of these two points, then the slope, m, of the line joining the two points is defined as $m = \dfrac{\Delta y}{\Delta x}$. If the coordinates of the two points are represented by (x_1, y_1) and (x_2, y_2), then the slope may also be defined as $m = \dfrac{y_2 - y_1}{x_2 - x_1}$. The slope is the rate of change of y with respect to x.

Example: Find the slope of the first two points plotted to draw the graph of the line $x + 4y = 8$ in the section preceding this. These are the points $(-4,3)$ and $(0,2)$.

Let $(-4,3)$ be (x_1,y_1) and $(0,2)$ be (x_2,y_2). Then $y_2 - y_1$ or Δy is $2 - 3$ or -1, and $x_2 - x_1$ or Δ_x is $0 - (-4)$ or 4. $m = \dfrac{-1}{4}$: The slope is $-\dfrac{1}{4}$.

The Slope-Intercept Form of a Straight Line: In the last example, notice that the slope of the line is $-\dfrac{1}{4}$ and that $-\dfrac{1}{4}$ (or m) is also the coefficient of x in the equation

$$y = -\frac{1}{4}x + 2.$$

The constant term $+2$, which we denote by b, is the y-intercept, that is, the value of y where the graph crosses the y-axis. By solving the equation of a line for y, we can put it in the form $y = mx + b$, which tells us immediately the slope and y-intercept of the line. For example, the line $y = \dfrac{2}{3}x - 4$ has a slope of $\dfrac{2}{3}$ and a y-intercept of -4. This information can be used to draw the graph of the equation instead of plotting points. Begin with the y-intercept (at the point $[0,-4]$), and move 3 units to the right and 2 units up to locate the next point on the line; continue this process for more points on the line.

Graphs of equations other than first degree do not appear as straight lines. The graphs of such equations may be drawn by preparing a table of corresponding values of x and y (obtained by substitution in the equation). These values are used to plot points whose coordinates they are; joining the points with a smooth curve produces the graph representing the equation. Figure 1 shows the graph of the equation $xy = 12$. An equation of the form $xy = k$ where k is a constant is a relationship between two variables that are *inversely proportional;* this type of relationship and its characteristic graph is common to many natural physical phenomena. Figure 2 illustrates the graph of $y = 2^x$ which is an *exponential function;* an exponential function and its characteristic graph is common in many medical and scientific areas, such as the growth of bacteria in a culture or the decay of a radioactive substance. The graphs in both Figures 1 and 2 approach certain lines but never actually reach them; such lines are called *asymptotes.* In Figure 1, both the x- and y-axes are asymptotes; in Figure 2, the x-axis is an asymptote.

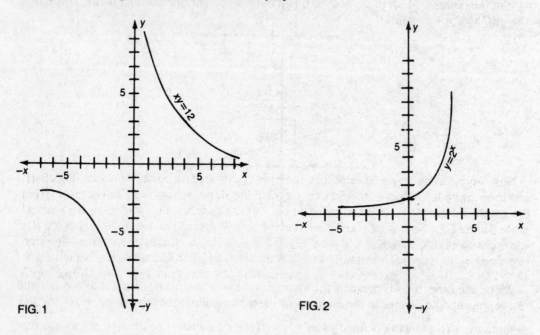

FIG. 1   FIG. 2

Finding the Equation from a Graph

Suppose that readings from experiments are taken on two variables, say blood clotting time and the quantity administered of a certain anti-clotting substance. If these data are used as coordinates of points plotted on a rectangular coordinate chart, and if the points turn out to lie in a straight line, then we know that we can represent the relationship between the two variables by a first degree algebraic equation. In fact, we can write the equation; all we need do is read the value of the y-intercept, b, from the graph and figure the slope, m, by noting the Δy and the Δx between two of the points; substituting the values of m and b in the slope-intercept form, $y = mx + b$, gives the equation.

But suppose that points plotted from experimental data readings do not lie in a straight line. Then the equation of the graph is not a first degree equation. To find out what it is, we use other types of coordinate systems. Two of those that are especially useful with the types of equations and graphs common in medicine and other sciences are the semi-log scale and the log-log scale.

Semi-log Graphs: The rectangular coordinate system uses scales on the x- and y-axes that are arithmetic, that is, the distances on the scale from 0 to 1, from 1 to 2, from 2 to 3, etc., are always the same. The semi-log coordinate system uses an x-axis that has an arithmetic scale, but the distances from the origin along the y-axis represent the values of the logarithms of the numbers instead of the numbers themselves. Thus, the y-axis scale begins at 1 (since log 1 = 0). Since log 10 = 1 and log 100 = 2, the distance on the scale from 1 to 10 is the same as the distance from 10 to 100. It is also the same as the distance from 100 to 1000, etc.

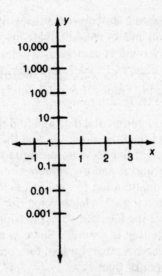

Now suppose that experimental data readings are plotted as points on a semi-log chart, and they turn out to lie in a straight line. Reading the slope, m, and the y-intercept, b, from the graph will enable us to write an equation, but the variable represented on the vertical scale will be log y instead of y and the intercept, b, will actually be log b. Note that log b is some constant. The equation will then be log $y = mx + \log b$. Since the common logarithm is defined as the exponent to which 10 must be raised to give the number, we can write $y = 10^{mx + \log b}$. Thus we have found an exponential function from the data plotted on a graph.

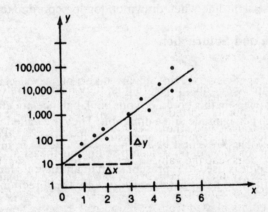

Example: The graph above, drawn on semi-log coordinate paper, shows a line obtained by plotting a scattering of points from experimental data. Find the equation of the line.

Read the y-intercept, b, from the graph: $b = \log 10 = 1$. Calculate the slope, m:

$$m = \frac{\Delta y}{\Delta x} = \frac{\log 1000 - \log 10}{3 - 0} = \frac{3 - 1}{3} = \frac{2}{3}$$

Using the slope-intercept form of the straight line, $y = mx + b$:

$$\log y = \frac{2}{3}x + 1$$

Since log y is the exponent to which 10 must be raised to equal y:

$$y = 10^{2/3x + 1}$$

Note that although for simplicity this discussion involves a y-axis scale which is for common logs (base 10), semi-log scales used in medicine could be scaled for natural logarithms (base *e*).

Log-log Graphs: In semi-log graphs, the x-axis has an arithmetic scale and the y-axis has a scale that is logarithmic. In log-log graphs, both the x-axis and y-axis have scales that are logarithmic.

Suppose we plot points from experimental data and find that they lie in a straight line on a log-log chart. As before, we can read the slope, *m*, and the y-intercept, *b*, and use them in the $y = mx + b$ form of the straight line to write the equation. However, the variables are now log y and log x instead of y and x, and the value we read for the y-intercept is actually log b. Thus, we can write an equation, $\log y = m \log x + \log b$. Making use of the laws of logarithms, $m \log x = \log x^m$, and $\log x^m + \log b = \log (bx^m)$. Thus, our equation becomes $\log y = \log (bx^m)$. Since we have the logs of two expressions equal, the expressions themselves are equal. Thus, our equation is $y = bx^m$. Since *m* may be any positive or negative integer or even a fraction, we have a powerful tool for converting data readings into complicated equations of degree greater than 1.

A first degree equation in two variables can always be rewritten in the form $y = mx + b$, and its graph is *always* a straight line on rectangular coordinate graph paper. The MCAT candidate should know that one type of exponential equation is of the form $y = a^{bx + c}$, where *a, b,* and *c* are constants, and that its graph is *always* a straight line when drawn on semi-log coordinate paper. In scientific work the "*a*" of $y = a^{bx + c}$ is frequently equal to *e*, the natural number, and *c* is frequently equal to 0, so that the most common form of an exponential equation in medicine or other sciences is $y = e^{bx}$.

MCAT candidates should also know that an equation of the form $y = ax^n$ where *a* and *n* are constants and *n* may be positive, negative, or a fraction, is known as a power law; its graph is *always* a straight line when drawn on log-log coordinate paper.

Vector Addition and Subtraction

Vectors

Most quantities are *scalar* quantities, that is, they have magnitude only. The length of a line, the number of pages in this book, or your bank balance are all scalar quantities. Some quantities have both a magnitude and a direction. They are called *vector* quantities. Examples are a wind velocity of 15 mph in an easterly direction, a downward (vertical) water pressure of 20 lb/in², or the motion of a ship sailing northeast at 23 knots. A directed line segment called a *vector* is used to represent such quantities; its length represents the magnitude of the quantity and its orientation represents the direction.

Vector Addition

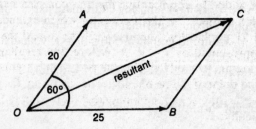

Suppose that two forces, one of 20 lb and one of 25 lb act simultaneously on a body at an angle of 60° to each other. We may represent the 20 lb force by vector $\overrightarrow{OA}$ and the 25 lb force by the vector $\overrightarrow{OB}$. Complete the parallelogram of which $\overrightarrow{OA}$ and $\overrightarrow{OB}$ are two sides. The diagonal of the parallelogram, $\overrightarrow{OC}$, is a vector which is called the sum of the vectors $\overrightarrow{OA}$ and $\overrightarrow{OB}$. $\overrightarrow{OC}$ is also called the *resultant* of the two vectors, $\overrightarrow{OA}$ and $\overrightarrow{OB}$, and $\overrightarrow{OA}$ and $\overrightarrow{OB}$ are the *components* of the force represented by $\overrightarrow{OC}$. If the object on which forces $\overrightarrow{OA}$ and $\overrightarrow{OB}$ are acting is free-moving, the object will move in the direction represented by $\overrightarrow{OC}$ and with a force whose magnitude is represented by the length of $\overrightarrow{OC}$.

If it is desired to compute the magnitude of $\overrightarrow{OC}$ in the above example, $\triangle OBC$ must be solved. Since $AOBC$ is a parallelogram, $BC = OA = 20$, and $\angle B \stackrel{\triangle}{=} 120°$. By the Law of Cosines, $(OC)^2 = (OB)^2 + (BC)^2 - 2(OB)(BC)\cos \angle B$. All the quantities on the right side of the equation are known, so $(OC)^2$, and hence $\overrightarrow{OC}$, can be calculated.

Questions on the MCAT involving vector addition could involve simpler cases than the above, usually those in which the two component forces are at right angles to each other.

Example: Find the resultant force and the angle it makes with the larger component, if two component forces, one of 10 lb and one of 20 lb, act at 90° to each other.

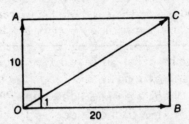

Draw vectors representing the two forces and complete the parallelogram of which they are sides. The diagonal of this parallelogram, which comes from their common origin, is the resultant or sum of the two forces. Vector $\overrightarrow{OC}$ is the resultant. In right $\triangle OBC$, $OB = 20$ and $CB = OA = 10$. By the Pythagorean Theorem, $(OC)^2 = 20^2 + 10^2$ or $(OC)^2 = 400 + 100$; since $(OC)^2 = 500$, $OC = \sqrt{500}$ or $10\sqrt{5}$. In right triangle OBC, $\tan \angle 1 = \dfrac{\text{opposite leg}}{\text{adjacent leg}} = \dfrac{10}{20} = \dfrac{1}{2} = 0.5000$. From the Tables of Trigonometric Functions, the angle whose tangent is 0.5000 is 27° to the nearest degree, so the resultant makes a 27° angle with the larger component.

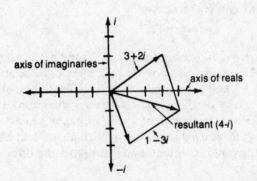

Vectors may also be added by representing them as complex numbers. The vector represented by the complex number $3 + 2i$ is the vector which extends from the origin to the point representing $3 + 2i$ graphically. Suppose we wish to add the vector represented by $3 + 2i$ to the vector represented by $1 - 3i$. As before, the resultant can be drawn as the diagonal of the parallelogram formed by using the two given vectors as sides. The complex number which is the end point of the resultant can be read from the graph; it represents the resultant vector. However, the sum can be obtained more simply by adding the two complex numbers algebraically:

$$\begin{array}{r} 3 + 2i \\ 1 - 3i \\ \hline 4 - i \end{array}$$

The resultant is $4 - i$.

Subtraction of Vectors

To subtract one vector from another, we simply add the additive inverse of the vector to be subtracted. If the complex number representation of the vectors is used, this simply means that the signs of the vector being subtracted are changed and the resulting complex number is then added to the other vector. If the parallelogram method is used, the vector being subtracted is replaced by a vector of the same magnitude but extending in the opposite direction. This new vector is then added to the other vector by forming a parallelogram and finding the diagonal which is the resultant (see diagram).

SUBTRACTING $\vec{OB}$ FROM $\vec{OA}$

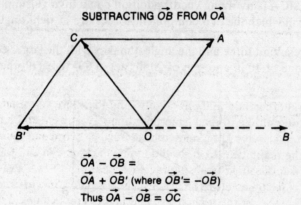

$\vec{OA} - \vec{OB} =$
$\vec{OA} + \vec{OB}'$ (where $\vec{OB}' = -\vec{OB}$)
Thus $\vec{OA} - \vec{OB} = \vec{OC}$

Verbal Reasoning— Test-Taking Strategies

This portion of the book will focus on various techniques to help you get the most out of reading.

You can learn to read efficiently and effectively, and the more you read the better you will read. People who do not like to read generally do not read well, and most people who do not read well read too slowly. They read almost word by word and must consequently backtrack to capture the main idea. You should read as fast as you can think without the loss of comprehension, misreading or losing facts or ideas.

Learning to read rapidly takes effort, willpower and a plan. Success depends on your interest and the effectiveness of the techniques and habits you acquire. Find the time for the activities that are necessary for academic success: first things first!

A great deal of your success depends on your frame of mind. You must develop confidence in your own ability. Believe in yourself. You have been successful in the past and will be successful in the future. Confidence comes with knowledge, experience and practice.

In the MCAT Examination, reading skill or verbal reasoning is assessed by presenting to the examinee one or more paragraphs of material. The selection is followed by a variable number of questions pertaining to it. Subjects from a wide variety of areas are used to test the student's ability to analyze data accurately. The information necessary to answer the questions is in the selection, and no prior knowledge is necessary to arrive at a correct answer.

Approach to the Reading Questions

There is no one correct way to handle this section. Some people routinely read the selection first, and some read the questions first. With either approach, rapid processing of information and maximum retention are key elements. The techniques of underlining (described later in this chapter) are useful here.

If you prefer to read the selection first, use the underlining technique to highlight the details. When you finish the selection, you should immediately move on to the questions and answer them one by one while the information is still fresh in your mind.

Some people read the questions first since they feel that they have better attention to details when they know what to expect. If you choose this approach, you read the passage with specific questions in mind. Then you can either answer the questions as a group when you have finished the passage, or answer the questions as the answers appear in the selection. Whichever way you proceed, we still advocate the underlining method. If you have to go back later, the material is already grouped and easier to work with. This will make backtracking more efficient.

Do not, however, leave questions blank in the hope of returning to them later. This could be costly since rereading the entire passage may require a great deal of time. (In the knowledge sections of the examination this is not a problem because the questions are units in themselves and not based on paragraphs.) Answer all questions as best you can, marking those you are not certain of for checking if you have time at the end. Please remember that you must base your answers on the material presented in the passage, not on your own knowledge or experience.

Quantitative questions should be approached in the same way as Reading questions. The only difference is that the information is presented in tables, graphs, charts, maps and other

204 • VERBAL REASONING

quantitative forms instead of straight prose. The student's ability to read and analyze the material is tested by the questions. There is no single perfect approach to this type of material. However, it is important to be sure you know what each number, axis, line or graph means before proceeding to answer the questions. Make sure that you are aware what information has been presented, what the limitations of the data are and what reasonable conclusions may be drawn from it. Do not base your answer on information that isn't there.

Ways and Means

Reading experts seem to agree that the rapid reader's comprehension is usually excellent, and the slow reader's comprehension is usually poor. This does not mean that the rapid reader never slows down for difficult material. It does mean that the rapid reader is able to find the right speed for the material, while the slow reader habitually reads more slowly than the occasion or subject matter demands.

Word-by-Word Reading: Word-by-word reading does not improve comprehension and makes concentration more difficult. Understanding and comprehension demand that you read groups of words, or ideas. As you read, you must analyze, think, group ideas and topics, spot relationships, and see similarities and differences in the passage. The word-by-word reader sees only the trees and misses the forest.

Backtracking: Most readers backtrack occasionally. This technique is not only acceptable but also part of efficient reading. All of us look back and reread a word or several words now and then. The good reader, however, does it less frequently than the poor reader. The efficient reader basically looks back only when he needs to, while the slow reader does it mechanically and out of habit. The inefficient reader usually reads most words, phrases, sentences and paragraphs more than once since he often misses the central idea or meaning the first time. The first time through, he has merely read the words and must therefore reread the selection to see how they are connected. The habit of reading single words rather than groups usually keeps you from grasping the central theme. Grouping words, sentences, and paragraphs as you go along allows you to make sense of the material and to focus on the theme and idea.

Pausing and Stopping: Inefficient readers usually allow long and frequent pauses as they proceed. This not only hinders concentration but also makes it difficult to absorb the ideas presented. If you pause after reading only a few sentences, you lose track of the author's train of thought. You may remember certain details, but the connections get lost.

Quick Skimming to Elicit the General Theme: This technique involves reading rapidly and concentrating on the key words and phrases that develop and support the theme. One might think that in this approach, the main point could be missed; however, nothing could be further from the truth. This is purposeful reading for comprehension, since its object is to grasp the central point and carefully note the key elements that support that point.

Key Words That Announce Conditions and Should Be Kept in Focus!

1. again, also, accordingly, just as
2. therefore, thus, hence, henceforth
3. for example, for instance, in other words
4. nevertheless, however, notice, but
5. always, at all times, under all circumstances, every time
6. finally, in conclusion, in brief, at last
7. never, not, no, none
8. only, specifically, significantly, importantly, decidedly
9. first, another, and, likewise, as well as, besides
10. despite, although, regardless

How is Material Usually Organized?

1. Most selections have a *central subject* (main idea) which could be used as the *title*. In many instances, the first sentence of a paragraph will tell you this main idea.
2. The material is usually presented in a fashion that answers a question, poses one, gives a solution, or gives a non-committal statement of fact.
3. Key words and facts should substantiate and solidify the main idea of the reading. These are the details. Always look for key words. If you go back and read the key words, you should be able to get the essence of the passage.
4. The details are usually of two types. The main details are directly related to the central theme, and are used to develop it. The subordinate details break down and clarify the main details, to further develop the theme. Breaking the material down this way can help you to understand it.
5. Read in a questioning manner. This will ensure that you are actively involved. Ask *who, what, when* and *where* to elicit key elements. Ask *how* and *why* to determine reasons.

Suggested Method for Efficient Analysis of Reading Material

1. Identify the topic or main theme and underline it with a *straight* line.
2. Find the main details about the topic and underline the key words or phrases with a curved line.
3. As you read the subordinate details about the details bracket them with (curved brackets).
4. Extraneous elements or qualifiers should be bracketed with [square brackets] as they are encountered.

Don't go overboard! Focus on key elements only. This simple method will allow you to backtrack if needed, and will help you answer the questions at the end of a selection. Your information is now arranged to highlight the interrelationships of facts. While you have read, you have been forced to think and organize the material. You have formed associations that will foster recall.

A Plan for Self-Improvement

1. Set aside a time and place specifically for reading every day even if it is only 10 minutes. You know the conditions under which you function best. No one can set them for you.
2. Develop the habit of reading for ideas. After you have read a passage, ask yourself what the central theme was and verbalize it. The verbalization will quickly synthesize the material and draw upon relationships (similarities, differences) in the passage. The central idea will not only be highlighted but also be substantiated and amplified. Picture yourself as a critic who is writing a review that will evaluate the material for a potential reader.
3. Read different material; become a versatile reader.
4. Keep a record of your progress and be optimistic. A positive attitude is half the battle. Don't be discouraged by plateaus; they are common.

The Do's and Don'ts

1. Even though *scientific* reading, unlike pleasure reading, often involves word-by-word reading, you should coordinate speed and thought processes, and you should read as fast as you think. Backtracking usually interferes with efficient assimilation and processing of information.
2. Even though word-by-word reading is slower and more tedious, eliminate irrelevant thoughts. You don't want them to intrude just because you believe you must have something to think about. Irrelevant thoughts make concentration impossible.
3. Usually, poor concentration will lead to poor comprehension, and unnecessarily slow reading can lead to poor concentration and poor comprehension. Read as rapidly as you can without losing comprehension. Adapt speed as necessary.

4. Don't hold back your thinking processes by unnecessarily slow reading. Do not create a gap between reading and thinking. In the same vein, do not stop and pause frequently since this also will allow gaps in your thinking to occur.

5. Remember, it's a poor reader who stops too often and pauses too long at each stop.

6. Apply the same concentration whether a selection is long or short.

7. Look for a general impression, main thoughts, and implications so that you may draw inferences. Read ideas rather than words. Identify your topics, the details about them and the details about the details. Above all, don't fail to note the important ideas.

8. Whether you are the original writer or the reader of a selection, you must approach it with the thought of a distinct design and technique to present a specific subject matter and topic. Look for special effects and results.

9. You can usually identify the main topic of a paragraph by key words or phrases that could serve as possible titles. Concentrate on why certain words are used and how they are used. By concentrating on why and how, you can establish and follow the main idea. During your reading, you should realize that the paragraph is merely a sum of its parts. In turn, look at paragraphs as key elements in the development of the ideas of the passage. Don't let minor details or sentences overshadow paragraphs or the whole selection. Where there are paragraph headings, these usually lead you to main ideas.

10. Central thoughts are usually found in the lead sentence or in the summary sentence, but they may be located in other places and may, at times, be implied rather than stated. Read to understand by focusing on central ideas and units of thought.

11. Exhibit versatility, and adjust to the material. Don't use the same technique for all material; be pliable, adapt, use common sense.

12. Most of the material you confront will be familiar and understandable to you. Don't stick too closely to the particular selection; always associate present material with previous material. Nothing is ever completely new. In this context, you must focus on detail and read for specific comprehension and specific meanings to see what is new. Whether you read for general or specific ideas, use your previous knowledge. Read for meaning. Try to determine the meaning of unfamiliar words as you reason through a selection. Don't let an unfamiliar word stump you and worry you unduly; the context will often help you determine the meaning.

13. Do not decrease speed because of fear that you might miss something, and do not fall into the trap of reading each sentence twice before you proceed. Don't reread material unless necessary, but if you need to reread, do not hesitate to spend the time to clarify meaning.

14. Do not read each sentence as a distinct unit, but use each unit to build the paragraph and the selection to create the whole.

15. As you read a selection composed of several paragraphs, reflect whether succeeding paragraphs amplify the ideas or points raised in the preceding paragraphs or whether they provide an example or illustration of them. Is a qualifier of a point introduced, or is another aspect of the same subject considered?

16. Before you answer the whole battery of questions, quickly review your underlinings to make sure you understood the point.

17. Under no circumstances should you get yourself involved more deeply than necessary with the reading selection and with the task. Don't read more into it than is there; answer the questions on the basis of only what is presented.

18. Be critical when you read; extract the important facts and see relationships and associations. Visualize descriptions accurately. Avoid misreading.

19. Avoid superficiality when you consider the selection. Don't come to a conclusion before you have read the whole passage and without sufficient thought. Don't jump to a conclusion.

Practice Reading Exercises

Exercise 1

Identify the central theme or topic, details, and details about details.

DIRECTIONS: Read the sample and underline the topic, the details of the topic, and bracket (the details about the details).

Example: Following the work of Chalmers and others, 831 geriatric and orthopedic patients in West London were reviewed for osteomalacia.

(a)   The topic deals with osteomalacia.
(b)   Details or key words are geriatric and orthopedic patients.
(c)   Details about details are (831 patients) and (West London).

DIRECTIONS: Read the sample paragraph and underline the topic, the details about the topic, and bracket the (details about details). Use square brackets for [extraneous material].

Example: Following the work of Chalmers and others, 831 geriatric and orthopedic patients in West London were reviewed for osteomalacia. History, relevant blood tests (calcium, phosphate, alkaline phosphatase, 24-hour urinary calcium) and radiology were assessed. Thirty-eight bone biopsies were performed. Thirty-three were positive (32 female, 1 male). Average age was 73.4 years. None had a history of gastric surgery. Twenty-eight were widows living alone. Three were sisters (spinsters) living together. Twenty-two lived on their own property. Average weekly income was $25.00. Average weekly food bill, $9.00 (mostly bread, canned meat and canned fruit). The minimum for a balanced diet was thought to be $18.00. Average milk consumption was one pint per week. None of the patients cooked regularly. Twenty-six never cooked at all. None had sought the assistance of any of the welfare organizations, through either pride, ignorance, or apathy. All showed subjective and objective improvement following calcium and Vitamin D supplementation and dietary improvement.

Method: Following the work of Chalmers and others, (831) geriatric and orthopedic patients in [West London] were reviewed for osteomalacia. History, relevant blood tests (calcium, phosphate, alkaline phosphatase, 24 hour urinary calcium) and radiology were assessed. Twenty-eight bone biopsies were performed. (Thirty-three were positive) ([32 female], 1 male). Average age was (73.4) years. [None] had a history of [gastric surgery]. (Twenty-eight) were (widows) living alone. Three were sisters (spinsters) living together. [Twenty-two] lived on their [own property]. Average weekly income was $25.00. Average weekly food bill, $9.00 (mostly bread, canned meat and canned fruit). The minimum for a balanced diet was thought to be $18.00. Average milk consumption (one pint) per week. None of the patients cooked regularly. (Twenty-six never) cooked at all. None had sought the assistance of any of the welfare organizations, through either pride, ignorance, or apathy. All showed subjective and objective improvement following calcium and Vitamin D supplementation and dietary improvement.

Method in Outline Form

(a) The topic: <u>osteomalacia</u>

(b) Details or key words:
1. geriatric, orthopedic patients
2. history, blood tests, radiology, bone biopsies
3. age, milk consumption, week
4. none cooked regularly, none assistance
5. improvement, calcium, Vitamin D, dietary

(c) Details about details:
1. (831)
2. (33 positive)
3. (73.4 years)
4. (twenty-eight widows)
5. (one pint)
6. (twenty-six never)

(d) Extraneous material:
1. [West London]
2. [32 female]
3. [None gastric surgery]
4. [Twenty-two own property]

Having used the underlining technique, let us use this information to answer the type of questions used in the examination.

DIRECTIONS: Choose the best answer.

1. Osteomalacia:

   A. has a predilection for males.
   B. occurs more frequently in females.
   C. can only be diagnosed by bone biopsy.
   D. has a predilection for apartment dwellers.

2. The average weekly income did not allow these people to buy more food.

   A. True
   B. False
   C. They needed to save for their old age.
   D. They spend their money on the little luxuries of life.

3. From these data we may conclude that:

   A. homeowners are more likely to develop osteomalacia than are renters.
   B. spinsters will not develop osteomalacia if they live alone.
   C. consumption of bread is a consistent factor in the development of osteomalacia.
   D. there seems to be a correlation between an unbalanced diet, irregular meal consumption, and osteomalacia.

4. Given a greater income, these individuals would have:

   A. eaten more nutritious meals.
   B. cooked at least two meals a day.
   C. spent a greater percentage of their income on food.
   D. the passage does not give enough information to answer this question.

5. This study:

   A. indicated that dietary supplementation is beneficial.
   B. utilized every technique available.
   C. utilized a great variety of patients.
   D. showed that at least ten percent of the elderly suffer from osteomalacia.

Answers

1. Answer **B**
   Statement A: The numbers (32:1) clearly show that males are not prone to osteomalacia.
   Statement B: Explained above.
   Statement C: History, relevant blood tests, and radiological examination can be used to diagnose osteomalacia, as well as a bone biopsy.
   Statement D: Living in an apartment is not mentioned; however, the paragraph does mention that 22 of 33 lived on their own property.

2. Answer **B**
   Statement A: The average weekly income is stated as $25.00 and a minimum considered necessary for a balanced diet was $18.00.
   Statement B: Explained above.
   Statement C: These were elderly individuals and the issue of saving is not addressed.
   Statement D: The passage does not comment on the luxuries of life.

3. Answer **D**
   Statement A: There is no discussion of homeowners vs. renters in the passage as far as disease is concerned.
   Statement B: The paragraph does not differentiate between spinsters living alone or infer that widows are more prone to the disease because they might live alone.
   Statement C: Although bread was a high intake item, no relationship to the disease was implied.
   Statement D: An unbalanced diet and the irregular consumption of food are definite contributory factors.

4. Answer **D**
   Statement A: Income ($25.00) exceeded expenditures ($18.00) for a necessary balanced diet.
   Statement B: The passage states that most did not cook at all.
   Statement C: There is no issue of income and expenditure; income was adequate to live on a balanced diet.
   Statement D: This is the best answer since the passage truly does not discuss the issue of greater income and a person's spending habits.

5. Answer **A**
   Statement A: Improvement was noted after dietary supplementation.
   Statement B: Only three techniques were mentioned and no reference was made to limitations of techniques.
   Statement C: Only registered, orthopedic patients of West London were used; this is certainly not a great variety.
   Statement D: Of the 831 patients, 33 were diagnosed to have osteomalacia; this figure is not even 5 percent.

Exercise 2

Identify the central theme or topic, details, and details about details.

DIRECTIONS: Read the sample and underline the topic, the details about the topic, and bracket the (details about the details). Use square brackets for [extraneous material].

Example: The orbit is a cone-shaped bony structure with an apex directed posteriorly and a large anterior opening.

(a) The topic deals with the orbit.
(b) Details or key words are bony, apex posteriorly, anterior opening.
(c) Details about details are (cone shaped).

DIRECTIONS: Read the sample paragraph and underline the topic, the details about the topic, and bracket the (details about the details). Use square brackets for [extraneous material].

Example: The orbit is a cone-shaped bony structure with an apex directed posteriorly and a large anterior opening. It may be described as having a floor, a roof, and medial and lateral walls. The roof is formed mainly by the frontal bone anterior to a small portion of the sphenoid bone. The floor of the orbit from anterior to posterior is composed of the zygomatic, maxillary, and palatine bones. The lateral wall consists of portions of the zygomatic bone anteriorly and the sphenoid bone posteriorly. The medial wall from anterior to posterior is formed by the frontal process of the maxilla, the lacrimal bone, the ethmoid bone, and the sphenoid bone. Besides the anterior opening, the orbit communicates with other regions via nine openings. The infraorbital nerve enters the orbit through the infraorbital foramen. On its medial wall the anterior and posterior ethmoidal foramina transmit the anterior and posterior ethmoidal nerves, respectively. Posteriorly, near the apex of the orbit, the optic nerve and the ophthalmic artery enter via the optic canal. Also located near the apex, the superior orbital fissure transmits cranial nerves III, IV, and VI and the opthalmic division of cranial nerve V.

Method: The orbit is a (cone-shaped) bony structure with an apex directed posteriorly and a large anterior opening. It may be described as having a floor, a roof, and medial and lateral walls. The roof is formed mainly by the frontal bone anterior to a small portion of the sphenoid bone. The floor of the orbit from (anterior to posterior) is composed of the zygomatic, maxillary, and palatine bones. The lateral wall consists of portions of the zygomatic bone anteriorly and the sphenoid bone posteriorly. The medial wall from anterior to posterior is formed by the frontal process of the maxilla, the lacrimal bone, the ethmoid bone, and the sphenoid bone. Besides the anterior openings, the orbit (communicates) with other regions via (nine openings). The infraorbital nerve enters the orbit through the inferior orbital fissure, then lies in the infraorbital groove in the floor and exits anteriorly through the infraorbital foramen. On its medial wall the anterior and posterior ethmoidal foramina transmit the anterior and posterior ethmoidal nerves, respectively. Posteriorly, near the apex of the orbit, the optic nerve and the ophthalmic artery enter via the optic canal. Also located near the apex, the superior orbital fissure transmits the (cranial nerves) III, IV, and VI and the (ophthalmic division) of cranial nerve V.

Method in Outline Form

(a) The topic: orbit

(b) Details or key words:
1. bony, apex posteriorly, anterior opening
2. floor, roof, medial, lateral walls
3. roof, frontal, sphenoid floor, zygomatic, maxillary, palatine lateral, zygomatic, sphenoid medial, frontal, maxilla, lacrimal, ethmoid, sphenoid
4. infraorbital nerve, infraorbital foramen
5. medial, anterior, posterior ethmoid foramina, nerves
6. optic nerve, ophthalmic artery, optic canal
7. supraorbital fissure, III, IV, VI, V

(c) Details about details:
1. (cone shaped)
2. (communicates)
3. (nine openings)
4. (cranial nerves)
5. (ophthalmic division)

Having read the passage and used the underlining technique, let us use this information to answer the type of questions used in the examination.

DIRECTIONS: Choose the best answer.

1. Which of the following statement(s) is/are neither supported nor contradicted by the information in the passage?

   A. The apex of the orbit is located posteriorly.
   B. The superior orbital fissure is located antero-laterally.
   C. The superior ophthalmic vein exits the orbit via the superior orbital fissure.
   D. The optic nerve has a relationship to the ophthalmic artery.

2. Which of the following concerning the bony orbit is/are correct?

   A. It is formed by seven bones.
   B. The anterior margin, or entrance of the orbit, is bounded by parts of the frontal, zygomatic, and maxillary bones.
   C. The roof is formed mainly by the frontal bone.
   D. All of the above.

3. Which of the following statement(s) is/are neither supported nor contradicted by the information in the passage?

   A. The superior ophthalmic vein anastomoses with the angular vein, which is a tributary of the the facial vein.
   B. The anterior ethmoidal foramen is located between the ethmoid and frontal bones.
   C. The ophthalmic artery is a branch of the internal carotid artery.
   D. All of the above.

4. Concerning the nine openings of the orbit:

   A. They are mostly cone-shaped.
   B. They are unique structures and highly specialized in man.

    C. Traversing the infraorbital foramen is the supraorbital nerve.
    D. Cranial nerves III, IV, V, and VI are in relationship to each other.

5. Concerning the orbit, which statement(s) is/are neither supported nor contradicted by the passage?

    A. The optic nerve supplies the retina.
    B. The trigeminal nerve supplies the conjunctiva.
    C. The superior rectus muscle elevates the eye.
    D. All of the above.

Answers

1. **Answer C**
   Statement A. The paragraph in the description of the boundaries of the orbit states that the apex is located posteriorly.
   Statement B. The passage places the position of the superior orbital fissure near the apex and so the statement is contradicted.
   Statement C. There is no mention of the superior ophthalmic vein, which incidentally does exit the orbit via the superior orbital fissure. This is an example of truly focusing on the information of the passage only and not depending on prior knowledge.
   Statement D. The passage mentions that both the optic nerve and ophthalmic artery enter the orbit via the optic canal and have a relationship to each other.

2. **Answer D**
   Statement A. The orbit is made up of the frontal, sphenoid, zygomatic, maxillary palatine; lacrimal and ethmoid bones.
   Statement B. As the walls are described from anterior to posterior one can easily determine that the frontal, zygomatic, and maxillary bones contribute to the anterior margin.
   Statement C. The passage describes that the roof is formed mainly by the frontal bone.
   Statement D. All statements were correct and supported by the passage. It is important to completely read the question and focus on the details presented since a scant reading could have led you to choose answer A only.

3. **Answer D**
   Statement A. This is a true statement, however, the passage does not comment at all on this matter.
   Statement B. Again a true statement, but no mention of the fact in the paragraph.
   Statement C. This is another true statement, but not commented upon in the passage.
   Statement D. Although every choice is correct, the passage did not support nor reject the information provided and careful scrutiny of the material presented was absolutely essential.

4. **Answer D**
   Statement A. It is mentioned that the orbit is a cone-shaped opening, but no reference is made as to the shape of the openings and communications of the orbit.
   Statement B. In this passage, no reference is made to man. An orbit is described and specialization is not commented upon.
   Statement C. The infraorbital fissure is traversed by the infraorbital nerve, which is the continuation of the maxillary division of the trigeminal nerve.
   Statement D. Since cranial nerves III, IV, V, and VI traverse the superior orbital fissure they have a relationship to each other; the correct answer.

5. Answer **D**

Statement A. This is a true statement, but the facts are not presented in the passage.

Statement B. It is true that the ophthalmic division of the trigeminal nerve supplies the conjunctiva its sensory innervation; however, no reference is made to that fact in the paragraph.

Statement C. The superior rectus muscle by its action is an elevator of the eye; the passage does not comment on the above.

Statement D. Although all of the answers are correct statements, none is supported nor contradicted by the passage. All answers must be based on the information presented.

Exercise 3

Identify the central theme or topic, details, and details about details.

DIRECTIONS: Read the sample and underline the topic, the details of the topic, and bracket the (details about the details).

Example: Just about anyone you talk to nowadays complains about the cost of his automobile insurance. It's about time that someone came to the defense of the insurance companies.

(a) The topic deals with automobile insurance.
(b) Details or key words are complains, cost, defense, companies.

DIRECTIONS: Read the sample selection and underline the topic, the details about the topic, and bracket the (details about the details). Use square brackets for [extraneous material] if desired.

Example: Just about anyone you talk to nowadays complains about the cost of his automobile insurance. It's about time that someone came to the defense of the insurance companies.

We are all familiar with the effects of inflation, but most people forget that the insurance companies are affected too. An interesting point should be noted. Even though the total costs of producing a policy have been increasing because of increased salaries, paper cost, equipment replacement, etc., the insurance companies' expense ratios have been going down.

If expenses are reduced, then why are premiums going up? Let's look at what makes up the rates that the insurance companies must charge. Automobile repair rates for labor have risen about 20 percent in the last year and a half. In addition, it has been shown that a new automobile costing $5000 would cost $20,000 if it were to be repaired with replacement parts (not including the engine). During this same period, a semiprivate hospital room has increased in cost over 22 percent and physicians' and surgeons' fees have increased 20 percent. Lawyers continue to ask for larger awards, and the courts are granting them. How can insurance companies continue to pay amounts inflated in this manner without reflecting the increase in their rates?

It is a real shame that the insurance companies don't make these facts known more widely to their customers. A widespread advertising campaign would help to explain their position and make it more tolerable when that next bill comes and has once again increased.

Method: Just about anyone you talk to nowadays complains about the cost of his automobile insurance. It's about time that someone came to the defense of the insurance companies.

We are all familiar with the effects of inflation, but most people forget that the insurance companies are affected too. An interesting point should be noted. Even though the total costs of producing a policy have been increasing because of (increased salaries, paper cost, equipment replacement, etc.) the insurance companies' expense ratios have been going down.

If expenses are reduced, then why are premiums going up? Let's look at what makes up the rates that the insurance companies must charge. Automobile repair rates for labor have risen about (20 percent) in the last year and a half. In addition, it has been shown that a new automobile costing ($5000) would cost ($20,000) if it were to be repaired with replacement parts (not including the engine). During this same period, a semiprivate hospital room has increased in cost over (22 percent) and physicians' and surgeons' fees have increased (20 percent). Lawyers continue to ask for larger awards, and the courts are granting them. How can insurance companies continue to pay amounts inflated in this manner without reflecting the increase in their rates?

It is a real shame that the insurance companies don't make these facts known more widely to their customers. A widespread advertising campaign would help to explain their position and make it more tolerable when the next bill comes and has once again increased.

Method in Outline Form

(a) The topic: automobile insurance
(b) Details or key words:
1. complains, cost
2. defense, companies
3. inflation, policy, increasing
4. expense ratios, down
5. premiums, up
6. repair, risen, replacement parts
7. hospital, physicians, increased
8. lawyers, awards, courts, granting
9. advertising campaign, tolerable, next bill, increased
(c) Details about details:
1. (20 percent)
2. ($5000), ($20,000)
3. (22 percent), (20 percent)

Having read the passage and used the underlining technique, let us use this information to answer the type of questions used in the examination.

DIRECTIONS: Choose the best answer.

1. The main point of the passage is to

A. come to the aid of the insurance companies.
B. write your representatives to curb the rise of insurance rates.
C. start a widespread advertising campaign to curtail insurance costs.
D. imply that insurance premiums are based on many factors and are a complex issue.

2. Which of the following is contradicted by the passage?

    A. Many people complain about their insurance rates.
    B. Insurance companies' expense ratios are continuing to rise with inflation.
    C. Insurance companies are affected by the inflationary features of the economy.
    D. Salaries affect policy costs.

3. The main topic of the passage is

    A. public awareness.
    B. advertising strategy.
    C. automobile insurance rates.
    D. expense ratios.

4. Which of the following is supported by the passage?

    A. A car repaired with replacement parts would cost four (4) times as much as a new car.
    B. The public is fully aware of why their insurance premiums are increasing.
    C. Insurance premiums have risen mainly because of larger awards in lawsuits.
    D. Inflation has little effect on insurance rates.

5. Factor(s) affecting the overall pricing structure of rates could be considered as

    A. paper costs.
    B. equipment replacement.
    C. hospitalization costs.
    D. all of the above.

Answers

1. Answer **D**
Statement A: No aid to insurance companies is advised, but it is suggested that the companies communicate to the public how rates are derived and what affects them.
Statement B: No campaign is suggested that involves elected officials.
Statement C: It is suggested that insurance companies explain their position on rates, but that certainly is not the main thread of the passage.
Statement D: This is the best answer since it addresses the complex factors upon which rates are based.

2. Answer **B**
Statement A: The passage implies that a lot of people comment on the high cost of insurance.
Statement B: It clearly is stated in the passage that insurance companies' expense ratios have been dropping and so the statement is contradicted by the passage.
Statement C: The key element of the passage is that insurance companies, just like the public, are affected by many economic parameters.
Statement D: Salaries are mentioned as one factor playing a role in rate determination.

3. Answer **C**
Statement A: The point of public awareness concerning factors affecting premiums is expressed; however, the issue is more specific.
Statement B: Insurance companies are advised to inform the public about rate determinants, but that certainly is not the key element or topic.

Statement C: Rates and what affects the rates and their impact on the public generally are addressed.
Statement D: Expense ratios were commented on specifically and were made the key issue.

4. Answer **A**
Statement A: The passage mentions that a car costing $5,000 new would cost $20,000 if it were repaired with replacement parts.
Statement B: Although public awareness is an issue, the passage neither implies nor states the level of awareness.
Statement C: Awards due to legal procedures are clearly only one factor of this complex issue.
Statement D: Inflation is an important factor and greatly influences the rate structure.

5. Answer **D**
The passage clearly identifies paper costs, equipment replacement costs, and hospitalization costs as factors that affect premiums.

Exercise 4

Identify the central theme or topic, details, and details about details.

DIRECTIONS: Read the sample and underline the topic, the details of the topic, and bracket the (details about the details).

Example: The blood vessels of the mammalian brain normally provide a barrier that blocks the passage of certain molecules which readily penetrate other body tissues.

a) The topic deals with blood vessels, brain, barrier.
b) Details or key words are passage, molecules, other, tissues.

DIRECTIONS: Read the sample selection and underline the topic, the details about the topic, and bracket the (details about the details). Use square brackets for [extraneous material].

Example: The blood vessels of the mammalian brain normally provide a barrier that blocks the passage of certain molecules which readily permeate other body tissues. This unique property of the brain vasculature is referred to as the blood-brain barrier and in normal functional states this property prevents the entrance of numerous intravascular probes such as horseradish peroxidase into the substance of the brain. However, in experimental studies of brain dysfunction, such as seen in mechanical brain injury, a disruption of the blood-brain barrier occurs, and experimental probes such as horseradish peroxidase can enter the brain's substance. The mechanism of this blood-brain barrier dysfunction in brain injury is poorly understood. Some contend that the mechanical stress of the injury physically disrupts the vessels and permits peroxidase leakage through defects in the vascular walls. Others argue that brain injury activates cellular mechanisms which allow the blood vessels to rapidly take up substances such as horseradish peroxidase, and then deposit them within and ultimately flood the substance of the brain tissue.

To date few substantive experimental data have been advanced to support any of the above-stated theories of blood-brain barrier dysfunction in instances of mechanical brain injury. However, research continues, for medical scientists realize that any rational therapeutic treatment of brain-injured patients is totally dependent upon the elucidation of those mechanisms involved in blood-brain barrier dysfunction.

Method: Example: The blood vessels of the mammalian brain normally provide a barrier that blocks the passage of certain molecules which readily permeate other body tissues. This unique property of the brain vasculature is referred to as the blood-brain barrier and in normal functional states this property prevents the entrance of numerous (intravascular probes) such as horseradish peroxidase into the substance of the brain. However, in (experimental studies) of brain dysfunction, such as seen in mechanical brain injury, a disruption of the blood-brain barrier occurs, and experimental probes such as horseradish peroxidase can enter the brain's substance. The (mechanism) of this blood-brain barrier dysfunction in brain injury is poorly understood. Some contend that the mechanical stress of the injury physically disrupts the vessels and permits peroxidase leakage through defects in the vascular walls. Others argue that brain injury activates cellular mechanisms which allow the blood vessels to rapidly take up substances such as horseradish peroxidase and then deposit them within and ultimately flood the substance of the brain tissue.

To date few substantive experimental data have been advanced to support any of the above-stated theories of blood-brain barrier dysfunction in instances of mechanical brain injury. However, research continues, for medical scientists realize that any rational therapeutic treatment of brain injured patients is totally dependent upon the elucidation of those mechanisms involved in blood-brain barrier (dysfunction).

Method in Outline Form

(a) Topic: blood vessels, brain, barrier
(b) Details or key words:
   1. certain molecules, readily permeate, other tissues
   2. unique, vasculature, prevents, entrance horseradish peroxidase
   3. injury, disruption, barrier, horseradish peroxidase
   4. barrier, poorly understood
   5. mechanical stress, disrupts, permits leakage
   6. injury, cellular mechanisms, allow, deposit, flood tissue
   7. few data, support
   8. treatment, injured, totally dependent, mechanisms
(c) Details about details:
   1. (intravascular probes)
   2. (experimental studies)
   3. (mechanisms)
   4. (dysfunction)

Having read and used the underlining technique let us use this information to answer the type of questions used in the examination.

DIRECTIONS: Choose the best answer.
  1. This passage implies that

    A. the blood-brain barrier is a structural rather than a physiological barrier.
    B. the mechanism of the barrier generally is agreed upon.
    C. the appropriate therapeutic management of the head-injured patients awaits the elucidation of the mechanism for blood-brain barrier dysfunction in brain trauma.
    D. mankind is unique to possess this barrier.

2. Which of the following is contradicted by the information in the passage?

   A. Brain injury activates mechanisms affecting the blood-brain barrier.
   B. The mechanisms responsible for blood-brain barrier dysfunction in brain injury have been identified and it is apparent that it is related to vasogenic shock.
   C. Experimental data to date cannot definitely support any specific theory.
   D. Only certain molecules are blocked normally.

3. Mechanical brain injury may physically disrupt the integrity of the brain's vasculature.

   A. This statement is supported by the information in the passage.
   B. This statement is contradicted by the information in the passage.
   C. This statement is neither supported nor contradicted by the information in the passage.
   D. Only circumstantial evidence is presented.

4. Horseradish peroxidase is a major therapeutic agent utilized after head trauma.

   A. This statement is supported by the information in the passage.
   B. This statement is contradicted by the information in the passage.
   C. This statement is neither supported nor contradicted by the information in the passage.
   D. Horseradish peroxidase is not mentioned in the passage.

Answers

1. Answer C
   Statement A: Although the passage comments that physical disruption certainly plays a role, it does not rule out physiological phenomena governing cell and membrane permeability.
   Statement B: Several theories exist concerning this barrier, but in all likelihood a blending of thought will evolve as more factors are elucidated.
   Statement C: Therapeutic management is hampered by our lack of complete understanding of the blood-brain barrier; this fact clearly is established in the passage.
   Statement D: Mankind is not unique; however, since this phenomenon is confined to mammals we are benefiting from its effect.

2. Answer B
   Statement A: After injury there is a breakdown in the blood-brain barrier that allows certain substances to pass.
   Statement B: Several theories have been advanced for dysfunction of the barrier, but the exact mechanisms have not been elucidated.
   Statement C: Hard experimental data to support one specific theory is still scarce.
   Statement D: The passage clearly states that only certain molecules are affected by the barrier.

3. Answer C
   The passage stresses that the blood-brain barrier is a complex phenomenon and that probably both physical and physiological factors are involved.

4. Answer C
   Horseradish peroxidase is used as a marker in experimental probes that are investigating the mechanisms of the blood-brain barrier. The passage does not comment as to a therapeutic value of this compound.

Exercise 5

Identify the central theme or topic, details, and details about details.

DIRECTIONS: Read the sample and underline the topic, the details of the topic, and bracket the (details about the details).

Example: Evolutionary evidence supports the freshwater theory of origin of the chordates. Some scientists believe that the ancestors of the chordates migrated from the sea to a freshwater or brackish water habitat during the Cambrian period.

a) The topic deals with the freshwater origin of the chordates.
b) Details or key words are evidence, supports, migrated, sea, freshwater.
c) Details about details are (Cambrian period).

DIRECTIONS: Read the sample selection and underline the topic, the details about the topic, and bracket the (details about the details). Use square brackets for [extraneous material].

Example: Evolutionary evidence supports the freshwater theory of the origin of the chordates. Some scientists believe that ancestors of the chordates migrated from the sea to a freshwater or brackish water habitat during the Cambrian period.

Prochordate ancestors of these early vertebrates inhabited the oceans of the pre-Cambrian period. They were in a state of constant osmotic equilibrium with their environment, which had a salinity equivalent to about one-half the salinity of the present-day oceans. Since these prochordates were in equilibrium with the surrounding environment, they did not face a problem of internal water regulation, and the kidney of these forms was principally concerned with regulation of nitrogenous wastes.

Migration of the earliest chordate ancestors into fresh water was the result of an attempt on their part to escape the giant marine cephalopods which ruled the oceans of the Ordovician period. Concomitant with their migration into a freshwater habitat, these early vertebrate ancestors were faced with a two-fold problem: (1) dilution of body fluids through absorption of excess water from a hypo-osmotic environment and (2) retention of physiologically important materials that were not readily obtainable from the environment. Whereas chordate ancestors could remove nitrogenous wastes by merely secreting these substances into a tubular excretory network, migration of early chordate forms into fresh water necessitated the development of a pressure system for removal of excess water. In these forms the glomerular filtration system evolved as a means of coping with the problem of excess dilution of body fluids. However, the glomerulus did not provide a perfect osmoregulatory mechanism. In addition to its ability to filter out excess water from body fluids, it also removed a number of metabolically important substances such as glucose, phosphates, etc. Thus the problem of removal of water and retention of important elements developed secondarily as a result of glomerular evolution. The problem of conserving important substances in the glomerular filtrate was solved with the evolution of tubular reabsorptive mechanisms capable of selective reabsorption of metabolites, through the reabsorption of salt and the elaboration of urine that was hypotonic to the blood.

In early anamniotes, the primitive kidneys were relatively inefficient when some species attempted to move into a more isosmotic or hyperosmotic environment. Thus these early vertebrates were confined to an entirely freshwater habitat.

With the evolution of the Agnathostomes (lampreys, hagfish, and slime eel) during the Silurian period, the crust of the earth was undergoing a major diastrophic change which compelled the freshwater vertebrates to diverge along two courses of evolution. Some forms became trapped in a freshwater habitat and became the ancestors of the freshwater fish and higher vertebrates. Others moved back to the oceans and became ancestors of marine teleosts. Movement of the ancestors of the marine teleosts back into a hypertonic environment forced new osmotic problems on these species. Having evolved osmoregulatory mechanisms designed to cope with a hypo-osmotic environment, they were faced with a problem of dehydration from osmotic loss of water through the glomerulated excretory system and the body surface. The result of their secondary invasion of a marine habitat was the evolution of two means of coping with the extremes of the environment. A number of species of ancestral marine teleosts underwent degeneration of the glomerular portions of the excretory system and retention of an aglomerular system that evolved specialized secretory mechanisms for removal of wastes and ingested inorganic materials. Another regulatory mechanism evolved through specialization of cells in the gill surfaces to secrete salts but retain water and thereby reduce the tendency of body fluids to become hypertonic to the body tissues.

The results of the digression of teleost ancestors into freshwater and saltwater species has been the basis for the wide diversity in the morphology of the renal system of this class of vertebrates.

Method: Evolutionary evidence supports the freshwater theory of origin of the chordates. Some scientists believe that ancestors of the chordates migrated from the sea to a freshwater or brackish water habitat during the Cambrian period.

Prochordate (ancestors) of these (early) (vertebrates) inhabited the oceans of the pre-Cambrian period. They were in a state of constant osmotic equilibrium with their environment, which had a salinity equivalent to about one-half the salinity of the present-day (oceans). Since these prochordates were in equilibrium with the surrounding environment, they did not face a problem of internal water regulation, and the kidney of these forms was (principally) concerned with regulation of nitrogenous wastes.

Migration of the (earliest chordate) ancestors into fresh water was the result of an attempt on their part to escape the (giant marine) cephalopods which ruled the oceans of the [Ordovician] period. Concomitant with their migration into a freshwater habitat, these early vertebrate ancestors were faced with a two-fold problem: (1) the dilution of body fluids through absorption of excess water from a (hypo-osmotic) environment and (2) retention of physiologically important materials that were not readily obtainable from the environment. Whereas chordate ancestors could remove nitrogenous wastes by merely secreting these substances into a (tubular excretory network), migration of early chordate forms into fresh water (necessitated) the development of a pressure system for (removal of excess water). In these forms the glomerular filtration system evolved as a means of (coping) with the problem of (excess dilution) of body fluids. However, the glomerulus did not provide a perfect osmoregulatory mechanism. In addition to its ability to filter out excess water from body fluids, it also removed a number of metabolically important substances such as (glucose, phosphates, etc.). Thus the problem of removal of water and retention of important elements developed (secondarily) as a result of the glomerular evolution. The problem of conserving important substances in the glomerular filtrate was solved with the evolution of tubular reabsorptive mechanisms capable of (selective) reabsorption of metabolites, through the reabsorption of salt and the elaboration of urine that was (hypotonic to the blood).

In early anamniotes, the primitive kidneys were relatively inefficient when some species attempted to move into a more (isosmotic or hyperosmotic) environment. Thus these (early) vertebrates were confined to an entirely freshwater habitat.

With the evolution of the (Agnathostomes) (lampreys, hagfish, and slime eel) during the (Silurian period), the crust of the earth was undergoing a major diastrophic change which compelled the freshwater vertebrates to diverge along two courses of evolution. Some forms became (trapped) in a (freshwater habitat) and became the ancestors of the freshwater fish and higher vertebrates. Others (moved back) to the oceans and became ancestors of marine teleosts. Movement of the ancestors of the marine teleosts back into a (hypertonic environment) forced new osmotic problems on these species. Having evolved osmoregulatory mechanisms designed to cope with (a hypo-osmotic environment), they were faced with a problem of dehydration from (osmotic loss of water) through the glomerulated excretory system and the body surface. The result of their secondary invasion of a marine habitat was the evolution of two means of coping with the extremes of the environment. A number of species of ancestral marine teleosts underwent degeneration of the glomerular portions of the excretory system and retention of an aglomerular system that evolved specialized secretory mechanisms for removal of wastes and ingested inorganic materials. Another regulatory mechanism evolved through specialization of cells in the gill surfaces to secrete salts but retain water and thereby reduce the tendency of body fluids to become hypertonic to the body tissues.

The result of the digression of teleost ancestors into freshwater and saltwater species has been the basis for the wide diversity in the morphology of the renal system of this class of vertebrates.

Method in Outline Form

(a) Topic: fresh-water, origin, chordates
(b) Details or key words:

1. evidence, support, migrated
2. sea to freshwater
3. prochordate, inhabited, oceans
4. constant osmotic equilibrium
5. one-half, salinity, present-day
6. did not, problem, water, regulation
7. kidney, regulation, nitrogenous
8. migration, fresh water, escape, cephalopods
9. migration, dilution, body fluids, excess water
10. chordate ancestors, remove, nitrogenous
11. migration, chordate, fresh water, development, pressure system
12. glomerulus, filtration, evolved
13. glomerulus, not, osmoregulatory
14. removed, substances
15. removal, water, retention, elements
16. solved, tubular, mechanism
17. reabsorption, metabolites, salt
18. elaboration, urine
19. anomniotes, kidneys, inefficient
20. vetebrates, confined, freshwater
21. freshwater, vertebrates, two courses

22. ancestors, freshwater fish, higher vertebrates
23. oceans, ancestors, marine teleosts, dehydration
24. secondary invasion, degeneration, glomerular, retention, aglomerular
25. gill, secrete salts, reduce body fluids, hypertonic
26. diversity, renal system, vertebrates

(c) Details about details:

1. (ancestors), (early), (vertebrates), (principally oceans)
2. (earliest chordate), (giant marine)
3. (hypo-osmotic)
4. (tubular excretory network)
5. (necessitated), (removal of excess water)
6. (coping), (excess dilution)
7. (glucose), (phosphates)
8. (selective), (hypotonic to the blood)
9. (early vertebrates), (entirely freshwater)
10. (Agnathostomes)
11. (Silurian period)
12. (trapped), (freshwater habitat)
13. (moved back), (hypertonic), (hypo-osmotic environment), (osmotic loss of water)

Having read the passage and used the underlining technique, let us use this information to answer the type of questions used in the examination.

DIRECTIONS: Choose the best answer.

1. Concerning the origin of chordates,

   A. all scientists have embraced the theory of the origin of chordates.
   B. life originated in the sea.
   C. ancestors of chordates potentially migrated from the sea.
   D. migration took place during the Ordovician period.

2. Concerning the kidney of prochordates,

   A. the kidney of prochordates faced severe fluid regulation problems.
   B. prochordates were in osmotic equilibrium with their surroundings.
   C. the kidneys were principally concerned with nitrogenous waste regulation.
   D. choices B and C are correct.

3. Which of the following statement(s) is/are contradicted by the passage?

   A. Small cephalopods ruled the oceans.
   B. Glomerular filtration provided complete osmoregulation.
   C. Glomerular filtration did not affect glucose.
   D. All of the above.

4. Concerning vertebrates,

   A. early vertebrates were confined to a freshwater environment.
   B. vertebrates diverged along many avenues of evolution.
   C. all left the freshwater environment.
   D. most went back to the oceans and became ancestors of marine teleosts.

5. Which of the following statements is neither supported nor contradicted by the information in the passage?

    A. The glomerular filtration apparatus evolved as a result of chordate migration into a freshwater environment.
    B. Gills played an important role in the evolution of vertebrates.
    C. Selectivity of tubular reabsorption solved many evolutionary filtration phenomena.
    D. The morphology of the kidney is relatively similar in all living forms.

6. Which of the following is not supported by the passage?

    A. Specialized cells in gills secrete salts.
    B. Hogfishes are considered Agnathostomes.
    C. Chordate ancestors could remove nitrogenous wastes.
    D. Teleosts inhabit mainly freshwater bodies.

Answers

1. Answer C
   Statement A: This answer is contradicted by the passage, which indicates that "some" scientists have embraced the theory.
   Statement B: It is neither supported nor contradicted.
   Statement D: The passage states that migration took place during the Cambrian Period while the cephalopods ruled the oceans of the Ordovician period.

2. Answer D
   Statement A: The paragraph clearly states that since prochordates were in a constant state of osmotic equilibrium, fluid regulation was not a factor.
   Statement B: It is supported by the information in the passage.
   Statement C: Clearly stated in the passage; therefore, the best answer is D.

3. Answer D
   Statement A: The passage mentions that giant marine cephalopods ruled the oceans.
   Statement B: The passage states that the glomerulus did not provide a perfect osmoregulatory mechanism.
   Statement C: According to the passage, glomerular filtration removed metabolically important substances such as glucose and phosphates.
   Statement D: All of the above statements were not supported by the passage.

4. Answer A
   Statement A: The passage mentions that the primitive kidney confined the early vertebrates to an entirely freshwater habitat.
   Statement B: Vertebrates diverged along two courses of evolution and not along many.
   Statement C: The passage indicates that some vertebrates became trapped in the freshwater habitat.
   Statement D: Only some went back to the oceans; the passage does not quantify.

5. Answer B
   Statement A: It is supported by the passage.
   Statement B: It is not discussed in the passage.
   Statement C: Selectivity and specialization were a key element in evolutionary success and this is supported by the passage.

Statement D: The paragraph contradicts this statement when it mentions that the results of the digression of teleost ancestors into freshwater and saltwater species has been the basis for the wide diversity in the morphology of the renal system.

6. **Answer D**
    Statement A: Specialized cells in the gill surfaces secrete salts and retain water.
    Statement B: Lampreys, hogfishes, and slime eel are Agnathostomes.
    Statement C: By secreting these substances into a tubular excretory network, chordate ancestors could remove nitrogenous wastes.
    Statement D: Teleosts live in freshwater and saltwater, and no quantification is expressed in the passage.

Writing the Essay

Since 1985, the Association of American Medical Colleges (AAMC) has been trial-testing an essay topic on the MCAT. This project was in response to a study about the professional preparation of the physician. The 1989 administrations of the MCAT included 60 minutes for the writing of two essays. In 1991 the essay became a permanent part of the MCAT.

Medical school faculties have long felt that writing skills are essential for a physician. Many have expressed the opinion that present-day students are somewhat weak in these skills. The goal of the essay topic is to see if the student has the ability and skill to write under standardized conditions. The students should be able to:

1. develop a central theme
2. synthesize material
3. separate major from minor issues
4. propose alternative solutions
5. present a theme in a flowing and logical manner
6. write in correct English, timed, at a first-draft composition level

No specific college courses to obtain essay writing skills have been advocated by anyone. The essay portion (two topics) of the examination will take 60 minutes (30 minutes/topic). It will be administered after the lunch break.

The AAMC has proposed the following guidelines for topic developments:

1. The topic should have *no* relationship to the application process or the candidate's career choice.
2. The topic should not deal with health care or religious themes.
3. Social subjects that may prejudice an evaluator due to opinions or judgmental statements made by the examinee should be avoided.
4. Questions should come from sources which would allow any candidate to respond fully despite recognized differences in social, ethnic and geographic background.
5. Formal course content, especially in the sciences, should be avoided.

Scoring Method

All essays will be scored by an experienced group of readers. A minimum of four readers will rate each essay on a six-point scale. An additional reader will be used if the four original scores differ by more than one point. For reporting purposes, the scores will be averaged and converted to an alphabetical score, with the scale ranging from J to T.

An essay that *exhibits* the major characteristics of logical analysis and presentation would fall in the range from J to Q, with J representing a percentile score between 0–8 and Q representing a range of 54–65. Essays in the Q and above range clearly should display a *grasp* of the material under discussion. The T range will represent the 91–100 percentile. Papers falling into this range definitely must *demonstrate* facets essential to good writing such as purpose, goal, and conviction.

Medical schools will receive the alphabetical score, but may also obtain writing samples. Both the examinee and the schools will receive percentile data, score distribution characteristics, and confidence bands.

Plan for Writing an Acceptable Essay

There are proper ways to present material in essay form. A person who has mastered the basic techniques will generally be successful while one who has not, usually does not give the reader an accurate representation of his basic fund of knowledge.

Several techniques should be considered:

1.   Read every essay question asked before you develop a game plan and start to answer. Note what is included and excluded in the questions.

2.   Decide exactly what is being asked. Are you asked to describe, discuss, compare, illustrate or give an opinion?

3.   Formulate your plan and make an outline, preferably in writing. The outline will help you to organize your presentation. It will aid you in including relevant material and minimize the tendency to forget important points in the heat of battle. Most importantly, it will provide you with a coherent train of thought that will aid in the recall of material.

4.   Write to the point, stress your key facts, and be specific.

5.   Present your ideas clearly and organize them to show that you understood the question.

Pay attention to key words that guide your answer.

1.   Words that require a specific answer are: state, cite, name, list, mention, identify, give, define.

2.   Words that require a certain amount of description are: describe, discuss, review, illustrate, develop, outline.

3.   Words that should focus your attention on associations, similarities and differences are: differentiate, compare, contrast, analyze, distinguish.

4.   Words that suggest that an opinion is desired are: assess, evaluate, comment, criticize, interpret.

Practice Essay Topics

1.   John F. Kennedy made the following comment: "The credit belongs to the man who is actually in the arena. Whose face is marred by dust, sweat and blood: who knows the enthusiasm, the great devotion, and spends himself in a worthy cause. Who at best if he wins knows the thrill of high achievement and if he fails at least fails while daring greatly so that his place shall never be with those cold and timid souls, who know neither victory nor defeat."

Explain what the author means when he comments on the man in the arena. Relate the concept of the passage to an area with which you are familiar.

2.   An American statesman said: "In matters of principle, stand like a rock; in matters of taste, swim with the current."

Explain what the statesman means. Include a description of a situation in which it is hard to distinguish between principle and taste. What criteria should one use to distinguish between matters of principle and matters of taste?

(Topics used by AAMC in seminars to pre-med and medical school faculties.)

The MCAT
Model Examination A

ANSWER SHEET

DIRECTIONS: After locating the number of the question to which you are responding, fill in the circle containing the letter of the answer you have selected. Use pencil (not a ballpoint pen) to completely blacken the circle.

VERBAL REASONING

1. Ⓐ Ⓑ Ⓒ Ⓓ
2. Ⓐ Ⓑ Ⓒ Ⓓ
3. Ⓐ Ⓑ Ⓒ Ⓓ
4. Ⓐ Ⓑ Ⓒ Ⓓ
5. Ⓐ Ⓑ Ⓒ Ⓓ
6. Ⓐ Ⓑ Ⓒ Ⓓ
7. Ⓐ Ⓑ Ⓒ Ⓓ
8. Ⓐ Ⓑ Ⓒ Ⓓ
9. Ⓐ Ⓑ Ⓒ Ⓓ
10. Ⓐ Ⓑ Ⓒ Ⓓ
11. Ⓐ Ⓑ Ⓒ Ⓓ
12. Ⓐ Ⓑ Ⓒ Ⓓ
13. Ⓐ Ⓑ Ⓒ Ⓓ
14. Ⓐ Ⓑ Ⓒ Ⓓ
15. Ⓐ Ⓑ Ⓒ Ⓓ
16. Ⓐ Ⓑ Ⓒ Ⓓ
17. Ⓐ Ⓑ Ⓒ Ⓓ
18. Ⓐ Ⓑ Ⓒ Ⓓ
19. Ⓐ Ⓑ Ⓒ Ⓓ
20. Ⓐ Ⓑ Ⓒ Ⓓ
21. Ⓐ Ⓑ Ⓒ Ⓓ
22. Ⓐ Ⓑ Ⓒ Ⓓ
23. Ⓐ Ⓑ Ⓒ Ⓓ
24. Ⓐ Ⓑ Ⓒ Ⓓ
25. Ⓐ Ⓑ Ⓒ Ⓓ
26. Ⓐ Ⓑ Ⓒ Ⓓ
27. Ⓐ Ⓑ Ⓒ Ⓓ
28. Ⓐ Ⓑ Ⓒ Ⓓ
29. Ⓐ Ⓑ Ⓒ Ⓓ
30. Ⓐ Ⓑ Ⓒ Ⓓ

31. Ⓐ Ⓑ Ⓒ Ⓓ
32. Ⓐ Ⓑ Ⓒ Ⓓ
33. Ⓐ Ⓑ Ⓒ Ⓓ
34. Ⓐ Ⓑ Ⓒ Ⓓ
35. Ⓐ Ⓑ Ⓒ Ⓓ
36. Ⓐ Ⓑ Ⓒ Ⓓ
37. Ⓐ Ⓑ Ⓒ Ⓓ
38. Ⓐ Ⓑ Ⓒ Ⓓ
39. Ⓐ Ⓑ Ⓒ Ⓓ
40. Ⓐ Ⓑ Ⓒ Ⓓ
41. Ⓐ Ⓑ Ⓒ Ⓓ
42. Ⓐ Ⓑ Ⓒ Ⓓ
43. Ⓐ Ⓑ Ⓒ Ⓓ
44. Ⓐ Ⓑ Ⓒ Ⓓ
45. Ⓐ Ⓑ Ⓒ Ⓓ
46. Ⓐ Ⓑ Ⓒ Ⓓ
47. Ⓐ Ⓑ Ⓒ Ⓓ
48. Ⓐ Ⓑ Ⓒ Ⓓ
49. Ⓐ Ⓑ Ⓒ Ⓓ
50. Ⓐ Ⓑ Ⓒ Ⓓ
51. Ⓐ Ⓑ Ⓒ Ⓓ
52. Ⓐ Ⓑ Ⓒ Ⓓ
53. Ⓐ Ⓑ Ⓒ Ⓓ
54. Ⓐ Ⓑ Ⓒ Ⓓ
55. Ⓐ Ⓑ Ⓒ Ⓓ
56. Ⓐ Ⓑ Ⓒ Ⓓ
57. Ⓐ Ⓑ Ⓒ Ⓓ
58. Ⓐ Ⓑ Ⓒ Ⓓ
59. Ⓐ Ⓑ Ⓒ Ⓓ
60. Ⓐ Ⓑ Ⓒ Ⓓ

61. Ⓐ Ⓑ Ⓒ Ⓓ
62. Ⓐ Ⓑ Ⓒ Ⓓ
63. Ⓐ Ⓑ Ⓒ Ⓓ
64. Ⓐ Ⓑ Ⓒ Ⓓ
65. Ⓐ Ⓑ Ⓒ Ⓓ

PHYSICAL SCIENCES

66. Ⓐ Ⓑ Ⓒ Ⓓ
67. Ⓐ Ⓑ Ⓒ Ⓓ
68. Ⓐ Ⓑ Ⓒ Ⓓ
69. Ⓐ Ⓑ Ⓒ Ⓓ
70. Ⓐ Ⓑ Ⓒ Ⓓ
71. Ⓐ Ⓑ Ⓒ Ⓓ
72. Ⓐ Ⓑ Ⓒ Ⓓ
73. Ⓐ Ⓑ Ⓒ Ⓓ
74. Ⓐ Ⓑ Ⓒ Ⓓ
75. Ⓐ Ⓑ Ⓒ Ⓓ
76. Ⓐ Ⓑ Ⓒ Ⓓ
77. Ⓐ Ⓑ Ⓒ Ⓓ
78. Ⓐ Ⓑ Ⓒ Ⓓ
79. Ⓐ Ⓑ Ⓒ Ⓓ
80. Ⓐ Ⓑ Ⓒ Ⓓ
81. Ⓐ Ⓑ Ⓒ Ⓓ
82. Ⓐ Ⓑ Ⓒ Ⓓ
83. Ⓐ Ⓑ Ⓒ Ⓓ
84. Ⓐ Ⓑ Ⓒ Ⓓ
85. Ⓐ Ⓑ Ⓒ Ⓓ
86. Ⓐ Ⓑ Ⓒ Ⓓ
87. Ⓐ Ⓑ Ⓒ Ⓓ
88. Ⓐ Ⓑ Ⓒ Ⓓ

89. Ⓐ Ⓑ Ⓒ Ⓓ
90. Ⓐ Ⓑ Ⓒ Ⓓ
91. Ⓐ Ⓑ Ⓒ Ⓓ
92. Ⓐ Ⓑ Ⓒ Ⓓ
93. Ⓐ Ⓑ Ⓒ Ⓓ
94. Ⓐ Ⓑ Ⓒ Ⓓ
95. Ⓐ Ⓑ Ⓒ Ⓓ
96. Ⓐ Ⓑ Ⓒ Ⓓ
97. Ⓐ Ⓑ Ⓒ Ⓓ
98. Ⓐ Ⓑ Ⓒ Ⓓ
99. Ⓐ Ⓑ Ⓒ Ⓓ
100. Ⓐ Ⓑ Ⓒ Ⓓ
101. Ⓐ Ⓑ Ⓒ Ⓓ
102. Ⓐ Ⓑ Ⓒ Ⓓ
103. Ⓐ Ⓑ Ⓒ Ⓓ
104. Ⓐ Ⓑ Ⓒ Ⓓ
105. Ⓐ Ⓑ Ⓒ Ⓓ
106. Ⓐ Ⓑ Ⓒ Ⓓ
107. Ⓐ Ⓑ Ⓒ Ⓓ
108. Ⓐ Ⓑ Ⓒ Ⓓ
109. Ⓐ Ⓑ Ⓒ Ⓓ
110. Ⓐ Ⓑ Ⓒ Ⓓ
111. Ⓐ Ⓑ Ⓒ Ⓓ
112. Ⓐ Ⓑ Ⓒ Ⓓ
113. Ⓐ Ⓑ Ⓒ Ⓓ
114. Ⓐ Ⓑ Ⓒ Ⓓ
115. Ⓐ Ⓑ Ⓒ Ⓓ
116. Ⓐ Ⓑ Ⓒ Ⓓ
117. Ⓐ Ⓑ Ⓒ Ⓓ
118. Ⓐ Ⓑ Ⓒ Ⓓ

119. Ⓐ Ⓑ Ⓒ Ⓓ
120. Ⓐ Ⓑ Ⓒ Ⓓ
121. Ⓐ Ⓑ Ⓒ Ⓓ
122. Ⓐ Ⓑ Ⓒ Ⓓ
123. Ⓐ Ⓑ Ⓒ Ⓓ
124. Ⓐ Ⓑ Ⓒ Ⓓ
125. Ⓐ Ⓑ Ⓒ Ⓓ
126. Ⓐ Ⓑ Ⓒ Ⓓ
127. Ⓐ Ⓑ Ⓒ Ⓓ
128. Ⓐ Ⓑ Ⓒ Ⓓ
129. Ⓐ Ⓑ Ⓒ Ⓓ
130. Ⓐ Ⓑ Ⓒ Ⓓ
131. Ⓐ Ⓑ Ⓒ Ⓓ
132. Ⓐ Ⓑ Ⓒ Ⓓ
133. Ⓐ Ⓑ Ⓒ Ⓓ
134. Ⓐ Ⓑ Ⓒ Ⓓ
135. Ⓐ Ⓑ Ⓒ Ⓓ
136. Ⓐ Ⓑ Ⓒ Ⓓ
137. Ⓐ Ⓑ Ⓒ Ⓓ
138. Ⓐ Ⓑ Ⓒ Ⓓ
139. Ⓐ Ⓑ Ⓒ Ⓓ
140. Ⓐ Ⓑ Ⓒ Ⓓ
141. Ⓐ Ⓑ Ⓒ Ⓓ
142. Ⓐ Ⓑ Ⓒ Ⓓ

WRITING SAMPLE
Use separate ruled sheets of paper.

BIOLOGICAL SCIENCES

143. Ⓐ Ⓑ Ⓒ Ⓓ
144. Ⓐ Ⓑ Ⓒ Ⓓ
145. Ⓐ Ⓑ Ⓒ Ⓓ
146. Ⓐ Ⓑ Ⓒ Ⓓ
147. Ⓐ Ⓑ Ⓒ Ⓓ
148. Ⓐ Ⓑ Ⓒ Ⓓ
149. Ⓐ Ⓑ Ⓒ Ⓓ
150. Ⓐ Ⓑ Ⓒ Ⓓ
151. Ⓐ Ⓑ Ⓒ Ⓓ
152. Ⓐ Ⓑ Ⓒ Ⓓ
153. Ⓐ Ⓑ Ⓒ Ⓓ
154. Ⓐ Ⓑ Ⓒ Ⓓ
155. Ⓐ Ⓑ Ⓒ Ⓓ
156. Ⓐ Ⓑ Ⓒ Ⓓ
157. Ⓐ Ⓑ Ⓒ Ⓓ
158. Ⓐ Ⓑ Ⓒ Ⓓ
159. Ⓐ Ⓑ Ⓒ Ⓓ
160. Ⓐ Ⓑ Ⓒ Ⓓ
161. Ⓐ Ⓑ Ⓒ Ⓓ
162. Ⓐ Ⓑ Ⓒ Ⓓ
163. Ⓐ Ⓑ Ⓒ Ⓓ
164. Ⓐ Ⓑ Ⓒ Ⓓ
165. Ⓐ Ⓑ Ⓒ Ⓓ
166. Ⓐ Ⓑ Ⓒ Ⓓ
167. Ⓐ Ⓑ Ⓒ Ⓓ

168. Ⓐ Ⓑ Ⓒ Ⓓ
169. Ⓐ Ⓑ Ⓒ Ⓓ
170. Ⓐ Ⓑ Ⓒ Ⓓ
171. Ⓐ Ⓑ Ⓒ Ⓓ
172. Ⓐ Ⓑ Ⓒ Ⓓ
173. Ⓐ Ⓑ Ⓒ Ⓓ
174. Ⓐ Ⓑ Ⓒ Ⓓ
175. Ⓐ Ⓑ Ⓒ Ⓓ
176. Ⓐ Ⓑ Ⓒ Ⓓ
177. Ⓐ Ⓑ Ⓒ Ⓓ
178. Ⓐ Ⓑ Ⓒ Ⓓ
179. Ⓐ Ⓑ Ⓒ Ⓓ
180. Ⓐ Ⓑ Ⓒ Ⓓ
181. Ⓐ Ⓑ Ⓒ Ⓓ
182. Ⓐ Ⓑ Ⓒ Ⓓ
183. Ⓐ Ⓑ Ⓒ Ⓓ
184. Ⓐ Ⓑ Ⓒ Ⓓ
185. Ⓐ Ⓑ Ⓒ Ⓓ
186. Ⓐ Ⓑ Ⓒ Ⓓ
187. Ⓐ Ⓑ Ⓒ Ⓓ
188. Ⓐ Ⓑ Ⓒ Ⓓ
189. Ⓐ Ⓑ Ⓒ Ⓓ
190. Ⓐ Ⓑ Ⓒ Ⓓ
191. Ⓐ Ⓑ Ⓒ Ⓓ
192. Ⓐ Ⓑ Ⓒ Ⓓ
193. Ⓐ Ⓑ Ⓒ Ⓓ

194. Ⓐ Ⓑ Ⓒ Ⓓ
195. Ⓐ Ⓑ Ⓒ Ⓓ
196. Ⓐ Ⓑ Ⓒ Ⓓ
197. Ⓐ Ⓑ Ⓒ Ⓓ
198. Ⓐ Ⓑ Ⓒ Ⓓ
199. Ⓐ Ⓑ Ⓒ Ⓓ
200. Ⓐ Ⓑ Ⓒ Ⓓ
201. Ⓐ Ⓑ Ⓒ Ⓓ
202. Ⓐ Ⓑ Ⓒ Ⓓ
203. Ⓐ Ⓑ Ⓒ Ⓓ
204. Ⓐ Ⓑ Ⓒ Ⓓ
205. Ⓐ Ⓑ Ⓒ Ⓓ
206. Ⓐ Ⓑ Ⓒ Ⓓ
207. Ⓐ Ⓑ Ⓒ Ⓓ
208. Ⓐ Ⓑ Ⓒ Ⓓ
209. Ⓐ Ⓑ Ⓒ Ⓓ
210. Ⓐ Ⓑ Ⓒ Ⓓ
211. Ⓐ Ⓑ Ⓒ Ⓓ
212. Ⓐ Ⓑ Ⓒ Ⓓ
213. Ⓐ Ⓑ Ⓒ Ⓓ
214. Ⓐ Ⓑ Ⓒ Ⓓ
215. Ⓐ Ⓑ Ⓒ Ⓓ
216. Ⓐ Ⓑ Ⓒ Ⓓ
217. Ⓐ Ⓑ Ⓒ Ⓓ
218. Ⓐ Ⓑ Ⓒ Ⓓ
219. Ⓐ Ⓑ Ⓒ Ⓓ

The MCAT
Model Examination A

VERBAL REASONING

9 PASSAGES
65 QUESTIONS
85 MINUTES

DIRECTIONS: The questions are based on the accompanying passages. Read each passage carefully, then answer the following questions. Consider only the material within the passage. For each question, select the *ONE BEST ANSWER* and indicate your selection by marking the corresponding letter on the Answer Form.

Passage I (Questions 1–9)

Periodic demands for educational reform, in conjunction with the corresponding efforts of the nation's public school systems to improve their instructional programs, are not an unusual phenomenon in the annals of this country's history. The most recent reform movement, however, which is viewed by many as a demand on the part of legislatures and the public for more effective schools, might be classified as unique. During the last 20 years, monumental amounts of research and discussion have been generated regarding all facets of public education.

The outcry was created in part by declining economic conditions and by the publication of such exhaustive studies of school resources and their impact as the Coleman et al., (1966) report on the *Equality of Educational Opportunity* and others (Jensen, 1969; Jenks et al. 1970; Rist, 1970; Avech, 1974), which seemed to point to the failure of the American educational system. The results of their findings caused considerable dismay in the educational community and the population at large, since they suggested that schools make little, if any, difference in the lives of the children who attend them. The socioeconomic status of the individual's family (Hodgson, 1975) as well as a measure of "pure luck" (ERIC Action Brief, 1981) were credited with influencing student achievement and other educational outcomes to a much greater degree than a pupil's school experiences.

Adapted from E. E. Seibel, "Principal Change Facilitator Style: Its Relationship to School Climate and Student Achievement." Doctoral Dissertation, Virginia Commonwealth University, 1986.

After the initial reaction of shock, neither researchers nor practitioners were content to stand by and accept the pessimistic picture that had been painted for them as a final verdict. In response, literally hundreds of studies have been conducted in schools across the country that focus on every aspect of public education.

Researchers have gone into the field in great numbers to obtain a firsthand view of the educational process in action. One early example of a now classic study that made an attempt to overcome the existing attitude of fatalism was that conducted by Weber (1971) in four Washington, D.C. schools. The results indicated that by placing a consistent school-wide emphasis on the teaching of basic skills, school leaders could be influential in improving the reading achievement of disadvantaged inner-city youngsters.

Many other research efforts, both ethnographic and quantitative in nature, have produced positive results and have infused practitioners with a new hope and a renewed belief that what takes place in schools can indeed make a significant difference in both the academic lives and the personal development of the pupils that they serve.

Although the negative effects of the early findings have been lessened, they have not been wiped away. The call for further reform continues, as evidenced by the continuing wave of national, state, and public demands contained in such reports as *A Nation at Risk* (Goldberg & James, 1983) and *Making the Grade* (Graham, 1983). Consequently, the research effort has intensified and has resulted in the translation of many of its findings into positive plans of action.

1. The central thesis of the passage is:

   A. schools do not make a difference in the lives of the students who attend them.
   B. instructional programs must always be improved and updated so that educational critics will be satisfied.
   C. although the call for educational reform in the United States has been an ongoing process, the past 20-year period has been an extremely research-oriented time in the public education arena.
   D. middle class parents should consider providing academic instruction for their children in the home setting.

2. According to this passage, what factors were partially responsible for triggering the educational reform movement that is discussed therein?

   A. The fact that the majority of citizens in the United States have attended the public schools themselves and therefore knew that instructional programs needed to be changed.
   B. The fact that many people wanted to teach their children at home and did not want to pay taxes to support the public school system.
   C. Anger over the implication that the amount of money a family has, as well as the amount of "luck" they encounter, can make a difference in a child's education.
   D. A decline in the national economy and the publication of exhaustive school resource studies.

3. The demand for educational reform and the resulting research that has been conducted over the past 20 years has been centered on:

   A. public schools.
   B. private schools.
   C. home education.
   D. correspondence courses.

4. The fourth paragraph states: "Researchers have gone into the field in great numbers to gain a firsthand view of the educational process in action." Which of the following statements would be reasonable assumptions to make as a result of that sentence?

   I. Many studies have been conducted in school settings.

II. The persons conducting the research are not simply basing their results on educational theories.
III. There appears to be a great deal of interest in the educational process.

   A. I only   C. I and II only
   B. II only   D. I, II, and III

5. What groups might the word "practitioners," used in paragraph three, stand for?

   A. doctors, dentists, lawyers
   B. educators
   C. superintendents, principals, teachers
   D. both B and C

6. The author of this passage gives the impression that:

   A. there is little hope for the successful future of public education in the United States.
   B. although serious problems exist in the educational arena, progress is being made, partially, as a result of the hands-on involvement of researchers.
   C. the field of education is so large that effective change cannot occur.
   D. too many people are involved in doing educational research.

7. Based on the information presented in the final paragraph, it probably is reasonable to conclude that:

   A. private schools provide students with a higher quality education than public schools.
   B. research efforts on effective schools will continue as plans of action are implemented and evaluated.
   C. the public is satisfied with the results of the effective schools movement.
   D. the problem of educational reform is finite.

8. Which of the following statements is *supported by* the information presented in this passage?

   A. Education reform in the United States has been ongoing.
   B. Researchers clearly have shown that public education in the United States has failed.
   C. Private education has taken the lead over public education.

D. Home teaching is becoming more and more popular with families who cannot afford to send their children to private schools.

9. Which of the following statements is *contradicted by* the information presented in this passage?

   A. A student's family income is the major factor in determining his success in school.
   B. As a result of the hundreds of studies that researchers have done in schools, they have been able to restructure public education and stop the demand for reform.
   C. The negative effects of the early research (1966–1974) have been completely erased as a result of later studies, thus restoring the taxpayers' faith in public education.
   D. All of the above.

Passage II (Questions 10–16)

The fairy tale of Cinderella is one of the most widely known folk stories in the world. In its various versions it captures the struggle for the young girl's passage into womanhood. It covers, in its scope, several of Karen Horney's ideas, as well as the trials, totems, and family patterns found in primitive cultures. The Cinderella story chronicles the transformation of the girl into the woman, the profane into the spiritual; ending in the heroine's resolution of her feminine powers.

The Cinderella story goes back as far as seventh century China. It is classified among the most well-known folktales in the world, and there is a version in nearly every language. The plot is universal: Cinderella, a beautiful, kind, and loving girl, suffers within her family, and is aided by some form of magic, through which she meets the man she is destined to marry. After the initial meetings with this man, she loses some article symbolic of the womb, and the man uses this article to find and betroth her.

Several of Karen Horney's theories from "The Distrust Between the Sexes" are evident in this folktale. One of the main ideas in Cinderella is the concept of the evil stepmother or foster mother. Even in instances where Cinderella's father is still living, the stepmother is allowed to abuse her. Her elder sisters are also given this privilege. This is because the moth-

Adapted from Heather Tuttle, "If the Shoe Fits," VCU, 1990.

er and sisters are older and less attractive than the heroine. Cinderella's persecution is permitted because, as Horney says, ". . . it is only the sexually attractive woman of whom [man] is afraid and who . . . has to be kept in bondage." In the cultures from which the story derives, old women are not sexually threatening to men and so the stepmother is given the power (by the father) to make the heroine submissive. Horney continues: "Old women, on the other hand, are held in high esteem, even by cultures in which the young woman is dreaded and therefore suppressed." Not only is the stepmother granted more power over Cinderella due to her position, but she feels her power potentially jeopardized by the sway that Cinderella's beauty may have over men. The sisters also feel jeopardized by the heroine's sexual attractiveness, which leads to greater resentment and cruelty on their part.

Another of Horney's theories prevalent in the story is the duality of motherhood. There are two aspects of motherhood, the virgin mother who is self-sacrificing, nurturing, and selfless, and the mother goddess, warm, earthy, sensual, and fertile. Both aspects are visible in the heroine. Cinderella, as she is first seen, sleeps in the cold, empty hearth, reflective of the virgin's womb, empty until acted upon by some outside force. She is covered in ashes, dressed in rags; in general a picture of self-effacing humility. Despite the hardships put upon her by her family, she is kind to them and even tries her best to beautify her stepsisters for the ball. She is virtuous, in contrast to her stepsisters and stepmother. After marriage to the prince, in the end, the heroine does not seek any revenge on her persecutors. In some renditions, she actually invites her family to come live with her and her new husband. Further evidence of this virginal mother aspect is the part that the prince plays in her life at this point. Like the ultimate example of nurturing motherhood, Mother Mary, who waits for the male god to act upon her, Cinderella lies in wait for the prince to come and save her. He is the aid she needs to be freed of her harsh life.

The other aspect of motherhood is revealed in her when magic help arrives from the outside. She is bestowed with sensual, material things: beautiful clothes, ornaments, cosmetics; things to make her desirable to men. The heroine is also gifted with the famous shoes, reflective of the womb. This prince is usually attracted to her for her physical appearance. She is displaying her sensual, seductive, earthy side and the prince is a reward for her power to act on him with her seductive ability. This dichotomy provides some confusion to the heroine, her family, and her suitor. The journey to resolve the puzzle of her two-fold womanhood is a main theme in this folktale.

The passage from a girl to a woman is only one of the several transitions that take place within our heroine. She also undergoes a spiritual transformation. In the beginning of every account, the heroine is dirty and ragged. In at least three versions, she is made to wear animal skins. These things are representative of the material, animalistic, profane world. As she is put through the trials for entering into adulthood, she is also put through trials to test her spirituality. In spite of hardships, she manages to remain pious, loving, and kind. These trials come to an end and she becomes clean and well dressed. She is described as radiant, angelic, and fairylike. The heroine is then presented to the prince. The image of the prince embracing the servant girl is heavily laden with religious meaning, especially during the period when this story became popular. This analogy was very often used by the convents of the Middle Ages to relate the relationship of the nuns to Jesus Christ. Cinderella's spiritual ascent is completed with her royal wedding.

The heroine's time of testing is not completely at an end until the two sides of her femininity merge. They have been in the process of merging since the time of her totem's arrival. Since the arrival of the totem, she has actively struggled with her two female aspects, the virginal/nurturing and the earthy/seductive. The heroine in each version of the tale is given a womb symbol: either a shoe or a ring. This symbol accompanies her when she meets the prince in her state of beauty and sensuality. She then loses this article with the prince, who uses it to find her. When he sees her again, she is once more virginal, modest, covered in dirt and ashes, yet she is missing this symbol of her womanhood. The prince is confused; this is not quite the girl he thought he came for. After he places the shoe on her foot (or the ring on her finger, as the case may be) he sees her as whole: sensual, earthy, yet loving and virginal. She no longer runs from him as she did in earlier encounters, when things became too intimate with the prince.

This is also a moment of recognition for Cinderella. She has discovered a unity of both female forces within her. There were clues previously as to the wholeness of her nature, but she ignored them. She managed to overlook the times when she was sensual, at the ball, and was still kind to her family, generously giving them jewelry. She failed to see her true nature when she was beautiful and yet very humble in the presence of nobility. Now she can no longer hide herself. The prince has seen her spiritual, virginal, and sensual facets and her true nature is revealed to all, including her astonished family. She has found strength in her wholeness, and the prince is both her aid in discovering herself and her reward for being discovered.

10. This passage asserts that:
   I. only those versions of the story that are American can be used to illustrate Horney's theories.
   II. regardless of the version of the Cinderella tale, the story tells of a young girl's passage into womanhood.
   III. the concept of the evil stepmother or foster mother is a main ingredient in the Cinderella story.
   IV. Cinderella's sisters typically are older than she and less attractive.
   V. the prince finally sees only one facet of Cinderella.

   A. I, II, and III   C. II, III, and IV
   B. I and IV   D. IV only

11. According to this passage, Cinderella:

   A. contemplates revenge on her sisters and mother but doesn't carry through with it.
   B. does not seek revenge at all.
   C. gives up her need for revenge after she marries the prince.
   D. cannot bring herself to completely forgive her persecutors.

12. The author of this passage concludes the following from the fact that in at least three versions of the story, Cinderella is made to wear animal skins.

   A. She needs the warmth that these skins provide.
   B. The animal skins have nothing to do with the rites of passage that she is going through.
   C. The animal skins symbolize the profane animal world that she figuratively is leaving.
   D. She may decide to keep the animal skins.

13. Throughout the essay, but especially in the concluding paragraphs, the author suggests that Cinderella:

   A. is less complex than she had originally thought herself to be.
   B. is moving psychologically toward a condition of wholeness.
   C. intentionally exploits the prince to bring about her own growth.
   D. is weakened by her newly discovered wholeness.

14. One might draw the following conclusions from this passage:

    A. Horney probably had the Cinderella story in mind when she formulated her theories.
    B. Folktales and fairy tales such as Cinderella can be useful in illustrating aspects of psychological theories such as those of Horney.
    C. Horney's theories are valid because the plots of the various versions of the Cinderella story bear them out.
    D. Horney altered the story to make it fit her theories.

15. An appropriate title for this essay would be:

    A. "If the Shoe Fits": Horney's Theories and the Cinderella Story.
    B. The Narcissism of Cinderella.
    C. The Stepmother as Heroine.
    D. The Varieties of Magical Experience: The Shoe that Fit.

16. If one were to write an essay that used logic similar to that in this essay, that study might be called:

    A. Fairy Tales of the Western World.
    B. Jack and the Beanstalk and the Theories of Sigmund Freud.
    C. Little Red Riding Hood and Snow White.
    D. Cinematic Interpretations of Eastern and Western Folktales.

Passage III (Questions 17–24)

Probably most people enter medical school driven in large measure by their desire to help their fellow humankind. Although the prospects of achieving substantial wealth and reasonably high public esteem may be related motives, most consider that the search to live some form of the Golden Rule is an important reason for entering medical school. There is a growing perception among the general public, however, that many physicians are more interested in themselves and their families than in their patients. An understanding of the role conflicts experienced in medical school, residency training, and professional

Adapted from addresses of Dr. Stephen M. Ayres, Dean, School of Medicine, Medical College of Virginia, Virginia Commonwealth University, 1990.

practice must begin in the earliest days of medical education.

The sociologist, Wendy Carlton, studied the development of medical students and concluded that three rather distinct perspectives, the moral, clinical, and legal, directly affect decision making by physicians. Her extensive observation suggested to her that "medical students are being socialized into using the clinical perspective to resolve clinical problems with little or no regard for the ethical aspects of their professional behavior. In particular there is a striking absence of both discussion of and concern with ethical issues, despite a growing body of literature that argues for the relevance of training in ethics for physicians in an age of technological medicine." The clinical perspective, to Carlton, meant the traditional evaluation of the patient to create a "clinical picture" and, indeed, she entitled her book *In Our Professional Opinion*.

Carlton found that medical students upon entering medical school use the moral, clinical, and legal perspectives in that order. After acquiring clinical experience they apply the ranking used by physicians: clinical, legal, and then the moral. Hospital administrators invoke the legal, the clinical, and then the moral. "Laypersons," she contended, "use the moral perspective and depend on professionals to provide the clinical and legal perspectives, though they may use information from the media in an attempt to address the clinical and legal aspects of problem solution."

There is considerable concern on the part of many that the clinical perspective described by Carlton can degenerate into a callous regard for patient interest. Shem, in 1978, presented a satirical view of the brutal world of the intern in his book, *The House of God*. Terry Mizrahi, a sociologist who observed medical house staff behavior in a large urban teaching center, felt that Dr. Shem's book "verified the overall detachment and dehumanizing resulting from the training process." Her book, *Getting Rid of Patients*, "substantiated a world of contradictions wherein the patient was oppressed while being characterized as the oppressor."

Melvin Konner, an anthropologist who entered medical school in his mid-thirties after a variety of experiences (including a two-year stint with faith-healers from the hunter-gatherers of the Kalahari desert in Africa), described his educational experiences in *Becoming A Doctor*. He characterized physicians as "tough, brilliant, knowledgable, hardworking, and hard on themselves. They are reliable and competent in situations ranging from 18-month-long management of cancer chemotherapy through 18-hour-long brain surgery to emergencies in which life may hinge on what they can do in 18 seconds. They have experienced many things that are closed to others. With very few exceptions, they are professionals.''

''Perhaps they have earned the right to arrogance; they certainly feel that they have. But one wonders if they can see the self-serving aspects of their behavior.'' Konner goes on to emphasize the importance of ''a nonphysical aspect to healing, which I am prepared to call spiritual. It relates to heart and mind, hope and will, love and courage, values and ideas, social and cultural—including religious—life. In the hospital, I learned to keep my thoughts to myself about all such matters. There, the pretense is that everyone knows about them, and it is unnecessary to talk of them. In reality, everyone 'knows' about them but practically nobody cares, except insofar as finding them the source of a good laugh. Such cynicism, which increases during the medical school years, deeply affects the young physicians' view of life—not just of illness but of the whole human experience. They have trained themselves to participate just so far and no farther with, say, a terminal cancer patient in his or her search for personal meaning; but then they cannot simply slough off this habit of diffidence when it comes to their own search for meaning, when they contemplate the course of their own lives. It is less than appealing, what this makes of them; yet I love them in some crazy way ... I would not want my daughter or son to be one or to marry one ... Yet of course, when I am in trouble—and notice that I do not say 'if'—I will go to them, and they will improve my chances.''

The life of the medical student is challenging and at times frustrating. While intelligence and good undergraduate preparation are essential, they are not enough. Medicine is really the study of the human condition. What was once called ''bedside manner'' or ''attitude,'' really means an understanding of the ingredients of human happiness. Although good health seems essential for the enjoyment of life, it is clearly not enough. And the advantages of good health frequently must be tempered by the need for reasonable diet, reasonable shelter, and love and understanding. The practice of medicine is a calling, not a business. Physician-healers must know the science of health and disease but must also know what comprises the total experience that generally is called ''being human.'' The first year of medical education, and part of the second, emphasizes the science of medicine. The patient experience towards the end of the first year of medical education, and the remaining years of education, are designed to help the student internalize the view that the practice of medicine must be based on the broadest possible understanding of the human condition. ''The secret of the care of the patient is in caring for the patient.''

17. The author could have chosen as a title for this passage:

A. Professional Growth of the Practicing Physician.
B. The Development of Medical Students.
C. The Life of the Medical Student.
D. The Development of the Physician.

18. The medical student of today:

A. is greatly concerned with achieving high public esteem.
B. needs only superior intelligence and a good undergraduate education to succeed.
C. hopes to marry a classmate in order to have a more congenial marriage.
D. is concerned and wants to serve humanity.

19. Carlton suggests that as medical students undergo their training:

A. the ethical and moral issues predominate their decision making process.
B. socialization elevates clinical decision making as a predominant force.
C. are greatly influenced by hospital administrators who concentrate on legal issues.
D. they soon feel that they have earned the right to arrogance because of their thorough training.

20. Which of the following statement(s) is/are substantiated by the passage?

A. Good health is enough for the enjoyment of life.
B. Love and understanding of human emotions are not serious considerations in the overall scheme of a human being.
C. Bedside manner can be learned.
D. Medicine must use as its basis for practice a broad appreciation of life and mankind.

21. Which of the following statement(s) is/are contradicted by the passage?

A. Medical education should not consider the role conflicts experienced by students of medicine.
B. Laypersons focus quickly on the clinical and legal perspectives.

C. Physicians concentrate on their own happiness and are not hard on themselves.

D. All of the above.

22. The passage presented would be most suitable:

   A. at a tenth year reunion of a class.
   B. at a faculty meeting.
   C. at an administrative council meeting.
   D. as an introductory lecture to freshmen medical students.

23. Decision making by physicians is influenced by:

   A. moral issues.
   B. clinical phenomena.
   C. legal opinions.
   D. all of the above.

24. Which of the following statements are *supported by* the passage?

   A. The first two years of medical school are devoted to learning the necessary science.
   B. There is patient contact in the first two years.
   C. There is a spiritual part to healing.
   D. All of the above.

Passage IV (Questions 25–30)

Throughout the various phyla of the plant and animal kingdom, numerous species have evolved. It is apparent that sexual reproduction plays an important role in the continuation of the species and in the expression of different phenotypes within the species. This mode of reproduction is accomplished by the fusion of two gametes that will give rise to a zygote. In order for future generations to maintain the same number of chromosomes as their parents, the gametes must undergo a reduction in chromosome number. If the offspring express phenotypic traits that are different from those of their parents, there must be a rearrangement of the DNA within the chromosomes. The reduction of the number of chromosomes and mixing of the gene pool are accomplished by the process of meiosis.

The process of meiosis is characterized by a naturally occurring sequence of events that are usually artificially subdivided into ten different stages. The

From Huge R. Seibel and Kenneth E. Guyer, *How to Prepare for the Medical College Admission Test*, 6th ed. Hauppauge, New York: Barron's Educational Series, Inc., 1990.

first five stages comprise the first or reductional division of meiosis. At the end of the reductional division, the chromosomes are reduced to one-half their original number (haploid). The last five stages comprise the second or equatorial division of meiosis. Germ cells undergoing meiosis give rise to haploid gametes that contain one representative of each type of chromosome. The chromosomes of the gametes may also demonstrate variations in genetic composition due to crossing over that takes place during the first prophase.

Replication of DNA occurs during interphase before the process of meiosis begins. The condensation and coiling of chromatin to form chromosomes marks the beginning of prophase I, the first stage of meiosis. Homologous chromosomes pair with one another to form a structure called a bivalent. Next each chromosome splits lengthwise to form two chromatids. The homologous pairs of chromosomes are now composed of four chromatids that are referred to as a tetrad. The chromatids of tetrads become short and thick and breaks may occur in them. The breaks are eventually repaired but segments of different chromatids may be joined together. This process, referred to as crossing over, enables segments of two different chromatids to be joined together. This enables the gametes to receive chromosomes derived from segments of both homologous chromosomes. In the second stage of meiosis or metaphase I, the nuclear membrane disappears, a spindle apparatus forms, and the homologous pairs align along the equatorial plate of the cell. In anaphase I, the homologous chromosomes migrate to opposite poles of the cell. Telophase I is characterized by the complete separation of the homologous pairs, and the spindle apparatus disappears. The nuclear membrane begins to reform and in many organisms a cytoplasmic division may occur at this stage.

After a brief interphase, prophase II begins. Prophase II is the first stage in the second or equatorial division of meiosis. It is characterized by the condensing of chromatin to form the chromosomes. During metaphase II, the spindle apparatus forms and the chromosomes line up along the equatorial plate. In anaphase II, the daughter chromosomes migrate to opposite poles of the cell. Anaphase II differs from the first anaphase in that the centromere divides and the two chromatids now become the daughter chromosomes. The daughter chromosomes separate completely and reach opposite poles of the cell in telophase II. Subsequent divisions of the cytoplasm result in the formation of two daughter cells that have a haploid number of chromosomes.

The two divisions of the germ cell during meiosis produce four gametes with one-half the original number of chromosomes.

25. According to this passage, at the end of the reductional division of meiosis:

   A. four haploid sets of chromosomes are produced.
   B. the homologous pairs of chromosomes are completely separated.
   C. the chromatin duplicates and coils.
   D. the centromeres divide and daughter chromosomes move to opposite poles of the cell.

26. According to this passage, crossing over occurs:
   A. during the equatorial division.
   B. before the tetrad separates.
   C. during anaphase I.
   D. during prophase II.

27. According to this passage, duplication of the chromatin occurs during:

   A. metaphase I.
   B. anaphase II.
   C. telophase I.
   D. interphase.

28. According to this passage, variation in genetic composition is made possible by:

   A. the formation of homologous pairs.
   B. mitotic division of germ cells.
   C. crossing over.
   D. random mutations.

29. It can be inferred from this passage that:

   A. all species in both the plant and animal kingdom are capable of sexual reproduction.
   B. haploid cells are only found in animals.
   C. four functional gametes are always formed by the process of meiosis.
   D. zygote formation may produce an offspring that has the same number of chromosomes as its parents.

30. Which of the following statement(s) is/are *supported by* the passage?

   A. Meiosis is artificially subdivided into ten stages.
   B. Reproduction results in phenotypic expression.
   C. DNA duplicates before meiosis starts.
   D. All of the above.

Passage V (Questions 31–38)

Does the order of a child's birth in a family have a bearing on the type of adult he/she will grow up to be, or is the theory of ordinal position simply an interesting topic of cocktail party conversation? Although it has been the highlight of numerous debates and the subject of various studies, ordinal position remains a little-understood personality variable.

Consider the oldest child in a family of three children. Parents often claim that their firstborn has a solid head on his/her shoulders, behaves in a mature manner, and is capable of getting along with adults. This important family member often exhibits a quiet front, yet is able to take the lead, care for his/her siblings, and act like a miniature adult. Parents view the firstborn as an intelligent individual who will grow up to be a pillar of the community. A perfect illustration of the importance of being firstborn can be seen in the old custom of primogeniture that was particularly popular during the feudal period in Europe.

Primogeniture allowed the oldest member of a family, in most situations oldest male, to inherit all lands and possessions of his parents, to the exclusion of his siblings. The ordinal position of being the firstborn male therefore carried much power, as the firstborn was considered to be intelligent, level-headed, and capable of taking over as family protector and landlord once the father died. Theoretically the oldest would be unselfish and see to the care of the younger family members, but in actuality this was often not the case. Outlawed in the United States and no longer the mode of inheritance in Europe for today's population as a whole, primogeniture was in evidence as late as the 1920s and can still be seen in degree with some of Europe's royal families.

The second born child in a family of three is pictured quite differently from the oldest. This child is much more lively, less willing to take orders, does not show the same interest in adults, and often has difficulty communicating with them. He/she may even become a "problem" child in school. Teachers have been heard to complain that "B is not in the least like A was … ." Could it be that the second born is striking out in an attempt to find his/her own place? The problems of the second child in a family seem to intensify even more when the "baby" comes along and moves him/her into the "middle child" position. Now he/she has to contend not only with a successful older brother or sister, but also with the youngest who seems to be the favorite.

The youngest child appears not to feel the need to measure up to anyone and goes along his/her own

From Hugo R. Seibel and Kenneth E. Guyer, *How to Prepare for the Medical College Admission Test*, 6th ed. Hauppauge, New York: Barron's Educational Series, Inc., 1990.

way to develop into an often exuberant, well-rounded individual. Because he/she is the baby, the mother doesn't expect this third sibling to function like a miniature adult, and she considers "cute" a great number of the actions that were viewed as unsatisfactory in the case of the other children.

Personality traits are not the only topic of interest in the ordinal position arena. The academic ability of children in various birth positions has also received attention. One interesting study reported a comparison of mathematics grades between women who were separated into three groups: (1) firstborn, (2) at least second born but not last born, and (3) last born in a family. Women without siblings were excluded from the study. The results indicate a statistical difference in mathematics grades between groups (1) and (3) but no other significant differences. Group (1) achieved higher mathematics grades than group (3).

Theories of motivation and anxiety have been advanced to explain the difference in achievement. The motivation theory states that the oldest child receives more encouragement from the parents than is given to other children. For a time, the first child is the only child, an experience not shared by the other children. Particularly during this early period the parents may try very hard to help the child, thus striving to experience vicariously their own unfulfilled expectations. The anxiety theory adds another factor to try to explain the lower achievement of the youngest child. Not only is the youngest child not pushed, as was the case with his/her older siblings, but this lack of parental pushing may be interpreted as lack of parental interest. The youngest child may develop feelings of anxiety, and these may interfere with performance. Thus, the youngest child may suffer as a result of less parental pressure and expectations as well as suffering from self-imposed anxiety, both contributing to lower performance.

31. The central thesis of the passage is that:

    A. the motivational drive (as well as the anxiety level of children) is directly linked to the order in which they are born.
    B. the development of a child's personality may be affected by the ordinal position he/she holds in his/her family.
    C. primogeniture, which is the custom of passing on property to the oldest male member of a family, is the vehicle used by the royal families of Europe to ensure that their fortunes will remain intact.
    D. ordinal position remains a little understood personality variable despite the fact that it is a popular topic both at the research and at the debate level.

32. Based on the information given in the passage, it is reasonable to conclude that:

    A. the oldest child in a family is the child best equipped to handle stressful situations.
    B. more research needs to be conducted before any concrete judgments can be made regarding the effect that birth order has on an individual's personality.
    C. academically, the youngest child tends to be lazy because he/she has been babied by parents and siblings.
    D. married couples should become well versed in ordinal position literature so that they will have a guide to follow when they are ready to have children.

33. What is the probable reason that the author used the paragraph on primogeniture in this passage?

    A. As a means of making the passage more interesting for the reader by introducing a historical topic.
    B. In order to make the reader aware of the fact that the firstborn was expected to share his inheritance with his younger siblings.
    C. To make the reader aware of the fact that the custom was outlawed in the United States around 1920.
    D. As a means of illustrating the fact that ordinal position, especially the place of the firstborn, has been a topic of interest for a long period of time.

34. Which of the following statement(s) is/are *supported* by the information in the passage?

    I. Parents often claim that firstborn children behave in a more mature manner than laterborn.
    II. The "baby" of the family is often a child with an outgoing personality.
    III. By the time the third child comes along, mothers no longer seem to put the same emphasis on certain aspects of behavior that they did when raising their first.

    A. I only   C. I and II only
    B. II only   D. I, II, and III

35. Which of the following statements is *contradicted by* the information given in the passage?

    A. Comparison to older siblings, by teachers and other adults, is the best method for stimulating the middle child to work harder.

B. Second born children who later move into the "middle child" position achieve on a higher plane in school than do second born who remain in the same position.

C. The youngest child does not feel the need to measure up to anyone.

D. The second born child sometimes has a problem communicating with adults.

36. Information concerning the academic ability of children in various birth positions is presented in paragraphs seven and eight. This section of the passage deals primarily with:

A. differences in mathematics achievement between males and females.

B. differences in achievement of students between mathematics and other courses.

C. differences in mathematics grades of females according to birth order.

D. the effect of parental support on mathematics achievement.

37. In presenting the information in paragraph eight, the author suggests that anxiety:

A. has no effect on mathematics achievement.

B. decreases mathematics achievement.

C. increases mathematics achievement.

D. can only be imposed by others.

38. Which of the following statement(s) is/are *supported by* the passage?

A. The example uses a family unit of five people.

B. Being the youngest could be of advantage in becoming a well-balanced individual.

C. Performance is related to anxiety in the youngest child.

D. All of the above.

Passage VI (Questions 39–45)

Performance appraisals—"Who needs them? I'm doing a good job, so why does someone need to sit and put it in writing, then waste my time and theirs talking about it? If I'm doing something that they don't like, let them tell me about it when it happens." This is a typical comment heard from many employees.

From Hugo R. Seibel and Kenneth E. Guyer, *How to Prepare for the Medical College Admission Test,* 6th ed. Hauppauge, New York: Barron's Educational Series, Inc., 1990.

The performance appraisal, if completed properly, can be one of the most useful tools a manager can use in developing and training subordinates regardless of what some employees may express. It is a compilation of the employee's strengths and weakness in one concise form. It serves to show the employee the areas in which a good job is being done and also indicates which areas need improvement. The appraisal serves as a permanent record that documents the employee's growth and progress or shows why a promotion is not offered. A performance appraisal forces a manager to discuss an employee's performance on a one-to-one basis and find out more about what the employee's opinions and aspirations might be. This area is often overlooked in the busy day-in and day-out routine of business. It gives the employee a chance to see what the boss really thinks about his or her work.

An interesting and often very beneficial way of handling a performance appraisal is to give employees a blank evaluation form a few days before the appraisal interview and ask that they rate themselves. When the appraisal takes place, the manager and employee compare their evaluations and work out the areas of disagreement so that each understands the other's position. An unusual result often takes place. Not only do the manager and employee end up with a better knowledge of each other, but they often find that their evaluations are very close to being in agreement. If anything, the employees usually find that they have underrated themselves. An exception to this result, which the manager must be alert to recognize, is that an unsatisfactory performer may evaluate his or her performance higher than does the manager. The appraisal interview in this situation can often be more valuable than that of the satisfactory performer. It gives the manager an opportunity to counsel an already trained employee and turn around the performance rather than having to seek out and train a replacement. The manager must evaluate the time, expense, and attitude of the present employee against the time and expense of hiring and training a new employee.

Performance appraisals, properly administered, can cut down on turnover and greatly increase the morale of a department. The end result is increased productivity, which is really what we are all striving to accomplish.

Although standard procedure in industry for many years, performance appraisals have also reached higher education. In recent years college students have come to see themselves as purchasing a service, specifically that of education. They have demanded greater accountability, asking that the remuneration of faculty members be tied to teaching effectiveness.

Many faculty members agree with the concept in theory but feel that measurement of teaching effectiveness is flawed.

Teaching effectiveness is often determined through evaluations by administrators, faculty colleagues, or students, or by a combination of two or more of these evaluations. Students are usually most interested in evaluations by students, believing that they are the "consumers" who are most directly affected by the quality of the "product" called teaching. Faculty members counter that evaluations by students are flawed, in that they are affected by the charisma (or lack of it) of the instructor, the level of difficulty of the subject matter, and the grades given in the course.

A more objective method has been suggested by various groups—the student performance at the end of the course. All students taking a particular course could be given a standard test; mean scores in sections taught by different instructors could then be compared and related to each instructor's teaching effectiveness. The results could be affected, of course, by the students' IQs, motivation, and prior instruction in the material covered by the course.

39. Which of the following statement(s) is/are *supported by* the information in the passage?

A. The performance appraisal gives the employee and the manager a time to discuss the employee's future in private.
B. Employees and managers usually can work out their differences during the appraisal interview.
C. Performance appraisals often lead to a better understanding between managers and employees and eventually can lead to increased productivity.
D. All of the above.

40. Which of the following statement(s) is/are NOT *supported nor contradicted by* the information in the passage?

A. Most large companies are now using the performance appraisal method because it has been proven a highly effective tool for dismissing unsatisfactory employees.
B. All performance appraisals are preceded by giving employees blank forms to rate themselves.
C. Managers feel that performance appraisals are a waste of time.
D. All of the above.

41. Which of the following statement(s) is/are *contradicted by* the information in the passage?

A. A satisfactorily performing employee will rate himself or herself higher than the manager.
B. A performance appraisal only points out the weak areas of performance.
C. A performance appraisal is the most useful tool a manager uses in developing and training subordinates.
D. All of the above.

42. According to the passage:

A. all suggested methods of evaluation of teaching effectiveness are quite subjective.
B. the charisma of the instructor is a factor in evaluation of teaching effectiveness.
C. evaluations of an instructor's teaching effectiveness are unaffected by student grades.
D. evaluations of an instructor's teaching effectiveness are affected by the time of day when lectures are given.

43. According to the passage, greater difficulty of the course would have what effect on student ratings of teacher effectiveness?

A. lower ratings
B. higher ratings
C. no effect
D. the passage does not say

44. The author indicates that students are most interested in ratings of teaching effectiveness when determined by:

A. evaluation by faculty colleagues.
B. evaluation by administrators.
C. evaluation by students.
D. objectively determined progress of the performance of the class.

45. According to the passage:

A. students view themselves as consumers.
B. performance evaluations benefit the parties involved.
C. performance appraisals can lead to increased productivity.
D. all of the above are true statements.

Passage VII (Questions 46–51)

Paul Tillich, in his article "The Lost Dimension in Religion," asserts that in contemporary Western society there is an absence of spirituality; moreover, that in spite of a growing interest in religion, and because of it, the religious element as Tillich defines it has all but vanished. The popularity of "go-to-church-every-Sunday" and the tel-evangelism of the 80s belong to the "concrete religion" of literal hermeneutics (the science of interpretating an author's words or scriptures), rituals, and institutions.

The lost dimension as Tillich describes it is the loss of each individual's asking himself or herself basic and important existential questions such as: "What is the meaning of life? Where do we come from, where do we go to? What shall we do, what should we become in the short stretch between birth and death?" This spiritual "dimension of depth" is lost to modern man, he says, and "religion as the state of being grasped by an infinite concern" is absent.

Though written 30 years ago, this observation is still insightful today, perhaps even more so. Tillich explains how spiritual depth has become lost to contemporary Man. He traces the causes to Man's relationship with Nature and with himself, a relationship in which Nature is "subjected scientifically and technically" by the whims of Man, and self-knowledge is nearly nonexistent.

But, Tillich claims that, though today's generations lack the courage to ask themselves weighty eschatological questions (dealing with final matters, such as death), previous generations had the courage to do so. On this point, Tillich is slightly evasive. Does he mean that, say, a rise in materialism and technology parallels a drop in spirituality, and that previous generations who were less materialistic and technologically oriented were more spiritual? Perhaps, but he seems to rely heavily on our technologically-oriented lives as evidence of a decline in spirituality. One might agree with him on this point but still believe that the roots go much deeper, and that our technology-based living and subsequent relationship with Nature is indeed an effect of something else as much as it is a cause of a loss of spirituality. Might not the dualistic perspective implicit in our own philosophical heritage, which seeks to divide the whole into parts, be called into question, along with the scientific method and "value-free" science? The present-day relationship between Man and Nature may well be a cause of the "loss of the dimension of depth"; but one could also argue that the seeds were sown a long time ago, so long ago that a more appropriate discussion of the

loss of spiritual depth would include Man's relationship to technology as well.

The true religion, according to Tillich, moves vertically, hence "depth." It involves a personal dimension as well; personal existential questions ask for personal existential answers. And what Tillich sees in present-day religion (institutional and literalistic) is a horizontal aspect, a dimension that denies itself "basic and universal meaning" and the symbolic interpretation of sacred texts. This "horizontal" religion goes hand-in-hand with contemporary horizontal living, where technological/industrial society makes things " 'better and better,' 'bigger and bigger,' " there is "movement ahead without end," and "every moment is filled with something" whether it be television or a 40-hour-a-week job. In the horizontal dimension, "no one can experience depth ... [or start] becoming aware of himself." Symptomatic of this kind of life is the question of whether or not God exists, a "discussion in which both sides are wrong, because the discussion itself is wrong and possible only after the loss of the dimension of depth."

Tillich advocates a kind of personal inquiry, a soul-searching "in spite of the loss of the dimension of depth"; an asking of questions such as "What is the meaning of Life?" But Tillich, for all his discussion of spirituality, makes no reference to the intuitive side of Man's nature. Tillich seems to imply that existential questions and any answers they might find are rational in their relationship to one another, and that the latter follows logically from the former; that there is indeed an answer that can be articulated. I suspect that this perspective is still inside the cultural context that gave rise to the loss of the dimension of depth in the first place—perhaps Tillich needs to step out of that context and into a context that is intuitive and in which personal existential questions are acknowledged from a source much deeper than the rational mind. It is perhaps the intuitive/spiritual that is the true religious character that, as Tillich says, "in spite of the loss of dimension of depth, its power is present, and is most present in those who are aware of the loss ... ."

Adapted from Taylor Fleet, "A Critique of Paul Tillich," VCU, 1989

46. The author of this passage observes that according to Tillich, contemporary society:

 A. is no longer interested in religion.
 B. suffers from a loss of spirituality.
 C. is more than willing to ask itself weighty existential questions.
 D. none of the above.

47. The author suggests that, according to Tillich:

A. true religion moves vertically.
B. true religion is the same as present-day (institutional and literalistic) religion.
C. present-day society encourages individuals to ask deep questions about human existence.
D. true religion asks questions addressing whether or not God exists.

48. The author takes Tillich to task on the following point:

A. his assertion that modern man lacks true religion.
B. his belief that people are more materialistic today than in the past.
C. his definition of spirituality.
D. failure to take into account the intuitive side of Man's nature in discussing ways by which individuals can find answers to spiritual questions.

49. The author finds Tillich's ideas about the lost dimension in religion as:

A. less valid than they were when Tillich wrote them 30 years ago.
B. at least as insightful as they were 30 years ago.
C. interesting but too theoretical to be applied to actual human beings.
D. illustrative of T.S. Eliot's idea that modern man lives in a spiritual wasteland.

50. An appropriate title for this essay might be:

A. The Relevance of Tillich's Ideas Thirty Years Later.
B. The Optimism of Paul Tillich.
C. Tillich as Champion of Man's Intuition.
D. The Tillich that No One Knows.

51. In contemporary "horizontal" religion, according to Tillich, there is:

A. a de-emphasis on television in the lives of individuals.
B. an accentuation of the small.
C. a clear goal at the end of the individual's struggle.
D. an emphasis on better and better and on bigger and bigger.

Passage VIII (Questions 52–58)

The temporomandibular joint is characterized as a bilateral diarthroidal articulation; that is, it is capable of both rotary (hinge) and translatory (gliding) motion. This range of motion permits movement both bodily (side) and in an anterior-posterior direction of the mandibular condyle within the glenoid fossa or cavity of this joint. The functional articulation actually occurs when each condyle contacts the articular eminence of the squamous part of the temporal bone. Both the right and left joints function as one unit, but each may move somewhat independently.

Interposed between the condyle and fossa and eminence is an articular disk or meniscus which is attached to the head of the condyle posteriorly and to the joint capsule laterally. This arrangement produces upper and lower joint compartments lined by synovium. The disk consists of dense collagenous connective tissue or may be fibrocartilaginous in nature. It fuses with the joint capsule, which is composed of dense fibroelastic connective tissue. This capsule is attached to the concave surface of the fossa, the convex surface of the eminence, and inferiorly to the neck of the concave surface of the fossa, the convex surface of the eminence, and inferiorly to the neck of the condyle. The thickened lateral part of the capsule forms the temporomandibular ligament.

The temporomandibular ligament functions to prevent excessive retraction of the mandible and thus limits border movements. Other ligaments attached to the joint include the sphenomandibular, the stylomandibular, and the tiny Pinto's. The sphenomandibular ligament functions to limit closure of the jaws. It becomes taut if the vertical dimension is decreased. The stylomandibular ligament functions to limit extreme mandibular protrusion and overclosure of the jaws. The tiny ligament, attached to the capsule, disk, and sphenomandibular ligament, inserts on the malleus of the ear. Tension on it may cause some change in position of the malleus.

Each synovial compartment is lined with a vascular layer of connective tissue. In areas not exposed to pressure, the synovial membrane is thrown into numerous folds. There are two kinds of cells comprising the membrane. Type A cells are phagocytic in nature and are found among type B cells that are secretory in nature. The cavity is filled with synovial fluid, a transparent, yellowish, viscous material. The fluid is a dialysate of plasma and lymph consisting of a protein-mucopoly-saccharide complex. Debris is removed from this lubricating and nutritional fluid by the type A cells of the membrane.

From Hugo R. Seibel and Kenneth E. Guyer, *How to Prepare for the Medical College Admission Test*, 6th ed. Hauppauge, New York: Barron's Educational Series, Inc., 1990.

52. The main topic of this passage is:

A. the unlimited movement capabilities of the temporomandibular joint.

B. the description of the functional anatomy of the joint.

C. the role of the ligaments in movements of the joint.

D. the histological characterization of various anatomic controls.

53. According to the passage, the meniscus is best described as:

A. the layer internal to the synovial compartments.

B. the connective tissue separating the lower compartment from the condyle.

C. the fibrocartilage positioned above the upper synovial cavity.

D. the attachment for the head of the condyle.

54. Unlike the articular disk, the joint capsule:

A. contains some connective tissue.

B. forms laterally into ligamentous tissue.

C. makes attachment with the joint.

D. consists of fibers and cells.

55. It can be concluded from the passage that:

A. border movements made by the mandible are restricted by ligamentous attachments.

B. overclosure of the jaws occurs frequently.

C. slack in one of the ligaments leads to tension in other ligaments.

D. protrusion involves movement of the mandible posteriorly.

56. According to the passage, the following are correct EXCEPT:

A. Phagocytes remove foreign material from the synovial fluid.

B. Only Type B cells produce the synovial fluid.

C. Pressure flattens areas of the synovial membrane.

D. Blood vessels are found among the connective tissue of synovial compartments.

57. Which of the following statement(s) is/are *supported by* the passage?

A. The temporomandibular joint is a universal joint.

B. A fair percentage of people experience discomfort in this joint during life.

C. There is no connection between this joint and the middle ear.

D. None of the above.

58. Which of the following statement(s) is/are *contradicted by* the passage?

A. The synovial fluid has similar qualities as plasma.

B. The disk has an attachment to the joint capsule.

C. Joint function is synchronized.

D. None of the above.

Passage IX (Questions 59–65)

Studies of part-time and full-time faculty members in specific states and types of institutions are numerous. A review of the literature reveals specific issues as hinges on which the implementation of policy changes may turn. Recent studies clearly show the impact of the increasing use of part-time faculty in higher education institutions. Recommendations range from converting all part-time positions to full-time ones, save those made necessary by last-minute budget increases, to moves away from the traditional tenure system to alternative systems. Recommendations revolve around: employment security; participation of part-time, temporary, and full-time "teach only" faculty in academic governance; access to academic due process (as regards appointments that clearly specify nature and conditions of appointment, rights to confer over terms and conditions, timely settlement of grievances, fair evaluation by peers to which they may have opportunity to respond); and compensation including salary and benefits.

Institutions have continued to hire part-time faculty at a rate that shows a 164 percent increase (compared to a 37 percent increase in number of full-time faculty) from 1970 to 1988. "Part-timers" have been hired because of organizationally perceived financial necessity, the desire to maintain administrative and curricular "flexibility," and the availability of aca-

Adapted from A. Nancy Avakian, Ph.D and Margaret Martin, "The Issues: Viewpoints of the Academy about Nontenure-Eligible Faculty Members," 1990.

demics who do not have full-time positions in their fields for various reasons. Between 40 and 45 percent of all nontenure-track positions surveyed by AAUP in 1984–85 were filled by women, whereas they held only 25 percent of the total number of full-time faculty positions covered in the survey.

What purposes are served for the institution? The writers of the 1986 "Report on Full-Time Nontenure-Track Appointments" in *Academe* say it is questionable whether any real flexibility is achieved because a substantial portion of the nontenure-eligible appointments occur in fields that are central to the institution's academic program ("core" courses, such as English Composition). Part-time adjuncts and graduate assistants perform most lower division teaching and approximately 40 percent of the undergraduate instruction taking place in American colleges and universities (Nielsen and Polishook, 1990).

The continual hiring of nontenure-eligible faculty members creates a class of insecure teachers whose status is inferior to that of both their tenure-eligible and tenured colleagues and whose role in some respects does not differ from that of teaching assistants. On the one hand, many are not required or expected to advise students, to participate in faculty personnel and budget matters, or to be involved in the development of curricula and the formulation and implementation of academic policy. They tend to receive less desirable teaching assignments, larger classes, and heavier teaching loads. Their compensation remains low, no matter how well they perform(ed). Their performance may never be reviewed.

Specifics may change with part-time and full-time "teach only" faculty appointments, yet some of the same conditions apply. They cannot develop habits of the professional academic, which includes research and revision of courses and curricula. They frequently work in unprofessional conditions (some without offices, so unable to allot "office hours" to students) and are virtually isolated from the stimulation and support of their colleagues. Because of these conditions, these instructional faculty members may lack both access to institutional resources necessary for building a research career and the incentive or pressure to become (equally) productive scholars. Many, particularly full time "teach only" faculty members, are overworked and continually distracted by the efforts involved in looking for more secure employment conditions. Academic freedom of these teachers is also in question, as what they feel or what they may say could affect their ability to "serve the institution." To those whose appointment must be renewed at the discretion of the institution, expression of commitment to academic freedom may not be enough.

The contagion of insecurity restricts unorthodox thinking, while the rising number of those faculty reduces the cadre of those faculty, notably those with tenure, who are uninhibited in advocating changes in accepted ideas and in the policies and programs of the institutions at which they serve," (*Academe*, July/August 1986, p17a).

The presence of "temporary" faculty members who must concern themselves with their status in the institution while pursuing other employment is reflected in morale–theirs, the institution's, and that of everyone around them. The creation of this "two-tier class system" erodes sound governance practices and the fellowship of the faculty. As tenure-track faculty members perform more administrative duties, student advising, and committee work, they have less time for research and professional development. This atmosphere is generally less supportive of scholarly pursuits.

What some perceive as the increasing incidence and abuse of nontenure-track appointments when many of the best faculty recruits are choosing private sector positions instead of careers in higher education works against efforts to recruit and encourage the talented young scholars who might otherwise be more interested. These abuses may also contribute to the numbers of those who are leaving the ranks of academia. The writers who recognize this trend cite the proliferation of these temporary positions as evidence of "shortsightedness" and "unregulated growth."

59. Issues of concern regarding part-time faculty include:

   A. job security.
   B. academic governance.
   C. grievance procedures.
   D. all of the above.

60. The title of the passage could be:

   A. The Effect of Nontenure Track Faculty on the Educational System.
   B. Academic Freedom in Jeopardy.
   C. Viewpoints of the Academy About Nontenure-Eligible Faculty.
   D. Reforms due to the Increase in Nontenure-Eligible Faculty.

61. Which of the following statement(s) is/are *supported by* the passage?

   A. Most part-timers are women.

B. Part-timers have been hired at an increased rate.

C. Flexibility has been achieved in curriculum development.

D. Core courses are taught mainly by full-time faculty.

62. Which of the following statement(s) is/are *contradicted by* the passage?

A. Part-time faculty is never expected to take part in curriculum development.

B. Performance review of part-time faculty is questionable.

C. Full-time "teach only" faculty has a secure base from which to function.

D. A and C of the above.

63. Tenure-track faculty:

A. leave most of the advising to part-timers.

B. in the future will have more time for scholarly pursuits.

C. are apt to initiate changes.

D. are chosen from a large pool of the best recruits.

64. Concerning temporary faculty:

A. they have and create morale problems.

B. they help erode the governance system in higher education.

C. some view the hiring of this group as shortsighted.

D. all of the above statements apply.

65. Which of the following statement(s) is/are *supported by* the passage?

A. The theme of the discussion has been well investigated.

B. Many reasons explain the existence of part-time faculty.

C. Part-time faculty has had an impact on higher education.

D. All of the above.

PHYSICAL SCIENCES

10 PROBLEM SETS OF 5–10 QUESTIONS EACH
15 PROBLEMS FOLLOWED BY A SINGLE QUESTION
77 QUESTIONS
100 MINUTES

DIRECTIONS: The following questions or incomplete statements are in groups. Preceding each series of questions or statements is a paragraph or a short explanatory statement, a formula or set of formulas, or a definition. Read the written material and then answer the questions or complete the statements. Select the ONE BEST ANSWER for each question and indicate your selection by marking the corresponding letter of your choice on the Answer Form. Eliminate those alternatives you know to be incorrect and then select an answer from among the remaining alternatives. A periodic table is provided (see p467). You may consult it whenever you wish to do so.

Passage I (Questions 66–70)

A set of parallel metal plates is enclosed in a glass tube that is evacuated so that there is a good vacuum inside. Wires leading to the plates are attached to a battery of voltage *V* creating an electric field between the positive and negative plates. An electron, which starts from rest at the negative plate, accelerates uniformly and strikes the positive plate. At the same instant, a proton starts from rest at the positive plate and accelerates to the negative plate. It is also possible to apply a magnetic field between the plates by the use of externally mounted current-carrying coils of wire.

66. How do the kinetic energies of the electron and proton compare when each reaches its opposite plate?

 A. The electron has the greater KE because its small mass makes it easier to accelerate to high speed.
 B. The proton has the greater KE because of its larger mass.
 C. Both kinetic energies are reduced to zero.
 D. The kinetic energies are equal.

67. Assume that the original accelerating electric field points horizontally North. A horizontal magnetic field pointing West is now applied using the external coils. What are the paths of the electron and proton now?

 A. They both travel in a straight line (undeflected).
 B. The proton is deflected vertically upward and the electron downward.
 C. The proton is deflected to the West and the electron to the East.
 D. They are both deflected vertically upward.

68. The position of the magnetic coils is rotated so that the magnetic field is now parallel to the electric field (North). What are the paths of the electron and proton now?

 A. They both are deflected upward.
 B. The paths of both are not deflected at all.
 C. The proton deflects downward and the electron upward.
 D. The proton is now deflected to the East and the electron to the West.

69. What is the effect of the magnetic field on the speed of the proton and the electron?

 A. The speeds of both were not affected.
 B. The proton speeds up and the electron slows down.
 C. Both speed up due to the magnetic force on them.
 D. The electron speeds up and the proton slows down.

70. The magnetic field is turned off and an additional small set of parallel plates is mounted horizontally so that the proton and electron (which are traveling horizontally) enter the region between the small plates where a vertically upward *E* field exists. What effect does this second electric field have on the proton and electron paths?

 A. No effect; they are not deflected.
 B. The proton is deflected upward and the electron downward.
 C. They are both deflected upward.
 D. The proton is deflected horizontally East and the electron is deflected to the West.

Passage II (Questions 71–76)

A safety engineering firm is employed to produce a film for high school driver education classes. The firm uses skilled test drivers driving both small cars and larger vans. The vans weigh three times as much as the cars and have larger tires with twice the tread width. The engineers also design several remotely controlled cars and vans in order to film crash tests.

71. Drivers of a car and a van brake hard and skid to a stop from 50 mph. The skid marks are measured to be the same length for both. Why are the stopping distances the same length?

   A. The mechanical work done by friction to stop both is the same.
   B. The frictional force between tires and road is three times greater for the heavier van so it slides the same distance as the car.
   C. The frictional force for the car and van are the same.
   D. The wider tires on the van require less friction force than the narrow tires on the car.

72. Two drivers in identical cars skid to a stop from speeds of 20 mph and 40 mph. How do the lengths of the skid marks compare?

   A. They are the same length.
   B. The 40 mph mark is twice as long.
   C. The 40 mph mark is four times as long.
   D. The 40 mph mark is eight times as long.

73. A remotely controlled car and van are crashed head-on at the same speed. Why does the car suffer more damage in the collision?

   A. The car and van had the same momentum.
   B. The forces during collision are equal and opposite, so the smaller and weaker car suffers more damage.
   C. The van exerts a larger force on the car.
   D. The mechanical work done in stopping the car is greater.

74. The car and the van collide head-on. This time the car is going 60 mph and the van is going 20 mph. Examination shows that the car suffers more damage than the van. Why is this so?

   A. The car and van have equal magnitudes of momenta before the collision.

   B. The force exerted on the car by the larger van is larger.
   C. The forces exerted during the collision are equal and opposite, so the weaker car suffers more damage.
   D. The mechanical work to stop the car is greater.

75. A driver in a van skids to a stop from 20 mph and a driver in a car skids to a stop from 60 mph. How do the length of the skid marks compare?

   A. The van skids three times further than the car, because it is three times heavier.
   B. The car skids three times further because it is lighter and is going three times faster.
   C. The car will skid nine times as far as the van.
   D. They skid the same length because the speed ratio is 1:3, whereas the weight ratio is 3:1.

76. In an experiment designed to test reaction times and show them on the film, guns that fire a yellow paint onto the road are mounted on the bumpers. When the driver hears the report of the gun, he locks the brake and the touch of his foot on the brake fires a second paint pellet onto the road. When one driver is tested at 20 mph and 60 mph, the distance between the paint marks is three times farther for the 60 mph test. How do his reaction times compare at 20 and 60 mph?

   A. His reaction time at 60 mph was three times faster.
   B. His reaction times remain the same.
   C. His reaction time at 20 mph was three times faster.
   D. His reaction time at 20 mph was 1/3 as short.

Passage III (Questions 77–81)

An engineer is to design a small conveyor belt with attached buckets to carry fixed quantities of dog food from the first floor of the factory up to the second floor, 4.0 m above, where each sample of dog food is dumped into a sack that moves underneath the end of the conveyor belt as the bucket dumps the dog food into the sack (see the sketch below). The sacks then move to another part of the plant where they are sealed and packed for shipment to stores. The engineer wishes to determine the power rating of an electric motor that will drive the conveyor belt, and also needs to know what current will be drawn by the motor. Each bucket has a mass of 2 kg and can carry 10 kg of dog food. The conveyor belt should carry 30 buckets per minute to the top because that is how fast (30 sacks per minute) the sacks are moved. As a first approximation, the engineer will assume that the system is virtually frictionless. He will also assume that the mass of the buckets, themselves, can be ignored, because there are as many going down as going up at any time.

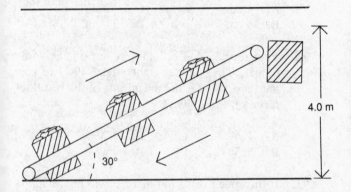

77. The engineer wants the angle of inclination to be 30°, as shown. How long should the conveyor belt be?

A. 3 m   C. 8 m
B. 6 m   D. 9 m

78. If the practical effect is to transport 30 buckets per minute from the bottom to the top of the belt, what power, in watts, is required?

A. 196 watts   C. 300 watts
B. 240 watts   D. 8800 watts

79. If an electric motor, operated at 120 volts, drives the conveyor belt, what current will it draw, in amperes? (Neglect losses.)

A. 1.6 amperes   C. 4.2 amperes
B. 2.0 amperes   D. 8.4 amperes

80. If the engineer now assumes that he should use a motor rated 45% higher in power (to allow for friction), what should the rated power (watts) of the motor be?

A. 240 watts   C. 420 watts
B. 290 watts   D. 12200 watts

81. If the conveyor belt runs faster so that 60 buckets per minute are raised rather than 30 buckets per minute, how should the rated power of the motor be changed?

A. It should be twice as large.
B. It should remain the same, since the mass carried in each bucket remains 10 kg.
C. It should increase by the square of 2.
D. It should increase by the square root of 2.

Passage IV (Questions 82–87)

A new experiment is designed to investigate the principle of conservation of momentum as well as energy transfers between colliding objects. An air track on which carts slide without friction is used. One end of the track is curved up so carts can be released at a height h. The carts slide down onto a horizontal section of the air track where the collisions occur. The collisions are always completely "elastic."

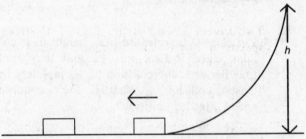

82. A cart (#1) of mass m is released at height h and collides elastically with an identical cart (#2), which is at rest on the flat horizontal section. What is the speed of cart #1 *just before* the collision?

A. $\sqrt{gh}$ C. gh
B. $\sqrt{2gh}$ D. $2gh$

83. What is the speed of the second cart, #2, *just after* the elastic collision?

A. $(\sqrt{gh})/2$ C. $\sqrt{2gh}$
B. $(\sqrt{2gh})/2$ D. gh

84. What is the speed of the first cart, #1, *just after* the elastic collision?

A. 0   C. $(\sqrt{2gh})/2$
B. $(\sqrt{gh})/2$ D. $\sqrt{2gh}$

85. Now cart #2 is replaced with a cart, #3, which is more massive. Cart #1 is released at height *h* and collides elastically with #3. How does the speed of cart #1, after the collision, compare with the result above when #1 collided with an identical cart?

    A. The speed of #1 is zero *after*.
    B. The speed is smaller in magnitude than before the collision.
    C. The speed is greater than before the collision.
    D. The speed remains the same, because the collision is elastic.

86. Suppose the collision of identical carts (#1 and #2) is "inelastic." How will the speed of cart #2 compare to the result above for an "elastic" collision?

    A. It will be the same, because total momentum is always conserved.
    B. It will be smaller.
    C. It will be zero.
    D. It will be larger.

87. Let cart #1 be released from height *h*. It collides with identical cart #2 and they stick together after the collision (a "completely inelastic collision"). What is their common speed after the collision?

    A. $1/2 \sqrt{2gh}$
    B. $1/2 \sqrt{gh}$
    C. $\sqrt{gh}$
    D. $\sqrt{2gh}$

    Questions 88–95 are independent of any passage and of each other.

88. A man 1.8 m tall stands 3 m in front of a plane mirror. How tall is his image?

    A. 0.6 m   **C.** 1.8 m
    B. 0.9 m   **D.** 3.6 m

89. A 4 kg object is slowly raised 4 m vertically. The mechanical work done is

    A. 16 joules.   **C.** 64 joules.
    B. 32 joules.   **D.** 157 joules.

90. A radioactive nucleus decays by the emission of a negative beta particle. What change does this cause in the nucleus?

    A. Its charge decreases.
    B. Its atomic mass number decreases.
    C. Its atomic mass number increases.
    D. Its charge increases.

91. A lens is used to form an image of an object located 12 cm in front of the lens. The image is projected onto a screen 12 cm behind the lens. What is the focal length of this lens?

    A. 4 cm   **C.** 12 cm
    B. 6 cm   **D.** 24 cm

92. Two forces of 3 N and 4 N act on the same object. They are at right angles (90°) to one another. What is the magnitude of the resultant force on the object?

    A. 1 *N*   **C.** 7 *N*
    B. 5 *N*   **D.** 25 *N*

93. If the speed of sound in air is 340 m/s, what is the wavelength of a 1200 Hz sound wave?

    A. 0.28 m   **C.** 3.5 m
    B. 0.56 m   **D.** 7.0 m

94. A ballet dancer weighing 110 pounds is standing on one toe. What is the pressure in pounds per square inch on the area of the floor under her toe, if the area of her toe is 3.5 in^2?

    A. 0.32 lb/in^2
    B. 31 lb/in^2
    C. 66 lb/in^2
    D. 390 lb/in^2

95. A temperature is measured to be 48°F. What is this temperature on the Celsius scale?

    A. 8.9°C   **C.** 32°C
    B. 16°C   **D.** 118°C

Passage V (Questions 96–105)

A class is to study electrical circuits. The laboratory portion is to be open-ended so that each pair of students does an experiment on their own, at their own pace. They are given resistors, batteries, voltmeters, ammeters, ohmmeters, oscilloscopes, capacitors, and inductance coils; as well as suitable general power supplies and function generators. The lecture portion covers the general theory including Ohm's law and Kirchhoff's laws for circuits, the operating properties of oscilloscopes, alternating current circuits (including RC, LC, and RLC series circuits), and the theory of induced *emf*'s using Faraday's law.

96. Two students are given three 2-ohm resistors and are to answer the following question: "How many *different* equivalent resistances can be constructed using three identical resistances in possible series and parallel arrangements?" The correct answer is:

A. four
B. five
C. seven
D. ten

97. What are the highest and lowest values of resistance (in ohms) that one can construct using the three 2-ohm resistors?

A. 3 ohms and 0.67 ohms
B. 6 ohms and 0.33 ohms
C. 6 ohms and 0.67 ohms
D. 6 ohms and 2 ohms

98. A battery of 4 volts is connected across the ends of a parallel connection of a 2-ohm resistor and a 1-microfarad capacitor. DC ammeters are connected so as to measure the current through the resistor and through the capacitor separately. What should the current be through the resistor and the capacitor respectively?

A. 0 A and 0 A
B. 0 A and 3 A
C. 2 A and 0 A
D. 2 A and 2 A

99. A 2-ohm resistor, a 2-millihenry inductor, and the 1-microfarad capacitor are connected in a series RLC circuit. The frequency of a function generator that supplies a sinusoidal signal to the circuit is adjusted until the circuit is *resonant,* which gives a maximum current in the circuit. What is the impedance of this circuit at the resonant frequency?

A. 0.46 ohms
B. 1.2 ohms
C. 2 ohms
D. 3.3 ohms

100. What is the AC current in this circuit, at resonance, if the function generator output is measured at 4 volts?

A. 0.3 A
B. 1.0 A
C. 2.0 A
D. 3.0 A

101. A small flat circular inductance coil of 100 turns has an area of 1 cm^2 (1×10^{-4} m^2). It is pulled out quickly from between the pole faces of a permanent magnet. The induced voltage is measured to be .01 V. What was the rate of decrease (in Tesla/s) of the magnetic field?

A. 0.5 T/s
B. 1 T/s
C. 2 T/s
D. 300 T/s

102. A battery of 6 volts is connected across the ends of a parallel connection of three 2-ohm resistors. What is the total current drawn from the battery?

A. 9 A
B. 3 A
C. 2 A
D. 1 A

103. When the 6-volt battery is connected across the three 2-ohm resistors in parallel, what is the current through each individual resistor?

A. 1 A
B. 0.33 A
C. 3 A
D. 9 A

104. Two 2-ohm resistors are connected in parallel and a third 2-ohm resistor is connected in series with the parallel combination. When a 6-volt battery is connected across this series-parallel combination, what total current is drawn from the battery?

A. 3 A
B. 6 A
C. 2 A
D. 0.5 A

105. The student is given an unknown resistance and a battery of unknown voltage. He connects an ammeter in series with the resistor to measure the current through it and connects a voltmeter in parallel with the resistor to measure the voltage across it. The battery is connected across the ends of the ammeter-resistor pair. The ammeter reading is 1.5 A and the voltmeter reading is 6 volts. What are the battery voltage and resistance respectively?

A. 6 V, 3 ohms
B. 3 V, 6 ohms
C. 6 V, 2 ohms
D. 6 V, 4 ohms

Passage VI (Questions 106–110)

Amino acids contain one or two amino functional groups and one or two carboxyl groups (depending on the particular amino aid). The first carboxyl group in a particular amino acid has a pK_a of about 2.1 and the second carboxyl group (if present) has a pK_a of about 4.0. The first amino group has a pK_a of about 9.0 and the second amino group (if present) has a pK_a of about 10.5. (The pK_a of the amino group relates to the ionization of the protonated $R-NH_3^+$ to form $H^+ + R-NH_2$.)

106. The isoelectric pH of an amino acid having two amino groups and one carboxyl group would be about:

    A. 3.05.   C. 6.50.
    B. 5.20.   D. 9.75.

107. The isoelectric point of an amino acid having two carboxyl groups and one amino group would be about:

    A. 3.05.   C. 6.50.
    B. 5.20.   D. 9.75.

108. At a pH of about 8, an amino acid with one carboxyl group and one amino group would:

    A. move toward the anode in an electrical field.
    B. move toward the cathode in an electrical field.
    C. exhibit no movement in an electrical field.
    D. probably move but in a direction that is not predictable.

109. Although not naturally occurring, an amino acid with two amino groups and two carboxyl groups would have an isoelectric point of about:

    A. 5.20.   C. 7.80.
    B. 6.50.   D. 9.75.

110. The change in net charge of amino acids from plus one or two to zero to negative one or two in response to different pH values in the medium is exploited in separation of amino acids by:

    A. electrophoresis.
    B. gas chromatography.
    C. ultracentrifugation.
    D. distillation.

Passage VII (Questions 111–115)

A balloon is filled with nitrogen gas (N_2) to a volume of 1000 mL at sea level at standard pressure. It is found that the volume of the balloon changes under a variety of conditions.

111. A decrease in volume to 900 mL would result from:

    A. a 10% decrease in °C.
    B. a 10% decrease in °K.
    C. a 10% decrease in °F.
    D. a 100% deccase in °F.

112. An increase of 10% in volume is noted in taking the balloon up a mountain; this is explained by:

    A. a 10% increase in atmospheric pressure.
    B. a conversion of 20% of N_2 molecules into N atoms.
    C. a 10% decrease in temperature (°C).
    D. a 10% decrease in atmospheric pressure.

113. Since H_2 has a molecular weight about one-fourteenth that of N_2, a similar balloon containing the same number of H_2 molecules at the same temperature and pressure would have a volume _____ that of the N_2-containing balloon.

    A. one-fourteenth
    B. fourteen times
    C. between three and four times
    D. equal to

114. If nitrogen existed in monoatomic form (i.e., N) rather than diatomic N_2 molecules, 0.05 moles of N would occupy _____ volume occupied by 0.05 moles of H_2 at the same temperature and pressure.

    A. twice the   C. the same
    B. one-half the   D. one-fourth the

115. If the balloon containing N_2 gas were simultaneously subjected to a 5% decrease in atmospheric pressure and a decrease in temperature from 27°C to 12°C, the volume of the balloon will:

    A. increase about 5%.
    B. increase about 10%.
    C. not change.
    D. decrease about 10%.

Passage VIII (Questions 116–120)

To each of two beakers is added 100 mL of distilled water. To one is added 0.01 mole of HCl and to the other is added 0.01 mole of acetic acid ($K_a = 1.8 \times 10^{-5}$ and $pK_a = 4.74$). The solution in each beaker is stirred well.

116. The initial pH of the distilled water is:

A. 5.0. C. 8.0.
B. 7.0. D. 9.0.

117. The beaker containing the solution of HCl will have a pH of about:

A. 1.0. C. 5.0.
B. 3.0. D. 7.0.

118. The beaker containing the solution of acetic acid will have a pH of about:

A. 1.0. C. 5.0.
B. 3.0. D. 7.0.

119. Addition of 0.01 mole of NaCl to the beaker containing HCl solution would bring about:

A. an increase of about 2 in the pH.
B. an increase of about 1 in the pH.
C. no change in the pH.
D. a decrease of about 1 in the pH.

120. Addition of 0.01 mole of sodium acetate to the beaker containing acetic acid solution would bring about:

A. an increase in pH to about 4.7.
B. an increase in pH to about 3.9.
C. no change in pH.
D. a decrease in pH to about 1.8.

Passage IX (Questions 121–125)

An aqueous solution of an inorganic acid is titrated with strong base to give the following titration curve:

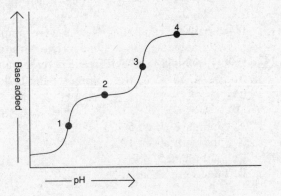

121. The pK_a with the lowest pH is at:

A. point 1.
B. point 2.
C. point 3.
D. point 4.

122. This acid appears to have _____ pK_a's.

A. 0 C. 2
B. 1 D. 3

123. Assuming we have covered the titration range from 0 to 14, this acid could be:

A. HF.
B. HCl.
C. H_3PO_4.
D. none of the above.

124. The greatest buffering is noted at:

A. points 1 and 2. C. points 1 and 3.
B. points 3 and 4. D. points 2 and 4.

125. Equal amounts of two species will be found at:

A. point 1 only.
B. point 2 only.
C. point 3 only.
D. more than one of the above.

Passage X (Questions 126–135)

A 0.01 mole of HCl is diluted to 1000 mL with water and mixed in a beaker to produce solution A. To this is added 1000 mL of water. After mixing, the resulting solution is solution B. To this is added 0.02 moles sodium propionate. After mixing, the resulting solution is solution C. To this is added 0.01 mole sodium propionate and 0.01 mole propionic acid. After mixing, the resulting solution is solution D. To this is added 1000 mL more water. After mixing, the resulting solution is solution E. To another beaker is added 0.005 mole of pyruvic acid. Water is added to a total volume of 500 mL. After mixing, the resulting solution is solution F. To solution F is added 0.005 mole of sodium pyruvate. After mixing, the resulting solution is solution G. K_a values are 1.3×10^{-5} for propionic acid, 1.4×10^{-4} for pyruvic acid, and 5.9×10^{-10} for boric acid. pK_a values are 4.89 for propionic acid, and 9.23 for boric acid. (For the purpose of this problem, assume no volume change occurs after the addition of small quantities of liquid or solid.)

126. The pH of solution A is:

    A. 2.0.   C. 4.0.
    B. 3.0.   D. 6.0.

127. The pH of solution B is:

    A. less than 2.
    B. between 2 and 3.
    C. between 3 and 4.
    D. between 4 and 7.

128. The pH of solution C is:

    A. 1.3.   C. 4.9.
    B. 3.8.   D. 9.2.

129. The pH of solution D is:

    A. between 1 and 2.
    B. between 3 and 4.
    C. between 4 and 5.
    D. greater than 5.5.

130. The pH of solution E is:

    A. between 2 and 3.
    B. between 4 and 5.
    C. between 5 and 6.
    D. greater than 6.5.

131. The pH of solution F is:

    A. between 2 and 3.
    B. between 4 and 5.
    C. between 5 and 6.
    D. greater than 6.5.

132. The pH of solution G is:

    A. 1.4.   C. 4.9.
    B. 3.8.   D. greater than 6.

133. The degree of ionization of pyruvic acid is:

    A. 0.012.   C. 1.2.
    B. 0.12.   D. greater than 2.

134. The percent ionization of pyruvic acid is:

    A. 0.12.   C. 12.
    B. 1.2.   D. greater than 20.

135. The pOH of solution C is:

    A. 4.8.   C. 10.2.
    B. 9.1.   D. 11.9.

Questions 136–142 are independent of any passage and of each other.

136. Often during the oxidation of coal which contains sulfur the anhydride of sulfuric acid is produced. Which of the compounds listed is that anhydride?

    A. SO_3 C. SO_4
    B. SO_2 D. H_2S

137. The sum of which of the following in the shells surrounding the nucleus is equal to the atomic number for an uncharged atom?

    A. protons   C. electrons
    B. neutrons   D. positrons

138. An atom that has lost two orbital electrons has a charge of:

    A. +1.   C. −1.
    B. +2.   D. −2.

139. An uncharged atom of a particular element has an electron distribution of $1s^2$, $2s^2$, $2p^5$. You would expect this to be a (an):

    A. metal.   C. metalloid.
    B. nonmetal.   D. amalgam.

140. The element above would most often be expected to gain or lose electrons and thus exhibit a valence of:

    A. +1.   C. −1.
    B. +3.   D. −2.

141. Which of the following will react with water to form an acidic solution?

    A. Na_2O C. CaO
    B. K_2O D. P_2O_3

142. Ionic bonding is seen in:

    A. O_2.   C. CIF.
    B. H_2.   D. KCl.

WRITING SAMPLE

2 ESSAYS
60 MINUTES (30 MINUTES/TOPIC)

DIRECTIONS: Your response must be a unified, organized essay; it should contain fully developed, logically constructed paragraphs. Remember quality is more important than length. Before you begin writing, make sure you have read the item carefully and understand what is being asked. Write as legibly as possible. Because your essays will be scored as first-draft compositions, you may cross out and make corrections on your response booklet as necessary. It is not necessary to recopy your essay.

Part 1

Consider this statement:

Men are dependent on circumstances, not circumstances on men.

Herodotus

Write a unified essay in which you perform the following tasks. Explain the meaning of the above statement. Describe a specific situation where circumstances might be dependent on men. Discuss what you think determines whether or not men are dependent on circumstances or vice versa.

Part 2

Consider this statement:

The voluntary death by which a man puts an end to intolerable suffering is really an act of redemption.

**Ernst Heinrich Haeckel
(German biologist)**

Write a unified essay in which you perform the following tasks. Explain what you think the above statement means. Describe a specific situation in which the voluntary death by which a person put an end to intolerable suffering would not be an act of redemption. Discuss what you think determines the choice of voluntary death in the face of human suffering.

BIOLOGICAL SCIENCES

10 PROBLEM SETS OF 5–10 QUESTIONS EACH
15 PROBLEMS FOLLOWED BY A SINGLE QUESTION
77 QUESTIONS
100 MINUTES

DIRECTIONS: The following questions or incomplete statements are in groups. Preceding each series of questions or statements is a paragraph or a short explanatory statement, a formula or set of formulas, or a definition. Read the written material and then answer the questions or complete the statements. Select the ONE BEST ANSWER for each question and indicate your selection by marking the corresponding letter of your choice on the Answer Form. Eliminate those alternatives you know to be incorrect and then select an answer from among the remaining alternatives.

Passage I (Questions 143–147)

A patient is brought into the emergency room and, upon examination, a thyroid goiter is discovered. You suspect that he is suffering from a thyroid disorder, and you ask the intern for a definition of *hypothyroidism.*

143. He responds that *hypothyroidism* is the general term for syndromes that reflect:

    A. increased secretion of thyroid hormones.
    B. decreased secretion of thyroid hormones.
    C. no change in secretion of thyroid hormones.
    D. increased secretion of thyroid stimulating hormone releasing factor.

144. A basal metabolism rate test is ordered that measures the rate of oxidative metabolism. In hypothyroidism, this rate is:

    A. above normal.
    B. normal.
    C. below normal.
    D. not significant in your diagnosis.

145. Because of the hypothyroidism that you suspect, you would also consider that this patient:

    I. has gained weight.
    II. converts less food into energy.
    III. stores more food as fat.
    IV. has an accelerated metabolic rate.

    A. I, III, and IV only
    B. II, III, and IV only
    C. I, II, and III only
    D. all of the above

146. The physical examination in this patient would also yield the following:

    A. The patient is mentally sluggish.
    B. The patient's skin is rough and dry.
    C. The patient's serum cholesterol level would be elevated.
    D. All of the above.

147. If hyperthyroidism were the diagnosis you would reason and find:

    A. a pituitary deficiency in TSH.
    B. a block in the oxidation of iodide to iodine.
    C. a phlegmatic patient.
    D. irritability.

Passage II (Questions 148–155)

The ABO blood group is transmitted in humans as alleles A and B that are codominant, occurring at the same autosomal locus as a recessive allele O. In some cases it may be utilized to assist in determining paternity or in reuniting a lost child with his or her biological parents.

148. A woman of blood type O claims a child of blood type AB, and alleges that the father is a man of blood type B. The most likely explanation is that:

    A. these are the biological parents.
    B. she is the mother but the man is not the father.
    C. neither is a possible parent of the child.
    D. she is not the mother but the man's blood type does not rule him out as the father.

149. If the man in question 148 is found to have previously fathered a child of blood type O, the chance that a child of the man and the woman in this question would be blood type O is:

A. zero.   C. 33%.
B. 25%.   D. 50%

150. With the information from the above question, the chance that any child of the man and woman would be a girl with blood type B is

A. zero.   C. 33%.
B. 25%.   D. 50%.

151. The above man with a phenotype B will possess which of the following genotype?

A. A/O   C. O/O
B. B/O   D. A/B

152. Phenotype may be defined as:

A. genetic makeup of an individual.
B. hidden traits of an individual.
C. unrelated characteristics.
D. visible expression of genotype.

153. Alleles are genes that:

A. arise during the cross-over process.

B. are linked to one chromosome only.
C. are always sex-linked and are transmitted from mothers to their sons.
D. occupy corresponding positions on homologous chromosomes.

154. Rh-related hemolytic anemia of the newborn (erythroblastosis foetalis) may result when the:

A. father, mother, and fetus are all Rh negative.
B. father and mother are Rh positive, but the fetus is Rh negative.
C. mother is Rh negative and the fetus is Rh positive.
D. mother is Rh positive and the fetus is Rh negative.

155. The czarina of Russia and Queen Victoria of England were normal women who produced sons suffering from hemophilia, a disease that is caused by a sex-linked recessive gene, h. The more common dominant gene, H, produces normal blood clotting. The genotype of these women must have been:

A. HH.   C. hh.
B. Hh.   D. none of the above.

Passage III (Questions 156–162)

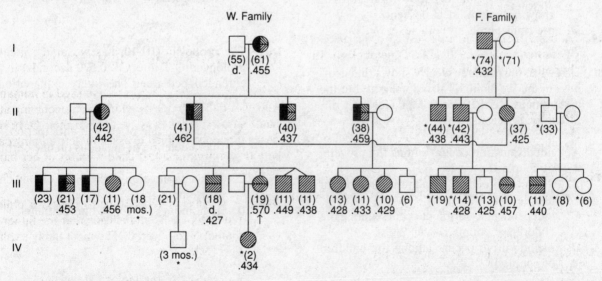

Study of *W* and *F* families showing presence of syncope, electrocardiographic evidence of prolonged Q-T interval and abnormal audiogram. The propositus (Case 1) is III-10 (**arrow**). Case 2 is her cousin (III-2). Figures in parentheses indicate subject's age. Intervals (in hundredths of a second) appear directly below each subject's age. **Black** symbols indicate abnormal audiogram; hatched symbols indicate prolonged QTc interval (0.425 second) (////) or syncope (\\\\); d = died. A history, physical examination and one or more electrocardiograms were obtained in all patients. An audiogram was obtained in all cases, except those marked by a star, in which hearing was only examined clinically.

Inheritance of Q-T prolongation (≥ 0.425 second) and cardiac arrhythmias in the W. and F. families is shown in the above pedigree, which was ascertained through the proposita, III-10, who suffered cardiac arrest and had to be resuscitated 12 hours after her first delivery following an uneventful pregnancy. A major objective of the study was the determination of whether prolonged Q-T interval in these families was (1) the autosomal recessive form, Jervell, Lang-Niel-sen syndrome, also characterized by high-frequency perceptive deafness, (2) Ward-Romano syndrome, an autosomal dominant form, not associated with deaf-ness, or (3) perhaps a third type, inherited in some other fashion.*

156. Prolonged Q-T interval and cardiac arrhyth-mias appear to be phenotypic manifestations of the same allele, a phenomenon known as

    A. genetic heterogeneity.
    B. genetic polymorphism.
    C. pleiotropism.
    D. phenocopies.

157. The pedigree clearly shows that the arrhyth-mias in the W. family are dominant because they

    A. affect both monozygotic twins in the third generation.
    B. are sometimes associated with deafness.
    C. show unbroken lineal descent.
    D. are transmitted by both sexes.

158. Likewise, the pedigree clearly shows that deaf-ness in the W. family is also dominant, but the arrhythmias are the result of an allele at a dif-ferent locus because:

    A. nondisjunction occurs among the progeny of couple II-1 @ 2.
    B. disjunction occurs among the progeny of couple II-1 @ 2.
    C. independent assortment occurs among the children of couple II-1 @ 2.
    D. meiotic drive occurs among the children of couple II-1 @ 2.

*Adapted by Dr. J. I. Townsend, Virginia Commonwealth University, from "Q-T Prolongation and Ventricular Arrhyth-mias With and Without Deafness in the Same Family;" E. C. Mathews, A. W. Blount, and J.I. Townsend, *The American Journal of Cardiology*, (1972): 29:702.

159. Careful comparative diagnostic studies of pro-longed Q-T interval and cardiac arrhythmias in the W. and F. families show the syndrome to be identical in both families, yet in the F. fam-ily this dominant trait skips a generation (II-11). This skipping is a phenomenon known as:

    A. reduced penetrance.
    B. unequal crossing over.
    C. transversion.
    D. variable expressivity.

160. That prolonged Q-T interval and the arrhyth-mias are autosomal is shown by:

    A. female to male transmission in both fami-lies.
    B. male to male transmission in the F. fami-ly.
    C. lack of male to male transmission.
    D. male to female transmission.

161. That deafness is autosomal is shown by:

    A. male to male transmission.
    B. lack of male to male transmission.
    C. two affected males (II-3 and II-5) have daughters whose hearing is normal.
    D. an affected female (II-2) has a daughter whose hearing is normal.

162. The proposita (III-10) has by far the greatest prolonged Q-T interval (0.570 seconds) in this extended pedigree. The likely explanation is that she:

    A. is an example of genetic anticipation.
    B. has a deletion of the locus on one chromo-some.
    C. has a duplication of the locus on one chro-mosome.
    D. is homozygous for the mutant allele.

Passage IV (Questions 163–169)

Oogenesis in oviparous vertebrates (such as am-phibians) is accompanied by extensive transcription. RNA is synthesized in the oocyte nucleus and subse-quently processed. The resultant mRNAs, tRNAs, and ribosomes (containing rRNAs) then accumulate in the oocyte cytoplasm. Most of these RNAs (referred to as oogenetic or maternal RNAs) and ribosomes do not function in translation until after embryonic development has been initiated. Although protein synthesis is detectable in the zygote prior to the beginning of cleavage, RNA synthesis is not detected in embryonic cells until later in development (as seen in the figure below). The RNA synthesized in embryonic cells is collectively referred to as embryonic RNA.

Transcriptional inhibitors, such as the antibiotic actinomycin D, are useful tools for studying patterns of RNA synthesis in development. When cells are treated with actinomycin D, actinomycin D binds to the guanine residues of DNA and blocks the subsequent synthesis of all types of RNA, without affecting DNA synthesis and cell division. Previously synthesized and processed RNAs are not affected by such inhibitors. The relative importance of oogenetic and embryonic RNAs in protein synthesis in embryos can be determined by blocking the synthesis of postfertilization RNA synthesis with a transcriptional inhibitor. When early cleavage stage amphibian embryos are exposed to a transcriptional inhibitor, development and protein synthesis continue until the blastula stage at which point development arrests.

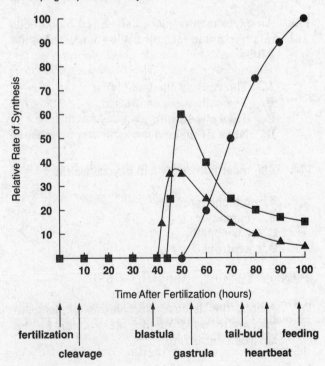

Relative Rate of mRNA (▲), tRNA (■), and rRNA (●) synthesis in developing amphibian embryos

163. Radiolabelled molecules are commonly used to monitor the amount and/or rate of synthetic processes in cells. A commonly employed radiolabel is tritum, H3. Which of the following tritiated molecules would be the most appropriate one for specifically monitoring RNA synthesis in amphibian embryos?

A. H3-adenine
B. H3-guanine
C. H3-thymidine
D. H3-uridine

164. Embryonic mRNA synthesis begins to be detected in amphibian embryos:

A. at the blastula stage.
B. during early cleavage.
C. at the gastrula stage.
D. during oogenesis.

165. An amphibian embryo at the gastrula stage would be actively synthesizing:

A. rRNA.
B. tRNA and rRNA.
C. mRNA and rRNA.
D. mRNA, tRNA, and rRNA.

166. Based on studies with actinomycin D, the development of amphibian embryos to the blastula stage is dependent on:

A. proteins synthesized using maternal mRNAs.
B. proteins synthesized using embryonic mRNAs.
C. the synthesis of mRNAs by embryonic cells.
D. the synthesis of tRNAs and rRNAs by embryonic cells.

167. Although actinomycin D treated embryos remain viable for a period of time and some protein synthesis can be detected in actinomycin D treated embryos, the embryos will not develop past the blastula stage. Which of the following would be the best explanation for the inability of the embryos to continue development.

A. In order to continue development the embryos need to synthesize more embryonic rRNAs and tRNAs.

B. In order to continue development the embryos need to synthesize more embryonic mRNAs and rRNAs.

C. In order to continue development the embryos need to synthesize more proteins using maternal mRNAs.

D. In order to continue development the embryos need to synthesize proteins using embryonic mRNAs.

168. Extensive stockpiling of developmentally important macromolecules (such as RNAs) prior to the initiation of development often shortens the time required for early developmental processes such as cleavage. In comparision to an organism with a similar body complexity, but which accumulated no maternal RNA in its eggs during oogenesis, the cleavage period in amphibians should be:

A. similar.
B. much longer.
C. slightly longer.
D. shorter.

169. In contrast to the situation in amphibians, only a small amount of RNA synthesis occurs during oogenesis in viviparous vertebrates (such as mammals) and the mammalian oocyte contains a minimal amount of oogenetic RNA. Synthesis of embryonic RNAs and ribosomes begins during the early cleavage stages. Therefore if mouse zygotes were exposed to a transcriptional inhibitor, development would probably arrest:

A. at the blastocyst stage.
B. at the blastula stage.
C. at the gastrula stage.
D. during the cleavage stage.

Passage V (Questions 170–176)

Blood is a fluid tissue consisting of numerous components such as red blood cells (RBCs), white blood cells, platelets, proteins and more. The cellular components comprise about 45% of whole blood, the remaining 55% is plasma.

One of the primary functions of blood is transport. Examples include nutrients, metabolic wastes, hormones, carbon dioxide and oxygen. RBCs play a major role in transport of CO_2 and O_2. The following questions center around the RBC.

170. All of the following are characteristics of an erythrocyte, EXCEPT:

A. contains a substance composed of four proteins and a prosthetic group.
B. biconcave disc shape.
C. made in the bone marrow of adults.
D. has a nucleus and cytoplasmic organelles.

171. Sometimes called the "graveyard" of the erythrocyte, the liver and spleen contain _____, which recognize and phagocytize red blood cells at the end of their approximate 120-day life span.

A. mast cells
B. platelets
C. macrophages
D. adipocytes

172. Sometimes referred to as a microscopist's "measuring stick," an erythrocyte is abundant in most tissues and can be utilized for size comparison in a viewing field. The approximate diameter of an RBC is:

A. 7 mm.
B. 7 μm.
C. 0.7 nm.
D. 70 nm.

173. An experimenter placed some red blood cells in a hypotonic medium. What happened to the RBCs?

A. The cells swelled and burst.
B. The cells were unaffected.
C. The cells shrunk.
D. None of the above.

174. The most numerous leukocytes are the:

A. lymphocytes.
B. monocytes.
C. eosinophils.
D. neutrophils.

175. Among the defense mechanisms available to humans to ward off their destruction by the environment is (are):

I. skin.
II. white blood corpuscles.
III. antibodies.
IV. sebaceous secretions.

A. III only   C. II and III only
B. II only   D. I, II, III, and IV

176. Blood pH is influenced by respiration; experimental hyperventilation in a physiology laboratory will result in the student's blood pH being:

A. lowered.   C. unaffected.
B. raised.   D. raised to pH6.

Passage VI (Questions 177–181)

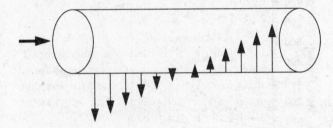

Above is a diagram of a typical capillary with a left to right blood flow as indicated. The arrows show the direction of fluid flow into and out of the capillary. On the left hand side of the capillary, the fluid flow is from the capillary to the interstitial space. On the right side, the fluid flow is from the interstitium to the capillary. Thus, there is a constant recirculation of the interstitial fluid.

In most cases, the fluid flow from the capillary to the interstitium and back again are closely balanced. The small excess of fluid remaining in the interstitium is eventually removed by the lymphatics. The net transport of fluid (Q) in the direction of the interstitium is governed by Starling's law

$$Q = K[(P_{cap} - P_i) - (\pi_{cap} - \pi_i)]$$

where P_{cap} and P_i are the hydrostatic pressures in the capillary and the interstitium respectively. The wall of the capillary acts as a permselective membrane, therefore osmotic pressures, π_{cap} and π_i, exist on the capillary and interstitial sides respectively and contribute to the driving force for fluid movement. K is the constant of proportionality relating the driving force to fluid flow and is known as the hydraulic conductivity of the capillary.

Choose the *one best* answer.

177. A patient develops a venous blood clot in one leg which blocks return of blood. What would you predict would happen to the net fluid flow in the capillaries?

A. Fluid flow in the direction of the interstitium increases.
B. Fluid flow in the direction of the interstitium decreases.
C. Fluid flow in the direction of the interstitium is unchanged.
D. The capillary osmotic pressure will increase.

178. A patient with protein malnutrition has a lower concentration of protein in his blood (The reflection coefficient (σ) of proteins is close to 1.) With all other things constant,

A. the hydrostatic pressure difference between the capillary and the interstitium will increase.
B. the fluid volume in the interstitium will decrease.
C. the net fluid flow will be in the direction of the interstitium.
D. the fluid volume in the interstitium stays constant.

179. An elastic bandage applied to the skin will result in

A. a larger hydrostatic pressure difference.
B. an increased interstitial volume.
C. an increase in flow into the capillary.
D. an increased oncotic pressure difference.

180. Assuming a steady state, an infusion of urea (a nonpolar solute with a reflection coefficient of 0) results in

A. an increase in the osmotic pressure difference.
B. an increased flow into the capillary.
C. a decrease in the interstitial volume.
D. no change in the interstitial volume.

181. The process by which a cell can move a substance from a point of lower concentration to a point of higher concentration (against the diffusion gradient) is called

A. osmosis.   C. turgor pressure.
B. plasmolysis.   D. active transport.

Passage VII (Questions 182–186)

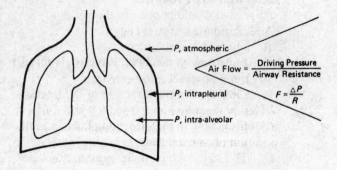

182. The driving pressure (ΔP) in breathing which causes air to flow into the lungs is:

    A. atmospheric pressure (*Patm*).
    B. the intra-alveolar (intrapulmonary) pressure (*Palv*).
    C. atmospheric pressure minus the intra-alveolar pressure.
    D. the intrapleural pressure (*Ppl*).

183. During inspiration, intra-alveolar pressure (*Palv*):

    A. transiently goes below atmospheric pressure (*Patm*).
    B. transiently goes above atmospheric pressure.
    C. equals atmospheric pressure.
    D. equals intrapleural pressure.

184. The alveolar ventilation per minute refers to the amount of fresh air that reaches the alveoli of the lungs per minute. Alveolar ventilation per minute equals the:

    A. functional residual capacity × frequency of breathing.
    B. physiologic dead space × frequency of breathing.
    C. anatomic dead space × frequency of breathing.
    D. (tidal volume − anatomic dead space) × frequency of breathing.

185. Hypoventilation produces which of the following changes in alveolar gas composition?

    A. The partial pressure of oxygen increases and the partial pressure of carbon dioxide decreases.
    B. The partial pressures of both oxygen and carbon dioxide increase.
    C. The partial pressure of oxygen decreases and the partial pressure of carbon dioxide increases.
    D. The partial pressures of both oxygen and carbon dioxide decrease.

186. Carbon dioxide is transported in the blood in all of the following forms, EXCEPT:

    A. carboxyhemoglobin.
    B. dissolved carbon dioxide.
    C. bicarbonate ions.
    D. carbamino-compounds.

Passage VIII (Questions 187–191)

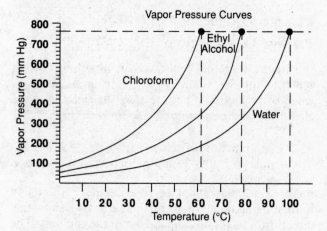

187. Compared to the vapor pressures of chloroform and water, the vapor pressure of ethyl alcohol is:

    A. constant.
    B. greater than either.
    C. greater than that of chloroform, but less than that of water.
    D. less than that of chloroform, but greater than that of water.

188. In degrees Celsius, the normal boiling point of chloroform is approximately:

    A. 61.   C. 100.
    B. 78.   D. 760.

189. The graph indicates that standard atmospheric pressure, in millimeters of mercury (Hg), is:

    A. between 0 and 100.
    B. less than 760.
    C. 100.
    D. 760.

190. At the top of a mountain where atmospheric pressure is less than standard atmospheric pressure, the boiling point of water is:

A. less than its normal boiling point.
B. more than its normal boiling point.
C. the same as that of chloroform and that of ethyl alcohol.
D. the same as that of chloroform.

191. At what atmospheric pressure would the boiling point of water equal the normal boiling point of ethyl alcohol?

A. 100   C. 500
B. 300   D. 700

Passage IX (Questions 192–196)

Toluene or methyl benzene is an important starting material for the synthesis of many aromatic compounds. In any of the reactions of toluene, assume that ortho and para isomers can be separated.

192. The reaction of toluene with Br_2 in the presence of $FeBr_3$ would be expected to produce primarily:

A. benzyl bromide, $C_6H_5CH_2Br$.
B. *m*-bromotoluene.
C. *o* and *p*-bromotoluene.
D. an equimolar mixture of *m*, *o*, and *p*-bromotoluene.

193. The compound that undergoes electrophilic aromatic substitution more readily than toluene is:

A. chlorobenzene.   C. acetophenone.
B. nitrobenzene.   D. phenol.

194. The best sequence of reagents for conversion of toluene to *m*-nitrobenzoic acid is:

A. HNO_3-H_2SO_4 then oxidation with hot $KMnO_4$ or $K_2Cr_2O_7$.
B. Oxidation with hot $KMnO_4$ or $K_2Cr_2O_7$ followed by HNO_3-H_2SO_4.
C. Bromination of toluene with Br_2-$FeBr_3$ followed by displacement with $NaNO_2$.
D. Reaction of toluene with Br_2-$FeBr_3$ followed by oxidation with $KMnO_4$ or $K_2Cr_2O_7$ and then displacement of Br by $NaNO_2$.

195. The major product of the reaction of *p*-nitrotoluene with Br_2-$FeBr_3$ is:

A. 2-bromo-4-nitrotoluene.
B. 3-bromo-4-nitrotoluene.
C. *p*-nitrobenzyl bromide, *p*-$NO_2C_6H_4CH_2Br$.
D. 2, 6-dibromo-4-nitrotoluene.

196. Which of the following resonance structures is a contributor to the intermediate formed in the nitration of toluene to form *p*-nitrotoluene?

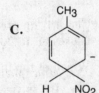

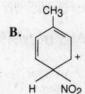

Passage X (Questions 197–204)

The categories of necessary dietary nutrients include the essential amino acids, essential fatty acids, essential elements, and the vitamins. The nine essential amino acids for humans are found in all dietary proteins. They are called: phenylalanine, valine, threonine, tryptophan, isoleucine, methionine, histidine, leucine, and lysine. All other amino acids that are found in proteins are nonessential and can be synthesized in the body from other dietary sources. The one true essential fatty acid is linoleic, however, linolenic and arachidonic acids can help meet the nutritional requirement for this category of nutrients. Because generally all of these essential fatty acids are found in combinations of oils and fats, all three can be viewed as "essential" in a practical sense. Along with carbohydrates, we obtain both essential amino acid and fatty acids from the macronutrients (i.e., large quantities) of protein and fat respectively in our diet.

The essential elements are subcategorized as the electrolytes sodium, potassium, and chloride; the bulk essential minerals—calcium, phosphorus, and magnesium and the trace essential minerals—iron, zinc, selenium, iodine, cobalt, molybdenum, manganese, copper, chromium, and fluoride. All of these are needed, but the amount we need each day varies from micrograms to hundreds of milligrams. Vitamins are found in foods in water soluble or fat soluble forms. The former includes vitamin C, thiamine, riboflavin, niacin, vitamin B_6, folacin, vitamin B_{12}, biotin, and pantothenic acid. The fat soluble vitamins are vitamins A, D, E, and K. These are all required in the diet in trace amounts (i.e., micrograms to milligrams).

Choose the *one best* answer for each of the following:

197. Which of the following is *not* an essential nutrient?

A. valine   C. glucose
B. linoleic acid   D. vitamin E

198. Which of the following is *not* a vitamin?

A. thiamine   C. niacin
B. biotin   D. arachidonic acid

199. Which of the following is *not* a fat soluble vitamin?

A. vitamin A   C. vitamin D
B. vitamin B_{12} D. vitamin E

200. Which of the following is a bulk essential element?

A. selenium   C. iron
B. copper   D. calcium

201. A macronutrient is:
  I. a carbohydrate.
  II. a protein.
  III. a fat.
  IV. a vitamin.

A. I only   C. I, II, and III
B. II only   D. I, II, III, and IV

202. Regulation of the resorption of calcium from bone is controlled by the:

A. thyroid gland.
B. parathyroid glands.
C. thymus.
D. adrenal glands.

203. Undigested food is eliminated from the body by the process of:

A. exocytosis.   C. egestion.
B. excretion.   D. catabolism.

204. The energy released from the anaerobic respiration of a glucose molecule is less than that released from the aerobic respiration of a glucose molecule because

A. aerobic respiration forms many more new, strong bonds than anaerobic respiration.
B. more enzymes are required for anaerobic respiration than for aerobic respiration.
C. anaerobic respiration occurs 24 hours a day, while aerobic respiration can occur only at night.
D. anaerobic respiration requires oxygen but aerobic respiration does not require oxygen.

DIRECTIONS: Read each passage carefully, study each table, chart, or formula, then answer the question following it. Eliminate those choices that you think to be incorrect and mark the letter of your choice on the answer sheet.

Blood samples from two groups of rats were assayed for luteinizing hormone (LH) in two separate radioimmunoassays. Half the rats were intact and half were orchidectomized. Some samples in each group were collected in the morning and some were collected in the afternoon. The data are summarized in the following table:

Assay 1

#	Intact or Orchid X.	Sampled AM or PM	LH ng/ml
1	I	AM	5.0
2	O	AM	50
3	I	PM	4.8
4	O	PM	480
5	I	AM	5.2
6	O	AM	52
7	I	PM	5.1
8	O	PM	350
9	I	AM	4.9
10	O	AM	100

Assay 2

#			
11	I	PM	7.5
12	O	PM	75
13	I	AM	7.7
14	O	AM	770
15	I	PM	7.3
16	O	PM	250
17	I	AM	7.4
18	O	AM	100
19	I	PM	7.6
20	O	PM	640

205. Based on the above table, which of the following statements is *not supported by* the information given?

A. Orchidectomy is followed by increased levels of LH in the blood.

B. Blood LH levels are higher in the afternoon than in the morning.

C. The differences between LH values in these two assays are probably explained by interassay variations because the ratios between intact and orchidectomized levels are similar.

D. LH release in the orchidectomized rats may be occurring episodically.

Ovulation in the rat can be blocked by systemic administration of drugs which depress neural function. However, ovulation depends on the response of the ovaries to LH released from the pituitary gland. In the following experiment, drug X was injected subcutaneously at 13:45 hours into several groups of rats and the presence or absence of ova in the oviduct determined on the following morning. In order to pinpoint the site of action of the drug, attempts were made to restore ovulation by stimulation of the brain; injection of LRF, the hypothalamic hormone which causes pituitary LH release; and injection of LH, which induces ovulation. The results are summarized below.

Treatment	Number of Rats Treated	Number of Rats Ovulating
Drug X	10	1
Drug X + LRF	10	5
Drug X + LH	10	5
Drug X + Brain Stimulation	10	1

206. The following statements are related to the above table. Select the statement *supported by* the information given.

A. The ovaries are responsible for the production of LH.

B. Drug X may be blocking the release of LRF from the brain and thereby preventing the activation of pituitary LH release.

C. Drug X may be preventing pituitary LH release in response to LRF.

D. The effect of Drug X on the brain is greater than its effect on the ovary.

Country	Crude Birth Rate Per Thousand/Year	Crude Death Rate Per Thousand/Year
Lebanon	54	26
Egypt	50	26
India	50	25
Pakistan	49	26
USSR	43	18
East Germany	18	10
West Germany	16	16
France	35	11
Spain	19	7
Holland	45	8
Luxemburg	17	11.8
Japan	15	13

207. Which of the countries in the table shows the most rapid population growth?

A. Spain   C. USSR
B. Holland   D. Lebanon

Female albino rats weighing between 170 and 230 g were housed in pairs in wire bottom cages and received a standard diet of rat pellets and chlorinated water *ad libitum*. Unanesthetized rats were restrained and shielded with lead so that only the head and neck regions were exposed. The animals received 6400 R of X-radiation in a single dose. Following irradiation careful check was maintained on the water and food consumption. Also, at varying intervals after exposure the animals were killed and the wet weights of their parotid salivary glands were determined. The results of these follow-ups are depicted below:

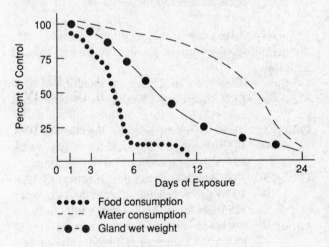

●●●●● Food consumption
– – – Water consumption
-●-● Gland wet weight

208. Which of the following statements is true concerning the data obtained from this experiment?

A. The animals continued to consume large

quantities of water up to the time of death.

B. An alteration in food consumption was already evident at 3 days after radiation.

C. Even though drinking and eating declined, the weights of the salivary glands remained unaffected until time of death.

D. Water consumption and wet weight of the glands first began to vary from control values at 8 days.

Levels of estrogens in the urine of the human female during the menstrual cycle, pregnancy, and the post-menopausal period were obtained from women during some routine work-ups during their visits to the ob-gyn clinic. The following data were obtained.

Time	Estriol μg/24 h	Estrone μg/24 h	Estradiol μg/24 h
Onset of menstruation	9	7	3
Ovulation peak	30	24	10
Luteal peak	20	18	9
Pregnancy, 150 days	10	1	.5
Pregnancy, term	35	4	2
Postmenopause	2	2	1

209. The second rise in all probability reflects an increased secretion of estrogens by the theca lutein cells of the corpus luteum.

A. This is a good assumption.
B. This is a bad assumption.
C. This is proven by the data.
D. There are no data available at all to make such an assumption.

Twenty male New Zealand albino rabbits were divided into four groups of 5 animals each and treated as follows:

Group 1: Received a subcutaneous injection of $10 \times 10^{\times 6}$ sheep red blood cells at two week intervals for a total of three injections.

Group 2: Received an intradermal injection of $10 \times 10^{\times 6}$ sheep red blood cells at two week intervals for a total of three injections.

Group 3: Received a subscapular injection of $10 \times 10^{\times 6}$ sheep red blood cells at two week intervals for a total of three injections.

Group 4: Received an intravenous injection of $10 \times 10^{\times 6}$ sheep red blood cells at two week intervals for a total of three injections.

During the six week immunization period antibody titers against sheep red blood cells were measured and the following results obtained:

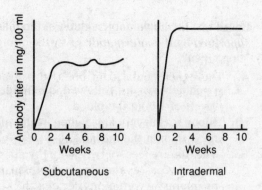

Subcutaneous   Intradermal

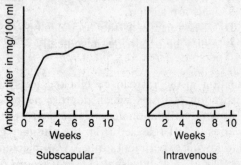

Subscapular   Intravenous

210. These data show that:

A. there is little difference in the results produced by the various routes of administration.

B. there is little difference between subscapular and subcutaneous injection routes.

C. the animals receiving intravenous red blood cells were immunologically incompetent.

D. antigen clearance was most rapid in the animals receiving intradermal injections.

An experimental drug, S24953, may maintain hepatic fatty acid oxidation at a normal rate in ethanol-treated rats. The following groups were studied at 8, 16, and 32 hours after administration of ethyl alcohol and glucose. Biochemically speaking a fatty liver is the end result of ethanol consumption.

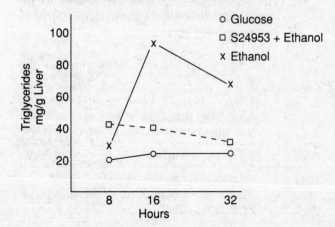

211. Based on the above data, select the statement(s) *supported by* the information given.

- **A.** The experimental data point to a nearly complete prevention of ethanol-induced fatty liver by S24953.
- **B.** The peak of the ethanol-induced fatty liver was observed around 16 hours after consumption.
- **C.** Ethanol caused a 300% increase in the concentration of liver triglycerides.
- **D.** All of the above are supported.

A blood sample was taken from a test subject. Then a masked man came in with a gun and appeared to murder 2 persons. The test subject was visibly upset. After 30 seconds, the "victims" stood up. The subject was told of the hoax, and blood samples were taken over a period of time for counting red blood cells (RBC).

Time	RBC/mm^3 of Blood
Control (before "murder")	5.5 million
30 seconds after "murder"	5.9 million
6.5 minutes after "murder"	7.0 million
14.5 minutes after "murder"	5.6 million
18.5 minutes after "murder"	5.5 million

212. Based on the above table, select the statement *supported by* the information given.

- **A.** There was an increase in the RBC/mm^3 of blood of the test subject a few minutes after he thought he witnessed murder.
- **B.** A larger change in the RBC/mm^3 of blood would have been noted if the test subject had been placed in greater fear for his own life.
- **C.** Having changed from the control value, there was no return to the control value for nearly 20 minutes.
- **D.** Although a return of RBC/mm^3 of blood to control value was noted, a rebound would be expected within an hour after the end of the experiment.

Production of organic compounds by photosynthesis was studied in Puerto Rico. The results are given in the table below with the theoretical yield based on percentage of light captured by the plant.

Plants	Carbohydrate Production (tons/acre) Present	Theoretical	Percentage of Sunlight Captured by Plant
Kelp	2.0	14	15
Cane	0.7	0.9	1.0
Plant Z	4.1	18	20

213. Within wide limits, the rate of carbohydrate production varies linearly with the incident light. If one doubled the incident light on an acre of cultivated kelp, how would the yield of kelp compare with the yield of an acre of plant Z on which the incident light was unchanged?

- **A.** It would surpass the carbohydrate yield per acre.
- **B.** It would approach the carbohydrate yield per acre.
- **C.** It would surpass the protein yield per acre.
- **D.** It would surpass the percentage of incident light captured.

MIDDLE INCOME PEOPLE

Samples	Mean Units of Major Food Categories Consumed Per Day Starchy Foods	Meaty Foods	Liquids
1	79	6.6	8
2	38	27	12
3	9	26	40

Samples	Incidence of Types of Tooth Decay (percent of sample) I	II	III	Type of Toothpaste Used (grams/ brushing) I	II
1	69	61	7	23	27
2	35	31	7	6	7
3	9	5	1	2	3

214. Based on the above table, select the statement *supported by* the information given.

- **A.** Considering the group classified as starch eaters, there does not seem a noticeable difference between the types of tooth decay and the sample of population.
- **B.** The average diet consumed results in less tooth decay.
- **C.** Reduced toothpaste use caused a reduction in all three types of cavities.
- **D.** Sample 3 exhibited less tooth decay.

Ten adult male guinea pigs were housed in individual cages in a room at 37°C. Five of the guinea pigs were fed an ascorbic acid deficient diet while the other five were fed standard guinea pig diet. Both groups were allowed access to water *ad libitum*. At weekly intervals the serum concentration of gamma globulin and lymphocyte reactivity were measured in both the experimental and control groups. The following graphs illustrate data collected from this experiment.

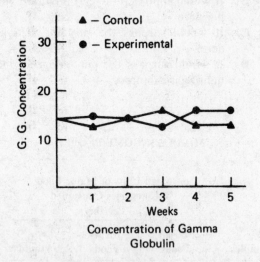

Concentration of Gamma Globulin

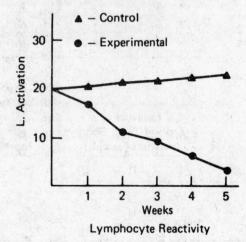

Lymphocyte Reactivity

215. A conclusion that can be reached from these data is

A. there are no sex differences in the response of guinea pigs to an ascorbic acid deficient diet.

B. temperature has a marked effect on gamma globulin concentration.

C. lymphocyte reactivity in the scorbutic guinea pig is independent of gamma globulin concentration.

D. gamma globulin concentration varies inversely with lymphocyte reactivity.

216. Which hydrocarbon is a member of the series with the general formula C_nH_{2n-2}?

A. butane   C. benzene
B. ethene   D. ethyne

217. Which class of compounds has the general formula R—O—R′?

A. esters   C. ethers
B. alcohols   D. aldehydes

218. Of the functional groups listed below, which is incorrectly identified?

A. —NH₂   amino group

B.
$$-\underset{\underset{O}{\|}}{C}-CH_3 \quad \text{acetyl group}$$

C.
$$-\underset{\underset{O}{\|}}{C}-NH_2 \quad \text{amide group}$$

D.
$$-\underset{\underset{O}{\|}}{C}-OH \quad \text{hydroxyl group}$$

219. An individual has at his disposal benzyl chloride, benzene, aluminum chloride, and sodium, and he wishes to synthesize diphenylmethane. He should react:

A. all four compounds
B. benzyl chloride and sodium.
C. benzyl chloride, benzene, and aluminum chloride.
D. benzyl chloride, benzene, and sodium.

Model Examination A Answer Key

VERBAL REASONING

1.	C	14.	B	27.	D	40.	D	53.	A
2.	D	15.	A	28.	C	41.	D	54.	B
3.	A	16.	B	29.	D	42.	B	55.	A
4.	D	17.	D	30.	D	43.	D	56.	B
5.	D	18.	D	31.	D	44.	C	57.	D
6.	B	19.	B	32.	B	45.	D	58.	D
7.	B	20.	D	33.	D	46.	B	59.	D
8.	A	21.	D	34.	D	47.	A	60.	C
9.	D	22.	D	35.	A	48.	D	61.	B
10.	C	23.	D	36.	C	49.	B	62.	D
11.	B	24.	D	37.	B	50.	A	63.	C
12.	C	25.	B	38.	D	51.	D	64.	D
13.	B	26.	B	39.	D	52.	B	65.	D

PHYSICAL SCIENCES

66.	D	82.	B	98.	C	113.	D	128.	C
67.	D	83.	C	99.	C	114.	C	129.	C
68.	B	84.	A	100.	C	115.	C	130.	B
69.	A	85.	B	101.	B	116.	B	131.	A
70.	B	86.	B	102.	A	117.	A	132.	B
71.	B	87.	A	103.	C	118.	B	133.	B
72.	C	88.	C	104.	C	119.	C	134.	C
73.	B	89.	D	105.	D	120.	A	135.	B
74.	C	90.	D	106.	D	121.	A	136.	A
75.	C	91.	B	107.	A	122.	C	137.	C
76.	B	92.	B	108.	A	123.	D	138.	B
77.	C	93.	A	109.	B	124.	C	139.	B
78.	A	94.	B	110.	A	125.	D	140.	C
79.	A	95.	A	111.	B	126.	A	141.	D
80.	B	96.	C	112.	D	127.	B	142.	D
81.	A	97.	C						

BIOLOGICAL SCIENCES

143.	B	159.	A	175.	D	190.	A	205.	B
144.	C	160.	B	176.	B	191.	B	206.	B
145.	C	161.	C	177.	A	192.	C	207.	B
146.	D	162.	D	178.	C	193.	D	208.	B
147.	D	163.	D	179.	C	194.	B	209.	D
148.	D	164.	A	180.	D	195.	A	210.	B
149.	D	165.	D	181.	D	196.	B	211.	D
150.	B	166.	A	182.	C	197.	C	212.	A
151.	B	167.	D	183.	A	198.	D	213.	B
152.	D	168.	D	184.	D	199.	B	214.	D
153.	D	169.	D	185.	C	200.	D	215.	C
154.	C	170.	D	186.	A	201.	C	216.	D
155.	B	171.	C	187.	D	202.	B	217.	C
156.	C	172.	B	188.	A	203.	C	218.	D
157.	C	173.	A	189.	D	204.	A	219.	C
158.	C	174.	D						

Explanation of Answers for Model Examination A

VERBAL REASONING

1. **C.** The central theme of the passage deals with the monumental amounts of research that have been done in the field of public education over the past 20 years. Mention of the vast research effort is made in paragraphs three, four and five, whereas paragraph six makes it clear that research will continue.

2. **D.** Paragraph two states that the outcry was created in part by declining economic conditions, as well as the publication of exhaustive studies of school resources and their impact.

3. **A.** Paragraph one makes it clear that the reform in question for this passage deals with the nation's public school systems.

4. **D.** All three statements are included in the answer. In education "the field" is considered the classroom (I). "Researchers" going into the field indicates that they are observing teachers and students in action (II). The fact that researchers have gone into the field in great numbers indicates that there is much interest in educational reform research (III).

5. **D.** The combination of **B** and **C** encompasses educators who are researchers as well as those who are practicing in the field at all levels, and names three specific sets of practitioners who are closest to school settings. The question asks, what groups, and a choice is provided to include all the combinations.

6. **B.** Paragraphs four and five discuss researchers in the field and some progress that has been made as a result of their efforts. The "tone" that the author sets in these paragraphs allows one to assume that she feels hands-on research is beneficial.

7. **B.** The paragraph states that research efforts have intensified as plans of action are *evaluat-*

ed. It is reasonable to conclude that the results of the evaluation process will lead to more specific questions that will then lead to further investigation.

8. **A.** The passage opens by telling the reader that *periodic* demands for educational reform are not unusual in this country's history. Examples of reform attempts are given throughout. The closing sentence makes it clear that researchers are continuing their efforts to find ways to improve public education.

9. **D.** Paragraph two shows that family income is a factor that influences success in school, but it is not the only factor. Although hundreds of studies have indeed been conducted, the cry for reform continues as evidenced in the last paragraph. The negative effects of the early research have been lessened as a result of recent studies, but paragraph six noted that they have not been eliminated.

10. **C.** Paragraph two traces the story back to seventh century China and goes on to state that the plot is universal. The central thesis of the passage is that all versions of the story share many ingredients, and the first paragraph asserts that one of these chronicles the transformation into womanhood. Paragraph three notes the evil stepmother as a feature common to various versions of the story.

11. **B.** A main point of the passage is that a consistent aspect of Cinderella's character is her loving and forgiving spirit.

12. **C.** No mention is made of Cinderella's need for warmth (**A** is incorrect). The skins clearly are important in a ritual sense (**B** is incorrect). Cinderella always returns to a clean, well-dressed state; and because it symbolically is essential that she give up the skins and there is no mention that she keeps them, **D** is incorrect.

13. **B.** Cinderella, as the author notes in the final paragraph, is moving toward a condition of wholeness. There is nothing to suggest, that she is less complex than she had thought (**A** is incorrect), that she exploits the prince (**C** is incorrect), or that her wholeness weakens her (**D** is incorrect).

14. **B.** A central purpose of the essay is to show how various versions of this tale make concrete various aspects of Horney's theories. Nowhere is there a suggestion that Horney had in mind the Cinderella story or that Horney altered the story in any way, thus **A** and **D** are incorrect. And, though one might find that the parallel between Horney's theories and the fairy tale provide one illustration of how the theories and the fairy tale provide one illustration of how the theories appear to be supported by their presence in a given story like *Cinderella*, nowhere is there a suggestion that the validity of a theory could be based on a single story application such as this one. Thus **C** is incorrect.

15. **A.** Although the first part of the title is a clever play on words, it also prepares the reader for the "fit" between Horney's theories and the Cinderella tale. The three other titles are not descriptive of the pattern of argument in the essay, and in the cases of **B** and **C**, contradict information in the text.

16. **B.** In **B**, the implication is that a fairy tale will be examined in view of a set of psychological theories. **C** is incorrect in that the comparison here is between two tales, not a tale and theory. **A** and **D** suggest studies that stray from the application of psychological theory to fairy tales.

17. **D.** The best and most encompassing title would be The Development of the Physician. The passage does not deal with professional growth and the development and training of the medical student exclusively. Although it is mentioned that the first two years of the study of medicine focus on the scientific aspects and thereafter the clinical practice predominates the life of the students, it is not examined specifically.

18. **D.** The passage makes it clear that most students enter this profession because they care for their fellow man and want to serve him; in fact the passage ends on the note that "the secret of the care of the patient is in caring for the patient." Achieving public esteem is a part of becoming a physician and certainly although intelligence and a good background help, they are not enough in the making of a physician. Marriage among classmates is not discussed.

19. **B.** Moral, clinical, and legal perspectives affect decision making and are in the order used upon first entrance into school. Socialization, however, elevates the clinical perspective to resolve the myriad of clinical situations. The issue of the influence of hospital administrators is not debated in the passage. The author quotes from Konner in respect to arrogance, but no conclusion is reached in respect to the statement that their extensive training gives anyone that right.

20. **D.** Good health, although essential, is not enough for medical practice; the article stresses continuously that the overall, the broad, the human, the appreciation of life, love, and mankind must be considered and held in focus in order to serve appropriately.

21. **D.** All the statements presented in this question are definitely contradicted by the information in the passage.

22. **D.** Because this passage basically describes the development and training—philosophical, ethical, legal, and clinical—of a student, the passage would be most appropriate if it were presented during a freshman orientation lecture.

23. **D.** In paragraph two it is made clear that the studies of Carlton showed that three rather distinct perspectives, the moral, clinical, and legal, directly affect decision making by physicians.

24. **D.** It is clearly pointed out in the last paragraph that most of the first two years is devoted to the science of medicine, but that there is patient contact towards the end of year one. In paragraph six, Konner mentions a nonphysical aspect of healing, which he calls spiritual.

25. **B.** The passage makes it clear that at the end of the reductional division the chromosomes are reduced to one-half their original number. Meiosis results in four gametes that possess one-half the chromosomal number of an adult.

The production of gametes, or sex cells—egg and sperm—is known as gametogenesis. Because an individual possesses an equal amount of genetic material from both parents and the same number of chromosomes as either parent, a reduction to one-half that number must be accomplished in the development of the egg and sperm.

26. **B.** During the process of meiosis, a recombination of genetic material is possible; this is effected through crossing over, as noted in paragraph three. In crossing over, comparable portions of chromatids are exchanged; crossing over is more the rule than the exception. Replication results during the first part of meiosis in four chromatids and two of them may exchange materials. This exchange occurs before the tetrads separate.

27. **D.** The third paragraph indicates that replication of DNA occurs during interphase before meiosis starts. Interphase is the time during which the cell grows and prepares itself for meiosis.

28. **C.** See the explanation for previous questions dealing with this passage.

29. **D.** Eggs and sperms are haploid; a fertilized egg (zygote) possesses the diploid number of the parent again. Also see explanations for previous questions.

30. **D.** The first sentence of paragraph two mentions ten stages. Paragraph one states that sexual reproduction plays an important role in the expression of different phenotypes, and paragraph three indicates that replication of DNA occurs during interphase before meiosis begins.

31. **D.** The fact that ordinal position remains a little understood personality variable is stated in the opening paragraph and sets the tone for the passage.

32. **B.** Although much research has been done on birth order, it is not possible to make *absolute* statements about any of the ordinal positions. It has not been proven, for example, that the oldest is *always* the most mature. The opening paragraph implies that more studies need to be conducted.

33. **D.** The author states that primogeniture is "a perfect illustration of the importance of being first born." Because the custom began in feudal times, it is reasonable for the reader to conclude that the paragraph was inserted to provide a sense that the subject of ordinal birth has been the subject of study for some time.

34. **D.** All statements made in the question are correct. Parents attach to their firstborn such characteristics as a solid head on his/her shoulders, a mature behavior, and the ability to associate with adults, to be able to lead, to care for siblings, and to grow up as a pillar of the community. The youngest child is freer to develop into an exuberant and free-spirited individual because mothers do not expect the youngest to function in an adultlike manner. Many actions that were frowned upon previously are now considered cute in nature.

35. **A.** Although a comparison of the middle child to the older child is made, no direct comment or evidence is presented that this helps him/her reach higher levels of achievement; in fact because of the comparison and the desire of the child to establish his own identity, he may even become a problem student. The passage makes it clear that the firstborn usually performs better, and that the youngest feels the least need to excel. It is also stated in the passage that communication with adults is typically a problem of the second born.

36. **C.** The last two paragraphs specifically deal mainly with a discussion of mathematics grades between women; three groups were analyzed: (1) firstborn; (2) second, but not last born; and (3) last born.

37. **B.** The anxiety theory tries to explain decreased achievement in mathematics of the youngest child. This child is not pushed by his parents, which could be interpreted as being due to lack of parental interest. Thus, the youngest may suffer from the lack of parental expectations as well as from a self-imposed anxiety. The combination of both factors contributes to lower performance.

38. **D.** Paragraph two cites a family with three children, and paragraph five states that the youngest child often develops into an exuberant and well-rounded individual. The last paragraph makes the point that the youngest may

develop feelings of anxiety, which may interfere with performance.

39. **D.** All the statements are supported by the information in the passage.

40. **D.** The author of the passage neither supports nor contradicts the statements presented in the question.

41. **D.** All three statements are clearly contradicted by the information presented in the passage.

42. **B.** The charisma of the instructor is a factor in the evaluation of teaching effectiveness. There are objective methods available and grades do play a role in student ratings. Time of day is not discussed in the passage.

43. **D.** The difficulty of subject matter material and its effect on student ratings is not discussed in the passage.

44. **C.** Students are usually most interested in evaluations by students, believing that they are the "consumers" who are most directly affected by the quality of the "product" called teaching.

45. **D.** Paragraph five visualizes students as purchasers. Paragraph two points out that employers and employees benefit from evaluations, and paragraph four states that the end result is increased productivity.

46. **B.** In paragraph one, the author plainly asserts that Tillich believes contemporary society is characterized by an absence of spirituality, whereas, ironically, there is a growing interest in religion.

47. **A.** Tillich, according to the author, sees true religion as moving vertically, and thus being characterized by "depth." Tillich's main thesis deals with the ways in which (1) present-day religion runs counter to true religion and (2) present-day society discourages people from asking weighty eschatological questions.

48. **D.** Although the author agrees with Tillich's assertions that modern man lacks true religion and is more materialistic now than in the past, he questions in his final paragraph the strictly "rational" ways that Tillich implies are the only ways of knowing spiritual truth. Nowhere in the essay does the author quarrel with Tillich's definition of spirituality.

49. **B.** In paragraph three, the author states plainly that Tillich's ideas are perhaps even more insightful or relevant than they were 30 years ago.

50. **A.** Though the author clarifies and qualifies Tillich's positions, he asserts that Tillich is still as relevant as he was "30 years ago."

51. **D.** These are the exact words that the author quotes Tillich as using. All other answers illustrate the opposite principle.

52. **B.** The main topic of this passage is to describe how a very specialized joint participates in the movement of the mandible functions. It is a two-joint proposition, which allows for opening and closing, protrusion and retraction, and lateral deviation movements.

53. **A.** Interposed between the condyle and fossa is the articular disk or meniscus. The meniscus divides the joint into two synovial compartments; in the upper compartment a gliding motion is allowed, whereas in the lower compartment a hinge motion prevails.

54. **B.** The paragraph states that the thickened lateral part of the capsule forms the temporomandibular ligament that prevents excessive retraction of the mandible.

55. **A.** It is stated in paragraph three that the temporomandibular ligament limits border movements.

56. **B.** Although the passage indicates that type B cells are secretory in nature, it does not limit this activity to type B cells. Phagocytes do remove foreign material, blood vessels supply the joint, synovial fluid is complex, and it is indicated that where there is a lack of pressure the membrane is thrown into folds.

57. **D.** Paragraph one describes this joint to be diarthroidal, capable of hinge and gliding movements. Although it is true that many suffer from temporomandibular joint problems, the passage does not address this issue. Paragraph three mentions the malleus, which is a middle ear bone, and the fact that one of the ligaments stabilizing the joint connects to the ossicle.

58. **D.** The last paragraph likens synovial fluid to plasma and lymph. Paragraph two states that the disk fuses with the joint capsule, and paragraph one states that both the right and left joints function as one unit.

59. **D.** Recent studies clearly show an impact of the increasing use of part-time faculty; and concerns are expressed about employment security, participation in governance, access to due process, grievances, evaluations, and fair compensation.

60. **C.** This is the best answer because the article covers many aspects of the impact of nontenure-eligible faculty on the educational mission of the university.

61. **B.** Part-time faculty has been hired at a rate that shows a 164 percent increase (compared to a 37 percent increase in number of full-time faculty) from 1970–1988.

62. **D.** The statements that part-time faculty is never expected to function in curriculum matters and that full-time "teach only" faculty has a secure base are contradicted by the passage.

63. **C.** The only statement supported by the passage is that tenure-track faculty are uninhibited in advocating changes in accepted ideas and in policies and programs of the institutions.

64. **D.** All choices represent correct statements. Temporary faculty foster morale problems among themselves, the institution, and everyone else. The two-tier system has eroded sound governance practices. Some writers view the hiring of temporary faculty as short-sighted and due to unregulated growth.

65. **D.** Paragraph one points out that many have studied the issues, and paragraph two states that various reasons exist for the presence of part-time faculty. It is clear from paragraph one that evidence exists and clearly shows the impact of the increasing use of part-time faculty in higher education institutions.

PHYSICAL SCIENCES

66. **D.** The work done on charged particles by electric fields depends on the charge on the particle and the voltage difference (not on the mass of the particle). The electric work, $W = qV$, increases the kinetic energy of the particles; in this case from zero to the final KE. Because the charges for electron and proton are equal, they have equal final kinetic energies (although the electron has a greater speed).

67. **D.** This question tests your knowledge of the force ($F = qvB \sin \Theta$) exerted on a moving charge by a magnetic field as well as the "right-hand rule" for positively charged particles, which relates the vector direction of the force to the vector directions of the velocity and the magnetic field. For a positive charge moving horizontally North through a magnetic field pointing horizontally West, the magnetic force is vertically upward. The negative electron is equivalent to a positive charge moving in the opposite direction so the force on *both* electron and proton is upward.

68. **B.** The proton and electron are now moving parallel to the magnetic field direction so that $\sin \Theta$ is zero in the magnetic force equation ($F = qvB \sin \Theta$). Thus the magnetic force on each is zero, and their paths are undeflected.

69. **A.** The magnetic force acts only at right angles to the velocity of a charged particle, so it can change the direction of the velocity vector but not its magnitude (speed *is* the magnitude of velocity).

70. **B.** The electric force, $F = qE$, shows that the direction of the force, F, is parallel to E for positive charges like protons and opposite (antiparallel) E for negative charges like electrons.

71. **B.** The frictional work uses up all the kinetic energy. Frictional force is μmg, and frictional work is μmgs. Thus:

$$W_f = KE_i - o = KE_i \quad \text{or} \quad \mu mgs = 1/2 \ mv^2$$

thus solving for skid length, s: $s = v^2/(2 \ \mu g)$, and the skid length is proportional to the *square* of the *speed*. The mass drops out of the equation.

72. **C.** Because the skid length depends on speed squared, a car with twice the speed of another will slide *four* times as far.

73. **B.** The forces during the collision *are* equal and opposite according to Newton's third law of motion. Each of the other responses is incor-

rect for the following reasons: **A.** The more massive van has *greater* momentum at the same speed. **C.** The forces are actually *equal* and opposite. **D.** It would require *more* mechanical work to stop the van because it has a larger mass. In this case, the vehicles do not stop. The large van would actually reverse the velocity of the small car and "drive" the car backwards.

74. **C.** As in explanation for question 73, the forces during collision are equal and opposite. The other responses are incorrect because: **A.** Equal and opposite magnitudes of momenta is not the explanation for the unequal damage. (In question 8, the momenta were *not* equal and opposite, and the car also suffered more damage in that collision!) **B.** The forces are actually equal and opposite. **D.** Is not a true statement.

75. **C.** As in explanation for question 72, the skid length depends on the square of the speed.

76. **B.** In this particular experiment, the paint marks are three times farther apart when the speed (60 mph) is three times greater. Thus the times to travel between paint marks, which is the reaction time, remains the same. (The reaction times could vary from one test to another. Here the two times happened to be identical.)

77. **C.** Elementary trigonometry states that the sine of an angle = (opposite side)/(hypotenuse). Sin 30° = 0.5, so the hypotenuse is two times as long as the opposite side.

78. **A.** The power is the work/(unit time) and the work done is equal to the total gain in gravitational potential energy. The time is 60 seconds. Thus:

P(watts) = (#buckets)(10kg/bucket)(g)(4.0m)/ (60s) = 196 watts.

79. **A.** Electric power, in watts, is related to voltage and current as follows:

$P = VI$. Thus $I = 196W/(120 V)$
= 1.6 amperes.

80. **B.** The higher power motor should have a power that is 1.45 times the smaller power, i.e.:

1.45 × 200 = 290 watts.

81. **A.** Because twice as much mass is raised through 4 m in one minute, the required work per minute, and thus the required power, is doubled.

82. **B.** The total mechanical energy is conserved on this frictionless track. The initial gravitational potential energy, *mgh,* is converted into kinetic energy in sliding down to the horizontal:

$$\frac{1}{2} mv^2 = mgh \quad \text{therefore } v = \sqrt{2gh}.$$

83. **C.** Because the total momentum and the total kinetic energy of the system of two carts both remain constant, the first cart gives up all its kinetic energy to cart #2. (cart #1 stops) (Both the conservation of kinetic energy equation and the conservation of momentum equations must be "satisfied" at the same time.) This can be done only by writing the equations in the following form:

$$\left(\frac{1}{2}mv^2\right) + 0 = 0 + \left(\frac{1}{2}mv^2\right)_2$$
$$(mv)_1 + 0 = 0 + (mv)_2$$

which is satisfied only if $v_1 = v_2$.

84. **A.** As shown above, the first cart is stopped by the collision, giving up all its momentum and energy to the second car. (The results of questions 17 and 18 are only correct for the case of *equal* masses for which the energy and momentum transfer are maximum.)

85. **B.** As above, only when the masses are equal, does the speed of #1 after the collision equal zero. Thus its speed is smaller because it *does transfer energy to #3.*

86. **B.** The transfer of energy to #2 will be smaller for the "inelastic" case where some energy is dissipated, and thus its speed will be smaller than for the elastic collision case.

87. **A.** The collision does conserve momentum so that the combined velocity of the carts after impact is $\frac{1}{2}$ the velocity of #1 before:

$$mv = (m + m)V. \quad \text{Thus: } V = \frac{V}{2} = \frac{1}{2}\sqrt{2gh}$$

88. **C.** The magnification of a plane (flat) mirror is 1.

89. **D.** The mechanical work done is equal to the gain in gravitational potential energy, *mgh*. ($g = 9.8$ m/s^2).

90. **D.** This question requires an understanding of the decay of radioactive nuclei. The negative beta particle is an electron (charge = $-e$). It is emitted from the decaying nucleus following the conversion of one of the neutrons into a proton (which remains in the nucleus) plus the emitted electron. The nucleus thus "gains" a proton and the nuclear charge increases by $+e$.

91. **B.** The thin lens formula is used to solve this problem:

$\frac{1}{f} = \frac{1}{p} + \frac{1}{q}$, where p and q are the object and image distances, respectively, and f is the focal length, thus:

$\frac{1}{f} = \frac{1}{12} + \frac{1}{12} = \frac{2}{12}$
$f = 24$.

92. **B.** This question requires a knowledge of the fundamental properties of forces as vectors (with both magnitude and direction). Because the two given forces act at right angles, they behave as the "components" of the resultant force and can be treated as the sides of a right triangle whose hypotenuse is the resultant force.

93. **A.** The speed of any wave is the product of its frequency and wavelength. $v = f\lambda$. This is true for *all waves*. (Light and radio waves, sound waves, waves on a string) Thus $\lambda = \frac{v}{f} = \frac{340 \text{ m/s}}{1200/s}$.

94. **B.** Pressure is force per unit area, that is:
$P = F/A = 110$ lb/3.5 in^2 = 31 lb/in^2.

95. **A.** The expression for converting degrees F to degrees C is:
T °C $= (T$ °F $- 32)5/9$. The student should remember that converting between the temperature scales is unlike the usual conversions, because the zeros of the scales do not agree. (0°C = 32°F)

96. **C.** The equivalent resistance of resistors connected only in series is: $R_S = R_1 + R_2 + R_3 +$

.... For a parallel connection: $\frac{1}{R_p} = \frac{1}{R_1} + \frac{1}{R_2} + \frac{1}{R_3}$, and so on. One can have (1) one resistor, (2) two in series, (3) three in series, (4) two in parallel, (5) three in parallel, (6) two in series with the third in parallel with the first two, and (7) one in series with a parallel connection of the other two. Thus there are only seven possible unique arrangements of three identical resistors. (If the three resistances were different, there would be more than seven possibilities.)

97. **C.** Three resistors in series yield an equivalent 6-ohm resistance and the same three in parallel yield a minimum resistance of 0.67 ohms. (It is not possible to have less than 0.67 ohms in any of the other six possible ways to arrange the three 2-ohm resistors.)

98. **C.** The capacitor cannot conduct a DC current after it is fully charged (which will take a very short time) so that an ammeter connected to read the current through only the capacitor will read zero. The 2-ohm resistor has a 4 volt potential difference across its terminals. Ohm's law for the resistor, $I = \frac{V}{R}$, shows that the current is 2 amperes. (Note that although there is no current through the capacitor, it does have the same potential difference of 4 volts.)

99. **C.** The impedance of the RLC series circuit is frequency dependent. It is given in general by:
$Z = \sqrt{R^2 + (X_L - X_C)^2}$. At the resonant frequency, the impedance is *purely resistive* because the inductive reactance, X_L, and the capacitive reactance, X_C, are equal. Thus $Z = R = 2$ ohms.

100. **C.** Because $Z = R = 2$ ohms at resonance, the AC form of Ohm's law gives the current very simply as:

$I = \frac{V}{Z} = \frac{V}{R} = \frac{4}{2} = 2.0$ A.

101. **B.** Faraday's law of induction states that the induced *emf* (voltage) is proportional to the rate of change of magnetic flux linking the circuit.

$\varepsilon = -N\frac{\Delta\phi}{\Delta t}$. Here the flux at any instant is given by $\phi = BA$, where A is the area of the coil. The expression then may be written as:

$\varepsilon = -NA\dfrac{\Delta B}{\Delta t}$. Solving for $\dfrac{\Delta B}{\Delta t}$, we have:

$\dfrac{\Delta B}{\Delta t} = \dfrac{(.01\ V)}{(100 \times 1 \times 10^{-4}\ m^2)} = 1\ \dfrac{T}{s}$.

102. **A.** The equivalent resistance of the three 2-ohm resistors in parallel is found first.

$\dfrac{1}{R_p} = \dfrac{1}{2} + \dfrac{1}{2} + \dfrac{1}{2} = \dfrac{3}{2}$

and $R_p = \dfrac{2}{3}$ ohm. Ohm's law is used to find the total current. $V = IR_p$ and thus

$I = \dfrac{V}{R_p} = \dfrac{6}{(2/3)} = 9$ amperes.

103. **C.** The junction current rule (Kirchhoff's first circuit law) states that the current into a junction in a circuit is equal to the current out of the junction. Because all three resistances are equal, the total current of 9 amperes splits up so that exactly one third flows through each of the resistors. Each resistor has a current of 3 A. One can also solve the problem by applying Ohm's law to one of the resistors noting that the full 6 volts appear across each resistor in parallel. Thus $I = \dfrac{V}{R} = 3$ A.

104. **C.** Again the series and parallel rules are used to calculate the equivalent total resistance. For the two resistors in parallel: $\dfrac{1}{R_p} = \dfrac{1}{2} + \dfrac{1}{2} = 1$, so that $R_p = 1$ ohm. This resistance is in series with the third 2-ohm resistor so that the equivalent resistance is:

$R_e = R_3 + R_p = 1 + 2 = 3$ ohms.

Ohm's law gives the total current through this equivalent resistance: $I = \dfrac{V}{R_e} = \dfrac{6}{3} = 2$ A.

105. **D.** In this circuit the full voltage drop due to the battery occurs across the single resistance, thus the voltmeter reading of 6 volts is also the battery voltage. The unknown resistance is found by once again using Ohm's law, $R = \dfrac{V}{I} = \dfrac{6}{1.5} = 4$ ohms.

106. **D.** The amino groups may exist as $R\text{-}NH_3^+$ with a charge of +1 or as $R\text{-}NH_2$ with a charge

of zero (0). The carboxyl group may exist as R-COOH with a charge of zero (0) or as R-COO$^-$ with a charge of -1. Thus, we might indicate the possible charged species of this amino acid at different pH's as

$(+\ +\ 0)\ \dfrac{pK_a = 2.1}{\text{(lowest pH)}}\ (+\ +\ -)\ \dfrac{pK_a = 9.0}{\cdots}\ (+\ 0\ -)\dfrac{pK_a = 10.5}{\text{(highest pH)}}\ (0\ 0\ -)$

We note that the third species $(+\ 0\ -)$ would have a net charge of zero. The pK$_a$'s that relate this species to those on both sides may be averaged to obtain the isoelectric point:

$\dfrac{9.0 + 10.5}{2} = 9.75$.

107. **A.** The reasoning is the same as in the above question, but the species are $(+\ 0\ 0)$, $(+\ 0\ -)$, $(+\ -\ -)$, and $(0\ -\ -)$. The pK$_a$'s on the two sides of the electrically neutral $(+\ 0\ -)$ are 2.1 and 4.0

$\dfrac{2.1 + 4.0}{2} = 3.05$.

108. **A.** The isoelectric point of such amino acid would be about $\dfrac{2.1 + 9.0}{2} = 5.55$. It would have a net charge of zero at that pH, increasingly positive net charge as the pH decreases, and increasingly negative net charge as the pH increases. Thus, at a pH of 8, this amino acid will consist of molecules most of which exist as the species having a net charge of -1.

109. **B.** As mentioned in explanations above, the isoelectric point would be the mean of the pK$_a$'s associated with the uncharged species. In this case:

$\dfrac{4.0 + 9.0}{2} = 6.5$.

110. **A.** Differences in the isoelectric points of various amino acids allow their separation in a buffer of appropriate pH in an electrical field (electrophoresis).

111. **B.** In applying the gas laws, only the Kelvin scale may be used because of the three, it is the only one with a natural zero.

112. **D.** When going up a mountain, we could expect the possibility of either a decrease in temperature or pressure. An increase in pressure is unlikely and would result in a decrease in volume. A decrease in temperature would result in

a decrease in volume. Because PV would remain constant, a 10% decrease in pressure would result in a 10% increase in volume.

113. **D.** $\dfrac{PV}{T} = nR$ Depending on the units of R, n can be the number of moles or the number of molecules (or atoms). Because R is a universal constant, the value of PV/T depends only on the number of molecules (or moles).

114. **C.** See explanation for question 113. Equal numbers of moles of any gas will occupy the same volume at equal temperatures and pressures.

115. **C.** $\dfrac{P_1V_1}{T_1} = \dfrac{P_2V_2}{T_2}$

$\dfrac{P_1V_1}{T_1} = \dfrac{(0.95)P_1V_2}{(0.95)T_1}$

$P_1V_1 = P_1V_2$ and thus $V_1 = V_2$
(Remember that T is calculated as °K (°C + 273). Thus the temperature decreased by 5%.)

116. **B.** The pH of distilled water is 7.0 and the hydrogen ion concentration is 1.0×10^{-7} moles/liter.

117. **A.** There is 0.01 mole in 100 mL or 0.1 mole/L. The HCl will be completely ionized and thus $[H^+] = 0.1$ mole/L.
$pH = -\log [H^+] = -\log (1.0 \times 10^{+1}) = 1$

118. **B.** $K_a = \dfrac{[H^+][Ac^-]}{[HAc]} = \dfrac{[H^+]^2}{[HAc]} = 1.8 \times 10^{-5}$

$= \dfrac{[H^+]^2}{0.1}$

$[H^+]$ would be between 1.2×10^{-3} and 1.5×10^{-3} by estimation of the square root.
$pH = -\log [H^+]$
$-\log (1.2 \times 10^{-3}) = -(-3) -\log 1.2$
Because log 1 = 0, log 1.2 would not be very different (about 0.08).
Thus. $-\log (1.2 \times 10^{-3}) = 3 - 0.08 = 2.92$, and $-\log (1.5 \times 10^{-3}) = 3 - 0.18 = 2.82$.
You could do the calculations with logarithm tables, but you should realize that the pH would be only slightly below 3.

119. **C.** A strong acid such as HCl is virtually completely ionized. The addition of a common ion (chloride in this case) causes no change in the pH.

120. **A.** The Henderson-Hasselbalch equation is used.

$pH = pK_a + \log \dfrac{[Ac^-]}{[HAc]}$

The assumption is that the salt is virtually completely ionized and that its contributes much, much more Ac^- than is contributed by the undissociated acid (HAc). Because the numerator and denominator of the fraction are equal, the fraction computes to unity. Because the log of 1 is zero, $pH = pK_a$ under these circumstances.

121. **A.** Points 1 and 3 are noted as showing buffering against pH change. Each of these is at the center of a range of buffering and would be a pK_a. Of these, point 1 is at the lower pH.

122. **C.** As noted in explanation for question 121, buffering is seen in two areas, indicating 2 pK_a's.

123. **D.** None of these would have 2 pK_a's. HF and HCl are strong acids and would not have a measurable pK_a. H_3PO_4 has 3 pK_a's.

124. **C.** Points 1 and 3, both pK_a's, show greatest buffering.

125. **D.** A and C are both correct, because equal amounts of two species will be found at a pK_a.

126. **A.** HCl in water is expected to be virtually 100% ionized into H^+ (or H_3O^+) and Cl^-.
$pH = -\log [H^+] = -\log (1 \times 10^{-2}) = 2$

127. **B.** Because the volume has doubled, [HCl] = 0.005 molar = 5×10^{-3}
Because HCl is virtually completely ionized,
$[H^+] = 5 \times 10^{-3}$ molar
$pH = -\log (5 \times 10^{-3})$
$\log 10^{-3} = -3$
$\log 5 = \underline{0.6990}$

$sum = -2.3010$
$-(-2.3010) = 2.3010$
Even if you are not provided with a calculator, you should recognize that the answer must be between 2 and 3 because log (5) is a positive number between zero and one.

128. **C.** The Henderson-Hasselbalch equation states

$pH = pK_a + \log \dfrac{[salt]}{[acid]}$

The strongly ionized HCl will react with sodium propionate to yield propionic acid. Thus 0.01 moles of HCl will react with 0.01 moles of sodium propionate to yield 0.01 moles of propionic acid (HPr). An additional 0.01 moles of NaPr will remain unreacted.

$$pH = pK_1 + \log\frac{[salt]}{[acid]} = 4.89 + \log\frac{(0.01)}{(0.01)}$$
$$= 4.89$$

(The concentrations should be expressed in molarities rather than simply total moles. Reflection allows us to recognize that the end result will be the same as long as we are consistent in a single set of computations.)

129. **C.** Because the solution was at the pK_a and we added equal quantities of salt and acid, it remains at the pK_a.

130. **B.** Look again at the Henderson-Hasselbalch equation. We have diluted [salt] and [acid] equally. Thus the pH remains at the pK_a.

131. **A.** $K_a = \dfrac{[H^+][Pyr^-]}{[HPyr]} = 1.4 \times 10^{-4} = \dfrac{[H^+]^2}{[HPyr]}$

$$= \frac{[H^+]^2}{0.01 \text{ molar}}$$

(Because HPyr ionized to give equal numbers of ions of H^+ and Pyr^-, their concentrations should be equal. Thus, substituting $[H^+]$ for $[Pyr^-]$ should introduce little error.)
$[H^+]^2 = (0.01) \times 1.4 \times 10^{-4} = 1.4 \times 10^{-6}$
$[H^+]$ would be approximately 1.2×10^{-3} by inspection.
$-\log (1.2 \times 10^{-3})$ is between 2 and 3.

132. **B.** The solution is at the pK_a value for the buffer pair because equal molar quantities of the buffer pair are present.

133. **B.** degree of ionization $= \dfrac{[H^+]}{[acid]}$
In an earlier problem in this set we calculated that when $[HPyr] = 0.01$, $[H^+] =$ about 1.2×10^{-3}
$$\frac{1.2 \times 10^{-3}}{0.01} = 0.12$$

134. **C.** Percent ionization $= 100$ (degree of ionization)
$100 \times 0.12 = 12$

135. **B.** $pH + pOH = 14$
$pOH = 14 - pH = 14 - 4.9 = 9.1$

136. **A.** Sulfur trioxide, SO_3, is often produced by the oxidation of any fuel that contains sulfur.
$SO_3 + H_2O \rightarrow H_2SO_4$ (sulfuric acid)
$SO_2 + H_2O \rightarrow H_2SO_3$ (sulfurous acid)

137. **C.** The atomic number represents the number of protons in the nucleus and (in the uncharged atom) the number of electrons in the shells surrounding the nucleus. Neutrons are found in the nucleus but have no charge.

138. **B.** An atom that has lost 2 electrons has a charge of $+2$; an atom that is electrically neutral has equal numbers of protons and electrons.

139. **B.** The K shell ($1s$) is filled with 2 electrons. The L shell (subshells $2s$ and $2p$) is filled with 8 electrons. This element, fluorine, is a nonmetal that is most likely to gain one electron and fill the L shell.
This will give the atom a charge (and valence) of -1.

140. **C.** See explanation for question 139.

141. **D.** A nonmetal oxide reacts with water to form an acid.
$P_2O_3 + 3H_2O \rightarrow 2H_3PO_3$ (Phosphorous Acid)

142. **D.** KCl is a salt. Salts contain ionic bonding between a metal and a nonmetal. The other compounds contain only covalent bonds between nonmetals.

WRITING SAMPLE

Part I, Essay

Herodotus's viewpoint here is clearly a fatalistic one. It is easy to see the logic behind it. Because mankind does not exist separately from either the rest of existence or the past, then every time that a man acts, he is in some ways also reacting to that surrounding existence and to the history that preceded that act. It is a frustrating point of view; and, in spite of its strange truth, it is probably a viewpoint best left without too much rumination. It is the given in life and the unchangeable. A resignation to this point of view would in some ways also be a voluntary denial of one's autonomy, of one's existence.

I say "voluntary" because I believe that the opposite viewpoint is, paradoxically, just as true. If I turn my head while driving in order to check my radio dial and in doing so also slightly turn my steering wheel causing an accident with an oncoming school bus, did not my act of turning my head create a circumstance whereby that accident occurred? Of course, it did. If I had not turned my head, then I would have not turned the wheel; and if I had not turned the wheel then the bus would not have hit my car. However, from Herodotus's viewpoint, my act did not exist by itself. Had the radio not been in the car, had a different song even been on the station, then I would perhaps not have turned my head to adjust the dial. Had the bus driver waited longer at her last stop or had she not stopped for a cup of coffee on her way to work, then perhaps she would not have been at that place at that specific time. The issue is as puzzling as the issue of whether the chicken appeared first or the egg. It is the question of the identification of an original cause in a long line of causes.

What a thinking person is most likely to conclude is that men and their circumstances are mutually interdependent rather than mutually exclusive and that therefore a statement like that of Herodotus is, in a sense, meaningless. His is only a statement of perspective and, further, a rather negative one. But to say the opposite, that circumstances are dependent on men and not vice versa would be naive and ignorant. A rational person would have to accept the interdependence of men and circumstances in order to live realistically and effectively in the world. He would then act carefully, remaining aware both that there are circumstances over which he has no control and that his act will be part of the circumstances to come.

Part 1
Explanation of First Response: 6

The paper focuses sharply on the statement and addresses each of the three writing tasks. Paragraph one explains what the statement means, paragraph two gives a specific situation in which men do, in fact, determine circumstances (a reversal of the assertion that "men are dependent on circumstances, not circumstances on men"), and in paragraph three reconciles the statement and the situation that illustrates that the opposite of the statement may also be true.

The paper provides an analysis of the potential dangers of all-or-none statements like the one in question. It does so by examining the logical extension of the idea that men are dependent on circumstances and by characterizing the implications of this assertion as "fatalistic." The logic of the paper's argument is sophisticated, on the one hand agreeing with the "strange truth" of Herodotus's point in paragraph one, but in paragraph two illustrating with a series of circumstances "dependent on men" that the reverse is also true. The final paragraph presents a balanced consideration of the interdependent relationship between individuals and the circumstances that they create and by which they are shaped.

The writing is clear and nicely controlled. The sentences are varied, containing simple (e.g., sentence one), compound (e.g., sentence four), and complex structures (e.g., sentence three). The first sentence of each paragraph serves as a topic sentence and gives unity to the paragraph that follows. Transitions, such as "however" in sentence five of paragraph two, provide coherence within the paragraph.

Part 2, Essay

Haeckel's quotation is an enigma because its meaning depends upon the interpretation of ambiguous words, "voluntary death," "intolerable suffering," and of course, "redemption." It is not clear whether the "voluntary death" is a suicide or a murder or any of the possibilities between these two extremes. So, even at the outset, the reader steps onto a shaky platform on which rests the remainder of Haeckel's statement. This "voluntary death" would specifically be the one that would put "an end to intolerable suffering." Because to "suffer" something is, in a sense, to "tolerate" it, then "intolerable suffering" would be an impossibility by definition. Finally, this enigmatic but "voluntary death," voluntary perhaps only because it is caused by a human act, is "an act of redemption." Naturally, one's thoughts might turn to the religious connotations of the word. In this case, it would mean a sort of act of deliverance from evil by sacrifice. If, however, you strip the mystery of religious aura from the word, it means simply a payback. Perhaps the redemption is the cashing in of the mortal life for freedom from human suffering. Keeping all of this in mind, Haeckel's statement, though still a puzzle of sorts, must mean that for a man to cause or to allow death in order to discontinue the suffering of pain (of one sort or another) is an exchange of the body, which is only loaned for the duration of mortality, in exchange for the freedom of the human spirit.

Now, one could argue (and people certainly have argued) endlessly about the moral right and/or wrong of this idea because it is at the core of the controversies over euthanasia, abortion, and the execution of criminals. The argument is over the "right" or "wrong" of this "redemption." Because "right" and "wrong" cannot really be defined but only agreed upon tentatively (as with laws), perhaps the literal meaning of the quote might be a better target for thought. The problem here is that it is not clear whose "intolerable suffering" is being referred to in the statement. For example, if I refuse to tolerate or to suffer the presence of my annoying little brother, is my killing him or allowing him to die an act of redemption? The thought is appalling, of course, but, according to Haeckel, it would, in fact, be a redemptive act (even if the sacrifice entailed is only that of my own innocence). The way that Haeckel's quotation is worded, there are no real exceptions.

Haeckel's quotation could be used to try to justify morally the act of taking a human life. But the statement does not morally justify anything; it merely defines a type of "voluntary death" as a sort of exchange. The end of a human's life is always an exchange of one state for another. So the moral question, the "choice" perhaps, is a personal one (or a legal one). Morality is not defined by absolute natural laws; it is rather defined personally (or, in a social situation, legally). What governs the choice maker or the potential actor consists of nothing more absolute and nothing less vague than his or her conscience and personal beliefs. Haeckel's quote could be used loosely to justify an act that results in death. But "used" is the key word here. Moral decision, decisions about right and wrong, are not that easy. Ultimately, the choice of a "*voluntary* death" in "the face of intolerable suffering" is determined only by the judgment and conscience of the individual, the mysterious "volunteer."

Part 2
Explanation of Second Response: 4

The paper focuses on the topic defined by the statement and addresses the three writing tasks. The first paragraph responds to the task of explaining the statement, in this case a task complicated by the need to clarify definitions of words that have multiple meanings. In the second paragraph, the paper provides what is clearly one of the most extreme examples imaginable to demonstrate that, given the phrasing of the quotation, there are no specific situations in which "voluntary death" would not be an act of redemption. Paragraph three explores the factors that determine the choice of voluntary death in the face of intolerable suffering.

There is no question that Haeckel's statement raises difficult problems, and it is clear that this essay constructs a sophisticated argument that explores the complexity of these problems. The strategy of defining ambiguous terms in paragraph one is a good one; the choice to explore the connotations of these words also is effective, though anyone who chooses to spend this much time on definition in the first paragraph should be aware of the danger of overdoing it. This essay stops just short of this. The reason that this essay received a 4 rather than a 5 or 6 is that the second task ("Describe a specific situation in which the voluntary death by which a person puts an end to intolerable suffering would not be an act of redemp-

tion") is not confronted as directly as it might be. The paper maintains that "there are no real exceptions," virtually by definition. The writer might have used his or her skill with definition clearly demonstrated in paragraph one to construct at least one hypothetical situation that would provide a conceivable exception to Haeckel's statement. In addition to the need for a specific "exceptional" situation in paragraph two, the paper could be strengthened by the use of other examples to illustrate the major points in paragraphs one and three. This paper in general, however, is tightly reasoned, and it moves logically toward the conclusion that the choice of voluntary death in the face of intolerable suffering is ultimately a moral decision, one based on conscience.

BIOLOGICAL SCIENCES

143. **B.** The thyroid hormones affect the rate of metabolism of all the tissues of the body; they control the growth, maturation, and differentiation of the organism. A goiter is any enlargement of the gland due to neoplasm or inflammatory disease. Endemic goiters are due to lack of iodine intake; this results in the increased production of TSH, compensatory hypertrophy and eventual exhaustion of the gland. Thyroxin deficiency leads to goiter; if the deficiency is not corrected cretinism in the young and myxedema in the adult may be a consequence.

144. **C.** Hypothyroidism would result in a patient who is fairly heavy, phlegmatic, is devoid of expression, and has rough and dry skin, and laboratory tests would show a low basal metabolic rate, low protein bound iodine, and a high serum cholesterol level.

145. **C.** The hypothyroid patient would have shown weight gain since less food is converted into energy and more food is stored as fat.

146. **D.** See explanations for questions 143–145.

147. **D.** A hyperthyroid patient would exhibit weight loss, nervousness, irritability, increased metabolic rate, rapid heart rate, sweating, and a protrusion of the eyeballs.

148. **D.** This woman is not the mother. She can contribute only the O gene, and this child must receive an A gene from one parent and a B gene from the other parent. The man cannot be ruled

out as the father with the limited information given, since he can contribute a B gene to a child.

149. **D.** If the man previously fathered a child with blood type O, then the man must have a genotype of BO. The woman can contribute only the O gene. Since the man has an equal chance of contributing the B or the O gene, there is a 50% chance of the child being type O (genotype OO) or type B (genotype BO).

150. **B.** The chance of any child of this couple being type B is 50% (see explanation for question 149). The chance that any child will be a girl is 50%. Since the blood type and the sex are independent of each other, multiply their individual chances (50% × 50% = 25%).

151. **B.** Phenotypic and genotypic characteristics may be expressed as follows:

Phenotype	Genotype
A	A/O
B	B/O
O	O/O
AB	A/B

152. **D.** Genotype refers to the genetic makeup of the organism. The genotype is expressed via phenotypic characteristics that are visible and observable under normal circumstances.

153. **D.** An allele is one of a pair of genes that occupies the same locus on homologous chromosomes.

154. **C.** Rhesus (Rh) agglutinogen is present in humans and is represented by a dominant gene R. The agglutinogen of an Rh positive fetus passes across the placenta, enters the maternal blood stream and elicits the production of an agglutinin (antibody) by the mother. The agglutinin passes into the circulation of the fetus and if present in sufficient concentration can produce agglutination, at times fatal to the developing fetus.

155. **B.** Hemophilia, a frequent disease of the royal houses of Europe, is a bleeding disorder transmitted through a sex-linked recessive gene. It results in abnormal coagulation; hemophilia A is the classical true hemophilia resulting from a deficiency of factor VIII. Both sexes carry a complete complement of sex-linked genes. A female, with the XX arrangement, will only exhibit a recessive gene if she has

received it from both parents (a rare event with an uncommon gene), whereas in the XY male the recessive gene cannot be masked because there is no partner X and so a larger number of recessive genes are expressed. A man receives his X from his mother and passes it on to his daughters. His daughters are the carriers of sex-linked traits and their sons may be affected.

156. **C.** Pleiotropism is defined as multiple phenotypic effects of a gene (allele).

157. **C.** I-2, who manifests prolonged Q-T interval, has 14 descendants who are also affected and six who are not. Each of the 14 affected descendants has an affected parent; both parents (II-3&10) of four are affected. The trait thus shows unbroken lineal descent and is, therefore, *dominant*.

158. **C.** Deafness *is not a pleiotropic affect of the gene producing prolonged Q-T*, for these abnormalities are observed *assorting* among the progeny of a male (II-1), who is doubly homozygous normal, and his wife (II-2), who is heterozygous for both abnormalities, that is, doubly heterozygous. Alleles segregate (Mendel's first law) from each other; non-alleles may assort. In the absence of linkage, *independent assortment* (Mendel's second law) of nonalleles occurs. Although the sample is not large enough to rule out weak linkage, it does rule out allelism.

159. **A.** Every affected descendant of the affected progenitor (I-3) of the F. family has at least one parent affected, except III-21, a son of II-11, who marks the only break in lineal descent of the trait. If the trait were recessive, the three normal mothers (I-4, II-9, and II-12) of affected children would have to be carriers. Because of the rarity of the defect and the lack of biological kinship between these women and their spouses, it is highly unlikely that they are carriers. It is probable that the trait is dominant and that the allele has slightly reduced penetrance and failed to manifest itself phenotypically in II-11.

160. **B.** If one were limited to the data on the W. family, it would be impossible to distinguish whether the defect is autosomal or X-linked. That is because we could not then rule out male-to-male transmission among the progeny of couple II-3&10, who have three arrhythmic

sons. Nonetheless, prolonged Q-T and the ar-rhythmias are clinically indistinguishable and almost certainly determined by the same *autosomal dominant* allele as in the F. family where male-to-male transmission shows that this dominant trait is autosomal. X-linked traits cannot be transmitted from father to son (male-to-male) because sons can receive their X chromosome (in which X-linked traits are transmitted) from only their mother, *not* from their father.

161. **C.** All of the daughters of affected males would be affected if the trait were X-linked because they received their father's X chromosome which would have contained the (dominant) mutant allele had it been X-linked. None of the daughters of the affected fathers (II-3 and II-5) are affected, thus the mutant allele is *not* in the X chromosome; the trait is autosomal.

162. **D.** Many autosomal dominant genes that produce rather mild phenotypic effects in the heterozygote produce much more extreme effects—in some cases, even lethality—in homozygotes. It is likely that *the proposita* (III-10) *is homozygous* for the prolonged Q-T allele and demonstrates the more extreme phenotype frequently manifested by homozygotes for rare autosomal dominant traits.

163. **D.** Developing embryos would be actively synthesizing both RNA and DNA (the latter would be associated with chromosome duplication prior to each cell division). Radiolabelled adenine, **A,** guanine, **B,** and uridine, **D,** would be incorporated into newly synthesized RNA. Radiolabelled adenine, guanine, and thymidine, **C,** would be incorporated into newly synthesized DNA. Because uridine is incorporated into RNA but not into DNA, radiolabelled uridine should be used to monitor RNA synthesis.

164. **A.** The correct answer is chosen after studying the graph. Note that the rate of mRNA synthesis begins to increase at the blastula stage, **A,** and reaches a peak just before the gastrula stage. As is stated in the passage and also illustrated in the graph, no RNA of any type is synthesized during cleavage. Because the question specifically asks about embryonic mRNA synthesis, **D,** is inappropriate.

165. **D.** Again the correct answer is chosen after

studying the graph. Embryonic RNA synthesis begins at the blastula stage. Initially mRNAs and later tRNAs begin to be synthesized. By the gastrula stage, rRNA synthesis has also begun. Therefore gastrula stage embryos would be synthesizing all types of RNA.

166. **A.** No synthesis of embryonic RNAs would occur in actinomycin D treated embryos. Because no embryonic mRNAs would be made, the proteins that these embryonic mRNAs would code for would also not be made. The proteins made by the developing embryos would be translated from the preexisting oogenetic or maternal RNAs.

167. **D.** Again actinomycin D treated embryos would be unable to synthesize embryonic RNAs. Because protein synthesis still occurs in these embryos, there must still be adequate rRNAs and tRNAs for translation of oogenetic or maternal mRNAs to continue. Therefore the best explanation is that continued development requires the synthesis of proteins using embryonic mRNAs (which would not be made in actinomycin D treated embryos).

168. **D.** Embryos with smaller stockpiles of maternal RNAs usually initiate synthesis of embryonic RNAs earlier in development and this usually results in a slower rate of cleavage. Embryos with a greater stockpile of maternal RNAs would undergo cleavage more rapidly than embryos with a smaller stockpile of maternal RNAs.

169. **D.** Because the mouse zygote contains a minimal amount of maternal RNAs and initiates synthesis of embryonic RNAs early in cleavage, one might expect actinomycin D treated embryos to arrest very early in development.

170. **D.** is the exception. A mature red blood cell does *not* have a nucleus or cytoplasmic organelles. They are lost during erythropoiesis. Choices **A, B,** and **C** *are* characteristics of an erythrocyte.

171. **C.** Macrophages residing in the liver and spleen engulf and break down the old erythrocyte, releasing hemoglobin, which is eventually broken down into iron and bilirubin; macrophage means "Big Eater."

172. **B.** This is a fact that needs to be committed to memory.

173. **A.** A *hypotonic* medium is one that has a lower osmotic pressure than the fluid of comparison in this example; the osmotic flow is from the solution *into* the cells, causing them to swell and ultimately burst. Remember osmotic water flow goes from regions of low to high osmotic pressure. The cells would shrink if placed in a hypertonic medium, that is, the fluid (water) in the cells would flow out into the surrounding medium.

174. **D.** The percentage of white blood cells varies as listed:
Agranular cells:
1. lymphocytes   20–25%
2. monocytes   3–8%
Granular cells:
1. neutrophils   65–75%
2. eosinophils   2–5%
3. basophils   0.5% or less

175. **D.** Humans are very well protected against the dangers of their surroundings. The external layer of skin is practically impermeable; it protects against trauma, bacteria, drying, water penetration, ultraviolet light, noxious agents, etc. White blood cells are influential in the mobilization of the immunological machinery of the body and also have the capability to engulf bacteria, etc., and destroy them. After an antigen enters the organism the immune system counters by producing antibodies to neutralize the effect and in many cases to protect the organism against susceptibility to the same agent in the future (the basis of immunization).

176. **B.** Hyperventilation is abnormally rapid, deep breathing resulting in a loss of CO_2 and an increase in blood pH. A person would be in the state of respiratory alkalosis since a decreased blood concentration of hydrogen ion is the result of pulmonary CO_2 elimination.

177. **A.** A reduction in venous blood return to the heart will result in an elevated P_{cap}. This increase in P_{cap} results in a larger driving force for fluid flow into the interstitium. There is no reason to believe that there would be a change in the osmotic pressures, which are largely due to proteins trapped on either side of the capillary wall. In fact, swelling of the leg secondary to the increased interstitial fluid is a common clinical finding.

178. **C.** Osmotic pressure (π) is equal to $\pi = \sigma RTC$, where R is the gas constant, T is the temperature, C is the concentration of solutes, and σ is the reflection coefficient. The reflection coefficient is an empirically determined constant that is inversely related to the permeability of a solute for the capillary wall. The lack of protein in the capillary will result in a decrease in the capillary osmotic pressure and will decrease $\Delta\pi$. This decrease will result in a net flow of fluid toward the interstitium increasing the total volume of fluid in the interstitium.

179. **C.** A constriction bandage increases P_i which results in a decreased ΔP and a net fluid flow into the capillary. P_{cap} is determined by the arterial pressures, and there is no reason for oncotic pressures to change significantly with externally applied pressure. A constriction bandage is a common form of treatment to reduce swelling (i.e. excess interstitial volume).

180. **D.** As explained in question 178, the reflection coefficient is a measure of how effectively a solute is confined by a membrane. The higher the coefficient, the greater is the solute's contribution to the osmotic pressure in that compartment. Because urea is a nonpolar solute with a reflection coefficient of 0, it is freely permeable to the capillary wall. Therefore in the steady state, the concentration of urea will be equal on both sides of capillary. Urea will contribute nothing to the difference in osmotic pressure or the net flux of fluid.

181. **D.** Active transport requires energy and allows a cell to move material from a point of lower concentration to a point of higher concentration.

182. **C.** The driving force (ΔP) causing air to flow into or out of the lungs is the pressure difference between the atmospheric pressure (*Patm*) and the intra-alveolar pressure (*Palv*). The absolute atmospheric or intra-alveolar pressures do not dictate air flow, it is the pressure difference that is important. Intrapleural pressure reflects lung elastic forces as well plus any smaller pressure difference between *Patm* and *Palv* while breathing. Thus, the absolute value of the intrapleural pressure has no bearing on inspiration.

183. **A.** During inspiration the chest wall enlarges, expanding the lungs and the intra-alveolar air.

Thus, the intra-alveolar pressure transiently drops below atmospheric pressure, pulling air into the lungs. During expiration the chest wall collapses causing the intra-alveolar pressure to transiently go above atmospheric pressure and air flows out of the lungs. When intra-alveolar pressure equals atmospheric pressure, no air will flow into or out of the lungs. The intrapleural pressure will always be lower than the intra-alveolar pressure by an amount equal to the elastic forces of the lungs. Thus, intra-alveolar pressure never goes below intrapleural pressure.

184. **D.** As defined, the alveolar ventilation equals the amount of fresh air which reaches the alveoli per minute. Thus, alveolar ventilation is the amount of fresh air reaching the alveoli per breath times the number of breaths per minute. Because part of the fresh air inspired gets no farther than the anatomic dead space (i.e. it doesn't reach the alveoli), the fresh air actually reaching the alveoli equals the tidal volume minus the volume of the anatomic dead space. The frequency of breathing times any other lung volume equals something other than the alveolar ventilation.

185. **C.** With hypoventilation, oxygen delivery to the alveolar gas is less than normal and the partial pressure of oxygen will decrease. Concurrently, the removal of carbon dioxide from the alveolar compartment is less than normal and the partial pressure of carbon dioxide will increase.

186. **A.** Most carbon dioxide is transported as bicarbonate ions. A portion is also bound to the amino groups of various proteins and transported as carbamino-compounds, mainly carbamino-hemoglobin. Some is transported in physical solution as dissolved carbon dioxide. Hemoglobin that has carbon monoxide bound to it is called carboxyhemoglobin and is unrelated to the transportation of carbon dioxide.

187. **D.** This question requires the ability to read a graph. The vapor pressure of any of the compounds at a given temperature can be found by (1) running a vertical line from that temperature on the scale of the horizontal axis (abscissa) to its intersection with the graph (curve) for that compound, (2) running a horizontal line from that point to its intersection with the vertical axis (ordinate), (3) reading or estimating

the vapor pressure from the scale on the ordinate. Because the curve for ethyl alcohol lies above the curve for water and below the curve for chloroform at every temperature on this plot, the vapor pressure of ethyl alcohol will always be read as lower than that of chloroform and higher than that of water, regardless of the temperature.

188. **A.** This question requires (1) the ability to read a graph, (2) a precise definition of the term "boiling point" as the temperature at which the vapor pressure of a liquid just equals the atmospheric pressure, (3) knowledge that standard atmospheric pressure (i.e., one atmosphere), which approximates atmospheric pressure at sea level is by convention 760 mm (Hg). (Knowing the boiling point of water [100° C], which is one of those reference points that everyone should know, one can deduce that the vertical dotted lines define the boiling points of the respective liquids, whereas the horizontal dotted line defines the vapor pressure at the boiling temperature.) Thus, the boiling point of any compound can be found by reading from the graph the temperature (boiling point) at which a vapor pressure of 760 mm (Hg) was attained. For chloroform, this is about 61° C.

189. **D.** This is the reverse of question 187. Knowing that the normal boiling point of water is 100° C, one can follow the perpendicular (vertical) dotted line from 100 on the abscissa to the point of intersection with the graph for water. This point coincides with the horizontal dotted line which obviously represents the vapor pressure for all of the liquids at their normal boiling points, i.e., the standard atmospheric pressure. The vapor pressure read from the ordinate is approximately 760 mm (Hg).

190. **A.** This question also requires the definition of boiling point as the temperature at which vapor pressure of a liquid equals atmospheric pressure. Although the pressure is not stated explicitly, it is stated that the pressure is less than standard atmospheric pressure. A cursory examination of the graph for water (or either of the other two liquids) reveals that vapor pressure increases as temperature increases and vice versa. Thus, if the vapor pressure required to equal atmospheric pressure is lower, the temperature (boiling point) required to attain that pressure should also be lower.

191. **B.** This question requires (1) determination of the normal boiling point of ethyl alcohol, (2) determination of the vapor pressure of water at that temperature, i.e., the atmospheric pressure at which water would boil at that temperature. As in the earlier examples, the normal boiling point of ethyl alcohol (about 78° C) can be read from the intersection of the graph for ethyl alcohol with the dotted line delineating 760 mm (Hg). The dotted line passing through this temperature intersects the graph for water at a point corresponding to 200–300 mm (Hg). This is the atmospheric pressure at which water would boil at 78° C. The only answer reasonably close to this value is **B**, 300.

192. **C.** The methyl group of toluene is an *o, p*-directing group.

193. **D.** The hydroxyl group is a highly activating group, whereas the chloro, nitro, and acetyl groups deactivate the ring towards electrophilic aromatic substitutions.

194. **B.** Oxidation of toluene yields benzoic acid. Nitration would yield the meta isomer because the carboxyl group is meta directing.

195. **A.** The methyl group activates the *o, p*-positions and directs the Br to the ortho position. The nitro group is a meta directing deactivating group.

196. **B.** The nitration of benzene involves the attack of a nitronium ion, NO^+_2, on toluene to form a cyclohexadienyl cation as the intermediate.

197. **C.** Valine is one of the nine essential amino acids, whereas linoleic acid is the only true essential fatty acid. Vitamin E is fat soluble and found in foods. Glucose is essential, but is obtained in other forms, such as polysaccharides. Polysaccharides contain many monosaccharide units joined in long chains and among the most important are starch and cellulose. Starch is the reserve carbohydrate in plants and on complete hydrolysis it yields glucose.

198. **D.** Linoleic, linolenic, and arachidonic acids (polyunsaturated) are listed as essential fatty acids, because they cannot be synthesized by the animal and must therefore be provided in the diet. Among the water soluble vitamins are thiamine, biotin, and niacin.

199. **B.** The fat soluble vitamins are vitamins A, D, E, and K. The water soluble vitamins are vitamin C, thiamine, riboflavin, niacin, vitamin B_6, folacin, vitamin B_{12}, biotin, and pantothenic acid.

200. **D.** The bulk essential minerals are calcium, phosphorus, and magnesium, whereas the trace essential minerals are iron, zinc, selenium, iodine, cobalt, molybdenum, manganese, copper, chromium, and fluoride.

201. **C.** Amino acids are derived from proteins; carbohydrates that are polyhydroxy aldehydes and the simplest carbohydrate units are known as monosaccharides. The most important monosaccharide is glucose; it is obtained by the hydrolysis of starch. Fat and oil comprise one of the three main classes of food. Fats and oils are esters of glycerol with carboxylic acids.

202. **B.** Parathyroid hormone acts upon bone, eliciting changes in calcium and phosphorus. Osteoclasts are the cells stimulated by parathyroid hormone to facilitate the resorption of calcium and phosphorus from bone. Administration of parathyroid hormone to animals without parathyroids results in an increase of phosphorus excretion in the urine, a fall in serum inorganic phosphorus levels, an increase in serum calcium, and an increase of calcium excretion in the urine.

203. **C.** Excretion concerns itself with the elimination of water (fluid) and metabolic wastes, whereas egestion is the process of eliminating undigested food materials. Catabolism is the chemical breakdown of molecules.

204. **A.** In anaerobic respiration, glucose is converted to two molecules of the 3-carbon compound pyruvic acid. In aerobic respiration, glucose is converted to six molecules each of carbon dioxide and water. Anaerobic respiration is only about 3% as efficient as aerobic respiration. The anaerobic pathway is the same as the aerobic to the pyruvic acid stage.

205. **B.** LH (luteinizing hormone) is secreted by the pituitary gland. In the male, it is also called ICSH (interstitial cell stimulating hormone) from its effects on the testes. In our case, half of each group had its testes removed. This eliminates the feedback from testes to pituitary. Comparison of AM and PM readings for

intact rats shows no significant differences in LH levels. For orchidectomized rats, levels vary widely, with no consistent AM–PM relationship.

206. **B.** Also see explanation for question 205, but note that hypothalamic areas of the brain secrete luteinizing releasing factor (LRF), which via the hypothalamo-pituitary portal system reaches the anterior pituitary to initiate luteinizing hormone production. LH then acts on the gonads to produce ova in the female. In this experiment Drug X probably blocks LRF because when LRF is administered with the drug, ovulation takes place. Statement **D** is neither supported nor contradicted by the information presented and has no impact.

207. **B.** It is obvious from the table that there is no population growth in West Germany and that the longest doubling time can be attributed to Japan; Holland has the largest excess of births over deaths, so it has the greatest rate of population growth.

208. **B.** Chemicals, X rays, cosmic rays, and so forth can exert an effect on tissues. Radiation supplemented by chemotherapy is used to treat patients with cancer, whereas ultraviolet rays may cause or facilitate the development of skin cancer. Our experiments were designed to determine if X-radiation causes an alteration in water consumption and volume of salivary glands in rats. The graph illustrates that the first parameter that was affected by 6400R was food intake; the above was evident at 3 days after irradiation. Water consumption was the least affected parameter.

209. **D.** Estrogen production by the corpus luteum diminishes drastically during pregnancy, and could stop altogether at or before parturition. There is no evidence to indicate whether the increased estrogen comes from reactivation of the corpus luteum or from some other follicle.

210. **B.** Injection routes are critical in the action of materials that stimulate immune responses. The purpose of the study was to determine the effect of different routes of administration on antibody titer. It is clear that intradermal administration produced the highest titer while there was little difference between subscapular and subcutaneous injection routes.

211. **D.** At 32 hours, liver triglycerides were little more for drug and ethanol than for glucose, so A is correct. B is correct because the ethanol graph peaks at 16 hours. C refers to the effects of ethanol, which produced three times as much triglycerides than glucose did.

212. **A.** The table shows that an increase in red blood cells was present at 6.5 minutes after the event. Statements **B** and **D** are neither supported nor contradicted by the data, but statement **C** is contradicted because there was a return to control values by 18.5 minutes.

213. **B.** Photosynthesis occurs in the chloroplasts of green plants, and sugars are formed from carbon dioxide and water in the presence of light and chlorophyll. During the process, light or radiant energy is converted to chemical energy in the form of carbohydrates. The basic reaction is:

$$6 CO_2 + 6 H_2O \rightarrow C_6H_{12}O_6 + 6 O_2$$

In our experiment without changing the incident sunlight, the largest percentage increase that is theoretically possible is predicted for kelp; if one doubled the incident light on kelp it most likely would approach the carbohydrate yield of plant Z.

214. **D.** Even though several variables are presented, sample 3 clearly shows the occurrence of less decay. Statement A is neither supported nor contradicted by the information. Statement B is contradicted by the information. Statement C is consistent with the information but includes an assumption of causation that cannot be assessed using the information given.

215. **C.** The object of this experiment was to determine the effect of ascorbic acid deficiency on the immunologic system. Two conclusions can be reached from an examination of the data: the scorbutic guinea pig probably has a partial immunologic deficiency and its lymphocyte reactivity is independent of gamma globulin concentration. There was no change in GG concentration, whereas lymphocyte reactivity dropped drastically.

216. **D.** The general formula C_nH_{2n-2} applies to all members of the alkyne series. The suffix for names in this series is "yne." Ethyne is the only choice that has the correct ending.

217. **C.** Ethers have the general formula R—O—R'. The other compounds have the following general formulas:

esters
$$R-C\overset{\textstyle O}{\underset{\textstyle O-R'}{\big<}}$$

aldehydes
$$R-C\overset{\textstyle O}{\underset{\textstyle H}{\big<}}$$

alcohols
$$R-OH$$

218. **D.** This configuration:
$$-\overset{\textstyle}{\underset{\textstyle O}{C}}-OH$$

is characteristic of carboxyl groups. A hydroxyl group is identified by—OH.

219. **C.** $\varnothing CH_2Cl + \varnothing \xrightarrow{AlCl_3} \varnothing-CH_2-\varnothing$
Friedel-Crafts Reaction

$\varnothing CH_2Cl + Na \longrightarrow \varnothing-CH_2CH_2-\varnothing$
Wurtz Reaction

The MCAT
Model Examination B

ANSWER SHEET

DIRECTIONS: After locating the number of the question to which you are responding, fill in the circle containing the letter of the answer you have selected. Use pencil (not a ballpoint pen) to completely blacken the circle.

VERBAL REASONING

1. Ⓐ Ⓑ Ⓒ Ⓓ
2. Ⓐ Ⓑ Ⓒ Ⓓ
3. Ⓐ Ⓑ Ⓒ Ⓓ
4. Ⓐ Ⓑ Ⓒ Ⓓ
5. Ⓐ Ⓑ Ⓒ Ⓓ
6. Ⓐ Ⓑ Ⓒ Ⓓ
7. Ⓐ Ⓑ Ⓒ Ⓓ
8. Ⓐ Ⓑ Ⓒ Ⓓ
9. Ⓐ Ⓑ Ⓒ Ⓓ
10. Ⓐ Ⓑ Ⓒ Ⓓ
11. Ⓐ Ⓑ Ⓒ Ⓓ
12. Ⓐ Ⓑ Ⓒ Ⓓ
13. Ⓐ Ⓑ Ⓒ Ⓓ
14. Ⓐ Ⓑ Ⓒ Ⓓ
15. Ⓐ Ⓑ Ⓒ Ⓓ
16. Ⓐ Ⓑ Ⓒ Ⓓ
17. Ⓐ Ⓑ Ⓒ Ⓓ
18. Ⓐ Ⓑ Ⓒ Ⓓ
19. Ⓐ Ⓑ Ⓒ Ⓓ
20. Ⓐ Ⓑ Ⓒ Ⓓ
21. Ⓐ Ⓑ Ⓒ Ⓓ
22. Ⓐ Ⓑ Ⓒ Ⓓ
23. Ⓐ Ⓑ Ⓒ Ⓓ
24. Ⓐ Ⓑ Ⓒ Ⓓ
25. Ⓐ Ⓑ Ⓒ Ⓓ
26. Ⓐ Ⓑ Ⓒ Ⓓ
27. Ⓐ Ⓑ Ⓒ Ⓓ
28. Ⓐ Ⓑ Ⓒ Ⓓ
29. Ⓐ Ⓑ Ⓒ Ⓓ
30. Ⓐ Ⓑ Ⓒ Ⓓ

31. Ⓐ Ⓑ Ⓒ Ⓓ
32. Ⓐ Ⓑ Ⓒ Ⓓ
33. Ⓐ Ⓑ Ⓒ Ⓓ
34. Ⓐ Ⓑ Ⓒ Ⓓ
35. Ⓐ Ⓑ Ⓒ Ⓓ
36. Ⓐ Ⓑ Ⓒ Ⓓ
37. Ⓐ Ⓑ Ⓒ Ⓓ
38. Ⓐ Ⓑ Ⓒ Ⓓ
39. Ⓐ Ⓑ Ⓒ Ⓓ
40. Ⓐ Ⓑ Ⓒ Ⓓ
41. Ⓐ Ⓑ Ⓒ Ⓓ
42. Ⓐ Ⓑ Ⓒ Ⓓ
43. Ⓐ Ⓑ Ⓒ Ⓓ
44. Ⓐ Ⓑ Ⓒ Ⓓ
45. Ⓐ Ⓑ Ⓒ Ⓓ
46. Ⓐ Ⓑ Ⓒ Ⓓ
47. Ⓐ Ⓑ Ⓒ Ⓓ
48. Ⓐ Ⓑ Ⓒ Ⓓ
49. Ⓐ Ⓑ Ⓒ Ⓓ
50. Ⓐ Ⓑ Ⓒ Ⓓ
51. Ⓐ Ⓑ Ⓒ Ⓓ
52. Ⓐ Ⓑ Ⓒ Ⓓ
53. Ⓐ Ⓑ Ⓒ Ⓓ
54. Ⓐ Ⓑ Ⓒ Ⓓ
55. Ⓐ Ⓑ Ⓒ Ⓓ
56. Ⓐ Ⓑ Ⓒ Ⓓ
57. Ⓐ Ⓑ Ⓒ Ⓓ
58. Ⓐ Ⓑ Ⓒ Ⓓ
59. Ⓐ Ⓑ Ⓒ Ⓓ
60. Ⓐ Ⓑ Ⓒ Ⓓ

61. Ⓐ Ⓑ Ⓒ Ⓓ
62. Ⓐ Ⓑ Ⓒ Ⓓ
63. Ⓐ Ⓑ Ⓒ Ⓓ
64. Ⓐ Ⓑ Ⓒ Ⓓ
65. Ⓐ Ⓑ Ⓒ Ⓓ

PHYSICAL SCIENCES

66. Ⓐ Ⓑ Ⓒ Ⓓ
67. Ⓐ Ⓑ Ⓒ Ⓓ
68. Ⓐ Ⓑ Ⓒ Ⓓ
69. Ⓐ Ⓑ Ⓒ Ⓓ
70. Ⓐ Ⓑ Ⓒ Ⓓ
71. Ⓐ Ⓑ Ⓒ Ⓓ
72. Ⓐ Ⓑ Ⓒ Ⓓ
73. Ⓐ Ⓑ Ⓒ Ⓓ
74. Ⓐ Ⓑ Ⓒ Ⓓ
75. Ⓐ Ⓑ Ⓒ Ⓓ
76. Ⓐ Ⓑ Ⓒ Ⓓ
77. Ⓐ Ⓑ Ⓒ Ⓓ
78. Ⓐ Ⓑ Ⓒ Ⓓ
79. Ⓐ Ⓑ Ⓒ Ⓓ
80. Ⓐ Ⓑ Ⓒ Ⓓ
81. Ⓐ Ⓑ Ⓒ Ⓓ
82. Ⓐ Ⓑ Ⓒ Ⓓ
83. Ⓐ Ⓑ Ⓒ Ⓓ
84. Ⓐ Ⓑ Ⓒ Ⓓ
85. Ⓐ Ⓑ Ⓒ Ⓓ
86. Ⓐ Ⓑ Ⓒ Ⓓ
87. Ⓐ Ⓑ Ⓒ Ⓓ
88. Ⓐ Ⓑ Ⓒ Ⓓ

89. Ⓐ Ⓑ Ⓒ Ⓓ
90. Ⓐ Ⓑ Ⓒ Ⓓ
91. Ⓐ Ⓑ Ⓒ Ⓓ
92. Ⓐ Ⓑ Ⓒ Ⓓ
93. Ⓐ Ⓑ Ⓒ Ⓓ
94. Ⓐ Ⓑ Ⓒ Ⓓ
95. Ⓐ Ⓑ Ⓒ Ⓓ
96. Ⓐ Ⓑ Ⓒ Ⓓ
97. Ⓐ Ⓑ Ⓒ Ⓓ
98. Ⓐ Ⓑ Ⓒ Ⓓ
99. Ⓐ Ⓑ Ⓒ Ⓓ
100. Ⓐ Ⓑ Ⓒ Ⓓ
101. Ⓐ Ⓑ Ⓒ Ⓓ
102. Ⓐ Ⓑ Ⓒ Ⓓ
103. Ⓐ Ⓑ Ⓒ Ⓓ
104. Ⓐ Ⓑ Ⓒ Ⓓ
105. Ⓐ Ⓑ Ⓒ Ⓓ
106. Ⓐ Ⓑ Ⓒ Ⓓ
107. Ⓐ Ⓑ Ⓒ Ⓓ
108. Ⓐ Ⓑ Ⓒ Ⓓ
109. Ⓐ Ⓑ Ⓒ Ⓓ
110. Ⓐ Ⓑ Ⓒ Ⓓ
111. Ⓐ Ⓑ Ⓒ Ⓓ
112. Ⓐ Ⓑ Ⓒ Ⓓ
113. Ⓐ Ⓑ Ⓒ Ⓓ
114. Ⓐ Ⓑ Ⓒ Ⓓ
115. Ⓐ Ⓑ Ⓒ Ⓓ
116. Ⓐ Ⓑ Ⓒ Ⓓ
117. Ⓐ Ⓑ Ⓒ Ⓓ
118. Ⓐ Ⓑ Ⓒ Ⓓ

119. Ⓐ Ⓑ Ⓒ Ⓓ
120. Ⓐ Ⓑ Ⓒ Ⓓ
121. Ⓐ Ⓑ Ⓒ Ⓓ
122. Ⓐ Ⓑ Ⓒ Ⓓ
123. Ⓐ Ⓑ Ⓒ Ⓓ
124. Ⓐ Ⓑ Ⓒ Ⓓ
125. Ⓐ Ⓑ Ⓒ Ⓓ
126. Ⓐ Ⓑ Ⓒ Ⓓ
127. Ⓐ Ⓑ Ⓒ Ⓓ
128. Ⓐ Ⓑ Ⓒ Ⓓ
129. Ⓐ Ⓑ Ⓒ Ⓓ
130. Ⓐ Ⓑ Ⓒ Ⓓ
131. Ⓐ Ⓑ Ⓒ Ⓓ
132. Ⓐ Ⓑ Ⓒ Ⓓ
133. Ⓐ Ⓑ Ⓒ Ⓓ
134. Ⓐ Ⓑ Ⓒ Ⓓ
135. Ⓐ Ⓑ Ⓒ Ⓓ
136. Ⓐ Ⓑ Ⓒ Ⓓ
137. Ⓐ Ⓑ Ⓒ Ⓓ
138. Ⓐ Ⓑ Ⓒ Ⓓ
139. Ⓐ Ⓑ Ⓒ Ⓓ
140. Ⓐ Ⓑ Ⓒ Ⓓ
141. Ⓐ Ⓑ Ⓒ Ⓓ
142. Ⓐ Ⓑ Ⓒ Ⓓ

WRITING SAMPLE
Use separate ruled sheets of paper.

BIOLOGICAL SCIENCES
143. Ⓐ Ⓑ Ⓒ Ⓓ
144. Ⓐ Ⓑ Ⓒ Ⓓ
145. Ⓐ Ⓑ Ⓒ Ⓓ
146. Ⓐ Ⓑ Ⓒ Ⓓ
147. Ⓐ Ⓑ Ⓒ Ⓓ
148. Ⓐ Ⓑ Ⓒ Ⓓ
149. Ⓐ Ⓑ Ⓒ Ⓓ
150. Ⓐ Ⓑ Ⓒ Ⓓ
151. Ⓐ Ⓑ Ⓒ Ⓓ
152. Ⓐ Ⓑ Ⓒ Ⓓ
153. Ⓐ Ⓑ Ⓒ Ⓓ
154. Ⓐ Ⓑ Ⓒ Ⓓ
155. Ⓐ Ⓑ Ⓒ Ⓓ
156. Ⓐ Ⓑ Ⓒ Ⓓ
157. Ⓐ Ⓑ Ⓒ Ⓓ
158. Ⓐ Ⓑ Ⓒ Ⓓ
159. Ⓐ Ⓑ Ⓒ Ⓓ
160. Ⓐ Ⓑ Ⓒ Ⓓ
161. Ⓐ Ⓑ Ⓒ Ⓓ
162. Ⓐ Ⓑ Ⓒ Ⓓ
163. Ⓐ Ⓑ Ⓒ Ⓓ
164. Ⓐ Ⓑ Ⓒ Ⓓ
165. Ⓐ Ⓑ Ⓒ Ⓓ
166. Ⓐ Ⓑ Ⓒ Ⓓ
167. Ⓐ Ⓑ Ⓒ Ⓓ

168. Ⓐ Ⓑ Ⓒ Ⓓ
169. Ⓐ Ⓑ Ⓒ Ⓓ
170. Ⓐ Ⓑ Ⓒ Ⓓ
171. Ⓐ Ⓑ Ⓒ Ⓓ
172. Ⓐ Ⓑ Ⓒ Ⓓ
173. Ⓐ Ⓑ Ⓒ Ⓓ
174. Ⓐ Ⓑ Ⓒ Ⓓ
175. Ⓐ Ⓑ Ⓒ Ⓓ
176. Ⓐ Ⓑ Ⓒ Ⓓ
177. Ⓐ Ⓑ Ⓒ Ⓓ
178. Ⓐ Ⓑ Ⓒ Ⓓ
179. Ⓐ Ⓑ Ⓒ Ⓓ
180. Ⓐ Ⓑ Ⓒ Ⓓ
181. Ⓐ Ⓑ Ⓒ Ⓓ
182. Ⓐ Ⓑ Ⓒ Ⓓ
183. Ⓐ Ⓑ Ⓒ Ⓓ
184. Ⓐ Ⓑ Ⓒ Ⓓ
185. Ⓐ Ⓑ Ⓒ Ⓓ
186. Ⓐ Ⓑ Ⓒ Ⓓ
187. Ⓐ Ⓑ Ⓒ Ⓓ
188. Ⓐ Ⓑ Ⓒ Ⓓ
189. Ⓐ Ⓑ Ⓒ Ⓓ
190. Ⓐ Ⓑ Ⓒ Ⓓ
191. Ⓐ Ⓑ Ⓒ Ⓓ
192. Ⓐ Ⓑ Ⓒ Ⓓ
193. Ⓐ Ⓑ Ⓒ Ⓓ

194. Ⓐ Ⓑ Ⓒ Ⓓ
195. Ⓐ Ⓑ Ⓒ Ⓓ
196. Ⓐ Ⓑ Ⓒ Ⓓ
197. Ⓐ Ⓑ Ⓒ Ⓓ
198. Ⓐ Ⓑ Ⓒ Ⓓ
199. Ⓐ Ⓑ Ⓒ Ⓓ
200. Ⓐ Ⓑ Ⓒ Ⓓ
201. Ⓐ Ⓑ Ⓒ Ⓓ
202. Ⓐ Ⓑ Ⓒ Ⓓ
203. Ⓐ Ⓑ Ⓒ Ⓓ
204. Ⓐ Ⓑ Ⓒ Ⓓ
205. Ⓐ Ⓑ Ⓒ Ⓓ
206. Ⓐ Ⓑ Ⓒ Ⓓ
207. Ⓐ Ⓑ Ⓒ Ⓓ
208. Ⓐ Ⓑ Ⓒ Ⓓ
209. Ⓐ Ⓑ Ⓒ Ⓓ
210. Ⓐ Ⓑ Ⓒ Ⓓ
211. Ⓐ Ⓑ Ⓒ Ⓓ
212. Ⓐ Ⓑ Ⓒ Ⓓ
213. Ⓐ Ⓑ Ⓒ Ⓓ
214. Ⓐ Ⓑ Ⓒ Ⓓ
215. Ⓐ Ⓑ Ⓒ Ⓓ
216. Ⓐ Ⓑ Ⓒ Ⓓ
217. Ⓐ Ⓑ Ⓒ Ⓓ
218. Ⓐ Ⓑ Ⓒ Ⓓ
219. Ⓐ Ⓑ Ⓒ Ⓓ

The MCAT
Model Examination B

VERBAL REASONING

9 PASSAGES
65 QUESTIONS
85 MINUTES

DIRECTIONS: The questions are based on the accompanying passages. Read each passage carefully, then answer the following questions. Consider only the material within the passage. For each question, select the *ONE BEST ANSWER* and indicate your selection by marking the corresponding letter on the Answer Form.

Passage I (Questions 1–8)

What is the essence of graphic design? How do graphic designers solve problems, organize space, and imbue their work with those visual and symbolic qualities that enable it to convey visual and verbal information with expression and clarity? The extraordinary flowering of graphic design in our time—as a potent means of communication and a major component of our visual culture—increases the need for designers, clients, and students to comprehend its essence.

Traditionally, graphic designers looked to architecture or painting for their model. Certainly, a universal language of form is common to all visual disciplines, and in some historical periods the various design arts have shared styles. Too much dependence upon other arts—or even on the universal language of form—is unsatisfactory, however, because graphic design has unique purposes and visual properties.

Graphic design is a hybrid discipline. Diverse elements, including signs, symbols, words, and pictures, are collected and assembled into a total message. The dual nature of these graphic elements as both communicative sign and visual form provides endless fascination and potential for invention and combination. Although all the visual arts share properties of either two- or three-dimensional space, graphic space has a special character born from its communicative function.

Perhaps the most important thing that graphic design does is give communications resonance, a richness of tone that heightens the expressive power of the page. It transcends the dry conveyance of information, intensifies the message, and enriches the audience's experience. Resonance helps the designer realize clear public goals: to instruct, to delight, and to motivate.

Most designers speak of their activities as a problem-solving process because designers seek solutions to public communications problems. Approaches to problem solving vary, based on the problem at hand and the working methods of the designer. At a time when Western nations are evolving from industrial to information cultures, a comprehensive understanding of our communicative forms and graphic design becomes increasingly critical.

The general public does not understand graphic design and art direction. Designers tell the story of a graphic designer trying to explain this job to Grandmother. The designer shows Grandmother a recent project and says, "You were asking me about what I do, Grandmother. I'm a graphic designer, and I designed this."

Pointing to the photograph in the design, the grandmother asks, "Did you draw that picture?"

"No, Grandmother, it's a photograph. I didn't draw it, but I planned it, chose the photographer, helped select the models, assisted in setting it up, art directed the shooting session, chose which shot to use, and cropped the picture."

"Did you write what it says, then?"

"Well, no," the designer replies. "But I did brainstorm with the copywriter to develop the concept."

Used with permission of Philip B. Meggs and John T. Bryan, *Type and Image*, 1989.

"Oh, I see. Then you did letter these big words?" asks the grandmother, pointing to the headline.

"Uh, no, a typesetter set the copywriter's words in type, but I specified the typefaces and sizes to be used," responds the designer.

"Well, did you draw this little picture down in the corner?"

"No, but I selected the illustrator, told her what needed to be drawn, and decided where to put it and how big to make it."

"Oh. Well, did you draw this little, what do you call it, a trademark?"

"Uh, no. A design firm that specializes in visual identification programs designed it for the client."

The grandmother is somewhat confused about just what it is that her grandchild does and why credit is claimed for all these other people's work.

1. The object of this passage is to:

   A. convince the reader that graphic designers are artists.
   B. illustrate the fact that the general public does not comprehend what graphic designers actually do.
   C. underscore the fact that understanding graphic design is essential in an information culture.
   D. provide the reader with a glimpse of the importance of graphic design in today's culture, as well as of its diverse nature.

2. According to this passage, graphic design today:

   A. is an important communication tool, as well as a major component of our visual culture.
   B. provides employment for people such as artists, directors, photographers, and writers.
   C. depends too much on other art forms.
   D. is a traditional discipline based on architectural design.

3. The author believes that the most important function of graphic design is to:

   A. provide attractive visual displays for the public.
   B. help Western culture make the transition from a technical to a communication oriented society.
   C. give communications resonance, thus helping the designer realize clear public

goals: to instruct, to delight, and to motivate.
   D. bring diversity to the art field.

4. Based on the information in the passage, what do graphic designers actually do?
   I. seek solutions to public communication problems
   II. organize space
   III. imbue their work with visual and symbolic qualities

   A. I only
   B. II only
   C. I and II only
   D. I, II, and III

5. Which of the following statements best supports the notion that graphic design is a *hybrid* discipline?

   A. The extraordinary flowering of graphic design in our time increases the need for designers who have the ability to problem solve.
   B. In graphic arts, diverse elements—including signs, symbols, words, and pictures—are collected and assembled into a total message.
   C. Graphic design transcends the dry conveyance of information.
   D. Graphic design has unique purposes and a special character.

6. The author feels that the general public does not understand the concept of graphic design. Which of the following reasons best describes why this confusion probably exists?

   A. Graphic designers confuse the general public because they have a difficult time describing what their actual role is in the production of a project.
   B. The general public is not really interested in a description of the makeup of graphic design.
   C. Confusion is caused by the fact that graphic designers do not single-handedly produce a product, such as a painting or a photograph. Their job is to *orchestrate* a variety of people and sources in order to creatively solve communication problems through visual means.
   D. The designer's end product is the only thing that the general public is concerned about.

7. Which of the following statements *least* supports the idea that graphic design is important in a communication culture?

   A. One important aspect of graphic arts is its ability to convey both verbal and visual information with clarity.
   B. Graphic arts heightens the expressive power of a page.
   C. Instruction and motivation are two goals that graphic designers have in mind when producing a piece of work.
   D. Architecture and painting were considered the traditional models for graphic design.

8. According to the passage, graphic design shares the following commonality with other visual disciplines:

   A. a dual nature and unique purpose.
   B. the expression of verbal information.
   C. heavy dependence on other art forms.
   D. a universal language of form.

Passage II (Questions 9–16)

Until recently, scientific data were a convenient tool in the scientific process, with the following steps: (1) formulating a question; (2) ascertaining what is known; (3) formulating a testable hypothesis; (4) conducting observations and collecting data; (5) analyzing the data and relating them to existing information; (6) formulating a new or modified hypothesis and (7) initiating a new round of studies until the question is answered, abandoned or restated. At various periods in the age of enlightenment, different components of the scientific method have been emphasized. Early on, propositions were formulated and debated with minimum organized observation or collection of data. The age of philosophers gave way to the age of observers, such as the astronomers who gazed at the sky and mapped the thousands of points of light, the naturalists who described and collected plants and animals, and the explorers who mapped rivers and oceans, coasts and mountains. Observers of nature gave way to the industrial age, during which inventors focused on solutions, oftentimes without well formulated questions, theory, or review of prior work. Naturalists and inventors recorded their observations in journals or log books as personalized memory aids. Inventors carried record keeping a step forward as a means of economy, to prevent repetition of failed

Adapted from *Basic Science*, S. Gaylen Bradley, 1990.

trials. In all of these circumstances, however, the records were a convenient tool of and for the individual. Data records of concepts and observations took on a new meaning during the age of inventions. Inventors sought to profit from their creations, not only by building and selling a better "mousetrap" but also by seeking legal protection under constitutionally guaranteed rights to patent intellectual property. Records of data became a part of the documentation for priority, due diligence and breadth of a claim. Record keeping for commercialization of intellectual property now has become formalized, standardized, and required.

During the past few decades, records of data have become essential components of the documentation for regulatory agencies approving utility, efficacy, or safety of new products or appliances. Progressively, regulatory agencies have extended the scope of their oversight, specifying some aspects of experimental design, data collection, and analysis. Most recently, regulatory agencies have insisted that all data collected be retained and made available for inspection, even data from aborted or defective studies. Data keeping and storage have become ends unto themselves, initially to ensure that work paid for was actually done and subsequently to ensure that unwanted results (e.g., toxicity of a drug) were not suppressed. It is perhaps a logical extension that managers of public funds have focused upon records of data as documentation that work paid for was actually done, much as an auditor of public accounts matches purchase orders, invoices, and disbursements. The managers of public funds, lacking the technical expertise to judge the quality and value of scientific investigations, have turned to process rather than product to demonstrate their diligence in protecting the taxpayers' money. The increased reliance on process rather than output measures reflects in part a loss of confidence by the public in the scientific community to have the ability and the will to judge and police itself. Regrettably, there are some bases for this loss of confidence in scientific peer review, and this loss of confidence permeates the scientific community itself as well as the managers of public funds.

Regardless of the cause, an increasing emphasis is now placed on data keeping and data storage. Any discussion on scientific data presupposes that there is general agreement on the definition of *data*. Unfortunately, there is no universally accepted definition of *data*. Perhaps the best we can do is conclude that, like pornography, we know *data* when we see them, or that data are defined by some unspecified *community standard*. Are data the holographic notes entered personally and immediately by the observer? Are data the printouts from apparatus? Are data the printouts of computers that accept input from the observer or directly from apparatus? Are data the embedded pieces of tissue from a treated animal, or the stained sections made from the tissue, or the notes of the observer examining the tissue, or all of these, or none of these? What are "materials and methods" as distinguished from "data" and from interpretation? How do we meet the demand that scientists must properly keep and store data, when we do not know what data are and whether or not they can be kept and stored other than by written notes of the observer or photographs of an event. Finally, who is responsible for keeping and storing data?

9. The passage could be entitled:

A. Scientific Experimentation.
B. Scientific Method.
C. Scientific Responsibility.
D. Scientific Data.

10. Throughout the history of experimentation and development of new knowledge:

A. the scientific method has been painstakingly applied and followed.
B. formulating a hypothesis has been a critical element in progress.
C. emphasis within the application of the scientific method has varied.
D. scientific data has been compared, analyzed, and scrutinized.

11. Which of the following statement(s) is/are NOT *supported by* the passage?
I. All scientific experimentation and observation throughout history was based on strict recording and analysis of data.
II. Philosophy about matter eventually turned to the scientific approach.
III. With industrialization came a method of solving questions utilizing the scientific approach.
IV. Industrialization was interested and emphasized practical solutions.

A. I, II, and III   C. II and IV
B. I and III   D. IV only

12. Which of the following statement(s) is/are NOT *supported by* the passage?
I. Inventors sought constitutional protection.
II. At the present, record keeping is an essential element of society.
III. Regulatory agencies can require complete documentation of data.

IV. Failed or aborted experiments do not need to be scrutinized because they are of little benefit.

A. I, II, and III   C. II and IV
B. I and III   D. IV only

13. Which of the following statement(s) is/are *supported by* the passage?
I. The criteria for a definition of data are fairly well established.
II. Data are verified by a computer printout.
III. Data must be recorded and stored.
IV. Responsibility for data storage rests upon the investigator.

A. I, II, and III   C. II and IV
B. I and III   D. none of the above

14. Which of the following statement(s) is/are *supported by* the passage?
I. There has been an evolution in the methodology of recording data.
II. After a foiled experiment, a modified hypothesis is part of the scientific approach.
III. Data storage has been utilized as an end unto itself in order to ensure completion of a project.
IV. Managers of public funds are usually well qualified to judge scientific work.

A. I, II, and III   C. II and IV
B. I and III   D. IV only

15. The passage argues that:

A. the public's money is well protected.
B. the public has trust in the scientific community.
C. the scientific community polices itself appropriately.
D. data collection and storage are increasingly stressed.

16. The passage would support the argument that:

A. scientific data are obtained after careful experimentation.
B. computerization will enhance the accuracy of data collection and keeping it appropriately.
C. regulatory agencies, the public, and the scientific community are working together in the venture to evaluate data and use it properly.
D. none of the above statements is addressed directly by the author.

Passage III (Questions 17–24)

It has become obvious in recent years that the decision-making power in many school districts is shifting, and is becoming more liberalized as both teachers and parents realize that they are an important facet in the total school operation. They know that without their support and cooperation the system cannot continue to function smoothly.

Consequently, today's educator is no longer content to sit in the background and let decisions be made and programs formulated. New teachers want a voice, they demand a piece of the action, and they are daring enough to question the judgments of the system in their desire to achieve a better educational experience for their students as well as a more economically realistic position for themselves.

Not too many years ago, perhaps as little as a decade in some areas, the decision making power in a school system could have been observed by quickly glancing at an organizational chart that would most probably have looked like this:

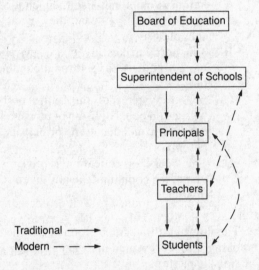

Although much simplified, the chart indicates a flow of power from the school board to the superintendent of schools down to the individual school principals and from there to the teachers and, finally, a minimal involvement of the students themselves.

The board of education was naturally found at the top, for it was assumed that this body represented the taxpaying community. Next in importance was the superintendent, whose word was considered to be law and who would, if so disposed, allow the principal some freedom to make decisions.

By the same token, those principals that prided themselves in being of a democratic nature, would

From Hugo R. Seibel and Kenneth E. Guyer, *How to Prepare for the Medical College Admission Test*, 6th ed. Hauppauge, New York: Barron's Educational Series, Inc., 1990.

then allow teachers to have a voice in selected matters and would even possibly afford students the opportunity of making minute decisions in appropriate areas.

Within the confines of the individual school, the principal was looked upon as the one person who knew more about educational matters than any other member of the staff. Therefore, he or she was spotlighted not only as the chief administrator, but as the supreme educational leader of the complex. Teachers occupied the place of facilitators, whose main job it was to take the programs that were handed down to them and see that they were carried out satisfactorily. The students were viewed as receptacles for receiving and digesting information. Their major contribution rested in being accepted to an institution of higher learning, thus making the system look good and giving the taxpayers the feeling that the money they spent was, after all, worthwhile.

The entire pattern of decision making, as presented, was based on the very real fact that the board of education controlled the purse strings of a school system. Because money has always been of supreme importance, it was considered the most logical path to follow. Few people thought to question its wisdom or bothered to seek alternatives.

The modern public has slowly come to realize that even though money is still the most crucial factor in operating an efficient school system, there are also other vital and important elements that contribute to its success.

For example, parents are demanding a voice in the operation of local schools. They favor an open door policy that affords them the opportunity to see what is going on in the classrooms and allows many of them to get involved on a parent-volunteer basis. Parents speak out in many cases by manipulating a very vital school input, over which they have strict control, namely their children. Thus we read of such things as parents keeping their offspring out of school to protest situations that they find unsuitable and intolerable. Even though these actions may not in themselves solve the problems, they do cause those in authority to sit up, take notice, and search for possible solutions at a speedy rate.

Every bit as important as the public's realization of its powers, is the teachers' realization that they too have a commodity that is of supreme importance to the system, and that is themselves. When teachers join forces and remove this vital input, school systems are forced to close and the educational machine comes to a halt. Teachers' strikes are now occurring more and more frequently in all areas of the country, and the threat of the entire profession becoming unionized is no longer a laughing matter.

Today's wise school systems have made note of

these developments and are attempting to deal with them reasonably. Sharing the decision-making power by allowing more realistic and meaningful input from both parents and teachers has become a reality in many districts. Although a revised look at the power flow chart today would probably show the players in the same basic positions, it would certainly have the arrows of decision coming not only down in a direct line, but also pointing up and out, allowing for a much more liberalized flow of communication and ideas.

17. The central theme of this passage deals with:

   A. the position of absolute power that is held by school boards in this country.
   B. the militant attitude that is displayed by many modern teachers.
   C. the shifting of decision making power in today's school systems from that of a top down, authoritarian model to one that is more decentralized in nature.
   D. increased parent interest in the public schools and the establishment of strong parent-volunteer programs.

18. The role of the teacher is presented by the author as changing from that of mere program facilitator to one of a vital voice in educational planning. This change has come about partially because:

   A. the National Education Association represents modern educators throughout the United States.
   B. teachers are more willing than ever to speak out concerning the development of new programs and policies.
   C. teachers often go on strike if their demands for new programs are not met.
   D. according to the modern side of the flow chart, teachers now discuss their ideas directly with the board of education.

19. Which one of the following statements contradicts the central theme of this passage?

   A. Today's students are radical and demand a share in the decision making process of local school boards.
   B. Principals are the instructional leaders in their schools.
   C. Students who get accepted to college make teachers look good.
   D. Because it has control over the purse strings, the board of education should have absolute power over all other facets of the educational machine within a school district.

20. Which of the following statements seems reasonable in light of the information presented in this passage?
   I. Parent-volunteer programs are one avenue of public involvement in local schools.
   II. Parents want to be placed above the board of education on the organizational chart.
   III. Parents are becoming a more powerful force in the operation of local schools.

   A. I and II   C. I and III
   B. II only   D. I, II, and III

21. Of the following statements, which one is NOT *supported nor contradicted by* the information presented in this passage?

   A. Parents sometimes use their children as tools for getting what they want in a school system.
   B. Teachers' strikes are taking place on a more frequent basis throughout the nation.
   C. School systems of the future probably will see an equal division of power among the board of education, principals, and parents.
   D. The board of education represents the taxpaying community in any given school district.

22. The flow chart that can be found after the third paragraph is presented in a very simplified version. It pictures:

   A. the traditional as well as the modern flow of power and communication of local school districts.
   B. teachers as being on a low rung of the educational totem pole.
   C. the superintendent as the most powerful figure in the school system.
   D. the fact that students often communicate with their teachers and the principal.

23. The power that parents are beginning to exert in school systems is an important strand in this passage. What is the probable reason that parents are not represented directly on the flow chart?

A. Parents operate as volunteers within the schools.

B. School systems resent the influence that parents are trying to exert on them.

C. Most organizational flow charts picture only those groups that are actual members of the organization.

D. Parents are represented indirectly though the board of education, because that board represents the taxpaying public.

24. As a result of the information presented in this passage, the reader might conclude that in the future:

A. the traditional decision-making power of public schools will continue to slip due to the demands made by parents and teachers.

B. public education will become more decentralized and parents might be involved in developing school policies.

C. it will become increasingly more difficult to determine who has the actual decision making power in a school district.

D. all of the above.

Passage IV (Questions 25–33)

Generally, state statutes grant school administrators the legal duty to establish, maintain, and protect the school's learning environment. It is a basic tenet of school law that school authorities may exclude from school any student whose conduct interferes with or in any way disrupts the operation of the school, or who openly defies school rules, or whose conduct is willfully insubordinate, or who poses a threat of harm to himself, to other persons, or to school property.

The terms used to characterize exclusion of students from school are suspension and expulsion. Generally, suspension denotes a temporary exclusion from school with a presumption that return to school is possible. Typically, by state code provision, school authorities possess the legal prerogative to suspend students from classes and from school. Expulsion denotes a longer term of exclusion from school with a presumption of finality regarding the termination of one's status as a student. Considered the most severe student punishment available to school authorities, state statutes and local policies usually provide that only a local school board has the prerogative to expel a student.

Adapted from H. G. Hudgins and Richard S. Vacca, *Law and Education: Contemporary Issues and Correct Decisions*, 2nd ed. Charlottesville, Virginia: The Michie Company, 1985.

In recent years, litigation has involved both the right of school authorities to suspend or expel, and the minimal procedural due process rights of students prior to suspension or expulsion. Following the landmark decision in *Gault,* in which the Supreme Court held that minor juvenile offenders in juvenile court were entitled to certain procedural due process protections, several lower courts began to clarify the procedural due process rights of students facing exclusion from school. The matter was ultimately treated by the United States Supreme Court in *Goss v. Lopez.*

Observing that a student possesses a property right to a public education, protected by the guarantees of the fourteenth amendment, the Supreme Court overturned an Ohio statute that allowed summary suspensions for up to ten days. In the Court's opinion, minimum procedures must be followed prior to exclusion from school. The Court held that in suspensions of ten days or less, notice of the charges and the right to be heard are required. And, if the student denies the charges, he or she must be informed of the evidence against him or her and be given the opportunity to present his or her side of the story. However, this requirement can be done informally and immediately after the incident. In *Goss,* the Supreme Court did not require that a public school system allow students to be represented by counsel, to present witnesses, or to confront and cross-examine witnesses. Nor did the Court rule on the elements of due process for suspensions of longer than ten days. The Court did observe that more procedural due process may be needed for longer suspensions.

Of major importance to the daily practice of school administrators is the Court's attitudes toward due process and school discipline, often missed by those who analyze this landmark case. First, the Court reemphasized the notion that procedural due process is a flexible legal standard, determined by the nature of the misconduct and the severity of the penalty. Second, the Court held that school officials are free to remove a student from school prior to a suspension if his or her presence is a danger to persons or property and/or is disruptive to teaching and learning.

Beyond the guidelines of the Supreme Court, a local school administrator is also bound by state statutory mandates and state court decisions, and these requirements vary. However, the following guidelines are generally accepted nationally and serve as excellent guidelines for school administrators: students must know in advance what standards of behavior are proscribed in their school and what modes of behavior are expected; they must know what specific disciplinary actions and punishments attach to violations of the rules; they must receive immediate and informed notice when they are accused of an infraction, and an opportunity to present his or her side of the story; and students must have an opportunity to appeal the decision to another administrative level within the school system. The administrator is reminded that these general elements become more formalized and technical when an expulsion is in process.

Two other student exclusion decisions from the United States Supreme Court should be briefly mentioned at this point because of their bearing on student procedural due process entitlements. The cases are *Wood v. Strickland,* and *Carey v. Piphus. Wood* involved the issue of students being allowed to sue local school board members for damages under Section 1983 for a denial of procedural due process in an expulsion hearing. In upholding the school board's actions, the Supreme Court held that individual board members could be sued if they knew or reasonably should have known that they denied students their constitutional rights or if board members acted with malicious intent.

Carey was a consolidation of two cases, both involving the suspension of a student from school. One student had violated a rule prohibiting the use of drugs at school, whereas the other student violated a rule against males wearing earrings at school. In rendering its decision in *Carey,* the Supreme Court held that students suspended from school without procedural due process are entitled to recover nominal damages of $1.00 and possibly extensive lawyers' fees. However, before any compensatory damages are awarded, a student must first submit proof of actual injury caused by the denial of due process. Punitive damages may be possible where a student can establish that school officials acted with the malicious intent to deprive him of his rights.

25. The main topic of this passage deals with:

    A. the duty that school administrators have to establish, maintain, and protect the school's learning environment.
    B. fourteenth amendment rights.
    C. due process rights.
    D. the exclusion of students from school by means of suspension and/or expulsion.

26. According to the information presented in this passage, exclusion from school refers to:

    I. any time-out procedure directed at a student as a result of a disciplinary infraction.
    II. a temporary removal from the educational setting by means of suspension.

    III. a longer term and possibly permanent removal from the educational setting by means of expulsion.

    A. I and II   **C.** II and III
    B. I and III   **D.** all of the above

27. According to the information given in this passage, most state statutes and local policies give the prerogative of expelling a student from school to:

    A. the classroom teacher.
    B. the building administrator.
    C. the school superintendent.
    D. the school board.

28. The issue of student expulsion has produced numerous court cases. Litigation in this area generally involves:

    A. the right of school authorities to suspend or expel, as well as the student's minimal due process rights prior to suspension or expulsion.
    B. the flexible standard of the due process right as well as the length of time of the expulsion.
    C. the past disciplinary record of a student as well as the type of punitive action that was taken previously.
    D. all of the above.

29. In which of the following cases did the United States Supreme Court first treat the issue of procedural due process rights for students?

    A. *Wood v. Strickland*
    B. *Brown v. Board of Education*
    C. *Goss v. Lopez*
    D. *Carey v. Piphus*

30. Which of the following statements concerning the right to a public education is the *most* significant in *Goss v. Lopez?*

    A. Every student has the right to a public education.
    B. Public education is an inalienable right.
    C. The right to a public education is a property right.
    D. The right to a public education is protected by the fourteenth amendment right.

31. Which of the following statements *contradicts* the holdings of the United States Supreme Court in *Goss v. Lopez?*

   A. Due process is a flexible standard.
   B. Due process is determined by the nature of the misconduct determined and the severity of the penalty.
   C. School authorities may not remove a student from school prior to a suspension.
   D. Minimal due process rights are required for suspensions of ten days or less, whereas more procedural due process might be needed for longer suspensions.

32. In which of the following student exclusion cases did the United States Supreme Court hold that an individual school board could be sued for knowingly denying a student his/her constitutional process rights?

   A. *Wood v. Strickland*
   B. *Brown v. Board of Education*
   C. *Goss v. Lopez*
   D. *Carey v. Piphus*

33. In which of the following student exclusion cases did the United States Supreme Court hold that suspension from school without procedural due process entitled a student to recover nominal damages and possibly extensive legal fees?

   A. *Wood v. Strickland*
   B. *Brown v. Board of Education*
   C. *Goss v. Lopez*
   D. *Carey v. Piphus*

Passage V (Questions 34–41)

Students in institutions of higher education hold diverse interests and backgrounds. There are average students as well as bright ones. Are the needs of average students different from those headed toward graduate school? Both need qualified and enthusiastic teachers.

When students evaluate teaching ability, they may or may not know a faculty member's academic qualifications or tenure status. Some nontenure-eligible faculty members have credentials comparable to tenure-track faculty members. The fact that a faculty member has a master's degree and teaches only lower level courses does not reflect on his or her teaching

Adapted from A. Nancy Avakian, "Some Reflections on Nontenure-Eligible Faculty Members." In *Role of Nontenure-Eligible Faculty in the Academy*, 1990.

ability. Yet criteria used to evaluate full-time faculty members are similar to those applied to part-time faculty members. In addition, there is often an abuse of nontenure-eligible faculty members who may be requested to teach five courses a semester while receiving only 20 percent of the pay of the full-time faculty member.

Some faculty members contend that tenure is the freedom to teach, speak and write. Both tenured and nontenure-eligible faculty members, in fact, enjoy these freedoms. Academic freedom is not necessarily contingent upon tenure because the university protects the constitutional right of freedom of speech for all faculty members.

Tenure means job security, and bonds an individual to the institution. Nontenure-eligible faculty members are expected to bond with the institution; yet how can this be accomplished when they often experience employment uncertainty? The response is that tenure is not the only way to achieve bonding. Long-term contracts or "rolling contracts" are alternatives. There are some faculty members who may not want or need job security.

These are individuals in business or technical and professional fields who want to bond with a scholarly community in order to teach. They may have a primary career elsewhere or they may be pausing between career moves.

Tenure affects attitude and morale. What makes so many nontenure-eligible faculty members feel they are second-class citizens? Often they do not have offices or have not been accorded recognition for their teaching excellence. Faculty attitudes are inhibitive of change as are economic considerations. Why do nontenure-eligible faculty have to teach only lower level courses? Many nontenure-eligible faculty members may, in fact, be better equipped to teach some upper level courses. In addition, as the pool of faculty members in certain disciplines, English, for example, diminishes, the salaries needed to hire nontenure-eligible faculty members will increase. This competitive situation will encourage nontenure-eligible faculty members to voice their complaints about the lack of diverse teaching assignments or the failure to be treated as professional equals.

Pay differential between tenure track and nontenure-eligible faculty members will vary, but issues of bonding will remain on the table.

There is a need to determine the role and purpose of research in the university. Although the tripartite foundation of teaching, public service, and research is espoused, the institution's reward system leans toward research. At the same time, legislators, students, and parents cry out for excellence in teaching in order to raise the standards of quality. This conundrum must be addressed.

298 • MODEL EXAMINATION B

Nontenure-eligible research faculty experience other concerns that are not necessarily bound to tenure. They want job security during the transitional periods, i.e., from receipt of one grant to another. They lose even their second class citizenship when job security is jeopardized. Long-term contracts are suggested in lieu of tenure.

Nontenure-eligible clinical faculty members practice usually in the medical and human services professions (dentistry, medicine, nursing, veterinary medicine, social work, clinical psychology, and counseling). In medicine and social work, much of the clinical teaching of patient care is delivered by nontenure-eligible faculty members who serve on a short-term basis. They represent the "off-site" faculty and serve as preceptors for clinical training of students. Their appointments cement the relationship between the practice and school. The clinical activities of nontenure-eligible faculty are not linked solely with the generation of income.

Tenure, for individuals in these disciplines, is usually accorded to individuals who have the M.D., Ph.D., or D.Ed. degrees. Lacking of tenure fosters the two-class system in which the vast majority of clinical care providers/teachers are, once again, made to feel they are relegated to the second class. Incentives and recognition of clinical performances are very important to clinical faculty members. Is it realistic to expect and demand excellence in all endeavors (teaching, research, public service) by the nontenure-track clinical faculty?

Usually complexity of clinical teaching and practice dictates the need for a large number of nontenure-eligible faculty members whose financial compensations vastly exceed the number of tenure positions and available resources. Does tenure have a place in clinical departments which have the potential to generate substantial income for the private practitioner?

34. Which of the following types of faculty is NOT discussed by the passage?

   A. research faculty
   B. clinical faculty
   C. part-time faculty
   D. administrative faculty

35. Which of the following statements is *contradicted by* the passage?

   A. Institutions should promote opportunities by which individuals may feel a bonding.
   B. Multiyear contracts would be beneficial to elicit identity with the institution.

C. There is a need to clarify the roles and differences of tenure and nontenure-eligible faculty.
D. Tenure is probably the only way to achieve bonding.

36. Issues of concern regarding nontenure-eligible faculty are:
   I. job security.
   II. compensation.
   III. evaluation.
   IV. academic freedom.

   A. I, II, and III   C. II and IV
   B. I and IV   D. I, II, III, and IV

37. Which of the following statements is *supported by* the passage?

   A. Responsibilities and qualifications of tenure and nontenure-eligible faculty are quite similar in many instances.
   B. There is a difference between undergraduate and graduate bond students and the instructors they need.
   C. Tenure-track faculty are apt to initiate changes.
   D. Students are knowledgeable about an instructor's status.

38. Which of the following statement(s) is/are NOT *supported nor contradicted by* the passage?
   I. Pensions should be reviewed as separate from issues of intellectual and academic freedom.
   II. State legislatures must be educated or reeducated about the role of faculty.
   III. Institutions should provide support for nontenure-eligible research faculty between receipt of grants.
   IV. Nontenure-eligible faculty members should have access to the institution's grievance procedures.

   A. I, II, and III   C. II and IV
   B. I and III   D. I, II, III, and IV

39. The functions of a university are:
   I. teaching
   II. research
   III. public service
   IV. protection of the constitutional right of freedom of speech

   A. I, II, and III   C. II and IV
   B. I and III   D. I, II, III, and IV

40. Which of the following statements is *supported by* the passage?

- **A.** Clinical faculty are greatly concerned with the generation of income for the institution.
- **B.** Many clinical faculty have long-term records of service.
- **C.** Nontenure-eligible faculty of both the undergraduate and professional schools feel like second class citizens.
- **D.** Clinical faculties do not require many incentives because they serve patients.

41. Which of the following is NOT *supported by* the passage?

- **A.** A number of nontenure-eligible faculty possess credentials comparable to tenure-track people.
- **B.** An advanced degree does not necessarily reflect upon a faculty member's teaching.
- **C.** Tenure does not mean bonding.
- **D.** The reward system usually favors the researcher.

Passage VI (Questions 42–47)

Herbert Hoover's initial reputation in public life arose from his legendary success in feeding the victims of World War I. Already established as a successful consulting engineer, he had responded to overwhelming human need at the outbreak of the war and had set up the Commission for Relief in Belgium to facilitate humanitarian responses to the dislocations of German occupation. From 1914 until the American declaration of war in April 1917, Hoover administered a complex organization to raise funds, obtain food, and transport it to the needy. Along the way, he negotiated and renegotiated with the warring governments, convincing them to permit his rescue operations. At the conclusion of the war, Hoover resumed international feeding with the American Relief Administration. And, during the 1920s, when he perceived need, he responded in the same fashion—in Russia from 1921–1923, for example, and again during the Mississippi floods of 1927.

The feeding, relief, and rescue operations made him one of the most beloved and admired men in the world. But that personal prestige was of small impor-

We gratefully acknowledge the help of Dr. Susan Esterbrook Kennedy, Professor of History and Geography, Virginia Commonwealth University, 1990.

tance to Hoover, compared with the sense of satisfaction at having "saved the lives of 1,400,000,000 human beings, mostly women and children, who otherwise would have perished."

In all of his rescue efforts, children represented Hoover's first concern. Orphaned himself by age ten, he showed a lifetime commitment to children—to making sure that all children should have the opportunity to grow up with adequately nourished bodies and minds. In public life, his efforts may be seen in the White House Conference on Child Health and Protection; in private life, he and Mrs. Hoover engaged in countless hidden charities, providing for destitute families and educating needy youngsters. Each of Hoover's relief operations also began with the concern for suffering children, and then expanded to include mothers, other women, the aged, and finally able-bodied men.

But Hoover's purpose stretched beyond mere feeding. He understood that the Four Horsemen of the Apocalypse rode together, and that Famine's grim companions could warp minds as well as bodies. Not often poetic, Hoover nevertheless printed this verse at the beginning of his great documentary study of his relief activities:

I am the stalking aftermath of all wars.
Pestilence is my companion.
Tumult and Revolution rise round my feet
We kill more than all of the guns.
I breed fears and hates that bring to man
  more wars,
From me comes no peace to mankind.
My legacy is to Children of Famine—
Stunted bodies and twisted minds.

The battle against starvation had critical long-term political and ideological aspects. The hungry could not long defend themselves—or defend Freedom.

The outbreak of World War II in Europe in September 1939 immediately raised the relief question again. Within less than two weeks, in conversations with representatives of the Franklin Roosevelt Administration, Hoover suggested centralizing all relief activities under a single agency, preferably the Red Cross. When invited to join the executive committee of the Red Cross, Hoover declared himself willing to accept only if the Red Cross would "take on the whole job," dealing with food, clothing, medicine, and other aspects of relief. Norman Davis, head of the Red Cross, defined its role more narrowly, arguing that there was a fundamental difference between emergency relief that had been the normal function of the Red Cross and that could be financed by private contributions, and the mass feeding and relief over an extended period that would require government financing. Hoover and Roosevelt's emissaries had reached an impasse.

42. In this passage the Red Cross:

    A. pictured itself as a broad-based, capable relief organization.
    B. viewed its role as supplying emergency relief.
    C. wanted Hoover to lead the organization.
    D. depended on government to finance its operation.

43. It is quite clear from the passage that Hoover's passion was:

    A. the hungry.
    B. the homeless.
    C. the children.
    D. the indigent.

44. Hoover was trained as:

    A. a politician.
    B. a businessman.
    C. a relief specialist.
    D. an engineer.

45. Which of the following is *contradicted by* the passage?

    A. Roosevelt supported Hoover's efforts.
    B. Hoover was active in negotiating between warring governments.
    C. Hoover's efforts were broad based.
    D. Hoover helped natural disaster victims.

46. Which of the following is/are *supported by* the passage?
    I. Hoover believed that a centrally coordinated effort would serve best.
    II. Deprived people will rise to the occasion and defend their liberties.
    III. Hoover was quick to act.
    IV. Hoover did not have his family's support.

    A. I, II, and III
    B. I and III
    C. II and IV
    D. none of the above

47. Which of the following would describe/fit Herbert Hoover best?

    A. He was a socialist.
    B. He was a republican.
    C. He was a globalist.
    D. He was a humanitarian.

Passage VII (Questions 48–53)

Aristotle believed that "right reasoning" or ethical thinking could best be taught by tragedies. He particularly liked *Antigone* in this regard. He pointed out that tragedies first capture the heart of the reader by having a hero (or someone with whom we can associate) and then showing that this likable person committed an "error in judgment" *(hamartia)*. Aristotle believed in training the *heart* as well as the *mind* and that pity and fear *(pathos)* can best be aroused by a hero's downfall that is actually his fault. The "error in judgment" is all the more terrifying when we realize that it could have happened to us just as easily. Tragedies show our worst fear: good and logical people can fail!

Tragedies can test the limits of a culture to function; they can depict institutional and national failures. Tragedies can also show a particular culture to be the source of error. For instance, in the historical examples, unchecked scientific research and religious proselytizing resulting from a cultural misjudgment. Modern cultural misjudgments are the Catholic persecution in Ireland, black slavery in America, and the Jewish holocaust in Germany. Yet, in these three modern cases, it is important to realize the role of *pathos,* or empathy, in teaching wisdom. The reader must *identify with those who made the error in judgment* to be motivated toward determining right reasoning. For instance, white Americans can feel guilt, humility (the "beginning of wisdom"), and uncertainty by studying slavery, whereas black Americans will feel mostly anger and resentment. Black Americans, for instance, should be introduced to the persecutions of other groups in other settings to obtain "true" or underlying wisdom about man's capacity for logical errors. Similarly, the holocaust is not a Jewish tragedy nor is the Irish persecution a Catholic tragedy in the classical sense of motivating the reader towards wanting to make good judgments. For such motivation, a person must "see" himself making the logical error, not just being a victim.

Tragedies can also show conflicts in values within one group or even within one person. Samuel Johnson criticized Shakespeare for a lack of morality in his plays; the hero often was a liar or an adulterer. What Shakespeare was actually so good at was showing the complexity of judgments in clear ways.

If tragedies are potentially effective for developing ethics and even wisdom, how can they be used in the educational arena? In his 1908 book, *Ethics,* John Dewey pointed out the "danger of either dogmatism or a sense of unreality when students are introduced

Adapted from material by Dr. James J. McGovern, Virginia Commonwealth University. Presented at the Conference on Educating the Gifted for the 21st Century (1990).

abruptly to theoretical ideas.'' Dewey went on to propose an efficiency: ''... he is encouraged to try them on simple problems before attempting the problems of the present.'' Following his lead, I propose to first introduce students to simple cases and then proceed to the more complex. Across the grades, this means beginning with picture books and one-page examples and eventually progressing to case studies in college. Of course, care must be taken to have the necessary elements of a empathetic character, moral dilemma, and mistake in judgment at all of these levels.

Sources for ethical tragedies are the Bible, classical literature, history, newspapers, books, and actual experiences. Shorter versions and profiles must be developed to make an ethical lesson in a reasonable amount of time. Uses or formats are Xerox pages, pamphlets, published articles, workbook, and computer ''what if'' simulations with or without video accompaniments.

The main idea is that all these tragedies, regardless of format, must be short but not too short. For instance, John F. Kennedy wrote a book called *Profiles in Courage,* which contained about a dozen stories of U.S. senators faced with ethical dilemmas. The stories are short in length, but long enough in description to capture the heart of the reader to wish the hero well. In this way, we can take the need for such virtues as wisdom and courage ''to heart.''

The renewal of ethical *skills* to each generation can be helped by understanding capitalistic and market mechanisms. (Notice I did not say ethical *knowledge* because we are not trying to transmit facts but to develop right reasoning.) For instance, if teachers at a certain grade level or in a certain subject area have a case study or pamphlet ''fair'' where their works are displayed, the better works will become known and used increasingly. A school district, university, or state education department could encourage development, publication, and ''survival of the fittest'' of ethical tragedies by similar display mechanisms, sales shows, or annotated bibliographies. Eventually, a *general* curriculum could be prescribed by the state education department.

Ethical pamphlets or booklets are being proposed instead of textbooks because of the modular or ''mix and match'' possibilities that they allow. For instance, a high school teacher can use a pamphlet to supplement a history course at a strategic point, whereas a business teacher in college can allow students to choose among some case studies and compare one of them to a recent event. The combination of student feedback and teacher rewriting should produce better case studies for the future. In this way, we can develop a naturally self-improving mechanism or *Tao* in this important area.

Encouraging teachers in various fields to write,

desktop publish, and trade ethical cases has another advantage. It not only keeps the cases current, but it encourages teachers in the present generation to put the ''key ideas'' together to allow wise leadership to be ''unlocked'' in individuals in the next generation. In many ways, our teachers determine and give birth to the future.

It is primarily through education that the process of heredity, which from the beginning has caused the world to rise to higher zones of consciousness, is furthered in a reflective form and in its social dimensions. The educator, as an instrument of Creation, should derive respect and ardor for his efforts from a profound, communicative sense of the development already achieved or awaited. ...

Pierre Teilhard de Chardin
The Future of Man

48. The material in this passage is an excerpt from a longer selection. Based on the tone of the content, which of the following statements describes the probable communication vehicle of the original piece?

A. The material comes from a methods textbook on education.
B. The material is part of a talk presented at a conference on educating gifted students.
C. The material comes from a theatrical article.
D. The material is taken from a speech given to college graduates.

49. The main theme of this passage is that:

A. studying plays or stories that have a tragic ending tends to make the reader view the lead character as a hero despite any judgment errors that he may be responsible for.
B. tragedies, such as those created by Shakespeare lack moral character because the hero generally is a liar or an adulterer.
C. the skills needed to develop ethical thinking in new generations can be fostered by studying tragedies.
D. an understanding of market mechanisms is needed to understand ethics.

50. The author's sense of the Greek word *hamartia* is:

    A. unavoidable mistakes.

    B. faulty logic.

    C. major injustices.

    D. personal grief.

51. In his book *Ethics,* John Dewey cautioned teachers to:

    A. avoid dogmatism.

    B. begin with theoretical overviews.

    C. start with simple cases.

    D. limit discussions to current situations.

52. Having teachers write their own ethical case studies:

    A. allows a standard curriculum to be developed.

    B. provides a free market mechanism.

    C. keeps the cases current.

    D. allows the writer to identify with the victim.

53. Passing on a sense of ethics from one generation to another can be accomplished by:

    A. teaching a basic body of knowledge.

    B. inspiring students to live good lives.

    C. teachers formulating good and humane reasoning, and this skill being picked up by students.

    D. reading about tragedies and other cases where evil doers suffer.

Passage VIII (Questions 54–59)

"I left home when I was 16 when my mother tried to kill me with a butcher knife. All I took with me was what I was wearing: a white T-shirt, bluejeans, and socks." Thomas Ashely Daniel's eyes are ablaze—as they almost always are—now 20 years later as he talks about his life.

"I lived part of the next two years in an abandoned car and played guitar in a blues band. I also lived in a sort of boarding house with a bunch of homosexuals and prostitutes. They were some of my best friends; they weren't complicated."

Thomas Daniel's severely personal photographs have won significant awards all over the country,

Used with permission of Thomas A. Daniel and John. T. Bryan, *VCU School of the Arts Journal,* 1986.

have been featured in three books, and have just earned a place for him in the nation's most important war-photography exhibition to data: "The Indelible Image: Some War Photographs, 1846 to the Present."

"It was an early morning prank that put me in the army. I was driving around the wealthy part of town at 6 o'clock in the morning, and I saw this guy carry his golf clubs out of the house and lean them against the trunk of his car. When he went back inside I drove by and grabbed the clubs and then drove up on an overlooking hill and watched. He looked everywhere for those clubs—twice in his trunk. I sold the clubs to a guy who later turned me in to the cops. He said he got to feeling guilty because he was a born-again Christian. My prostitute friends bailed me out, and rather than a jail sentence I was given a military option." Tom's eyes widen and shift rapidly. He breathes quickly and wipes his hand across his cheek. "Pretty smart. What does society do with the misfits? Send them to war."

Now Thomas Daniel teaches part-time in VCU's Department of Photography. He has a B.F.A. in Design from VCU, an M.A. in Photography from Goddard. He's won three Fellowship Grants from the Virginia Museum of Fine Arts. He has three dozen photographs in Doubleday's *The Virginians.* His list of exhibitions includes solo shows at Princeton and the Southeastern Center for Contemporary Art.

In Vietnam, Tom saw, photographed, and experienced most of the horrors of war. Shortly after he'd bought his first camera at the PX, the company photographer was killed. Tom volunteered to be the replacement. "I didn't know a thing about a darkroom or photography, but I told them I knew everything in the world." His eyes sparkle as he recollects. "I found the batallion photographer and gave him a pound and a half of pot to teach me."

After the war, and an army commendation medal in 1968 for the Tet Offensive, Tom pursued an education: first at Chowan, then the B.F.A. from VCU, and finally the M.A. from Goddard. His photographs continued to display the kind of human intensity he'd seen in Vietnam. "I have to have the human element in my photographs. I don't find that in nature—I could never be a nature photographer. I like confrontations."

54. The passage could be labeled as:

    A. fiction.

    B. a mystery.

    C. a biography.

    D. an autobiography.

55. The story deals with a man in his:

A. teens. C. thirties.
B. twenties. D. forties.

56. Which of the following statements is *contradicted by* the passage?

A. The artist's career was planned.
B. The artist's career evolved in a haphazard fashion.
C. The artist is not overly enthusiastic about nature.
D. The artist enjoys action.

57. One can deduce from the passage that the terminal degree in the artist's field could be the:

A. associate degree. C. B.F.A. degree.
B. PX degree. D. M.A. degree.

58. The artist:

A. left home to pursue a career.
B. joined the army of his own free will.
C. learned his trade in school.
D. probably has an interest in war photographs in general.

59. One result of the episode involving the theft of the golf clubs for the individual who took them was:

A. he was able to learn to play golf.
B. he became close friends with the golfer from whom he took the clubs.
C. he wound up in the army.
D. he was able to exchange the clubs for his first camera.

Passage IX (Questions 60–65)

As the strategic importance of an information systems component within an organization grows, so does the need for the ability to continue data processing operations in the wake of a disaster. Preparation falls into two categories: (1) backup and recovery procedures to minimize risks due to storage media or other types of hardware failure, as well as loss of data due to program errors, and (2) contingency planning to provide the capability to maintain an adequate

Adapted from Ben Owen, "Systems Performance Evaluation," MCV/VCU, 1990.

level of support, despite a prolonged lack of resources. However, experts have estimated that less than 50 percent of central data processing sites in the United States have an adequate contingency plan, largely due to its lack of immediate corporate benefit.

Cost/benefit analysis can be used to determine which disaster planning control measures an organization should consider. The framework of the analysis is based on the expected benefit of a control used for a specific threat. Obviously, the benefit must be positive (cost of control is less than expected value of control), and the cost must also be considered in conjunction with financial analysis for other unrelated corporate projects.

Determination of cost of control is done by adding the initial costs of the control measure to the present value of recurring costs over a three to five year period, based on the company's borrowing rate.

Derivation of expected value of control is less straightforward. It is the product of expected loss × control effectiveness. Expected loss is calculated by multiplying the cost of total or partial damage to a specific hardware or software component by the probability of a specific threat. This probability must be annualized by calculating the expected occurrences of the threat per year. Statistical means, consensus of experts, or use of consultants are techniques a company might use to establish this type of probability.

After all threats are determined, the ones with the greatest likelihood should receive the highest planning priority. Again, each scenario must be financially analyzed and only controls with positive payback should be weighed against competing corporate projects for possible implementation.

Various strategies for disaster recovery include: (1) no action, (2) the fortress, (3) the commercial hot site, (4) the commercial cold site, (5) the warm site, (6) reciprocal processing agreements, and (7) privately owned sites.

The fortress represents the centralized data center that has taken extreme preventive measures to ward off disaster. They do not use alternate site plans, and are therefore jeopardized in the event of a major catastrophe, such as a destructive tornado. On the other hand, they are probably very well prepared for the occurrence of disasters with higher probabilities, such as equipment failure or data loss.

The commercial hot site leases space to companies charging monthly fees for a specified number of years, including a maximum available number of weeks of usage during that time period. All computing equipment necessary for critical operations is provided. The hot site offers the advantage of being able to reestablish processing operation very quickly, but drawbacks include the high cost and the possibility that another firm who also has membership at the same site may have a disaster just before you do.

The commercial cold site leases building space only; no computing equipment is included. It is less expensive than a hot site lease, but may not provide proper coverage because of possible inability to lease necessary computer equipment in a widespread disaster. The shared membership arrangement could also put a firm at a disadvantage.

The warm site is a service bureau with which one contracts for specified processing time when necessary. The primary advantages of the warm site are that the equipment is already in place, and most store backups for firms in time of need, making the recovery time even faster than the hot site. The primary disadvantage of the warm site is the high cost for general services that are not well suited for specialized processing requirements.

The reciprocal agreement involves two companies who provide backup capability for one another during a disaster. This arrangement has the advantage of providing more specialized equipment, assuming that reciprocating firms have similar hardware and software processing requirements. The cost is much lower than that of commercial solutions, and the only competition comes from the host site itself. The disadvantages of this setup include the two firms possibly growing apart in terms of compatibility, and potential contract violations.

Privately owned sites are used by some large firms, and involve a private hot or cold site that is used in emergencies. The same advantages and disadvantages exist for these as do for commercial hot or cold sites, except that they are more available, and in the case of the hot site, more responsive. However, they are obviously more expensive to own.

Two of the most important management issues involved in disaster planning are who is responsible and which applications get top priority. Ideally, a disaster recovery team is formed with members representing the entire corporation, who are part-time members of this project. The leader need not necessarily be from the Information Systems area. The prioritization of application recovery can be decided by this team, or by the Disaster Planning steering committee, but should be formalized. The vehicle for this is the disaster recovery plan.

60. According to the passage:
    I. program errors may result in data loss.
    II. the majority of data processing centers have inadequate contingency plans.
    III. corporations see no immediate benefit derived from data processing.

A. I only   C. I and II only
B. II only   D. I, II, and III

61. This passage summarizes planning considerations for computer disaster recovery. The passage deals with issues, such as:
    I. benefits versus costs of recovery.
    II. identification of quantitative techniques employed by management.
    III. comparisons of strategies for emergency operation sites.

A. I only   C. I and II only
B. II only   D. I, II, and III

62. Among major management issues to be considered were:
    I. responsibility for planning.
    II. prioritization of critical applications.
    III. formalization of a plan.

A. I only   C. I and II only
B. II only   D. I, II, and III

63. Which of the following statement(s) is/are *supported by* the passage?
    I. Statistics may be used to establish priorities in planning.
    II. Planning contingency systems must be analyzed in the total schema of a corporation's operation.
    III. Most organizations have adequate plans in case of an emergency.

A. I only   C. I and II only
B. II only   D. I, II, and III

64. Cost control must consider:

    A. the initial costs of measures.
    B. a time span of three to five years.
    C. the borrowing rate of a company.
    D. all of the above.

65. Which of the following statement(s) is/are *supported by* the passage?

    A. The fortress type of data storage is quite safe in most emergencies.
    B. Hot sites are quite costly.
    C. Cold sites seem to be most disadvantageous.
    D. All of the above are supported.

PHYSICAL SCIENCES

10 PROBLEM SETS OF 5–10 QUESTIONS EACH
15 PROBLEMS FOLLOWED BY A SINGLE QUESTION
77 QUESTIONS
100 MINUTES

DIRECTIONS: The following questions or incomplete statements are in groups. Preceding each series of questions or statements is a paragraph or a short explanatory statement, a formula or set of formulas, or a definition. Read the written material and then answer the questions or complete the statements. Select the ONE BEST ANSWER for each question and indicate your selection by marking the corresponding letter of your choice on the Answer Form. Eliminate those alternatives you know to be incorrect and then select an answer from among the remaining alternatives. A periodic table is provided (see p467). You may consult it whenever you wish to do so.

Passage I (Questions 66–70)

Several rooms with audio equipment are to be used to test human hearing, including auditory discrimination, as well as the properties of sound deadening materials, sound baffles, and so on. The temperature of the room can be varied so that the sound speed can be varied. The speakers can be operated from a variety of sound sources but the most common source will be function generators that generate pure sine tones over a reasonably large frequency range. Audio amplifiers will be used to produce rather high sound levels. Several different speakers operating from separate sources can be used at one time.

66. The function generators are used to produce sine tones with a frequency range of 30 Hz to 28 KHz (kilohertz). About what percentage of human beings can hear this entire range of 30–28000 Hz?

   A. 0%
   B. 15%
   C. 50%
   D. 70%

67. One speaker is used to produce a sound level of 40 dB (decibels). A second identical speaker operating at the same power level is then switched on. What is the decibel level of the two speakers operating together?

   A. 40 dB
   B. 43 dB
   C. 60 dB
   D. 80 dB

68. The speaker amplifier draws a current of 2.2 A rms, when driving the speaker at 40 dB. What power does the amplifier require when operated at 120 V rms?

   A. 55 watts
   B. 88 watts
   C. 120 watts
   D. 264 watts

69. What is the impedance, in ohms, of the above speaker amplifier in question 3?

   A. 0 ohms
   B. 54.5 ohms
   C. 88 ohms
   D. 264 ohms

70. One speaker operates at 450 Hz and a second operates at 456 Hz. A listener located about midway between the speakers hears what beat frequency?

   A. 3 Hz
   B. 6 Hz
   C. 450 Hz and 456 Hz
   D. 906 Hz

Passage II (Questions 71–76)

A pendulum system is devised to study the properties of oscillating systems. The pendulum consists of a bob of 2 kg mass on the end of a very light rod 80 cm long (as shown in the sketch). If one displaces the pendulum through a small angle of less than about 10° from the vertical, it behaves as a simple pendulum of length L with a period of oscillation given by $T = 2\pi\sqrt{L/g}$.

The instructor also wishes to use this system to study energy interchanges, from potential energy to kinetic energy, and so on. The pendulum is made so that it can be connected to an escapement mechanism with a set of falling weights (similar to the grandfather clock) for the purpose of replacing the small amount of energy lost to friction during each oscillation cycle. When the weights fall through their entire vertical displacement, it is the same as if a mass of 1.2 kg fell through 40 cm. The speed of the pendulum bob can be measured at any point along its arc by the use of a photogate timer.

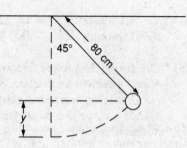

71. The bob is first raised to the position shown where the rod makes an angle of 45° with the vertical. What is its height y above the lowest position?

A. 0.14 m   C. 0.40 m
B. 0.23 m   D. 0.60 m

72. Ignoring the small amount of energy lost to friction, use the principle of conservation of mechanical energy to calculate the expected speed of the bob as it passes through the lowest point of its swing (when released from the 45° position).

A. 2.12 m/s   C. 4.84 m/s
B. 3.05 m/s   D. 8.12 m/s

73. The bob is now released when the rod makes an angle of about 8° from the vertical. What is the period of oscillation?

A. 0.9 s   C. 2.4 s
B. 1.8 s   D. 4.6 s

74. What is the frequency of oscillation with the bob released from the 8° position as in the preceding question?

A. 0.55 Hz   C. 2.30 Hz
B. 1.11 Hz   D. 2.40 Hz

75. The rod is now replaced with a rod of a length such that the period of the pendulum (for the small angle case) is exactly 2 s. It is found that the falling weight of mass 1.2 kg takes 54 minutes to fall through the 40 cm height. Calculate how much energy is lost to friction during *each* cycle.

A. 0.0006 joules   C. 0.240 joules
B. 0.003 joules   D. 1.240 joules

76. The rod is released from the smaller angle of 4° with the vertical. What is the period of oscillation?

A. 1.8 s   C. 2.5 s
B. 3.6 s   D. 0.9 s

Passage III (Questions 77–81)

A physics instructor devises a simple electrical circuit setup in which one can easily insert various resistors and capacitors in series and parallel combinations. One can have only resistor combinations, only capacitor combinations, or capacitor-resistor combinations. The circuit is usually used for DC (direct current) studies but can also be used for AC (alternating current) studies. The DC battery voltage is 6 volts. The AC rms voltage is 120 volts (at 60 Hz). The student inserts the resistors and/or capacitors as instructed and has available suitable ammeters and voltmeters for both the DC and AC experiments. (There are three resistors, each of 2 ohms resistance. There are also three capacitors, each of 1 microfarad capacitance.)

77. All three resistors are connected in series and the combination is connected to the 6-volt DC battery. What voltage drop occurs across each individual resistor as measured by the voltmeter?

A. 0.33 V   C. 2.0 V
B. 1.0 V   D. 6.0 V

78. One capacitor and one resistor are connected in parallel. The ends of this combination are then connected to the 6 V DC battery. What are the final current and voltage, respectively, across the 1 microfarad capacitor?

A. 0 A, 6 V   C. 0.33 A, 6 V
B. 0.33 A, 3 V   D. 6 A, 6 V

79. Two of the 2-ohm resistors are connected in parallel and the 120 V AC voltage is applied to the ends of this parallel combination. What current will the AC ammeter measure if connected so it measures only the current through one of the resistors?

A. 1 A   C. 60 A
B. 2 A   D. 120 A

80. Two resistors are connected in parallel and the set of parallel resistors is then connected in series with the third resistor. If this series-parallel combination is connected across the 6-volt battery, what total DC current is drawn from the battery?

A. 0.5 A	C. 3 A
B. 2 A	D. 6 A

81. One capacitor and one resistor are connected in series. The 120 V, 60 Hz AC voltage is then applied to this series "RC" circuit. What is the AC current through this series circuit?

A. .045 A	C. 0.72 A
B. 0.50 A	D. 40.0 A

Passage IV (Questions 82–87)

An air track with carts is used as an (almost) frictionless system to study both elastic and inelastic collisions. The purpose is to understand the principle of conservation of linear momentum as well as the conservation of energy principle. It is assumed that total kinetic energy is conserved for the collision of air track carts with spring steel bumpers. The velocities of the carts are determined by the use of photogate timers, both before and after collisions. Carts with masses of 150 g and 450 g are available. Some carts have "sticky" bumpers so that they stick together after colliding (in "completely inelastic" collisions). The total kinetic energy is not conserved (constant) in these latter collisions. Two of the different mass carts have a spring that can be compressed between them. A taut string tied between the carts keeps the spring compressed. The string is burned with a match and the two carts fly apart in opposite directions.

82. When the string is burned, the 150 g cart is observed to have a velocity of 3 m/s. What is the magnitude of the opposite velocity of the 450 g cart?

A. 0.33 m/s	C. 3 m/s
B. 1 m/s	D. 9 m/s

83. Two of the 150 g carts with the spring steel bumpers collide. One is at rest before the collision. The second has a velocity of 2 m/s just before they collide. What is the velocity of the second cart just after the collision?

A. 1 m/s in the opposite direction
B. 1 m/s in the same direction
C. 2 m/s in the same direction
D. 2 m/s in the opposite direction

84. A 450 g cart passes through two photogates that are 2 m apart. It has a speed of 4.0 m/s through the first photogate and a speed of 3.0 m/s through the second photogate. About how much energy was lost to air friction during the passage between the gates?

A. 1.1 joules	C. 2.3 joules
B. 1.6 joules	D. 8.8 joules

85. The energy lost to air friction is also the work done "against" air friction. From the result of the preceding question, calculate the average retarding force due to air friction over the 2 m distance.

A. 0.8 N	C. 3.2 N
B. 1.6 N	D. 4.9 N

86. One end of the air track is now elevated. A 450 g cart is given a push and then passes through a photogate. It ascends the track and comes to rest at a point that is measured to be a vertical height of 0.5 m above the photogate. Ignoring air friction, what was the speed of the cart through the photogate?

A. 1.24 m/s	C. 4.55 m/s
B. 3.13 m/s	D. 6.26 m/s

87. Two of the different mass carts are tied together with the compressed spring between them. When the string is burned the 150 g cart is observed to have a velocity of 3 m/s. What is the magnitude of the opposite velocity of the 450 g cart?

A. 3 m/s	C. 9 m/s
B. 1 m/s	D. 0.33 m/s

Questions 88–95 are independent of any passage and of each other.

88. In order to do a blood transfusion, a container of blood of density 1050 kg/m^3 is placed 1 m higher than the level of the patient's arm. How much greater is the pressure of the blood as it enters the arm than if the container were at the same level as the arm?

A. 9.8 N/m^2	C. 10300 N/m^2
B. 1050 N/m^2	D. 12000 N/m^2

89. Liquid flows at a velocity of 2 m/s through a tube of diameter 1 cm. It then flows through a constricted part of the pipe of diameter 0.5 cm. What is the flow velocity in the constriction?

A. 1 m/s	C. 4 m/s
B. 2 m/s	D. 8 m/s

90. An automobile tire has a radius of 35 cm and a mass of 6 kg. It rotates at an angular velocity of 3 rev/s. What is the linear speed of a point on the rim of the tire?

A. 1.05 m/s   C. 6.3 m/s
B. 2.10 m/s   D. 6.6 m/s

91. Monochromatic light of wavelength 620 nanometers falls on a transmission diffraction grating with 600 lines per mm. What is the diffracted angle for the second order image? (1 nm $= 10^{-9}$ m)

A. 24°   C. 48°
B. 32°   D. 82°

92. Ball #1 of mass 2 kg is thrown horizontally from the edge of a building of height 2 m with an initial velocity of 4 m/s. At the same instant ball #2 of mass 1 kg is dropped from the same height. What are the respective times for #1 and #2 to reach the ground?

A. 0.64 s, 0.64 s   C. 1.28 s, 0.64 s
B. 0.64 s, 1.28 s   D. 3.46 s, 0.64 s

93. A convex-convex lens of focal length 10 cm is used as a simple magnifier. The magnified image is seen by looking through the lens. If the object is 4.0 cm from the lens, where is the image with respect to the lens?

A. 2.9 cm on same side as the object.
B. 2.9 cm on opposite side from the object.
C. 6.7 cm on same side as the object.
D. 6.7 cm on the opposite side from the object.

94. A net force of 5 N acts on a mass of 3 kg, accelerating it from rest. If the force acts over a distance of 3 m what is the final speed of the mass?

A. 3.2 m/s   C. 15 m/s
B. 6.2 m/s   D. 30 m/s

95. A patient is injected with a solution of Technicium-99m, which is radioactive with a half-life of 6 hours. If the injection originally contained 100 millicuries of Tc-99m, how much of the Tc-99m is left after 24 hours?

A. 0.08 millicuries   C. 12.5 millicuries
B. 6.3 millicuries   D. 25 millicuries

Passage V (Questions 96–105)

Students in a medical physics class are given the assignment of planning a nuclear medicine facility. They not only design the rooms and choose the major equipment, they also will have to solve elementary problems dealing with treatment, doses, radiation protection and safety, and the general principles of the physics of typical isotopes that might be used in diagnostic nuclear medicine. They are required to be familiar with concepts of half-life, half-thickness for shielding, and the decay schemes of representative isotopes.

96. The most common isotope used in diagnostic work is Technicium. It is furnished from a generator or "cow" in which the negative beta decay of Molybdenum-99 produces the desirable metastable isotope of Technicium according to the following decay scheme:
$$_{42}Mo^{99} \rightarrow {}_ZTc^A + {}_{-1}e^0.$$
What are the atomic number, Z, and mass number, A, of the Tc isotope?

A. 41, 99   C. 43, 98
B. 42, 99   D. 43, 99

97. If the Mo^{99} has a physical half-life of 67 hours, about what fraction is left after 5.5 days?

A. 0.10   C. 0.40
B. 0.25   D. 0.45

98. This isotope of Technicium has a physical half-life of 6 hours. When it is tagged onto a polyphosphate carrier used for a certain procedure there is a biological half-life of 12 hours (for the biological excretion of the carrier). What is the "effective half-life" in this case?

A. 4.0 hours   C. 10 hours
B. 7.5 hours   D. 14 hours

99. The "cow" was milked at 8:00 AM. At 2:00 PM the activity of the milked sample is measured by a technician and found to be 200 millicuries. What was the activity of the Technicium at 8:00 AM?

A. 100 mCi   C. 300 mCi
B. 150 mCi   D. 400 mCi

100. Thallium-201 is used for myocardial perfusion studies of the heart. It decays by electron capture when the nucleus captures one of the atom's own orbital electrons (converting a proton in the nucleus into an uncharged neutron), with the emission of gamma rays used for the imaging. What are the atomic number, Z, the mass number, A, of the Mercury isotope produced in the decay of the Thallium-201?

$$_{81}Th^{201} + _{-1}e^0 \longrightarrow {}_Z Hg^A + \Gamma s$$

A. 80, 201   **C.** 81, 201
B. 80, 202   **D.** 81, 203

101. The Thallium-201 half-life is 74 hours. If the sample has an activity of 80 millicuries initially, what will be the activity after 9.25 days?

A. 2.5 mCi   **C.** 10 mCi
B. 5 mCi   **D.** 20 mCi

102. One advantage of the Thallium isotope is the "low whole body absorbed dose per millicurie," which, for T1-201 is 70 millirads/millicurie. If the recommended amount to be injected for a heart scan is 10 microcurie per Kg of body mass, what would be the whole body dose in millirads for a 70 Kg person?

A. 340 mrad   **C.** 720 mrad
B. 490 mrad   **D.** 1340 mrad

103. Another feature that makes Technicium a desirable isotope for diagnostic nuclear medicine use is that it is a "pure gamma emitter." What is the meaning of the terminology "pure gamma emitter?"

A. The gamma radiation stays in the patient's tissue while the electrons are detected.
B. Particles emitted cannot escape tissue while the gamma radiation escapes.
C. The isotope decay emits only penetrating gamma radiation that can escape from tissue and be detected.
D. The isotope decay emits energetic electrons that act like gamma rays.

104. A patient is injected with Technicium and is estimated to have received a whole body dose of 400 millirads. If the "Quality Factor" is 1 for gamma radiation and 3 for low energy neutrons, what was the dose received by the patient in rem units?

A. 4 mrems   **C.** 1200 mrems
B. 400 mrems   **D.** 4000 mrems

105. The half-thickness of lead for the absorption of the gamma radiation from a particular isotope is 0.4 cm of lead. How many half-thicknesses are necessary to reduce the radiation penetration to less than 1% and how thick would the lead be?

A. 2 half-thicknesses, 1.2 cm
B. 4 half-thicknesses, 3.2 cm
C. 7 half-thicknesses, 2.8 cm
D. 11 half-thicknesses, 4.4 cm

Passage VI (Questions 106–110)

One mole each of CO_2, H_2O_2, and O_2 are in a closed container at 25°C and standard pressure.

106. The molar percentage of CO_2 is:

A. 25%.   **C.** 40%.
B. 33%.   **D.** 55%.

107. The weight percentage of CO_2 is:

A. 25%.   **C.** 40%.
B. 33%.   **D.** 55%.

108. The number of molecules of CO_2 is:

A. 1.8×10^9.   **C.** 9.3×10^{18}.
B. 1.0×10^{14}.   **D.** 6.0×10^{23}.

109. If the compounds should break down to the elements, the number of total moles of gas would be:

A. three.   **C.** five.
B. four.   **D.** six.

110. At standard temperature and pressure, the original CO_2, H_2O_2, and O_2 would occupy a volume of:

A. 1 liter.   **C.** 25 liters.
B. 10 liters.   **D.** 45 liters.

Passage VII (Questions 111–115)

Separate beakers are used for the preparation of 1 M solutions of $NaNO_3$, $BaCl_2$, $NaCl$, and sodium acetate.

111. The lowest pH will be:

    A. $NaNO_3$.
    B. $BaCl_2$.
    C. NaCl.
    D. sodium acetate.

112. The highest pH will be:

    A. $NaNO_3$.
    B. $BaCl_2$.
    C. NaCl.
    D. sodium acetate.

113. The closest pH's of any two of these solutions will be:

    A. NaCl and $NaNO_3$.
    B. NaCl and $BaCl_2$.
    C. $BaCl_2$ and sodium acetate.
    D. $BaCl_2$ and $NaNO_3$.

114. If the solutions of NaCl and $NaNO_3$ are mixed in one beaker and the temperature adjusted to 383°K, the contents of the beaker will most likely:

    A. freeze.
    B. boil.
    C. exhibit precipitation of $NaNO_3$.
    D. exhibit a marked color change.

115. Dilution of the $NaNO_3$ solution to 0.5 molar will bring about:

    A. an increase of pH by about 2.
    B. no significant change in pH.
    C. a decrease of pH by about 2.
    D. a decrease of pH by about 4.

Passage VIII (Questions 116–120)

The resident starts a fire in the fireplace in an apartment at 15°C. After a few minutes, he stirs his 90°C coffee with a silver spoon and quickly notes a substantial increase in the temperature of the handle of the spoon. He removes the silver spoon and stirs the coffee with a stainless steel spoon. He stands facing the fire and notes that the front of his body is becoming warm. He moves behind a screen and is much cooler. After about 45 minutes, he finds that the temperature has increased behind the screen.

116. Heat is transferred through the silver spoon by:

    A. consolidation.
    B. conduction.
    C. convection.
    D. coordination.

117. The handle of the stainless steel spoon will:

    A. become as hot as quickly as is true of the silver spoon.
    B. become hotter or will reach the same temperature more quickly than is true of the silver spoon.
    C. not become hot as quickly as is true of the silver spoon.
    D. become colder while in the coffee.

118. Heat reaching the resident while standing in front of the fire is most likely accomplished by:

    A. consolidation.
    B. conduction.
    C. convection.
    D. radiation.

119. Increase in temperature behind the screen is most likely explained by:

    A. consolidation.
    B. conduction.
    C. convection.
    D. radiation.

120. In general, the fastest transfer of heat from a heat source to another object through a gas is by:

    A. coordination.
    B. conduction.
    C. convection.
    D. radiation.

Passage IX (Questions 121–125)

The LeChatelier principle states roughly that when stress is placed upon an equilibrium system, the system will react in a direction to relieve the stress.

121. In the equilibrium reaction
    $$CO(g) + Cl_2\ (g) \rightleftharpoons COCl_2\ (g),$$
    the imposition of higher pressure will result in increased percentage(s) of:

    A. CO.
    B. Cl_2.
    C. $COCl_2$.
    D. A and B.

122. In the equilibrium reaction
    $$2H_2S\ (g) \rightleftharpoons 2H_2\ (g) + S_2\ (g),$$
    an increase in the applied pressure will result in (a) higher percentage(s) of:

    A. H_2S.
    B. H_2.
    C. S_2.
    D. B and C.

123. In the equilibrium reaction
    $$H_2\ (g) + Cl_2\ (g) \rightleftharpoons 2\ HCl\ (g),$$
    imposition of increased pressure would result

in a higher percentage of:

A. H_2.   C. HCl.
B. Cl_2.   D. none of the above.

124. To an equilibrium mixture of H_2, Cl_2, and HCl in the equation in question 123, is added additional Cl_2. The result will be a (an):

A. increase in the amount of HCl.
B. decrease in the amount of H_2.
C. increase in the amount of H_2.
D. more than one of the above.

125. $X(g) + Y(g) \rightleftharpoons 2Z(g)$
If the above hypothetical reaction is at equilibrium, addition of more Z (without changing pressure or temperature) will result in:

A. presence of more X.
B. presence of less X.
C. a change in K_{eq}.
D. more than one of the above.

Passage X (Questions 126–135)

Ionization constants for weak bases may be dealt with in the same way as the ionization constants for weak acids.
$B + H_2O \rightleftharpoons BH^+ + OH^-$

$K_b = \dfrac{[BH^+][OH^-]}{[B]}$ and $pK_b = -\log \dfrac{[BH^+][OH^-]}{[B]}$

126. Ammonia has a K_b of 1.8×10^{-5}. Its pK_b would be:

A. between 2 and 3.
B. between 3 and 4.
C. between 4 and 5.
D. greater than 5.5.

127. A 0.01 molar solution of ammonia in water would have a pOH of:

A. between 2 and 3.
B. between 3 and 4.
C. between 4 and 5.
D. greater than 5.5.

128. The pH of the above solution would be:

A. between 3 and 5.
B. between 6 and 8.5.
C. between 10 and 11.
D. between 12 and 14.

129. Hydrazine has a K_b of 1.7×10^{-6}. Its pK_b would be:

A. between 3 and 4.   C. between 5 and 6.
B. between 4 and 5.   D. between 6 and 7.

130. A 0.001 molar solution of hydrazine in water would have a pOH:

A. between 3 and 4.
B. between 4 and 5.
C. between 5 and 6.
D. between 6 and 7.

131. The above solution would have a pH:

A. between 3 and 4.
B. between 5 and 6.
C. between 6 and 8.
D. of none of the above.

132. Assuming equal concentration (and solubility) the highest pH will be observed with an aqueous solution of a base having a pK_b of:

A. 3.5.   C. 6.2.
B. 4.8.   D. 6.8.

133. A theory of acids and bases that does NOT necessarily involve hydrogen or hydroxyl ions was developed by:

A. Arrhenius.
B. Brønsted and Lowry.
C. Gordon.
D. Lewis.

134. The base NaOH would be expected to have a pK_b of:

A. 2 ± 1.   C. 9 ± 1.
B. 5 ± 1.   D. none of the above.

135. The pH of a 0.001 molar aqueous solution of NaOH would be:

A. 3   C. 9
B. 5   D. 11

Questions 136–142 are independent of any passage and each other.

136. Which is the oxidizing agent in the reaction:
$2Fe^{2+} + Cl_2 \rightarrow 2Fe^{3+} + 2Cl^-$?

A. Fe^{2+} C. Cl^-
B. Fe^{3+} D. Cl_2

137. Which molecule is nonpolar and contains a nonpolar covalent bond?

A. F_2 **C.** HF
B. CCl_4 **D.** H_2O

138. Which compound reacts with an acid to form a salt and water?

A. CH_3Cl **C.** KCl
B. CH_3COOH **D.** KOH

139. Which bond is formed by the transfer of an electron from one atom to another?

A. ionic bond   **C.** peptide bond
B. covalent bond   **D.** hydrogen bond

140. The maximum number of electrons that a single orbital of the $3d$ sublevel may contain is:

A. 1   **C.** 3
B. 2   **D.** 4

141. Given the following K_{sp} values, which compound will be the least soluble in water?

A. $AgBr = 5.0 \times 10^{-13}$
B. $AgCl = 1.8 \times 10^{-10}$
C. $Ag_2CrO_4 = 1.1 \times 10^{-12}$
D. $AgI = 8.3 \times 10^{-17}$

142. Which could act either as an oxidizing agent or a reducing agent?

A. Fe^0 **C.** Fe^{3+}
B. Fe^{2+} **D.** Cu^0

WRITING SAMPLE

2 ESSAYS-TOPICS
60 MINUTES (30 MINUTES/TOPIC)

DIRECTIONS: Your response must be a unified, organized essay; it should contain fully developed, logically constructed paragraphs. Remember quality is more important than length. Before you begin writing, make sure you have read the item carefully and understand what is being asked. Write as legibly as possible. Because your essays will be scored as first-draft compositions, you may cross out and make corrections on your response booklet as necessary. It is not necessary to recopy your essay.

Part 1

Consider this statement:
It is no wise man that will quit a certainty for an uncertainty.

Samuel Johnson

Write a unified essay in which you perform the following tasks. Explain what you think the above statement means. Describe a specific situation in which a wise man would quit a certainty for an uncertainty. Discuss the circumstances that you think determine whether or not one should or should not give up certainty for uncertainty.

Part 2

Consider this statement:
Destruction is, after all, a form of creation.

Graham Green

Write a unified essay in which you perform the following tasks. Explain what you think the above statement means. Describe a specific situation in which an act of destruction is not a form of creation. Discuss what you consider to be the circumstances that determine the relationship between destruction and creation.

BIOLOGICAL SCIENCES

10 PROBLEM SETS OF 5–10 QUESTIONS EACH
15 PROBLEMS FOLLOWED BY A SINGLE QUESTION
77 QUESTIONS
100 MINUTES

DIRECTIONS: The following questions or incomplete statements are in groups. Preceding each series of questions or statements is a paragraph or a short explanatory statement, a formula or set of formulas, or a definition. Read the written material and then answer the questions or complete the statements. Select the ONE BEST ANSWER for each question and indicate your selection by marking the corresponding letter of your choice on the Answer Form. Eliminate those alternatives you know to be incorrect and then select an answer from among the remaining alternatives.

Passage I (Questions 143–147)

The diagram below represents three generations of a human family, some of whose members have a non-lethal birth defect. Individuals 1, 3, and 4 are distantly related and come from a family in which the defect has occurred for many generations. Information on the occurrence of the defect among the ancestors of individual 2 is unavailable. The preceding four generations of the family and the siblings of individual 19 included no individuals who expressed the defect. The defect is caused by a single gene for which new mutations are very rare. The individuals with birth defects are represented by solid black symbols while the individuals who have a normal phenotype are represented by open symbols. Males are represented by squares and females are represented by circles.

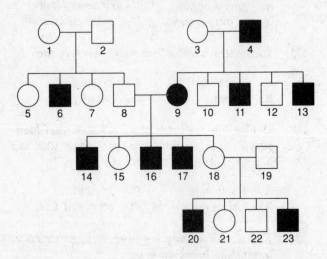

143. The defect is most likely caused by:

A. an autosomal gene for which the defective allele is recessive to the normal allele.

B. an X-linked gene for which the defective allele is recessive to the normal allele.

C. an autosomal gene for which the defective allele is dominant to the normal allele.

D. An X-linked gene for which the defective allele is dominant to the normal allele.

144. The genotype of individual number 1 in the family:

A. is most likely to contain only normal alleles.

B. is most likely to contain only defective alleles.

C. is most likely to contain both normal and defective alleles.

D. cannot be determined from the pedigree.

145. The genotype of individual number 6 in the family:

A. is most likely to contain only normal alleles.

B. is most likely to contain only defective alleles.

C. is most likely to contain both normal and defective alleles.

D. cannot be determined from the pedigree.

146. The genotype of individual number 8 in the family:

A. is most likely to contain only normal alleles.

B. is most likely to contain only defective alleles.

C. is most likely to contain both normal and defective alleles.

D. cannot be determined from the pedigree.

147. The genotype of individual number 9 in the family:

    A. is most likely to contain only normal alleles.

    B. is most likely to contain only defective alleles.

    C. is most likely to contain both normal and defective alleles.

    D. cannot be determined from the pedigree.

Passage II (Questions 148–157)

Many scientists think of the pituitary gland as the master gland responsible for the secretion of many different hormones. A reciprocal relationship operates between the hormones secreted by the pituitary and the hormones produced by the target organs; this delicate control of balance of production of secretory product between the pituitary and the target organs is known as "negative feedback." Among the many hormones produced by the pituitary gland are ACTH, FSH, LH, TSH, and STH. The following experiments were set up to demonstrate the actions of some of the above factors. Twenty-five day-old immature male and female rats were subjected to the following treatment for 10 days: Group 1 was given a 0.5 cc saline injection; Group 2 was given a 0.5 cc FSH injection; and Group 3 was given a 0.5 cc crude pituitary extract injection. The results were recorded in table form.

MALE RATS

Groups	Body Weight grams	Testes mg	Seminal Vesicles mg	Prostate mg	Thyroid mg	Adrenals mg
1	86	3750	18	71	6.0	20
2	82	5310	57	176	6.1	21
3	83	4830	24	163	7.5	27

FEMALE RATS

Groups	Body Weight grams	Ovaries mg	Uterus mg	Thyroid mg	Adrenals mg
1	83	20	25	5.9	22
2	82	43	83	5.7	21
3	84	33	61	7.1	37

148. Based on the information provided, which of the following statement(s) is/are supported by the data?

    A. From the table it seems as if the crude pituitary extract had a lesser effect on the sex organs than did FSH.

    B. Pituitary extract affected every organ under investigation.

    C. Hypophysectomy probably would have resulted in a decreased weight of the organs under investigation.

    D. All of the above.

149. Based on the information provided, which of the following statement(s) is/are supported by the data?

    A. The administration of FSH alone to an immature rat will produce follicular growth, but uterine and vaginal configurations will remain infantile since LH is also needed. The experimental data indicate uterine growth, casting doubt on the purity of the FSH preparation.

    B. Both FSH and LH are necessary for the production of estrogen.

    C. FSH has as its target organs the organs of reproduction.

    D. A and C of the above.

150. Based on the information provided, which of the following statement(s) is/are contradicted by the data?

    A. FSH in the male had the greatest effect on the weight of the prostate gland; the tissue is therefore most reactive to it.

    B. The adrenal weight probably would drop if the animals were deprived of ACTH.

    C. In these experiments, none of the hormones in the pituitary extract probably were as effective as a purified fraction of them might have been.

    D. Body weights were not a significant experimental parameter.

151. Housed in the sella tursica is the:

    A. pineal organ.   **C.** olfactory bulb.
    B. pituitary gland.   **D.** optic chiasm.

152. Social stress will affect most severely the:

    A. pancreas.   **C.** adrenal.
    B. pineal.   **D.** parathyroid.

153. During the follicular phase of a normal menstrual cycle, ovarian changes occur that are due to pituitary secretions of:

    A. FSH only.   **C.** oxytocin.
    B. LH only.   **D.** FSH and LH.

154. Follicle-stimulating hormone is to estrogen as luteinizing hormone is to:

    A. progesterone.

    B. testosterone.

    C. vasopressin.

    D. luteotrophic hormone.

155. The pituitary (master) gland releases a gonadotrophic hormone that stimulates the production of testosterone by:

    A. spermatogonia.
    B. interstitial cells of Leydig.
    C. Sertoli cells.
    D. epididymis.

156. Each of the following is under control of the adenohypophysis EXCEPT the:

    A. thyroid.   C. testis.
    B. adrenal medulla. D. adrenal cortex.

157. The sperm count of a normal 25-year-old male would be

    A. one million/ml.
    B. one hundred million/ml.
    C. one hundred thousand/ml.
    D. four million/ml.

Passage III (Questions 158–165)

The diagram illustrates a typical single neuron; the basic unit of the nervous system. Neurons connect with each other and in that manner an impulse is conducted and transmitted throughout the body. Two types of cell processes are indicated.

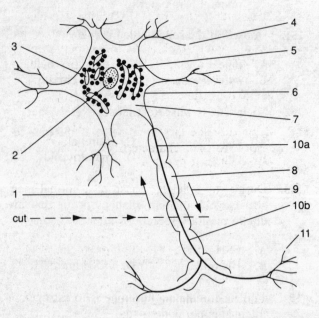

158. An impulse would be transmitted to another neuron by:

    A. 4.   C. 10a.
    B. 6.   D. 11.

159. Protein synthesis is carried out mainly by:

    A. 2.   C. 5.
    B. 3.   D. 7.

160. Cellular "digestive" or "suicide" packages is a common description or name for:

    A. mitochondria.
    B. Golgi zones or Golgi bodies.
    C. lysosomes.
    D. centrosomes.

161. The neurotransmitter acetylcholine is released by:

    A. axon terminals.
    B. dendrite terminals.
    C. Golgi apparatus of neuron cell bodies.
    D. Schwann cells.

162. We speak in terms of an aggregation of nerve cell bodies in the central nervous system as the site of a (an):

    A. ganglion.   C. cranial nerve.
    B. nucleus.   D. association area.

163. The neurolemma of an axon is part of the:

    A. nerve cell body.   C. node of Ranvier.
    B. Schwann cell.   D. axoplasm.

164. Which of the following germ layers gives origin to the nervous system?

    A. ectoderm   C. endoderm
    B. mesoderm   D. ectoderm and
                        endoderm

165. The cell bodies of the motor neurons are located in the spinal cord in the :

    A. intermediolateral cell column.
    B. dorsal root ganglia.
    C. dorsal horn (gray matter).
    D. ventral horn (gray matter).

Passage IV (Questions 166–173)

In order for a thoracic surgeon to visualize the heart he or she must open up the pericardium which is a sac that covers the heart. A human heart is four-chambered and is composed of right and left atria which are separated by an interatrial septum that is frequently marred by defects. In the fetus the foramen ovale is an opening in this septum and blood passes from the right atrium to the left atrium so that the pulmonary circulation may be bypassed. A patent foramen ovale may contribute to the condition known as "blue baby." Two ventricles are also present; specifically we can speak of a right ventricle that pumps deoxygenated blood to the lungs and a left ventricle that pumps oxygenated blood to the tissues of the body. Between the ventricles is located the interventricular septum.

The superior and inferior vena cava and the coronary sinus empty into the right atrium. From here blood passes into the right ventricle to be pumped into the lungs via the pulmonary arteries. Blood from the lungs is returned to the left atrium by the pulmonary veins; it then passes into the left ventricle to leave upon its contraction via the aorta to supply the arterial system of the body. The heart alternately contracts and relaxes, and this cardiac cycle is repeated about 75 times per minute; the duration of one cycle is about 0.8 second. Atrial systole (contraction) which takes about 0.1 second is followed by ventricular systole lasting about 0.3 second and absolute diastole (relaxation) follows lasting about 0.4 second.

The heart has an automatic rhythmic beat, but it is also under the influence of nerves which, however, serve only to change the force or frequency of the contractions of the muscle in accordance with the physiologic needs of the organism. The modification of the intrinsic rhythmicity is by way of the two parts of the autonomic nervous system; stimulation occurs through the sympathetic portion while homeostatic maintenance is mainly a function of the parasympathetic portion. Stimulation through the sympathetic nerves increases the rate and force of the heart beat; while slowing and reduction in force are the result of parasympathetic stimulation. Vasodilation of the coronary arteries is brought about by sympathetic stimulation while vasoconstriction is elicited by parasympathetic stimulation.

166. When a physician informs a patient that his blood pressure reading is 160/90, she refers respectively to:

A. systolic blood pressure of the left ventricle.
B. blood pressure in the veins of the arm.
C. systolic and diastolic pressures of the brachial artery.
D. systolic pressure of the aorta and diastolic pressure in the superior vena cava.

167. The vital centers for control of heart rate, respiratory rate, and blood pressure are located in the:

A. pons.   C. cerebellum.
B. medulla.   D. hypothalamus.

168. Blood in the pulmonary veins is rich in:

A. oxyhemoglobin.   C. hemoglobin.
B. carbaminohemoglobin.   D. uric acid.

169. Running to catch the bus to go to work has produced a rapid heart rate, an increase in the respiratory rate, and an increase in blood pressure in an individual. We can attribute these changes to:

A. the peripheral nervous system.
B. the central nervous system.
C. the parasympathetic component of the autonomic nervous system.
D. the sympathetic component of the autonomic nervous system.

170. Which of the following muscle types is NOT under the control of the autonomic (involuntary) nervous system?

A. heart (cardiac)   C. skeletal (striated)
B. smooth   D. arrector pili

171. The functional unit of a striated muscle is known as the sarcomere. A sarcomere on an electron micrograph is the region between:

A. two A bands.   C. two H bands.
B. two I bands.   D. two Z bands.

172. If we examine the three types of muscles in respect to their characteristics, which of the series below is false?

	Characteristic	Cardiac	Skeletal	Smooth
A.	No. of Nuclei	One-Several	Many	One
B.	Position of Nuclei	Central	Central	Central
C.	Striations	Present	Present	Absent
D.	Control	Autonomic	Voluntary	Autonomic

173. Heart beat is initiated by the:

A. vagus nerve.
B. sympathetic nervous system.
C. A-V (atrio-ventricular) node.
D. S-A (sino-atrial) node.

Passage V (Questions 174–178)

Human immunodeficiency virus type-1 (HIV-1) initiates infection of a cell by binding of a viral envelope protein (gp120) to a cell surface glycoprotein (CD4) on the cell. CD4 is found primarily on a subset of T lymphocytes. The CD4 molecules on these T lymphocytes normally function as receptors for the class II major histocompatibility complex molecules on the surfaces of antigen-presenting cells. Some cultured cell lines [including HSB(CD4+)M.23 and H9 cell lines] express CD4 and can therefore bind gp120 protein and can be infected by HIV-1. One possible strategy for inhibition of the spread of HIV-1 infection would be treatment with small molecules that resemble the region of CD4 molecules that binds gp120 and that would therefore bind to gp120 molecules on virus particles and prevent the virus particles from binding to cells.

A series of experiments in which a class of modified dipeptides called CPFs were evaluated is shown in Figures 1 and 2. Two different CPFs (CPFDD and CPFDF) were tested. Figure 1 describes the effects of pretreatment of HSB(CD4+)M.23 cells with CPFs on the subsequent binding of fluorescent-labelled gp120. Figure 2 describes the production of HIV-1 virus (measured as viral p24 protein production by the cells) by H9 cells which were exposed to HIV-1-infected T lymphocytes in the presence of various concentrations of CPFs.

Data modified from Finberg et al, *Science* (1990): 249:289-291.

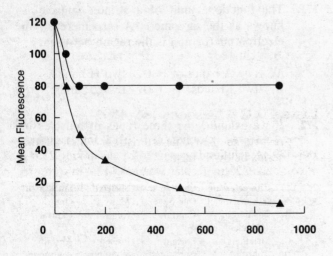

Binding of gp120 (visualized with fluorescent antibody staining) to HSB(CD4+)M.23 cells after incubation of the gp120 with CPFDF (●) or CPFDD (▲).

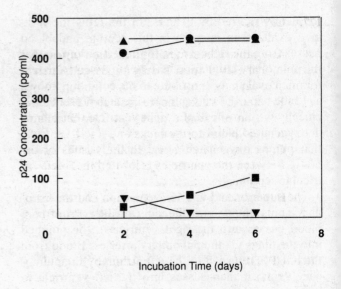

Virus production (measured as p24 protein production) by H9 cells exposed to HIV-1 infected T cells.

174. CPFDD:

   A. inhibited gp120 binding to CD4 more strongly than CPFDF.
   B. inhibited gp120 binding to CD4 less strongly than CPFDF.
   C. stimulated gp120 binding to CD4 more strongly than CPFDF.
   D. stimulated gp120 binding to CD4 less strongly than CPFDF.

175. CPFDF:

   A. inhibited gp120 binding to CD4 more strongly than CPFDD.
   B. inhibited gp120 binding to CD4 less strongly than CPFDD.
   C. stimulated gp120 binding to CD4 more strongly than CPFDD.
   D. stimulated gp120 binding to CD4 less strongly than CPFDD.

176. According to the data presented in Figure 1, a 50 μM/L increase in the concentration of CPFDD caused the largest increase in inhibition of the binding of gp120 to CD4 when the initial concentration of CPFDD was:

   A. 0.
   B. 150 μM/L CPFDD.
   C. 300 μM/L CPFDD.
   D. 800 μM/L CPFDD.

177. CPFDD:

A. caused total (>95%) inhibition of transfer of HIV-1 from T cells to H9 cells after 6 days.

B. caused strong (approximately 75%) inhibition of transfer of HIV-1 from T cells to H9 cells after 6 days.

C. caused weak (approximately 25%) inhibition of transfer of HIV-1 from T cells to H9 cells after 6 days.

D. caused no (<5%) inhibition of transfer of HIV-1 from T cells to H9 cells after 6 days.

178. CPFDF:

A. caused total (>95%) inhibition of transfer of HIV-1 from T cells to H9 cells after 6 days.

B. caused strong (approximately 75%) inhibition of transfer of HIV-1 from T cells to H9 cells after 6 days.

C. caused weak (approximately 25%) inhibition of transfer of HIV-1 from T cells to H9 cells after 6 days.

D. caused no (<5%) inhibition of transfer of HIV-1 from T cells to H9 cells after 6 days.

Passage VI (Questions 179–184)

The A B O blood grouping system is explained on the basis of a single triallelic system with genes A, B, and O operating at a single genetic locus. Phenotypic and genotypic characteristics may be expressed as follows:

Phenotype	Genotype
A	A/A; A/O
B	B/B; B/O
O	O/O
AB	A/B

The A and B genes appear to be codominant; they are dominant over O, which is recessive.

179. Utilizing this system, transfusions have become relatively safe. The universal recipient is considered to be type:

A. A. C. O.
B. B. D. AB.

180. Which of the following agglutinogens do these individuals carry on their red blood cells?

A. A C. O
B. B D. A,B

181. A person of blood type A can receive blood of type(s):

A. A. C. O.
B. B; A. D. A; O.

182. Two people are planning to have a family. The woman has blood type A/A and the man B/B. Their children might have the following:

A. A and B.
B. B only.
C. A/B only.
D. A and B and A/B.

183. A man with blood cell genotype B/O marries a woman with type A/B. Their offspring could have any of the following:

A. A/B, B/B, A/O, B/O.
B. A/B and B/O only.
C. A/O and B/B only.
D. none of the combinations above.

184. A foreign protein, when introduced into the body, is recognized and elicits an immunologic response; this substance is known as a (an):

A. antigen. C. complement.
B. antibody. D. vitamin.

Passage VII (Questions 185–189)

The following information is used for questions 185–189. A solution is prepared by dissolving 25.0 g of compound X (molecular weight of 125) in water to make a solution of 100 ml. The density of the solution is 1.15 g/ml.

185. The molality (m) of X is:

A. 1.0 m. C. 2.0 m.
B. 2.2 m. D. 0.20 m.

186. The molarity (M) of X is:

A. 1.00 M. C. 0.100 M.
B. 0.200 M. D. 2.00 M.

187. The % (w/w) of the solution of X is:

A. 20%.   C. 25%.

B. 21.7%.   D. 28.8%.

188. The number of moles of X in 20 ml of this solution is:

A. 0.04 moles   C. 5 moles

B. 2 moles   D. 10 moles

189. If X reacts with compound Y in a molar ratio of 1:1, the volume of this solution which would react with 20 ml of a 0.4 M solution of Y is

A. 4 ml

B. 20 ml

C. 40 ml

D. 200 ml

Passage VIII (Questions 190–194)

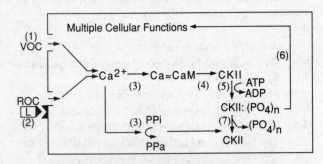

Many of the physiological functions of neurons are mediated by signal transduction systems. By way of intermediate messengers, transduction systems relay extracellular signals to intracellular effector elements which produce a physiologic response. Depending on their position in the relay chain, the intermediate relay elements are known as second messengers, tertiary messengers, and so on.

In the stylized neuron above, the extracellular signal (a neurotransmitter) is signified by the letter "L" (ligand). When "L" binds to its receptor, it opens the associated channel which admits extracellular calcium into the neuron. This constitutes a Receptor Operated Channel (ROC). Admission of calcium via the ROC serves to depolarize the neuron. With depolarization, the Voltage Operated Channel (VOC) can also open to admit calcium. When the cell is sufficiently depolarized, both channels close and no more calcium is admitted.

An elevation of calcium within the cell serves to activate the calcium binding protein Calmodulin (CaM). Activated CaM, in turn, activates a Calcium/

Calmodulin-dependent Kinase (CKII). A kinase is a specialized enzyme that can transfer a phosphoryl group from a high energy donor such as ATP to an appropriate substrate phosphoprotein. CKII can transfer phosphoryl groups to itself in a process known as autophosphorylation. The autophosphorylated form of CKII is active and is able to carry out multiple cellular functions including increasing neurotransmitter synthesis and release.

CKII is inactivated by dephosphorylation. The initial calcium influx also serves to activate inactive Protein Phosphatases (PP), the enzymes that remove phosphoryl groups from phosphoproteins. The activity of these phosphatases is, however, somewhat slower than the other components in the system. Thus, the complete system contains all of the elements necessary for transducing an initial extracellular signal into a physiologic response. It also contains an internal mechanism for terminating the response.

190. Increasing the activity of CKII could be best achieved by blocking step(s):

A. 3.   C. 7.

B. 5.   D. 3 and 7.

191. Decreasing the activity of CKII could be achieved by blocking step(s):

A. 2 only.   C. 2 or 4 or 5.

B. 5 only.   D. 7.

192. An electrode is used to depolarize the neuron to the same extent as activation of the ROC. No neurotransmitter ligand (L) is present to bind to its receptor. Calcium, present in normal extracellular concentrations, would enter the cell through:

A. the ROC.

B. the VOC.

C. ROC and the VOC.

D. none of the above.

193. The enzyme responsible for transfer of a phosphoryl group from a high energy donor to a suitable substrate is known as a:

A. phosphatase.   C. transferase.

B. catalase.   D. kinase.

194. CKII can perform its multiple cellular functions because:

A. there is more kinase than phosphatase.

B. there is more phosphatase than kinase.

C. the inactivation pathway is slower than the activation pathway.

D. the activation pathway is slower than the inactivation pathway.

Passage IX (Questions 195–199)

A student is given four unknown clear colorless liquids, each having the molecular formula $C_5H_{10}O$. Assume that the compounds shown below are in bottles labeled I–IV. The contents of these bottles are to be associated with their chemical or physical properties.

$$\underset{\underset{CH_3}{|}}{CH_3\overset{\overset{O}{||}}{C}CHCH_3} \qquad \underset{\underset{CH_3}{|}}{CH_3CHCH_2CH{=}O}$$

I   II

$$\underset{\underset{CH_3}{|}}{CH_3C{=}CHCH_2OH} \qquad CH_3CH_2\overset{\overset{O}{||}}{C}CH_2CH_3$$

III   IV

195. The compound above that has the highest boiling point would be:

A. I.   C. III.
B. II.   D. IV.

196. The compound above that would react with 2,4-dinitrophenyl hydrazine to form a hydrazone and gives a positive Tollen's test with $Ag(NH_3)_2OH$ is:

A. I.   C. III.
B. II.   D. IV.

197. The compound above that on hydrogenation with H_2 in the presence of a catalyst, such as Pt or Ni, forms a chiral center, and which can be resolved into R and S enantiomers is:

A. I.   C. III.
B. II.   D. IV.

198. The reaction of acetaldehyde (ethanal) with isopropyl Grignard reagent, $CH_3CHMgBr$,

$$\underset{\underset{CH_3}{|}}{}$$

followed by hydrolysis and then oxidation with $K_2Cr_2O_7$ would be expected to produce:

A. I.   C. III.
B. II.   D. IV.

199. The name of the compound above that would rapidly decolorize Br_2 in CH_2Cl_2 is:

A. 3-pentanone.
B. 2-methyl-2-pentanone.
C. 3-methyl-2-buten-1-ol.
D. 2-methyl-2-buten-4-ol.

Passage X (Questions 200–204)

Ten milliliters of blood were removed from a patient, and centrifugation was utilized to separate 5 ml of plasma from the blood cells. A 3-ml sample of the plasma was extracted with 100 ml of an appropriate lipid solvent. The lipid solvent was then evaporated to 10 ml, and a 0.1 ml sample was analyzed for cholesterol. The color produced in the colorimetric analysis at 560 millimicrons was exactly equal to a standard in which 0.5 mg of cholesterol was known to be present.

200. The cholesterol concentration of the patient's plasma was:

A. 200 mg cholesterol/100 ml plasma.
B. 295 mg cholesterol/100 ml plasma.
C. 867 mg cholesterol/100 ml plasma.
D. 1667 mg cholesterol/100 ml plasma.

201. In order to make the above calculations it was *not* necessary to know:

A. the volume of plasma separated from the blood.
B. the volume of plasma subjected to extraction.
C. the solvent volume after evaporation.
D. the volume of sample that was subjected to colorimetric analysis.

202. If the addition of twice the volume of standard produces more than twice the absorbance at 560 millimicrons, this is probably best explained by:

A. exceeding the linear range of the method.
B. error in pipetting.
C. error in weighing to prepare the standard solution.
D. any or all of the above.

203. Cholesterol is an intermediate in the biosynthesis of:

    A. essential fatty acids.
    B. steroid hormones.
    C. essential amino acids.
    D. prostaglandins.

204. The essential fatty acids are required in the human body in the biosynthesis of:

    A. ascorbic acid.   **C.** estrogen.
    B. bile acids.   **D.** prostaglandins.

DIRECTIONS: Read each passage carefully, study each table, chart, or formula, then answer the question following it. Eliminate those choices that you think to be incorrect and mark the letter of your choice on the answer sheet.

A scientist sets up the following experiment. Ten male rats are placed in each of two cages. One cage is placed in a room regulated at a constant temperature of 37°C (group A) while the other cage is placed in a similar room kept at 45°C (group B). Food and water were provided *ad libitum* to both experimental sets. Food consumption, water consumption, ACTH blood level, and heart rate were determined for a period of ten days. The following bar graphs illustrate the results.

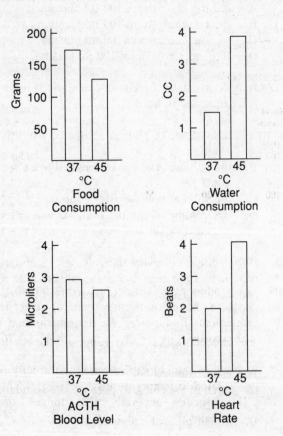

205. The investigator after examining the four graphs can report that:

    A. at a higher temperature the rats were more active.
    B. the rats maintained at 37°C developed a desire for water.
    C. ACTH level is not markedly affected by the experimental conditions.
    D. at higher temperatures more food is required.

Animals utilized in the following experiment were golden hamsters (*Mesocricetus auratus*). Normal diet consisted of Purina laboratory chow provided *ad libitum*. Animals were divided into three groups: group A—Control; group B—Cold exposed at 5°C ± 1°C for five days; group C—Cold exposed at 5°C ± 1°C for 30 days. Body weight (BW), thyroid weight (TW), ^{131}I uptake (^{131}I), and Serum Protein Bound Iodine^{-127} (PB ^{127}I) were measured.

Groups	BW grams	TW mg/100 g BW	^{131}I Uptake 24 hours	Serum PBI μg/100 ml
A	97	5.89	5.88	4.09
B	79	5.55	15.37*	5.27*
C	110	6.25	11.06*	5.02*

*Fisher's "T" significant to .001

206. The data suggest that:

    A. the morphology of the thyroid gland was not altered because no significant weight change was recorded.
    B. the thyroid gland is in a physiological state of hyperactivity in cold-exposed animals.
    C. hamsters in the cold are in great distress.
    D. the thyroid gland is in a physiological state of hypoactivity in cold-exposed animals.

An investigation was conducted to compare early host response to transplantable tumor, as manifested by mast cell adenine release, in golden hamsters with growing tumor and in golden hamsters immunized with tumor antigen and bacteria adjuvant. The following tables summarize the results.

Comparison of adenine release in hamsters sensitized with tumor antigen and bacteria adjuvant and adjuvant controls.

TABLE 1

Groups	No. of Animals	% Release
Tumor antigen and bacteria adjuvant	40	66.51
Bacteria adjuvant	40	11.13

Comparison of adenine release in the golden hamster with growing tumor and untreated controls.

TABLE 2

Groups	No. of Animals	% Release
Tumor transplant	40	33.50
Normal controls	40	7.50

207. Based on the information given, select the statement which is *not supported by* information in the above passage.

    A. While adjuvant controls had more adenine release than untreated controls, their group average was significantly below that of the animals actively sensitized to tumor.

    B. Animals that received transplants released half as much adenine as those given tumor antigen and bacteria adjuvant.

    C. There is a significant difference between the tumor-bearing animals and their controls indicating some degree of enhanced cellular sensitization.

    D. The experiments indicate that the immunological system of the golden hamster can respond with adenine release upon challenge with antigen prepared from that tumor.

This diagram represents fiber pathways by which impulses from the retina are carried to the brain. Note components of each optic nerve and which retinal

region, and corresponding visual field region, are carried by each optic nerve component.

Assume lesions 1-4 are functionally complete; that is, they result in complete sensory loss for a particular visual field region.

208. Based on location of the lesions in the previous diagram, predict what the *visual field deficit* (black region) would be for lesion #2.

Lesion 2

A.
B.
C.
D.

The life span of poikilotherms is related to the ambient temperature. In order to investigate the process of aging in these animals one must keep meticulous records of the temperature. Various parameters, other than temperature, have been introduced into aging studies which alter the life span, and one of these, ^{60}Co gamma rays, has been widely utilized with the following results.

No. of Animals	Temp. °C	Sex	Dose rads	Life Span days ± S.D.
100	18	M	0	55 ± 1
100	18	F	0	65 ± 2
100	18	M	10,000	40 ± 1
100	18	F	10,000	65 ± 2
100	20	M	10,000	55 ± 1
100	20	F	10,000	75 ± 2
100	20	M	0	65 ± 2
100	20	F	0	75 ± 2

209. The following statement(s) are related to the passage. Based on the information, select the statement(s) *supported by* the information in the passage.

    I. Life span of the animals is indirectly related to temperature.

    II. Females generally live longer than males.

III. Radiation affects the life span of males more than that of females.

A. I only   C. I and III only
B. III only   D. I, II, and III

The data below show the result of an experiment concerning cell cooperation in the immune response. The experiment attempts to determine if thymus and bone marrow cells are required for antibody to be produced against egg albumin. Various donor cells (thymus or bone marrow) are injected into recipient mice whose immune system has been rendered non-responsive by X-irradiation. Antibody levels were then determined in the serum of the recipient animals.

Donor Cells Injected	Antibody Production
1) Thymocytes + egg albumin	0
2) Thymocytes	0
3) Bone marrow + egg albumin	0
4) Bone marrow	0
5) Thymocytes + bone marrow + egg albumin	+++
6) Spleen cells + egg albumin	+++
7) Lymph node cells + egg albumin	+++

210. Based on the information given, select the statement which is *not supported by* information in the above passage.

A. In this system, bone marrow and thymus cells are required for a mouse to make antibody to egg albumin.
B. Thymus cells or cells derived from the thymus are probably found in the spleen.
C. Thymus cells or bone marrow cells or both are capable of synthesizing antibody.
D. In the intact animal, the thymus would probably be important as a source of antibody.

Days on Drug	Strength of Drug	Factor 1	Factor 2	Factor 3	Factor 4	Factor 5	Factor 6
0	0	12.5	33.0	26.5	9.3	6.2	71
6	0.05	10.7	17.0	47.0	9.6	5.0	73
6	0.10	3.0	9.8	64.0	7.0	4.8	80
6	0.20	4.8	8.9	49.2	2.4	4.6	62
6	0.50	12.0	7.9	55.8	10.7	6.6	73
12	0.05	12.5	9.8	23.1	12.9	11.0	45
12	0.10	4.4	7.9	40.7	8.3	9.1	49
12	0.20	6.8	7.2	43.0	5.9	16.7	54
12	0.50	3.9	5.7	34.2	5.3	23.0	43

211. Based on the information given, select the statement *contradicted by* the data in the above table.

A. The 12-day treatment period consistently produced a greater effect than the 6-day period.
B. The percentage of Factor 3 increased and that of Factor 2 decreased.
C. If there was an increase in Factor 3 and a decrease in Factor 2, there was a resultant rise in the Factor 3/Factor 2 ratio.
D. The proportion of isolated Factor 4 did not show any consistent trend.

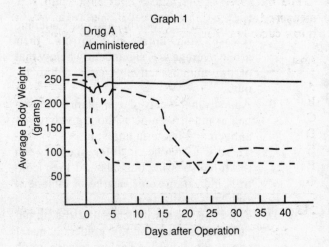

Graph 1

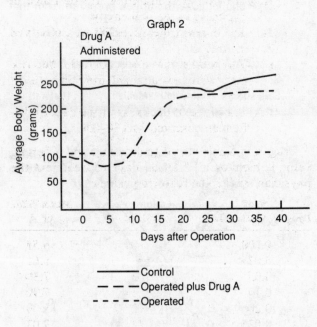

Graph 2

Control
— — Operated plus Drug A
— — — Operated

212. Based on the information given, select the statement(s) *supported by* the information in the above graphs.

A. In graph 1, the operated animals lacked a desire to eat for about one week, but then ate again to maintain their body weights at a reduced level.

B. In graph 1, the operated group that received drug A maintained their body weight while on the drug.

C. In graph 1, when the drug was discontinued, lack of desire to eat set in and remained until the animals' weights declined to the level of the animals that were operated on but did not receive the drug.

D. All of the above.

The thickness of the human oral epithelium was measured in seven different areas of the oral cavity in thirty cadavers. The results are tabulated below.

Area	Average	Range
A	500μ	125-950μ
B	362μ	178-780μ
C	254μ	130-489μ
D	238μ	156-320μ
E	204μ	135-270μ
F	68μ	30-146μ
G	123μ	35-260μ

213. Based on the above table, select the statement *contradicted by* the information given.

A. The oral epithelium has a wide range of thickness in the oral cavity.

B. The thinnest measurement was observed in Area G.

C. The results above are not valid because they were not attained from living subjects.

D. The range of thickness of the oral epithelium as observed was 30–950μ.

Drug X is administered to a patient and a certain value is monitored. After 30 days of treatment the physician studies the following values:

% of Drug X Administered	Days	Mean Value of Y
0.000	0	6.51
0.025	3	6.61
0.05	3	7.39
0.10	3	7.90
0.20	3	8.00
0.025	15	9.02
0.05	15	9.07
0.10	15	9.27
0.20	15	9.53
0.025	30	10.80
0.05	30	11.80
0.10	30	12.00
0.20	30	12.51

214. Based on the previous table, select the statement *not demonstrated by* the information given.

A. The drug has an effect.

B. There is a dose relationship to the response.

C. The dose administered is of critical importance as can be deduced from the values.

D. The physician can expect values of "Y" to continue to reflect dosage.

Distribution of relative amounts of radioiodinated amino acids in thyroid homogenates after administration of graded doses of PTU for three days.

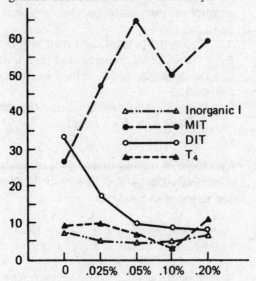

Distribution of relative amounts of radioiodinated amino acids in thyroid homogenates after administration of graded doses of PTU for six days.

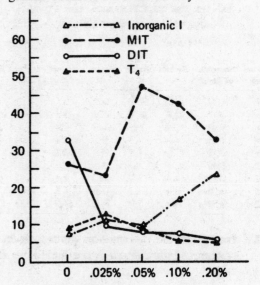

215. Based on the previous graphs, select the statement(s) *supported by* the information given.

    A. The percentage of labeled MIT increased and that of labeled DIT decreased; in the six-day treated group there is a rise and then a decline in the MIT detected.

    B. The amount of MIT rose from 26% in the controls to 64% in the three-day experimentally treated animals.

    C. A rise in the MIT/DIT ratio is observed.

    D. All of the above.

216. You have at your disposal benzene, bromine, nitric acid, and sulfuric acid. If you wish to produce *m*-bromonitrobenzene, you should:

    A. nitrate the benzene and then brominate.

    B. brominate the benzene and then nitrate.

    C. do either A or B. They work equally well.

    D. forget it. You cannot obtain the desired product with these materials.

217. One mole of methyl magnesium bromide will react with one mole of substrate to give the indicated product upon hydrolysis. Which substrate and product are correct?

    A. acetaldehyde → primary alcohol

    B. carboxylic acid → tertiary alcohol

    C. ester → ketone

    D. ketone → secondary alcohol

218.
$$A + B + C \xrightarrow{\text{E(enzyme)}} ABCD \rightarrow D + F + E$$
$$\quad (1) \qquad\qquad (2) \qquad (3) \qquad\qquad (4)$$

In the above reaction, the enzyme-substrate complex is represented by

    A. 1.   **C.** 3.

    B. 2.   **D.** 4.

219. Phenylamine is cooled to 0°C and treated with HCl and $NaNO_2$. After a few minutes of reaction time cuprous bromide is added, and the solution is heated.
What percent nitrogen is contained in the final aromatic product?

    A. 20   **C.** 8

    B. 15   **D.** 0

Model Examination B Answer Key

Verbal Reasoning

1.	D	14.	B	27.	D	40.	C	53.	C
2.	A	15.	D	28.	A	41.	C	54.	C
3.	C	16.	D	29.	C	42.	B	55.	C
4.	D	17.	C	30.	C	43.	C	56.	A
5.	B	18.	B	31.	C	44.	D	57.	D
6.	C	19.	D	32.	A	45.	A	58.	D
7.	D	20.	C	33.	D	46.	B	59.	C
8.	D	21.	C	34.	D	47.	D	60.	D
9.	D	22.	A	35.	D	48.	B	61.	D
10.	C	23.	C	36.	A	49.	C	62.	D
11.	B	24.	D	37.	A	50.	B	63.	C
12.	D	25.	D	38.	D	51.	C	64.	D
13.	D	26.	C	39.	D	52.	C	65.	D

Physical Sciences

66.	A	82.	B	98.	A	113.	A	128.	C
67.	B	83.	C	99.	D	114.	B	129.	C
68.	D	84.	B	100.	A	115.	B	130.	B
69.	B	85.	A	101.	C	116.	B	131.	D
70.	B	86.	B	102.	B	117.	C	132.	A
71.	B	87.	B	103.	C	118.	D	133.	D
72.	A	88.	C	104.	B	119.	C	134.	D
73.	B	89.	D	105.	C	120.	D	135.	D
74.	A	90.	D	106.	B	121.	C	136.	D
75.	B	91.	C	107.	C	122.	A	137.	A
76.	A	92.	A	108.	D	123.	D	138.	D
77.	C	93.	C	109.	B	124.	D	139.	A
78.	A	94.	A	110.	D	125.	A	140.	B
79.	C	95.	B	111.	B	126.	C	141.	D
80.	B	96.	D	112.	D	127.	B	142.	B
81.	A	97.	B						

Biological Sciences

143.	B	159.	C	175.	B	190.	C	205.	C
144.	C	160.	C	176.	A	191.	C	206.	B
145.	B	161.	A	177.	B	192.	B	207.	C
146.	A	162.	B	178.	D	193.	D	208.	B
147.	B	163.	B	179.	D	194.	C	209.	D
148.	D	164.	A	180.	D	195.	C	210.	D
149.	D	165.	D	181.	D	196.	B	211.	A
150.	A	166.	C	182.	C	197.	A	212.	D
151.	B	167.	B	183.	A	198.	A	213.	B
152.	C	168.	A	184.	A	199.	C	214.	C
153.	D	169.	D	185.	B	200.	D	215.	D
154.	A	170.	C	186.	D	201.	A	216.	A
155.	B	171.	D	187.	B	202.	B	217.	C
156.	B	172.	B	188.	A	203.	B	218.	C
157.	B	173.	D	189.	A	204.	D	219.	D
158.	D	174.	A						

Explanation of Answers for Model Examination B

VERBAL REASONING

1. **D.** At the end of the first paragraph, the author states the need for designers, clients, and students to understand the essence of graphic design. The remainder of the passage provides examples of the many objectives that this discipline accomplishes.

2. **A.** In sentence number two, the author speaks about the extraordinary flowering of this art form and describes it as a potent means of communication as well as a major component of our visual culture.

3. **C.** Paragraph four describes resonance as being the most important thing that graphic design provides. Resonance is viewed as a richness of tone that heightens the expressive power of a page.

4. **D.** Graphic design is a diverse field. The first five paragraphs include mention of each of the tasks given above. Problem solving can be found in paragraphs one and five; organization of space in paragraphs one and three; visual and symbolic qualities in paragraphs one, two, and three.

5. **B.** In paragraph three the author states that graphic design is a hybrid discipline in which, "Diverse elements, including signs, symbols, words, and pictures are collected and assembled into a total message."

6. **C.** The example of the designer explaining his job to his grandmother is used to illustrate the general public's confusion about graphic design. The answers he gives to her questions show that he has pulled together the talents of many people to produce his end result. The grandmother does not understand because she probably is used to an artist producing *a* work by himself rather than by coordinating the work of others.

7. **D.** Of all the statements listed, **D** has the least intense communication vocabulary in it. In a communication society, clear verbal and visual information are essential, expressive power in design conveys important messages, and instruction as well as motivation are important facets of keeping well informed.

8. **D.** In paragraph two the author says that a universal language of form is common to all visual disciplines, but that too much dependence upon other arts—such as architecture and painting—is unsatisfactory for graphic artists because their discipline has unique purposes and visual properties.

9. **D.** The passage clearly discusses all four answers to the question. The scientific method is detailed at the onset, scientific experimentation and responsibility are discussed, but definitely the author has written this text to debate and clarify the issues that surround the gathering, recording, and storing of scientific data.

10. **C.** The author makes the point that at various periods, different components of the scientific method have been emphasized. It is also emphasized that early on, propositions were formulated and debated with minimum organized observation or collection of data. The above statement would eliminate the several critical elements of the strict application of the scientific method as mentioned in **A**, **B**, and **D** of the question.

11. **B.** The passage makes it clear that throughout history a great deal of haphazard observing, recording, and analysis have occurred. It is stated in the article that with the coming of the industrial age, inventors focused on solutions, but that oftentimes they did not start with well formulated questions. The scientific method requires the above. Philosophers did give way to the age of the observers and observers gave way to the industrial age. There is no support in the passage for the claim that, as industrialization progressed, a clear scientific approach became standard for solving problems.

12. **D.** The passage does point out that inventors sought legal protection under constitutionally guaranteed rights to patent intellectual property. It is clearly stated at the end of paragraph one that record keeping now has become formalized, standardized, and required. Regulatory agencies not only can, but do require (according to the passage) that they be allowed to inspect complete records of product development. Statement IV is contradicted in paragraphs one and two; failed experiments should be recorded to eliminate repetition, and also unwanted results (e.g., toxicity of drug) should not be suppressed because harm might result.

13. **D.** None of the statements is supported by the passage. In paragraph three, the author makes the point that there is no universally accepted definition of data. The question asked in paragraph three is "are data the printouts of computers?" But no answer is provided, and this question is raised because we don't know what data are. Can we require scientists to record and store it? The paragraph ends asking who is responsible for keeping and storing data.

14. **B.** It is quite clear from the passage that an evolutionary process has been involved in the data collection process and that data keeping and storage have become ends unto themselves in order to ensure that work paid for was actually done. No mention is made regarding the must of a modified hypothesis, and the fact that managers of public funds are clearly inadequate to judge scientific work is inescapable.

15. **D.** The passage focuses on data collection and storage and makes it quite clear that the public's money is not well protected, that the public truly has no great trust in science, and that above all, scientific peer review and policing are flawed.

16. **D.** While all three statements are viable and reasonable, they are not discussed by the author.

17. **C.** The main theme of the passage deals with the shifting of decision-making power in school districts, from one where the board of education is the most important player to one where power is shared. Paragraph one states this in the opening sentence. The remainder of the passage goes on to name the parties that are becoming more powerful, especially teachers

and parents. The flow chart, which represents both traditional and modern decision-making power, graphically supports the information presented in the passage.

18. **B.** Paragraph two discusses the fact that today's teachers want to have a voice in program development as well as in determining salary scales. Later in the passage teachers are presented in an even more forceful light as their power to bring an educational system to a halt by means of strikes is noted.

19. **D.** Because the central theme of the passage discusses the fact that the board of education no longer holds absolute power in most school districts, **D** is a direct contradiction to the theme since it proposes that the power remain with the board.

20. **C.** Statement I, which talks about the emergence of parent volunteer programs in schools, and statement III, which claims that parents are becoming more powerful in schools, are both true according to the passage.

21. **C.** The *degree* of decision making power desired by the parties described in this passage is not mentioned and therefore **C**, which calls for *equality* of power, is not supported. The statement is not contradicted because a specific degree of power is not a topic of the passage.

22. **A.** The chart presents the traditional flow of power and communication by using a solid arrow that comes from the board of education down through the students. The modern flow is represented by the broken arrows, whose direction not only goes up and down but swings out between teachers and the superintendent and students and the principal.

23. **C.** The chart presented is a simplified version of a typical organizational flow chart. Parents operate outside of the organization in the sense that they are not elected or appointed to an official position, sign no contract, and receive no salary. Although the students represented on the chart also do not sign a contract and receive no salary, the implication of a contract exists. According to law, children must attend school until age 16.

24. **D.** All three statements are conclusions that reasonably could be drawn from this passage. Paragraphs one and two talk about the present

shift in decision-making power and allude to the fact that it will continue to occur. The chart shows how this has been liberalized. As parents become more involved in school affairs, the possibility of being a part of the policy making process may become a reality. As decision making becomes more decentralized and more site based, it will become harder to point to the decision maker because the latter process will be shared.

25. **D.** Although the fourteenth amendment is the vehicle that guarantees and protects a student's right to a public education, the main focus of this passage concerns expulsion from school, which would be a denial of that right.

26. **C.** Time-out procedures are not mentioned in this passage. Exclusion from school is the actual removal of a student from the educational setting. The difference between suspension and expulsion is described in paragraph two.

27. **D.** Expulsion from school generally is considered to be the most severe student punishment available to school administrators. In paragraph two of the passage, the author writes that state statutes and local policies usually provide that only a local school board has the prerogative to expel a student.

28. **A.** Paragraph three notes that in recent years litigation has involved both the right of school officials to exclude students as well as the rights that students have to due process prior to suspension and/or expulsion.

29. **C.** Although the matter had been treated in lower courts, *Goss v. Lopez* brought the exclusion question to the United States Supreme Court. The case is explained in paragraphs three through five.

30. **C.** Paragraph four points out that the right to a public education is a property right. Because the fourteenth amendment protects an individual's right to his/her property, the removal of a student from school would constitute an affront to his/her property.

31. **C.** Paragraph five explains that school officials *do* have the power to remove a student from the school setting, prior to suspension, if his/her presence constitutes a danger to persons or property and/or is disruptive to teaching and learning.

32. **A.** Paragraph seven discusses *Wood v. Strickland*. Although upholding the school board's actions in the case, the Court ruled that an individual member could be sued if he knew or reasonably should have known that a student's constitutional rights were denied.

33. **D.** The last paragraph discusses the fact that students have a right to nominal damages. In this case, *Carey v. Piphus,* punitive damages may also result if an official acted with malicious intent.

34. **D.** Paragraph two discussed the fact that criteria used in evaluations are similar for full-time and part-time faculty. Paragraphs seven and eight deal with research faculty, whereas the remaining paragraphs discuss clinical faculty. The issue of administrative faculty is not addressed specifically by the passage.

35. **D.** Paragraph four addresses the issues of bonding and identifying with an institution and also points out that long-term contracts would be one solution in the job security issue. The whole passage deals with the roles of several categories of faculty and the diverse issues posed and the need to find appropriate solutions. It is clearly stated in paragraph four that tenure is *not* the only way to achieve bonding.

36. **A.** Job security is discussed in paragraph four. The inequity of compensation and the evaluation criteria are addressed in paragraph two. Academic freedom is discussed in paragraph three and is a nonissue according to the author.

37. **A.** Paragraph two indicated that qualifications do not necessarily distinguish faculties and the level of the course taught does not reflect teaching ability. The argument that all students need qualified and enthusiastic instructors is made at the onset of paragraph one. Paragraph three indicates that academic freedom protects all faculty and introduction of changes is not limited. Paragraph two makes it quite clear that when students evaluate teaching, they may or may not know a faculty member's academic qualifications or tenure status.

38. **D.** None of the statements made is discussed in the passage.

39. **D.** Paragraph seven mentions the tripartite foundation of teaching, research, and public service. In paragraph three it is pointed out that the right of freedom of speech for all faculty members is guaranteed.

40. **C.** Paragraph nine makes the argument that much of clinical teaching is delivered by nontenure-eligible faculty who serve on a short-term basis and the activities are not linked solely with the generation of income. The passage is clear on the issue of relegation of nontenure-eligible faculty to second class citizenship. The last paragraph stresses that incentives and recognition are very important to clinical faculty members.

41. **C.** Paragraph two substantiates statements **A** and **B.** Paragraph four states that tenure means job security and bonds an individual to the institution. Paragraph nine makes it clear that the institution's reward system leans toward research.

42. **B.** Paragraph five makes it clear that the Red Cross believed that it should serve as an emergency relief organization and obtain its funds from private contributions. Hoover was invited to join the executive committee; Norman Davis was the head of the Red Cross.

43. **C.** Paragraph three points out that in all of Hoover's rescue efforts, children represented his first concern.

44. **D.** Paragraph one states that Hoover was a successful consulting engineer before he undertook his relief activities.

45. **A.** The last line of the passage leaves no doubt that Hoover's and Roosevelt's camps did not agree with each other. Paragraph one mentions that Hoover took an active part in negotiating between the warring factions and that his efforts were not limited to war victims. He helped handily the victims of the Mississippi floods of 1927.

46. **B.** Hoover (paragraph five), within less than two weeks of outbreak of hostilities, raised the relief question and suggested that one organization should provide a focal point. Paragraph four ends with the line that hungry people cannot defend themselves nor defend freedom. Paragraph three makes it clear that Mrs. Hoover supported her husband's efforts.

47. **D.** There can be no doubt in the reader's mind that Hoover was a humanitarian with an interest in helping victims.

48. **B.** This question truly should awaken the reader to the fact that the whole passage, including the references and credits, should be read. In the credit it is pointed out that the material was presented at a conference on education of the gifted for the twenty-first century.

49. **C.** Paragraph four states that tragedies are potentially effective for developing ethics and even wisdom. The last paragraph emphasizes that teachers can put key ideas together for wise leadership in individuals of the next generation. It is proposed that teachers determine and give birth to the future. **D** tries to mislead you drastically, but careful reading of paragraph seven points out that the author distinguishes between ethical skills and ethical knowledge, which is the development of right reasoning.

50. **B.** The author in paragraph one does not speak of unavoidable mistakes, major injustices, or personal grief. However, faulty logic is presented and associated with the word *hamartia*.

51. **C.** In paragraph four it is pointed out that Dewey feared a danger of either dogmatism or a sense of unreality when students are abruptly introduced to theoretical ideas. He proposes to first introduce students to simple cases and then proceed to the more complex.

52. **C.** Paragraph nine reasons that teacher preparation of material keeps the cases current, and in this way the cases help future generations.

53. **C.** Paragraphs seven through nine emphasize the combination of student feedback and teacher production of material (formulating good and humane reasoning) to be an essential skill in the passing on of a sense of ethics from one generation to another.

54. **C.** This passage is a biography because it is a history of a person's life written by someone else; an autobiography is written by the person himself/herself.

55. **C.** Paragraph one mentions that the artist left home at the age of sixteen and that the interview took place 20 years later.

56. **A.** It should be clear to the reader that most things concerning this artist's career evolved in a haphazard fashion. Because the artist concentrates on war pictures, mother nature takes on a minor role.

57. **D.** Because there is no evidence to the contrary and because the candidate has a respectable job and position, it is quite safe to assume that the M.A. in Photography is an appropriate terminal degree.

58. **D.** Paragraph one mentions that the artist was chased out of his home. After a theft, he was given an option of jail or the army (paragraph four). This photographer learned his trade in the army and probably has an interest in war photography in general because he enjoys confrontation.

59. **C.** One of the main points of the entire passage is that strange twists of fate that determine an individual's destiny often are the results of entirely unpredictable events. In this case, rather than going to jail the individual wound up in the army, a turn of events that led ultimately to his interest in photography.

60. **D.** Paragraph one makes it clear that all three statements in the question are true.

61. **D.** Paragraph two discusses the issue of cost/benefit in disaster planning measures. Paragraph three, four, and five deal with quantification, whereas paragraph six mentions the fortress, hot, warm, cold, and privately owned sites, and the reciprocal processing agreements.

62. **D.** The last paragraph mentions that the two most important management issues involved in disaster planning are who is responsible and which applications get top priority. It is also pointed out that a formal plan should be the final outcome of the process.

63. **C.** Paragraph four points out that statistical means are a technique used by a company to establish priorities. Paragraph five emphasizes that each scenario must be financially analyzed and weighed against competing corporate projects. It is pointed out in paragraph one that less than 50 percent of central data processing sites have adequate contingency plans.

64. **D.** Paragraph three deals with the determination of cost and mentions initial costs, costs over a three to five year period, and a company's borrowing rate.

65. **D.** Paragraph seven stresses that the fortress system is probably very well prepared for disasters. In paragraph eight it is mentioned that hot sites are associated with high costs. Paragraph nine states that cold sites provide space only, and there is concern about proper coverage and the shared membership arrangement.

PHYSICAL SCIENCES

66. **A.** Humans can only hear the range of frequencies from about 20 Hz to 20,000 Hz, thus no one can hear the upper end of the frequency range given.

67. **B.** A doubling of the intensity of a source of sound corresponds to an increase of 3 dB in the apparent loudness level. The dB level is given by: $dB_1 = 10 \log_{10}(I/I_o)$. The problem solution proceeds as follows:
$$40 \text{ dB} = 10 \log_{10} (I_1/I_o)$$
$$\text{or} \quad 4 = \log_{10} (I_1/I_o).$$
Then the dB level for two speakers (with $I_2 = 2I_1$) is:
$$\begin{aligned} dB_2 &= 10 \log_{10} (I_2/I_o) = 10 \log_{10} (2I_1/I_o) \\ &= 10 \log_{10} (2) + 10 \log_{10} (I_1/I_o) \\ &= 3 \text{ dB} + 40 \text{ dB} = 43 \text{ dB}. \end{aligned}$$

68. **D.** The power is given by $P = VI$ where V and I are the rms values for ac circuits. Note that the formula has the same form for direct current circuits.

69. **B.** The ac form of Ohm's Law is the same as for dc circuits,
$V = IZ$ where Z is the impedance in ohms.
$Z = 120 \text{ V}/2.2 \text{ A} = 54.5$ ohms.

70. **B.** The beat frequency one hears is given by the difference of the two frequencies ($f_b = 456 - 450 = 6$ Hz).

71. **B.** The result is obtained from the sketch by calculating
$$y = L - L\cos\emptyset,$$
where $L\cos\emptyset$ is the vertical side of the right triangle of acute angle 45° and hypotenuse $L = 0.8$ m.

72. **A.** In this question, one uses the conservation of energy principle, equating the loss of gravitational potential energy, mgy, to the gain of kinetic energy, $1/2\ mv^2$.
$1/2\ mv^2 = mgy$ or $v^2 = 2gy$
thus $v = \sqrt{2(9.8\text{m/s}^2)(0.23\text{m})}$.

73. **B.** The equation for the period is given. $L = 0.8$ m with $g = 9.8$ m/s^2.

74. **A.** The frequency, in Hz, is always the reciprocal of the period, in seconds.
$f = 1/T = 1/1.8$ s.

75. **B.** The falling weight of mass 1.2 kg loses potential energy, mgh ($h = 0.4$ m). Because 54 minutes (3240 s) is the time for $3240/2 = 1620$ cycles, the energy lost per cycle is:
$(1.2\text{ kg})(9.8\text{m/s}^2)(0.4\text{m})/(1620) = 0.003$ joules/cycle.

76. **A.** As long as the angle is a small angle, the period is independent of the angle of release. The answer is the same as for a release angle of 8° (1.8 seconds).

77. **C.** The equivalent resistance for series connections of resistors is equal to the sum of the individual resistances.
$R_s = R_1 + R_2 + R_3$, and so on. Then $I = V/R_s$ from Ohm's law; so I = 1 A.
The individual voltage drops are also found using Ohm's law,
V = 1 A × 2 ohm = 2 volts.

78. **A.** No DC current can flow through the capacitor. The 6 volts does appear across the capacitor (when it is fully charged).

79. **C.** For a parallel connection, the full 120 volt drop occurs across both resistors. Then
$I = V/Z = V/R = 120/2 = 60$ amperes AC, is the current through each resistor. (Note that $Z = R$ for a "pure" resistance.)

80. **B.** The rules for parallel and series combinations of resistors must be used to find the equivalent total resistance. ($1/R_p = 1/R_1 + 1/R_2 = 1/2 + 1/2$ and then $R_p = 1$ ohm) ($R_s = R_3 + R_p = 3$ ohms = the equivalent resistance) Using Ohm's law again,
$I = 6$ volts/3 ohms = 2 amperes.

81. **A.** The solution to this problem requires one to calculate the impedance Z for the RC series circuit. Here $Z = \sqrt{(X_c)^2 + R^2}$ where $X_c =$

$1/(2\pi\ fC)$ where f is the 60 Hz frequency and C is 1×10^{-6} Fd. The AC form of Ohm's law then gives $I = V/Z = 120/2653 = .045$ amperes.

82. **B.** The energy for the motion comes from the expanding compressed spring so that energy is not "conserved" here. However, the total momentum of the two cart system is constant. Because the initial total momentum was zero, the final momentum of the system is also zero, i.e. $P_i = P_f$, or
$0 = m_1v_1 + m_2v_2$
and $v_2 = -m_1v_1/m_2 = -1.0$ m/s.

83. **C.** Because of the spring steel bumper we may assume that the total kinetic energy of the two cart system is conserved as well as the total momentum. There are two equations that apply, namely:
$m_1v_1 + 0 = m_1v_1 + m_2v_2$ and
$1/2\ m_1v_1^2 + 0 = 1/2\ m_1v_1^2 + 1/2\ m_2v_2^2$.
All the m's are equal, so $V_1 + V_2 = 2$ m/s and $V_1^2 + V_2^2 = 4$ m^2/s^2. The equations are satisfied only if one of the V's is 0 and the other is 2 m/s. The solution of these two equations shows that the first cart stops, giving up all its kinetic energy to the second cart. Hence, $V_2 = 2.0$ m/s in the same direction as the original velocity of cart #1.

84. **B.** In this question the energy dissipated due to air friction is apparent because of the decrease in the kinetic energy of the cart.
$E_{\text{lost}} = 1/2\ mv_i^2 - 1/2\ mv_f^2 = 1.6$ joules
($m = 0.45$ kg, $v_f = 3.0$ m/s, and $v_i = 4.0$ m/s.)

85. **A.** If one equates the energy loss in explanation for question 84 to the (negative) work done by friction over the distance of x = 2.0 meters;
$F_f x = 1.6$ joules, then $F_f = 0.8$ N.

86. **B.** This question deals with the interchange of energy between the forms of kinetic energy and gravitational potential energy. The total energy is conserved but does change form.
$KE_i = PE_f$
$1/2\ mv^2 - 0 = mgh$. Solving this for $v = \sqrt{2gh}$ we find that $v = 3.13$ m/s.

87. **B.** As above we use the conservation of linear momentum principle with the initial momentum of the system equal to zero. $v_2 = -1.0$ m/s.

88. **C.** The added pressure caused by the height, y, of the blood of density d is $P = dgy = (1050$ $kg/m^3)(9.8 \ m/s^2)(1 \ m) = 10300 \ N/m^2$.

89. **D.** The flow rate is given by Av where A is the cross-sectional area and v is the fluid velocity. Because the flow rate is constant through both the wide and constricted portions of the pipe $A_1v_1 = A_2v_2$ and the area of the circular cross-section is $A = d^2/4 \ (d = 2r)$; $A_2 = 4A_1$ then v_2 is 4 times greater than v_1.

90. **D.** The linear velocity of a point traveling in a circle is related to its angular velocity by $v = Rw$ where w is the angular velocity in rad/s. For this problem $w = 3 \ rev \times 2\pi \ rad/rev$.

91. **C.** The diffraction grating formula gives the angular position of each diffracted image of order n for light of wavelength λ where the grating spacing is d.
    $n \lambda = d \sin\theta$.
    Here $n = 2$, $d = 10^{-3} \ m/600$ lines, and then, $\sin\theta = 0.74$, $\theta = 48°$.

92. **A.** The time for the vertical fall is the same for both balls:
    $y = 1/2 \ gt^2$ because the initial vertical velocity component is zero for both balls. The y and t values are the same for both balls. The problem can then be answered by inspection since only the first (A) answer has both times the same.

93. **C.** The thin lens formula is used to find the image distance. $1/f = 1/p + 1/q$, where p is the object distance and q is the image distance. f and p are positive so the formula gives $q = -6.7$ cm. The image is on the same side as the object and is virtual, upright, and magnified.

94. **A.** The concept used in this problem is that the work done by the force is equal to the gain in kinetic energy. $Fs = 1/2mv^2 - 0$, because the mass starts from rest. (Alternatively, one can calculate the acceleration using Newton's second law and then use the equation of uniformly accelerated motion, $v^2 = 0 + 2as$, for the case where the initial velocity is 0.)

95. **B.** In each half-life the activity will decay an additional fraction of 1/2. If the total time is an integer number of half-lives as it is in this problem (24 hours = 4 half-lives of Tc-99m) one can find the fraction remaining as follows:

$1/2 \times 1/2 \times 1/2 \times 1/2 = 1/16$.
Then: $A = 1/16 \times 100$ mCi $= 6.3$ mCi
(If the time is not an integer number of half-lives one must use the exact expression for exponential decay;
$A = A_o e -(0.693 \ t/T)$, where A_o is the initial activity and T is the half-life.)

96. **D.** Both the total nucleon number and the total charge are constant in a nuclear reaction. The number of nucleons is the sum of all protons and all neutrons, whereas the charge number is the sum of all proton charges. Here the total charge is 42 and the total number of nucleons is 99. Thus: $42 = Z - 1$ or $Z = 43$ for Tc and $99 = A + 0$ so that $A = 99$ for Tc.

97. **B.** Given that the half-life (the time for one-half the original nuclei to decay) is 67 hours for Mo^{99}, we find that 5.5 days is very nearly two half-lives. Thus after 5.5 days only 1/4 or 0.25 remains.

98. **A.** The effective half-life is given by the expression $1/Te = 1/T_{phy} + 1/T_{bio}$ so that the effective values is always less than either T_{phy} or T_{bio}. One should be able to answer the question without knowing the exact form of the above equation by realizing that biological excretion helps rid the body of the original radioactive material at the same time it is decaying. (There is only one answer, A, smaller than T_{phy}).

99. **D.** Because one half-life for Tc99m has elapsed since 8:00 the activity must have been two times larger at 8:00 AM. (The activity in curies is the number of decays per second, 1 Ci $= 3.7 \times 10^{10}$ dps.)

100. **A.** As in question 96 above, the total nucleon number and total charge on each side of the decay equation are constants. Thus the number of nucleons remains 201 $(201 + 0 = 201)$, whereas the charge on the nucleus decreases by 1 $(81 - 1 = 80)$

101. **C.** 9.25 days is equal to three half-lives for Tl-201. The fraction remaining is then:
    $1/2 \times 1/2 \times 1/2 = 1/8$. Thus 1/8 of 80 mCi remains.

102. **B.** This problem is simply a conversion problem in effect because all necessary information is given.
    $(70 \ mrad/mCi) \times (10 \ microCi/kg) \times 70 \ kg = ?$
    One must convert millicuries and microcuries

to the same units so that they will cancel. 10 microCi = 0.010 millicuries. The result is 490 millirads.

103. **C.** As the term implies, only gamma radiation is emitted in the decay. This is desirable because particle radiation, such as electrons and alpha particles, cannot escape the body tissue and thus cannot be detected. Such particles would expose the patient to radiation damage without any useful result.

104. **B.** Because Technicium-99m emits no particles, the whole dose is due to gamma radiation and the rem dose is the same as the rads. 400 mrads = 400 mrems.

105. **C.** The fraction penetrating must be less than 1%, i.e. less than 0.01. One can multiply 1/2 by itself until the result is less than 0.01. This requires 7 terms: $1/2 \times 1/2 \times 1/2 \times 1/2 \times 1/2 \times 1/2 \times 1/2 = 0.0078$. Thus 7 half-thicknesses $= 7 \times 0.4$ cm = 2.8 cm of lead is required.

106. **B.** One mole of three is 33%.

107. **C.** It is necessary to recall the approximate atomic weights: C—12; O—16; H—1. Thus the weights are 44g for CO_2, 34g for H_2O_2, and 32g for O_2. The total weight is 110g and 44/110 = 0.4 or 40%.

108. **D.** The number of molecules in a mole of any compound is 6.0×10^{23} (Avogadro's number).

109. **B.** The elements would be C, O_2, and H_2. By inspection there would be one mole of C, three moles of O_2, and one mole of H_2. The C would be a solid and there would be four moles of gas (3 + 1).

110. **D.** Under conditions of standard temperature and pressure, a mole of any gas will occupy 22.4 liters. Thus one mole each of CO_2 and O_2 will occupy a total of 2(22.4) = 44.8 liters. H_2O_2 is a liquid. One mole of H_2O_2 is only 34g and will occupy less than 0.05 liters.

111. **B.** $BaCl_2$ can reversibly hydrolyze to form 2 HCl and $Ba(OH)_2$. The HCl will be strongly ionized, providing large numbers of hydrogen ions. $Ba(OH)_2$ will be weakly ionized, providing few hydroxyl ions. There will be a net contribution of hydrogen ions. NaCl and $NaNO_3$

can each reversibly hydrolyze to form a strong base and a strong acid. There will be no net contribution of hydrogen or hydroxyl ions. Sodium acetate can reversibly hydrolyze to form a weak acid (acetic acid) and a strong base (NaOH). There will be a net contribution of hydroxyl ions.

112. **D.** See explanation for question 111. Sodium acetate can reversibly hydrolyze to form NaOH and acetic acid, producing a net contribution of hydroxyl ions.

113. **A.** NaCl and $NaNO_3$, each a salt of a strong acid and a strong base, will be essentially neutral.

114. **B.** The temperature of 383°K is equal to 110°C. Although the salts will increase the boiling point of water, it should boil at or below this temperature.

115. **B.** No significant change will be noted on dilution of this salt of a strong base and a strong acid.

116. **B.** Heat is transferred through the solid by conduction. Silver is a good conductor of heat.

117. **C.** Stainless steel is not as good a conductor of heat as is silver, and the handle of the stainless steel spoon will not become so hot or so quickly.

118. **D.** Transfer of heat through a gas or vacuum is quickly accomplished in line of sight by radiation. The heat is carried at the speed of light by infrared rays.

119. **C.** The screen would block transfer of heat by radiation. Instead, the heat would be more slowly transferred as the fire heats the air, producing convection currents.

120. **D.** Transfer of heat from a heat source to another body through a gas is quickly accomplished by radiation.

121. **C.** It is noted that there are two moles of gas on the left side of the equation and one mole on the right side. Considering the fact that one mole of gas occupies a volume of 22.4 liters at standard temperature and pressure, imposition of greater pressure should favor the shift of equilibrium to the right, thus reducing the total number of moles of gas.

122. **A.** Two moles of gas are noted on the left side of the equation and three moles on the right. Thus greater pressure should shift the equation to the left, favoring H_2S.

123. **D.** Because two moles of gas are noted on each side, a pressure change should not affect the equilibrium of the reaction.

124. **D.** A and B are both correct. Without a change in K_{eq}, the addition of either reactant on the left side will result in more of the product on the right side, which uses up some of the H_2.

125. **A.** Without a change in temperature or pressure, addition of material on one side of an equilibrium equation will result in more of a product or products on the other side. This will occur without a change in K_{eq}.

126. **C.** $pK_b = -\log K_b$ = between 4 and 5 (by inspection).

127. **B.**
$$K_b = \frac{[NH_4^+][OH^-]}{[NH_3]} = \frac{[OH^-]^2}{0.01}$$
$$= 1.8 \times 10^{-5}$$
$$[OH^-]^2 = (0.01)(1.8 \times 10^{-5})$$
$$= 1.8 \times 10^{-7}$$
$$[OH^-] = 4 \times 10^{-4}$$
$$pOH = -\log[OH^-] = \text{between 3 and 4}$$
(by inspection).

128. **C.** $pH = 14 - pOH = 14 - 3.40 = 10.60$.

129. **C.** $pK_b = -\log K_b$ = between 5 and 6 (by inspection).

130. **B.**
$$K_b = \frac{[HyH^+][OH^-]}{[Hy]} = \frac{[OH^-]^2}{0.001}$$
$$= 1.7 \times 10^{-6}$$
$$[OH^-]^2 = (0.001)(1.7 \times 10^{-6})$$
$$= 1.7 \times 10^{-9}$$
$$[OH^-] = \text{about } 4 \times 10^{-5}$$
pOH is between 4 and 5.

131. **D.** $pH = 14 - pOH = 14 - (\text{between 4 and } 5) = \text{between 9 and 10}$.

132. **A.** As the smallest pK_a will give the lowest pH, the smallest pK_b will give the lowest pOH and the highest pH.

133. **D.** The Lewis theory or concept does not deal specifically with hydrogen ions or hydroxyl ions.

134. **D.** NaOH is a strong base and is assumed to be virtually completely ionized.

135. **D.** $pOH = -\log[OH^-] = -\log(1 \times 10^{-3}) = 3$
$pH = 14 - pOH = 11$.

136. **D.** The half-reactions for the given reaction are as follows:
oxidation: $2Fe^{2+} \rightarrow 2Fe^{3+} + 2e^-$
reduction: $Cl_2 + 2e^- \rightarrow 2Cl^-$
An oxidizing agent is defined as the substance being reduced. In this redox equation, Cl_2 is being reduced and is the oxidizing agent.

137. **A.** Nonpolar covalent bonds are formed between atoms of the same element or atoms with the same electronegativity. The F_2 molecule has one nonpolar covalent bond only and is therefore a nonpolar molecule.

138. **D.** An acid reacts with a base to form a salt and water. KOH is a base.

139. **A.** This is a definition of an ionic bond. It results in two ions of opposite charge.

140. **B.** Although different sublevels have different maximum numbers of orbitals, any one orbital can hold a maximum of two electrons.

141. **D.** The smaller the K_{sp}, the less soluble the salt. Of the four choices, AgI has the smallest K_{sp} (the largest negative exponent).

142. **B.** A substance can act as both an oxidizing agent and a reducing agent only if the oxidation state of the element can become higher and lower than it is. There are no lower oxidation states for Fe^0 and Cu^0; there are no higher oxidation states for Fe^{3+}.

WRITING SAMPLE

Part 1, Essay

A wise man, according to Johnson, is one who knows that dreams and hopes are no substitute for reality. Though it may not always be pleasant or exciting to know what the next day will bring, there is no wisdom in reaching out for something exciting or pleasant when one cannot be sure that it is there. A realist has more hope to find happiness if he takes his reality and alters it than one who casts about in the dark hoping to find a pot of gold. A man may take his last dollar and buy a lottery ticket, hoping to win a jackpot, but the wise man will take his last dollar and use it to buy food. Though the foolish man may think that because he is desperate, good, and deserving and that God or fate will intervene on his behalf, the wise man knows that fate and God will do little to even the odds. The wise man knows he needs food more than he needs a one in seven million chance of becoming rich.

But what courage does it take to face each day that is the same as the last? Is it wise to keep one's feet firmly planted on the ground, taking no risks? To stay with what is certain out of fear of the unknown is certainly safe, but it may be unwise. Imagine a shoe retailer is approached by a partner who has developed a new last and leather that will make women's shoes more comfortable to wear, but they will appear just as stylish. The partner asks the store owner to place the new shoes in his front window, and for this favor the two will share whatever profits come from the venture in half. The shoe salesman refuses, knowing that the shoes he has shown in his window for the last five years have brought in a steady stream of customers. Though he is not getting rich, at least he is certain that his current display works. The partner sets off to find another store owner, discovering one only three doors down from the first shop he visited. The second owner takes the risk, for he knows that nothing great is achieved without some peril. For days the first shoe salesman sees streams of people walking by his store, and wondering where they are going, peeks outside to see them entering his competitor's shop. Word has spread, and even the first shopkeeper's regular male customers desert him for the shop down the street. Though women buy the new shoes for themselves, men pick them up for their wives; and while they are in the shop, they find it convenient to buy their own shoes there, too. The first shopkeeper goes out of business, blaming himself for not having the wisdom to have faith in a good, albeit unproved, idea.

Had the shopkeeper been wiser, perhaps what he would have seen was that this was not a matter of uncertainty. It is possible that had he been thinking, he would have recognized that it was a certainty that women would want to wear a more comfortable shoe, and that though it seemed new and risky to stock the new shoes, there was no risk involved at all. The wisdom is not in an unwillingness to make a change, it is in the unwillingness to make a change without considering the realistic possibilities of it. The chances involved in buying a lottery ticket make it such an impossible odd that the wise man will reject the notion of spending his last dollar on it. The chances that women will prefer comfortable and stylish shoes over uncomfortable and stylish shoes, however, is not a chance at all. It is reasonable to assume that given the choice between discomfort and comfort the customer will choose comfort. A wise man knows a certainty when he sees it, and he knows that sometimes what appears to be a risk is not a risk at all. By the same token, a wise man knows when a safe offer

is really a risk, and no matter how often he says, "I need this money, surely fate will let me have it. It is only fair that one who is as deserving as I should win" will not change the odds in a lottery. So the wise man is indeed one who will not quit certainty for uncertainty, but it is the same wise man who knows the difference.

Part 1
Explanation of First Response: 6

This essay focuses clearly on Johnson's statement and addresses each of the three writing tasks. Paragraph one explains what the statement means, paragraph two gives a specific situation in which men would not be wise to give up a certainty for an uncertainty, and paragraph three explores circumstances that determine whether it is wise or unwise to give up a certainty for an uncertainty.

The paper provides an explanation of the quotation by introducing "reality" as a qualifier for "certainty" and "dreams and hopes" for "uncertainty." This allows the author to cite concrete examples like the one that refers to the lottery to complete the explanation by referring to realistic and unrealistic acts. Through an effective example in paragraph two, the paper illustrates that safety, contrary to the implication of the quotation, may sometimes be unwise, as the first owner discovers. Finally the passage provides a balanced analysis of the things that determine whether quitting certainty for uncertainty is wise or unwise.

The writing in this essay is clear and controlled. The writer's use of concrete examples is one of the strongest features of the passage. They grow logically out of the main ideas of each paragraph and illustrate the ideas very effectively. The lottery ticket example is easy to relate to as an example of the uncertainty of taking a long shot, whereas the shoe shop example provides a clear example of a time when acting on at least mild uncertainty can be wise indeed. There is variety in the sentence structure, and the paper flows smoothly from one sentence to the next.

Part 2, Essay

Graham Green's definition of destruction is really only an argument of semantics. Because "create" only means to bring into being, to cause to exist, then any act of change is also an act of creation. The idea is not a new one and appears in even as ancient a myth as that of the phoenix, who rises again out of the ashes of its own funeral pile. What Green is suggesting is an alternative perspective by which one could view or interpret destruction. The connotations of "destruction" are generally negative ones. Green is offering another option and a more optimistic one, a view of destruction as a new beginning or a sort of rebirth.

Taken only at literal face value, Green's statement could be a dangerous one. It could be taken as an argument for anarchy, chaos, or, even more specifically, violence and murder. Of course, this would all depend on whether or not the interpreter sees "creation" as always a positive end. Further, it would depend on whether or not creation is viewed as an end or a means. For example, murder, for most people, is certainly not a positive thing. It is, however, undeniably an act of destruction. It is also undeniably an "end" of sorts, as an unalterable change. Murder is an act of destruction that separates the corporeal existence from the spiritual one. Because there is nothing really *new* that exists as a result, because it is not a means of propagating other possibilities, one could argue that murder is an act of destruction that is not, in fact, also an act of creation.

To destroy is to disintegrate or to demolish, to cause a cessation of one form of existence. What would follow would inevitably be another form of existence. For example, if I demolish my house, then I, by default, create a pile of rubble. I could even say that I have created that pile of rubble, because it did not exist before I demolished my house. To create is to bring into being. Because (granted that we are not dealing with the loss of matter) destruction is the ceasing of one thing to exist in its present state, then one is always creating a new state of being with every destruction. The taking of a life would be one possible exception because the dead body has not been created and there is no accounting for the spirit that has been "lost." In general, however, the relationship between destruction and creation is inevitable, as one necessitates the other.

Part 2
Explanation of Second Response: 4

This essay does a nice job with tasks one and three. Paragraph one explains the statement by giving a traditional definition of "create," commenting then on connotations of destruction, and finally suggesting how Green offers another option for seeing acts of creation. Paragraph two expands the explanation and moves toward a general example, murder, which might not, because it is not "positive," be considered an act of creation. The final paragraph examines the circumstances that determine the relationship between creation and destruction.

The paper has many strengths. The essay is thoughtful, and it flows smoothly from sentence to sentence, paragraph to paragraph. The use of transitions, such as "however" in the final sentence, pro-

vides coherence. The paper shows sensitivity to language, particularly in its examination of the denotation and connotation of creation and destruction. The paper would have received a rating of 5 or 6 if it had dealt more directly with the second task: that of providing a specific situation in which destruction is not a form of creation. The example of murder as such remains too general. The example of the demolition of the house in the final paragraph is effective in making the paper more concrete. Other such examples in the rest of the paper would be helpful.

BIOLOGICAL SCIENCES

143. **B.** Individuals 6, 20, and 23 could be produced by dominant defective alleles (either autosomal or sex-linked) only if all three cases resulted from new mutations since the parents in all three cases have only normal phenotypes. Because mutations are specified as rare, this is unlikely. A recessive autosomal defective allele could explain all observations down through individual 18, but the presence of a defective allele in individual 19 is unlikely due to no occurrences of the defect in that individual's ancestors and the low incidence of new mutations. The sex ratio of defective individuals (all male except for one female, and she had a defective father) is highly unlikely for an autosomal recessive defective allele. The expected probability of males among defective offspring is ½ for a recessive autosomal allele (i.e., normal chance of male offspring), so the probability of the observed sex ratio among defective offspring is very unlikely. For these reasons, a defective autosomal recessive allele is not a likely explanation. An X-linked recessive defective allele easily explains all observations. Defective male offspring received an X chromosome containing a recessive defective allele from their mothers (most of whom are normal due to a dominant normal allele on their other X chromosome) and the recessive allele determined their phenotype since the Y chromosome contained no allele for the characteristic. Most females were normal due to a normal allele on the X chromosome received from their fathers. The defective female (9) received a defective X from both parents.

144. **C.** Female 1 must contain one normal allele (because she has a normal phenotype and she produced normal male 8) and one defective allele (because she produced defective male 6).

145. **B.** Male 6 would contain only one allele for the characteristic since he (like all normal human males) has only one X chromosome. The Y chromosome from his father lacks an allele for the characteristic. His defective phenotype must be produced by a defective allele on his X, so he contains only defective alleles.

146. **A.** Male 8 would have one allele for the characteristics (on his single X chromosome—see explanation for question 3). Because his phenotype is normal, the allele must be normal, and he would contain only normal alleles.

147. **B.** Female 9 must have two X chromosomes (like all normal human females). Because her phenotype is defective, both X chromosomes must contain defective alleles. Female 9 would therefore contain only defective alleles.

148. **D.** All of the statements of the question were supported by the data. Although it would have been a good assumption that crude pituitary extract would have a lesser effect than pure FSH, one must examine the data. In our case the extract did affect every organ, however, the weight increase was less than when FSH was administered. With the data available concerning the effect of pituitary extract, it is safe to assume that hypophysectomy would have resulted in decreased organ weights. Remember, FSH in the female stimulates the growth of the ovarian follicle, whereas in the male it stimulates the testes to produce sperm.

149. **D.** FSH in the female stimulates the development of the ovarian follicle and the production of estrogen; LH and prolactin are responsible for the corpus luteum, which secretes progesterone and prepares the uterus for implantation of the fertilized egg. Because uterine growth was observed in our case, it is safe to assume that FSH was not of the highest purity. Our data neither supports nor contradicts the statement that FSH and LH are necessary for estrogen secretion. Because our data shows that FSH did not affect the thyroid and adrenal glands, the statement that FSH primarily affects the reproductive organs is supported.

150. **A.** The data shows that FSH in the male had its greatest effect on the seminal vesicles and not the prostate gland. Statements (B) and (C) are not supported nor contradicted, whereas statement (D) is a truism supported by the data; body weights did not vary significantly.

151. **B.** The pituitary gland is located within the sella tursica.

152. **C.** Stress and strain will have a pronounced influence on the output of epinephrine and norepinephrine by the adrenal medulla. Activation of the sympathetic portion of the autonomic nervous system will result in increased activity by the adrenal medulla which can be considered the site of the postganglionic cell bodies of that segment of the sympathetics.

153. **D.** The reproductive cycle is under hormonal regulation; gonadotropic hormones of the pituitary (anterior lobe) stimulate the ovaries to produce a mature egg. The pituitary and ovaries have a reciprocal effect upon each other. FSH (follicle stimulating hormone) from the pituitary elicits estrogen production from the developing follicle. When estrogen concentration reaches a certain blood level, it inhibits FSH production. At that time the egg is discharged and the cells lining the follicle come under the influence of another gonadotropin LH (luteinizing hormone), which influences the development of the corpus luteum. The corpus luteum produces the hormone progesterone which influences the wall of the uterus in preparation for implantation. As the concentration of progesterone rises, LH production is checked. If fertilization has occurred, the production of FSH is curtailed throughout the period of gestation through the production of estrogen by the placenta and ovary. If fertilization does not occur, the cycle begins anew.

154. **A.** FSH stimulates morphogenesis of the follicle primarily, whereas LH is required for either estrogen or progesterone synthesis. FSH and LH are required during the follicular phase.

155. **B.** The interstitial cells are stimulated by ICSH (interstitial cell stimulating hormone, which is identical with LH in the female) a gonadotrophin of the pituitary to produce androgens. Testosterone is an androgen.

156. **B.** The pituitary secretes ACTH, FSH, LH, TSH, and STH. ACTH acts on the adrenal cortex; FSH and LH on the gonads; TSH on the thyroid, and STH on the general system. The adrenal medulla can be considered to house the post ganglionic neurons for part of the sympathetic portion of the autonomic nervous system and is responsible for epi- and norepinephrine production.

157. **B.** Between 3 to 4 ml of semen comprise one ejaculate which contains between 300–400 million sperm cells.

158. **D.** Terminal branches transmit impulses to other neurons.

159. **C.** Protein synthesis is mainly carried out by the ribosomes. Let us identify the components of the neuron numbered: (2) nucleus with nucleolus, containing the genetic material of the cell and directing the synthetic activity of the cell; (3) Golgi apparatus (zone), the packaging and concentrating area of the cell's secretory activity; (4) dendrites, the processes that pick up an impulse and carry it towards the cell body; (5) endoplasmic reticulum (rough in this case—ribosomes are attached), the synthetic machinery of the cell (proteins etc.,); (6) cell membrane, semipermeable and the protector of the cell from its environment; (7) cytoplasm (specifically the area here is called the axon hillock); (8) myelin sheath (Schwann cell covered by its neurilemma, the insulator of the axon; (9) direction of conduction of an impulse; axons (10a) conduct impulses away from the cell body to the junction with the dendrites of another neuron. The junction point is known as the synaptic area; the impulse can cross the synapse only from the axon to the dendrite and no backflow is permitted; (11) terminal branches of the axon. In a lesion (cut) the process distal from the cell body would completely degenerate; retrograde degeneration would be detected in the proximal portion and the cell body, however, the proximal portion has the capacity to regenerate.

160. **C.** Lysosomes contain hydrolytic enzymes and are also known as digestive (suicide) bags.

161. **A.** The chemical mediator of cholinergic nerve impulses is acetylcholine and is released by the axon terminals.

162. **B.** The neuron is a cellular element; as a highly specialized cell, it carries out the function of neuronal transmission. A nucleus is a cluster of nerve cell bodies within the central nervous system (brain and spinal cord), whereas a ganglion is defined as a cluster of nerve cell bodies outside the central nervous system (sympathetic chain ganglia, celiac plexus, and so on).

163. **B.** The neurolemma of an axon is part of the Schwann cell (outer membrane).

164. **A.** Ectoderm is the germ layer of origin of the nervous system.

165. **D.** The gray matter of the spinal cord is divided into two (2) components: motor and receptor. The motor part is comprised of the ventral and intermediolateral columns and gives rise to the ventral roots. Ventral horn cells supply voluntary muscles; intermediolateral cells give rise to preganglionic sympathetic fibers of the thoraco-lumbar system. The receptor portion is located in the dorsal horn. The white matter of the spinal cord is composed of nerve fibers in a network of connective tissue.

166. **C.** Blood pressure is usually measured by placing the sphygmomanometer cuff around the arm compressing the brachial artery and vein. Maximum blood pressure is obtained during ventricular contraction (systole); in our case 160. Minimum blood pressure indicates ventricular rest (diastole); in our case 90.

167. **B.** The medulla is a part of the brain stem and connects to the spinal cord at the foramen magnum. The following cranial nerves are associated with the medulla: a, XII—hypoglossal nerve; b, XI—spinal accessory nerve; c, X—vagus nerve; d, IX—glossopharyngeal nerve; e, VIII—stato-acoustic nerve; and f, portions of the facial nerve (VII). The vagus nerve (X) is the most important parasympathetic nerve. Stimulation of vagal fibers slows the heart rate; constricts the smooth muscles of the bronchial tree; stimulates secretion by the bronchial mucosa; and promotes peristalsis, gastric, and pancreatic secretions. Blood pressure control also involves aortic body, carotid sinus, and carotid body receptor modulation by the glossopharyngeal (IX) and vagus (X) nerves.

168. **A.** From the right ventricle blood is sent to the lungs via the pulmonary arteries; this blood is rich in carbaminohemoglobin and the CO_2 will be exchanged for O_2. Blood returns from the lungs to the left auricle via the pulmonary veins; this blood has been oxygenated and is rich in oxyhemoglobin. Blood then passes to the left ventricle and then out via the aorta to supply the tissues of the body.

169. **D.** The sympathetic component of the autonomic nervous system mobilizes the body's reserves in case of emergencies.

170. **C.** Skeletal (striated) muscle is under volun-

tary control. The autonomic nervous system innervates cardiac muscle, smooth muscle, and glands. Arrector pili musculature is associated with skin and is smooth musculature.

171. **D.** A sarcomere is the region between two Z bands. In simple terms we are dealing with this unit: ZIAHAIZ. Contraction of the sarcomere is due to the fine filaments (actin) sliding between the thick filaments (myosin) pulling the Z bands to which they are attached. This pulls the Z bands closer together, and so the sarcomeres are shortened.

172. **B.** In skeletal muscle, the nuclei are found peripherally. To complete the chart, the speed of contraction should also be mentioned. Skeletal muscle is the fastest working, smooth the slowest, and cardiac muscle occupies an intermediate position.

173. **D.** Heart beat is initiated by the S-A (sinoatrial) node, which is also known as the pacemaker.

174. **A.** Incubation of gp120 with increasing concentrations of CPFDD reduced binding of the gp120 to CD4+ cells to nearly zero (see Figure 1), so CPFDD inhibited the binding. CPFDF caused partial inhibition at low concentrations, but caused much less inhibition at higher concentrations than CPFDD (see Figure 1).

175. **B.** See explanation for question 174.

176. **A.** In Figure 1, a 50 uM/L increase in CPFDD concentration caused the largest reduction in fluorescence at the beginning of the curve.

177. **B.** In Figure 2, p24 production by infected T cells + H9 cells + CPFDD was severely reduced, but was not totally prevented. After 6 days of incubation, p24 production is increasing and is greater than p24 production by infected T cells alone. Therefore the inhibition was strong but not total.

178. **D.** In Figure 2, p24 production by infected T cells + H9 cells + CPFDF was very similar to infected T cells + H9 cells. Therefore no inhibition was detectible in the experiment.

179–181. **(179-D) (180-D) (181-D).** As can be seen from the table, there are four major blood types and the explanation as to universal donor and recipient is based on the following:

Type	Agglutinogens on Cells	Agglutinins in Serum and Plasma
AB—can receive A, B, AB, or O (universal recipient)	A, B	none
A—can receive A, O	A	anti b
B—can receive B, O	B	anti a
O—can receive only O, but can give to all; therefore, O is the universal donor	O	anti ab

182. **C.** The ABO blood grouping system is explained on the basis of a single triallelic system with genes A, B, and O operating at a single genetic locus. Phenotypic and genotypic characteristics may be expressed as follows:

Phenotype	Genotype
A	A/A; A/O
B	B/B; B/O
O	O/O
AB	A/B

The A and B genes appear to be codominant; they are dominant over O, which is recessive.

183. **A.** See explanations for questions 179–182. One gene from each parent can produce any of the four combinations named.

184. **A.** Any substance that has the capability to elicit an immunological response, such as the production of antibody that is specific to that substance, is considered an antigen.

185. **B.** The molality (m) of a solution is the number of gram molecular weights (moles) in 1000 g of solvent. For the example given, the solution density is 1.15 g/ml—meaning that 100 ml weighs 115 g. This includes 25 g of compound X, so that the solvent weighs 90 g (115–25). The number of moles is 0.200 moles (25 g of X divided by molecular weight of 125). This number of moles (0.200) is in 90 g, so the molality is

$$\frac{0.200 \text{ moles}}{90 \text{ g}} = \frac{\text{number moles}}{1000\text{g}}$$

and that results in 2.2 m.

186. **D.** The molarity (M) of a solution is the number of gram molecular weight (moles) in 1 liter (1000 ml) of solution. For the example given here, 25.0 g of compound X (molecular weight 125) is 0.200 moles in 100 ml of solution. Therefore in 1000 ml there are 2.00 moles and this is 2.00 mole/liter, that is 2.00 M.

187. **B.** Percent is parts per hundred. The solution weighs 115 g (1.15 g/ml times 100 ml). Because 25.0 g of compound X is in this solution, the percent is $25/115 \times 100$ and therefore is 21.7%.

188. **A.** A 2 M solution contains 2 moles/1 of X. Thus 20 ml of solution would contain 20 ml × 2 moles/1000 ml = 0.04 moles.

189. **A.** 20 ml of Y solution contains 20 ml × 0.4 moles/1000 ml = 0.008 moles. The volume of X solution which contains the same number of moles = 0.008 moles × 1000 ml/2 moles = 4 ml.

190. **C.** Although blocking the activation of the phosphatases by blocking the effect of calcium (step 3), the CKII activation pathway would also be blocked. For this reason, (A) and (D) are incorrect. The autophosphorylation of CKII at step 5 is the final step in the activation of CKII. A block here, as suggested by **B**, would not increase but inhibit CKII activity; hence **B** is also a poor choice.

191. **C.** CKII activity could be decreased by blocking calcium influx, calmodulin activation of CKII, or autophosphorylation. There are more than the single sites suggested in (A) and (B). Blocking dephosphorylation by the phosphatase, step 7, **D**, would serve to *increase,* not decrease, CKII activity.

192. **B.** Only a Voltage Operated Channel (VOC) is opened by depolarization alone. As stated in the passage, a Receptor Operated Channel (ROC) is opened by the binding of an appropriate ligand. The question states that depolarization is produced and no neurotransmitter ligand is present, so **A** and **C** are incorrect.

193. **D.** This comes straight out of the reading: A kinase is an enzyme that transfers phosphoryl groups from a high energy donor to a suitable substrate. **A** is incorrect, because a phosphatase antagonizes the actions of a kinase by *removing phosphoryls* from phosphoproteins.

Catalases and transferase, **B** and **C,** are enzymes, but their specific functions are not phosphorylating phosphorproteins. If you chose one of these answers you attempted to address more than the question asked. Stick with the simple approach and do not read anything extraneous into the question.

194. **C.** The question requires that you synthesize two pieces of given information. First, that both the CKII activation and inactivation (phosphatase) pathways are activated by calcium and, second, that the phosphatase response to calcium is slower than other components of the system. **D** suggests the reverse of this situation and is therefore wrong. It is plausible that is less phosphatase than kinase (**B**), however, this is not addressed in the reading and you would have no basis for arriving at this interpretation. **A,** also not addressed in the reading, would not constitute a plausible mechanism for CKII to function. It would suggest a mechanism that would render CKII permanently nonfunctional.

195. **C.** All have the same molecular formula, and only III is capable of intermolecular hydrogen bonding.

196. **B.** II is the only aldehyde of the four. I and IV form hydrazones but do not give a positive Tollen's test.

197. **A.** On hydrogenation, I is converted to:

$$
\begin{array}{c}
OH \\
| \\
CH_3-C-CHCH_3 \\
|| \\
HCH_3
\end{array}
$$

in which the carbon with the hydroxyl group is chiral.

198. **A.** The reaction sequence is:

$$
CH_3CH{=}0 + CH_3CHMgBr \xrightarrow[\substack{H_3O^+}]{\text{then}} CH_3CHCHCH_3 \xrightarrow{K_2Cr_2O_7} I
$$

$$
\begin{array}{cc}
| & | \\
CH_3 & CH_3
\end{array}
$$

with OH over the central carbon.

199. **C.** Compound III has a double band to react with Br_2. The hydroxyl group is given priority in numbering.

200. **D.**
$$\frac{0.5 \text{ mg}}{0.1 \text{ ml}} = \frac{X}{10 \text{ ml}}$$

$$X = \frac{(0.5)(10)}{0.1} = 50 \text{ mg}$$

This 50 mg represents the total amount in the entire 3 ml of plasma that was extracted.

$$\frac{50 \text{ mg}}{3 \text{ ml}} = \frac{X}{100 \text{ ml}}$$

$$X = \frac{(50)(100)}{3} = 1667 \text{ mg}/100 \text{ ml}$$

201. **A.** See the explanation to answer 200. The calculation is based on 100 ml plasma, not on the total amount of plasma.

202. **B.** Exceeding the linear range would ordinarily lead to a lower absorbance than expected. An error in weighing to prepare the standard solution would introduce a constant error. The remaining possibility, a pipetting error, is most likely. Pipetting errors may be positive or negative.

203. **B.** Cholesterol is an intermediate in the biosynthesis of steroid hormones, bile acids, and vitamin D. Essential fatty acids and essential amino acids must be consumed by the organism in the diet.

204. **D.** Prostaglandins are potent compounds; they are structurally unique in the respect that they contain 20 carbon atoms and are formed from essential fatty acids. They affect the nervous system, circulation, reproductive organs, and metabolism.

205. **C.** Adrenocorticotropic hormone (ACTH) is produced by the beta cells of the pituitary and stimulates the adrenal cortex to produce glucocorticoids, which increase blood sugar and liver glycogen levels. The function of the adrenal medulla is to secrete adrenalin and noradrenalin. These compounds affect the vascular system, the heart, and respiration. One must assume that being housed in an elevated temperature setting is a stressful situation and, besides an increase in water consumption due to sweating, heart rate would be elevated. ACTH levels should remain fairly steady.

206. **B.** Thyroid hormones control the rate of metabolism and the growth, maturation, and differentiation of the organism, and influence nervous system activity. Five events are associated with thyroid hormone production: (1) trapping iodine; (2) oxidation of iodide to organic iodine; (3) hormone synthesis; (4) storage of thyroglobulin; and (5) release of hormone into the circulation. Increased activity by the organ is known as hyperthyroidism. The experimenter was interested in determining the influence of cold exposure on parameters used to assess thyroid function. Cold has a significant effect on ^{131}I uptake and serum PBI and the animals were in a hyperthyroid state physiologically.

207. **C.** The statement: there is a significant difference between tumor-bearing animals and their controls indicating some degree of cellular sensitization, is not investigated and this conclusion cannot be made from the data presented; all the other statements are supported by the data.

208. **B.** The visual system is made up of the eye and complex nerve pathways for interpretation by the cerebral cortex. Seeing starts with the ganglion cells of the retina, optic nerve, optic chiasma (nasal retinal field fibers cross), optic tract, lateral geniculate body, optic radiations, visual cortex (area 17 of occipital lobe of cerebrum). In lesion 2, the uncrossed fibers of the right optic nerve are affected and the patient would show a deficit in his/her medial optic field.

209. **D.** A careful look at the data shows that temperature could indirectly influence life span, that females tend to live longer, and that radiation has a more deleterious effect on males.

210. **D.** Bone marrow is the largest organ in the body (4.5% of total body weight); red bone marrow is hemopoietic, whereas fat is predominant in yellow bone marrow. Lymphopoiesis is a function of the thymus and occurs mostly during fetal and early postnatal life. The thymus produces circulating lymphocytes known as T cells, which migrate to lymph nodes and the spleen where they give rise to immunologically competent cells. The thymus also is thought to stimulate lymphocyte production and enhance immunological competence. Because in our experiment neither bone marrow nor thymus cells alone induced antibody production, the hypothesis of cell cooperation can be accepted. Because thymocytes did not produce a response statement, **D** is contradicted by the results.

211. **A.** Careful scrutiny of the data shows that the percentage of Factor 3 increased and that of Factor 2 decreased, with a resultant rise in Factor 3/Factor 2 ratio. No consistent trend could be seen for Factor 4. Factor 6 showed a decline in the 12-day group and that could be due to decreased amounts of Factors 2 and 3. For the various factors, the 12-day period sometimes produced more and sometimes less outcome than the 6-day period.

212. **D.** This problem can be solved easily by careful analysis as to what takes place under the three experimental conditions, comparing graph 1 to graph 2. All statements in the question are supported by the evidence.

213. **B.** Careful analysis shows that there exists a wide range of thickness in oral epithelium (30–950μ) lining the oral cavity. A quick calculation yields an average thickness of 238μ. The thinnest measurement was observed in area F and, therefore, statement **B** is contradicted by the results.

214. **C.** Examination reveals that statement **C** is neither supported nor contradicted by the information. That the drug has an effect and that a dose/response is present is clear, however, that the dose is of critical importance cannot be deduced from the values and, therefore, statement **C** is not demonstrated by the evidence.

215. **D.** The function of the thyroid is to produce the thyroid hormones T_3-triiodothyronine and T_4-tetraiodothyronine or the thyroxin. Iodine plus tyrosine yields monoiodotyrosine (MIT); the union of two units of MIT produces diiodotyrosine (DIT) and the adding of one more MIT yields triiodothyronine (T_3). If to T_3 an MIT is joined, thyroxin (T_4) is the product; if two DIT's unite, thyroxin also is formed. Scrutiny of the presented data shows that all three statements are supported by the information presented and that propylthiouracil (PTU) interferes with thyroid hormone production; PTU is an antithyroid compound used to treat patients.

216. **A.** Remember that nitro groups are deactivating, meta-directing substituents and that halogens are deactivating, ortho, para-directing substituents. If bromination precedes nitration, then very little m-bromonitrobenzene will result.

217. **C.** Under the stated conditions aldehyde (except formaldehyde) → secondary alcohol; carboxylic acid → methane + carboxylic acid; ester → ketone; ketone → tertiary alcohol.

218. **C.** Substrate(s) or reactant(s) react(s) with the enzyme to form an enzyme-substrate complex. This complex breaks down into product(s) and frees enzymes ready for formation of a new enzyme-substrate complex.

219. **D.** We have described conditions for the formation of a diazonium salt and then replacement of the diazonium salt by Br to produce monobromobenzene. (The replacement is known as the Sandmeyer reaction.) The intermediate diazonium salt is often unstable at room temperature, so a lower temperature is used.

The MCAT
Model Examination C

ANSWER SHEET

DIRECTIONS: After locating the number of the question to which you are responding, fill in the circle containing the letter of the answer you have selected. Use pencil (not a ballpoint pen) to completely blacken the circle.

VERBAL REASONING

1. Ⓐ Ⓑ Ⓒ Ⓓ
2. Ⓐ Ⓑ Ⓒ Ⓓ
3. Ⓐ Ⓑ Ⓒ Ⓓ
4. Ⓐ Ⓑ Ⓒ Ⓓ
5. Ⓐ Ⓑ Ⓒ Ⓓ
6. Ⓐ Ⓑ Ⓒ Ⓓ
7. Ⓐ Ⓑ Ⓒ Ⓓ
8. Ⓐ Ⓑ Ⓒ Ⓓ
9. Ⓐ Ⓑ Ⓒ Ⓓ
10. Ⓐ Ⓑ Ⓒ Ⓓ
11. Ⓐ Ⓑ Ⓒ Ⓓ
12. Ⓐ Ⓑ Ⓒ Ⓓ
13. Ⓐ Ⓑ Ⓒ Ⓓ
14. Ⓐ Ⓑ Ⓒ Ⓓ
15. Ⓐ Ⓑ Ⓒ Ⓓ
16. Ⓐ Ⓑ Ⓒ Ⓓ
17. Ⓐ Ⓑ Ⓒ Ⓓ
18. Ⓐ Ⓑ Ⓒ Ⓓ
19. Ⓐ Ⓑ Ⓒ Ⓓ
20. Ⓐ Ⓑ Ⓒ Ⓓ
21. Ⓐ Ⓑ Ⓒ Ⓓ
22. Ⓐ Ⓑ Ⓒ Ⓓ
23. Ⓐ Ⓑ Ⓒ Ⓓ
24. Ⓐ Ⓑ Ⓒ Ⓓ
25. Ⓐ Ⓑ Ⓒ Ⓓ
26. Ⓐ Ⓑ Ⓒ Ⓓ
27. Ⓐ Ⓑ Ⓒ Ⓓ
28. Ⓐ Ⓑ Ⓒ Ⓓ
29. Ⓐ Ⓑ Ⓒ Ⓓ
30. Ⓐ Ⓑ Ⓒ Ⓓ

31. Ⓐ Ⓑ Ⓒ Ⓓ
32. Ⓐ Ⓑ Ⓒ Ⓓ
33. Ⓐ Ⓑ Ⓒ Ⓓ
34. Ⓐ Ⓑ Ⓒ Ⓓ
35. Ⓐ Ⓑ Ⓒ Ⓓ
36. Ⓐ Ⓑ Ⓒ Ⓓ
37. Ⓐ Ⓑ Ⓒ Ⓓ
38. Ⓐ Ⓑ Ⓒ Ⓓ
39. Ⓐ Ⓑ Ⓒ Ⓓ
40. Ⓐ Ⓑ Ⓒ Ⓓ
41. Ⓐ Ⓑ Ⓒ Ⓓ
42. Ⓐ Ⓑ Ⓒ Ⓓ
43. Ⓐ Ⓑ Ⓒ Ⓓ
44. Ⓐ Ⓑ Ⓒ Ⓓ
45. Ⓐ Ⓑ Ⓒ Ⓓ
46. Ⓐ Ⓑ Ⓒ Ⓓ
47. Ⓐ Ⓑ Ⓒ Ⓓ
48. Ⓐ Ⓑ Ⓒ Ⓓ
49. Ⓐ Ⓑ Ⓒ Ⓓ
50. Ⓐ Ⓑ Ⓒ Ⓓ
51. Ⓐ Ⓑ Ⓒ Ⓓ
52. Ⓐ Ⓑ Ⓒ Ⓓ
53. Ⓐ Ⓑ Ⓒ Ⓓ
54. Ⓐ Ⓑ Ⓒ Ⓓ
55. Ⓐ Ⓑ Ⓒ Ⓓ
56. Ⓐ Ⓑ Ⓒ Ⓓ
57. Ⓐ Ⓑ Ⓒ Ⓓ
58. Ⓐ Ⓑ Ⓒ Ⓓ
59. Ⓐ Ⓑ Ⓒ Ⓓ
60. Ⓐ Ⓑ Ⓒ Ⓓ

61. Ⓐ Ⓑ Ⓒ Ⓓ
62. Ⓐ Ⓑ Ⓒ Ⓓ
63. Ⓐ Ⓑ Ⓒ Ⓓ
64. Ⓐ Ⓑ Ⓒ Ⓓ
65. Ⓐ Ⓑ Ⓒ Ⓓ

PHYSICAL SCIENCES

66. Ⓐ Ⓑ Ⓒ Ⓓ
67. Ⓐ Ⓑ Ⓒ Ⓓ
68. Ⓐ Ⓑ Ⓒ Ⓓ
69. Ⓐ Ⓑ Ⓒ Ⓓ
70. Ⓐ Ⓑ Ⓒ Ⓓ
71. Ⓐ Ⓑ Ⓒ Ⓓ
72. Ⓐ Ⓑ Ⓒ Ⓓ
73. Ⓐ Ⓑ Ⓒ Ⓓ
74. Ⓐ Ⓑ Ⓒ Ⓓ
75. Ⓐ Ⓑ Ⓒ Ⓓ
76. Ⓐ Ⓑ Ⓒ Ⓓ
77. Ⓐ Ⓑ Ⓒ Ⓓ
78. Ⓐ Ⓑ Ⓒ Ⓓ
79. Ⓐ Ⓑ Ⓒ Ⓓ
80. Ⓐ Ⓑ Ⓒ Ⓓ
81. Ⓐ Ⓑ Ⓒ Ⓓ
82. Ⓐ Ⓑ Ⓒ Ⓓ
83. Ⓐ Ⓑ Ⓒ Ⓓ
84. Ⓐ Ⓑ Ⓒ Ⓓ
85. Ⓐ Ⓑ Ⓒ Ⓓ
86. Ⓐ Ⓑ Ⓒ Ⓓ
87. Ⓐ Ⓑ Ⓒ Ⓓ
88. Ⓐ Ⓑ Ⓒ Ⓓ

89. Ⓐ Ⓑ Ⓒ Ⓓ
90. Ⓐ Ⓑ Ⓒ Ⓓ
91. Ⓐ Ⓑ Ⓒ Ⓓ
92. Ⓐ Ⓑ Ⓒ Ⓓ
93. Ⓐ Ⓑ Ⓒ Ⓓ
94. Ⓐ Ⓑ Ⓒ Ⓓ
95. Ⓐ Ⓑ Ⓒ Ⓓ
96. Ⓐ Ⓑ Ⓒ Ⓓ
97. Ⓐ Ⓑ Ⓒ Ⓓ
98. Ⓐ Ⓑ Ⓒ Ⓓ
99. Ⓐ Ⓑ Ⓒ Ⓓ
100. Ⓐ Ⓑ Ⓒ Ⓓ
101. Ⓐ Ⓑ Ⓒ Ⓓ
102. Ⓐ Ⓑ Ⓒ Ⓓ
103. Ⓐ Ⓑ Ⓒ Ⓓ
104. Ⓐ Ⓑ Ⓒ Ⓓ
105. Ⓐ Ⓑ Ⓒ Ⓓ
106. Ⓐ Ⓑ Ⓒ Ⓓ
107. Ⓐ Ⓑ Ⓒ Ⓓ
108. Ⓐ Ⓑ Ⓒ Ⓓ
109. Ⓐ Ⓑ Ⓒ Ⓓ
110. Ⓐ Ⓑ Ⓒ Ⓓ
111. Ⓐ Ⓑ Ⓒ Ⓓ
112. Ⓐ Ⓑ Ⓒ Ⓓ
113. Ⓐ Ⓑ Ⓒ Ⓓ
114. Ⓐ Ⓑ Ⓒ Ⓓ
115. Ⓐ Ⓑ Ⓒ Ⓓ
116. Ⓐ Ⓑ Ⓒ Ⓓ
117. Ⓐ Ⓑ Ⓒ Ⓓ
118. Ⓐ Ⓑ Ⓒ Ⓓ

119. (A) (B) (C) (D)
120. (A) (B) (C) (D)
121. (A) (B) (C) (D)
122. (A) (B) (C) (D)
123. (A) (B) (C) (D)
124. (A) (B) (C) (D)
125. (A) (B) (C) (D)
126. (A) (B) (C) (D)
127. (A) (B) (C) (D)
128. (A) (B) (C) (D)
129. (A) (B) (C) (D)
130. (A) (B) (C) (D)
131. (A) (B) (C) (D)
132. (A) (B) (C) (D)
133. (A) (B) (C) (D)
134. (A) (B) (C) (D)
135. (A) (B) (C) (D)
136. (A) (B) (C) (D)
137. (A) (B) (C) (D)
138. (A) (B) (C) (D)
139. (A) (B) (C) (D)
140. (A) (B) (C) (D)
141. (A) (B) (C) (D)
142. (A) (B) (C) (D)

WRITING SAMPLE
Use separate ruled sheets of paper.

BIOLOGICAL SCIENCES
143. (A) (B) (C) (D)
144. (A) (B) (C) (D)
145. (A) (B) (C) (D)
146. (A) (B) (C) (D)
147. (A) (B) (C) (D)
148. (A) (B) (C) (D)
149. (A) (B) (C) (D)
150. (A) (B) (C) (D)
151. (A) (B) (C) (D)
152. (A) (B) (C) (D)
153. (A) (B) (C) (D)
154. (A) (B) (C) (D)
155. (A) (B) (C) (D)
156. (A) (B) (C) (D)
157. (A) (B) (C) (D)
158. (A) (B) (C) (D)
159. (A) (B) (C) (D)
160. (A) (B) (C) (D)
161. (A) (B) (C) (D)
162. (A) (B) (C) (D)
163. (A) (B) (C) (D)
164. (A) (B) (C) (D)
165. (A) (B) (C) (D)
166. (A) (B) (C) (D)
167. (A) (B) (C) (D)

168. (A) (B) (C) (D)
169. (A) (B) (C) (D)
170. (A) (B) (C) (D)
171. (A) (B) (C) (D)
172. (A) (B) (C) (D)
173. (A) (B) (C) (D)
174. (A) (B) (C) (D)
175. (A) (B) (C) (D)
176. (A) (B) (C) (D)
177. (A) (B) (C) (D)
178. (A) (B) (C) (D)
179. (A) (B) (C) (D)
180. (A) (B) (C) (D)
181. (A) (B) (C) (D)
182. (A) (B) (C) (D)
183. (A) (B) (C) (D)
184. (A) (B) (C) (D)
185. (A) (B) (C) (D)
186. (A) (B) (C) (D)
187. (A) (B) (C) (D)
188. (A) (B) (C) (D)
189. (A) (B) (C) (D)
190. (A) (B) (C) (D)
191. (A) (B) (C) (D)
192. (A) (B) (C) (D)
193. (A) (B) (C) (D)

194. (A) (B) (C) (D)
195. (A) (B) (C) (D)
196. (A) (B) (C) (D)
197. (A) (B) (C) (D)
198. (A) (B) (C) (D)
199. (A) (B) (C) (D)
200. (A) (B) (C) (D)
201. (A) (B) (C) (D)
202. (A) (B) (C) (D)
203. (A) (B) (C) (D)
204. (A) (B) (C) (D)
205. (A) (B) (C) (D)
206. (A) (B) (C) (D)
207. (A) (B) (C) (D)
208. (A) (B) (C) (D)
209. (A) (B) (C) (D)
210. (A) (B) (C) (D)
211. (A) (B) (C) (D)
212. (A) (B) (C) (D)
213. (A) (B) (C) (D)
214. (A) (B) (C) (D)
215. (A) (B) (C) (D)
216. (A) (B) (C) (D)
217. (A) (B) (C) (D)
218. (A) (B) (C) (D)
219. (A) (B) (C) (D)

The MCAT
Model Examination C

VERBAL REASONING

9 PASSAGES
65 QUESTIONS
85 MINUTES

DIRECTIONS: The questions are based on the accompanying passages. Read each passage carefully, then answer the following questions. Consider only the material within the passage. For each question, select the *ONE BEST ANSWER* and indicate your selection by marking the corresponding letter on the Answer Form.

Passage I (Questions 1–7)

Before responsibility for preserving records of data can be placed, it is necessary to determine who owns scientific data. In industry, the ownership of data and records of data is well established, and formalized in employment contracts. In universities and research institutes, the matter is not so clearly defined although it is clear that the federal government expects an institution to exert ownership of data resulting from federally funded grants and contracts, and to be prepared to take immediate possession of data, and to store and preserve scientific data for some unspecified period. It is not the universal practice or culture of universities to claim ownership of scientific data. In fact, most investigators believe that they own the data derived from their investigations and plan to take their databooks with them in the event that they relocate. There is less consistency in perceptions of ownership of data of research trainees. Many research trainees feel that they own the data derived from their studies, whereas some preceptors are very clear that they expect the data to remain with them. Universities are confronted with a serious dilemma in that institutions of higher education have long acknowledged that members of the academy own their inspiration, concepts, and scholarly writings. Universities, however, have occasionally laid claims to the products of assigned projects, works of art, and computer programs created by members of the academy. Who then owns an application for a research grant or contract? This is not a matter solely for esoteric discourse, but a subject of faculty grievance and litiga-

tion. Federal granting agencies provide for the transfer of sponsorship of grants, grant applications, and equipment from one institution to another, but to date, federal agencies do not provide for the transfer of ownership of scientific data, with attendant rights and responsibilities, from one institution to another. This appears to be an inconsistency in federal policy and practice.

There remain the questions of custody and storage of data. Should custody of data records be vested in technicians, trainees, laboratory managers, or heads of laboratories? Who has the right of access to data records and under what circumstances? Can a laboratory head require trainees to share data, or conversely, forbid trainees and technicians from sharing data? Under what circumstances may an administrator seize custody of data records to measure progress, audit for quality, search for inventions, or search for breaches in scientific conduct? How are data records to be stored and for how long? Must chromatographic gels be preserved, or photographs of them or tracings and scans of them, or written notes describing noteworthy features of the gel? Who pays for preservation, storage, and cataloging of data records? What steps must be taken to prevent loss by deterioration, removal, or destruction (e.g. by fire)? How long must data records be kept and what is the temporal reference point: when the observations were made, when the source of funding ended, or when the data were last used in a claim, report, or publication?

It must be recognized that there are differences between discovery research and work performed to substantiate a claim made to a regulatory body. Much of scientific research lies somewhere between fundamental investigations and applied work for commercialization. There is no doubt that research training

---

Adapted from S. Gaylen Bradley, *Basic Sciences*, Vol. 1, no. 4, MCV/VCU, 1990.

today must include instruction on data collection and proper recording of data. There is a need for clear understanding among members of a research team about the custody of data records and the ownership of data. Institutions must establish and communicate policies about data storage and ownership. There may be a need for formal written agreements between investigators and the institution, and between the institution and sponsors. The scientific community and research institutions need to work with federal granting agencies and public policymakers to develop meaningful definitions, appropriate policies and guidelines, and practical strategies to address scientific data, their collection, recording, custody, ownership, storage, access, and cataloging. The problem requires immediate attention by scientists, administrators, regulators, and policymakers. The institution has the responsibility to assist investigators by providing resources, including a quality assurance unit, to provide guidance about these complex issues.

1. With regard to scientific data:

   A. ownership is clearly established.
   B. federal agencies lay immediate claim to data after a contract has expired.
   C. preserving it is a burden the investigator must bear.
   D. there remain questions of custody and storage.

2. Which of the following statements is *supported by* the passage?

   A. It really is not necessary to struggle with the questions as to who owns data.
   B. Industry has an informal agreement with employees and inventions stay with the company.
   C. Rules are quite clear as to the time factor involved concerning the preservation of data.
   D. Universities do not usually claim ownership of data.

3. The passage argues that:

   A. original data, no matter what form, must be preserved.
   B. the costs of preservation should be borne by the investigator.
   C. the time factor when preservation should start is determined by when the source of funding ended.
   D. custody of records is not a settled issue.

4. The author of the passage believes that:
   I. institutions must establish policies regarding data.
   II. research teams should discuss and clarify as to who controls the data.
   III. grants can be transferred.
   IV. federal agencies guide the transfer of data and ownership of it from institution to institution.

   A. I, II, and III   C. II and IV
   B. I and III   D. IV only

5. Which of the following statement(s) is/are *supported by* the passage?
   I. There are no differences between discovery and verification.
   II. Written agreements usually are not necessary to establish ownership.
   III. Public policymakers have defined the problem at hand.
   IV. Institutions should provide leadership concerning the data issue.

   A. I, II, and III   C. II and IV
   B. I and III   D. IV only

6. Which of the following is/are *neither supported nor contradicted* by the passage?

   A. The public feels that the scientific community has a good grasp of the issues.
   B. Regulatory agencies require complete documentation for their evaluation.
   C. Without data storage, projects would not be completed.
   D. All of the above.

7. The passage would support:

   A. a clarification as to the rights of trainees in respect to their findings.
   B. the right of an administrator to take control of documents and see to it that data is properly shared, stored, and utilized.
   C. regulations that data should be stored uniformly for seven years, just as is in the case for income tax documents.
   D. the view that although there is a problem, it should be resolved slowly.

Passage II (Questions 8–15)

The dependence process begins with an initial exposure to a psychoactive drug. The drug experience allows an individual to perceive two contrasting altered states of consciousness, the normal state versus the drug-induced state. If the drug state is perceived by an individual as more pleasurable (or producing a less painful state) than the nondrug state, then such an individual may make a choice of maintaining the drug state. The word pleasurable, however, has many meanings, and may not be related to "feeling good." Thus, someone may initiate smoking tobacco, for example, not because it makes him/her feel good (most times it doesn't) but because his/her specific peer group dictates tobacco use as a means of acceptance. Belonging to the group is pleasurable, not the use of tobacco; any drug can serve such a purpose. Many examples of this drug-human interaction can be noted, and the lesson learned, is that humans take drugs for many reasons that essentially meet their own individual needs, whether it be feeling good, peer pressure, or whatever.

Therefore, drugs may not always serve primarily as reinforcers of behavior but may have important secondary reinforcing qualities as well. Regardless of the reasons for using a specific chemical agent, however, it should be understood that most drugs produce their effects via an alteration of brain neurochemistry, which can lead to other more long-term problems, especially if the drug is consumed on a chronic basis.

Once an individual takes on the responsibility of using a given chemical agent chronically, then he/she is beginning to allow other variables to take over his/her own drug taking behavior, and to some degree will lose his/her ability to control this behavior. Taking drugs repeatedly means that one swallows, injects, sniffs, or smokes a given agent at certain times, in certain places and possibly with certain people. Each time a drug is taken all these events become cumulatively conditioned with the drug forming a conditioned-stimulus (cs) complex (learned associations). If repeated enough times, the drug takes on stimulus properties initiating certain effects psychologically. Thus, if one associates smoking behavior with feeling good with friends (peer control), then one may need to smoke when those friends are not present to feel good. Conversely, the presence of friends may also act as a stimulus to smoking. What occurs is that the use of the drug can come under environmental (stimulus) control and behavior comes under drug-induced stimulus control. Over time these events can merge to a point where drug taking becomes more and more contingent upon environ-

mental events. The example of this stimulus-complex may be too simplistic, but one may be able to significantly reduce his/her pain by going through the drug taking ritual without administering the drug. Thus, the pharmacological effects of morphine, for example, may be elicited by going through the ritual including an injection of water. Counselors feel that some heroin addicts may be addicted to the needle, and thus the term, "needle freaks." Much of these effects are difficult to detect but have been verified in controlled human experiments. We should not take these effects lightly and should suspect that similar CS complex can occur with most drugs we take.

Acute behaviorally effective doses of psychoactive drugs generally disrupt most learned behaviors. Thus, alcohol acutely disrupts the ability of any individual to drive an automobile. However, if the individual continues to drive under the influence of alcohol, then two things can occur. First, the individual will develop behavioral tolerance to the alcohol. That is, such a person will learn to adapt to the drug state and will learn how to manage his/her automobile in spite of the pharmacological effects of alcohol. As this process continues, the learning of how to drive the car and how to get to certain places (to the ABC store) can also become contingent upon the alcohol state. Thus, an individual may have difficulties finding the ABC store when sober. This phenomena is called *drug-induced state dependent learning*. Its premise is that the retention of information learned under the drug state is contingent upon the reinstitution of the drug state. There are many examples of this with most psychoactive drugs. In fact, one might consider this a form of dependence. Thus, a person may need to continue using a specific drug in order to perform specific tasks learned under the drug state.

Drugs that are abused by man appear to have very subtle but profound effects on specific neurotransmitter systems in the brain. In the normal state these chemicals, which are the means by which nerves communicate with each other, are in a very delicate balance allowing one to perceive his/her environment and make adjustments to act in accordance with his/her own needs. Psychoactive drugs tend to disrupt this balance, which in effect alters an individual's ability to respond in his/her environment.

At this point there is one theoretical model that suggests that the drug dependent person's neurochemical system is out of balance and that the individual uses a given drug to allow his/her neurochemical systems to function in a more normal fashion. This theory has been promoted as a mental health model in order to explain the success of chemotherapy in the control of several psychotic states. However, this has yet to be substantiated in the substance abuse area.

Adapted from John A. Rosecrans, "Psychological and Neurochemical Mechanisms Involved in the Maintenance of Chemical Dependencies" *Drug Dependence Outline*, MCV/VCU, 1990.

8. This passage deals with:
   I. the acute pharmacological experience.
   II. the habitual drug use: the condition of drug effects as a prelude to dependency.
   III. learning aspects.
   IV. neurochemical aspects.

   A. I, II, and III
   B. I and III
   C. II and IV
   D. I, II, III, and IV

9. Which of the following statements is *supported by* the passage?

   A. A drink here and there really does not hurt.
   B. Your first drink starts you on your way to drug abuse.
   C. A pleasurable state is associated with euphoria.
   D. Drug use follows certain patterns.

10. Human beings partake in drugs because of:

    A. peer pressure.
    B. psychological need.
    C. depression due to marital pressure.
    D. all of the above.

11. Chemical agents consumed chronically:

    A. alter the mind.
    B. seem to act in a predictable fashion.
    C. modulate neurochemical mechanisms.
    D. have relatively short-term effects.

12. Once an individual is addicted:

    A. ritual becomes the order of the day.
    B. environmental conditions may play a dominant role.
    C. injection of a placebo replaces the chemical.
    D. the side effects decrease and use becomes less harmful.

13. According to the author:

    A. certain tasks can be better learned while under the effects of drugs.
    B. certain tasks can be better performed while under the effects of drugs.
    C. certain tasks may be difficult to perform if not under the influence of drugs.
    D. behavioral tolerance will lessen the influence of drug affliction.

14. Which of the statements is *contradicted by* the passage?

    A. Many variables play a role in the effects exhibited by drugs.
    B. Drug users lose the ability to control their own drug taking behavior.
    C. Chemotherapy is the cure for drug use.
    D. Specific neurotransmitters are affected by drug use.

15. Drugs may often serve as:

    A. agents that make an individual feel that he/she "can take on the world."
    B. primary and/or secondary reinforcers of behavior.
    C. crutches for persons who have low self-esteem.
    D. all of the above.

Passage III (Questions 16–24)

For almost a thousand years Alexandria was the world's center of higher learning. The library eventually contained a half million scrolls, and the museum contained a zoo, botanical garden, astronomical observatory, anatomical exhibit, and treasures from around the world. Teaching was limited only to what was necessary to train researchers for the next generation. The main focus was on improving understanding so that each generation could inherit a more advanced civilization. Teaching was not an end or good in itself.

The school of Alexandria was modeled after the Lyceum of Aristotle. What Aristotle received from Plato and what passed to the school at Alexandria was a sense of optimism and dedication in seeking the truth. We know that Plato marveled at the underlying principles of mathematics, such as the Pythagorean theorem, and that he tried to find underlying principles or "truths" in other fields of study. Aristotle's improvement was to take this idea of generalization apart and show that when deduction and induction were used alternately, we had a *method* of finding underlying principles.

The first librarian was Herodotus of Ephesus, who with these new methods of logic, dared to edit Homer's *Iliad* and *Odyssey*. The second librarian was Eratosthenes of Cyrene who, to mention one specific item, measured the size of the earth. First, he measured the angle of the sun (six degrees) at midday on

Adapted from Dr. James McGovern, "Alexandria: The First Research University," MCV/VCU, 1990.

midsummer's day at Alexandria because he knew from previous trips to Syrene (near today's Aswan Dam) that the sun shone to the bottom of its wells (zero degrees) on that very day and time each year. Then, he only had to measure the distance between these two places to calculate the circumference of the earth (60/360 = distance/circumference).

The third librarian, Aristophanes of Byzantium, commissioned 70 scholars to translate the Bible into Greek; and this translation, used by Jesus Christ, became known as the *Septuagint*. (There is other evidence to suggest that the ''flight into Egypt'' took place in Alexandria.) The fourth librarian was Aristarchus of Samosthrace who developed the eight parts of speech and wrote commentaries on the works of Homer, Pindar, and Aristophanes of Athens.

Returning to the faculty, we should not fail to acknowledge what we owe to Euclid beyond geometry. Euclid, who was commissioned to start a school of mathematics around 300 B.C., established a mode of accumulating understanding by starting with a few axioms and theories, stacking conclusions into workable structures of knowledge. Examples today would be the Periodic Chart of Elements, the Myers-Briggs Personality Types, and the concept of management schools, to name a few structures or inferential models in different disciplines.

Apollonius and Archimedes were in the next generation of scholars. Whereas Apollonius gave us the conic sections, Archimedes gave us number systems (myriads) capable of counting the sands of the earth. That same generation included Aristarchus of Samos who taught that the earth moved around the sun and whose name appeared in the margin of a book used by Copernicus while studying at Bologna in the seventeenth century.

During the following century, Hipparchus of Nicea calculated the length of the year to within minutes and the length of the month to a few seconds. Around 150 A.D. Claudius Ptolemy wrote 13 books on astronomy, called the *Almagest*. This set also explained that finding a descriptive model for understanding was more important than accounting for every fact or observation. In his books on astrology, he summarized the beliefs of the Greeks, Egyptians, and Persians and gave us the horoscopes and Zodiac signs used today. Also around 150 A.D. Galen came to Alexandria to study. He was the authority on medicine for more than a thousand years; when physicians found parts of a body to differ from his descriptions, they concluded that the person was abnormal.

During the early days of Alexandria, prisoners were dissected alive. However, evil was not limited to ''pagans'' but discrimination and killing occurred between Jews and Greeks, Christians and Egyptians, and so on. Around 400 A.D., a Christian mob under Cyril ripped the flesh off the mathematician Hypatia because her beliefs were not like theirs.

Whereas understanding could be accumulated in libraries and transmitted by books from generation to generation, wisdom (seeing the importance of doing good for others, i.e. human truths) has to be reinspired again and again by individuals in each generation.

Through the centuries, religion and classical humanism have contended to underwrite the meaning of wisdom. Sometimes, religion (morality) provided the rationale for justice, at other times, humanism (ethics). Whatever, the lesson from Alexandria's past is that whenever a true sense of the underlying principles of morality *or* ethics was not present, minorities and individuals suffered. Thus, during periods of ebbing or pluralistic religious beliefs (like today), ethics becomes necessary to form a behavioral consensus, to ''hold these truths.'' Accordingly, the university's first mission is not to acquire new understandings nor to teach many students, but to reinspire wisdom at an effective level in each new generation.

16. Which statement best summarizes the attitude at the ancient library-museum at Alexandria?

   A. It was basically a teacher-training school.
   B. It was an academy of philosophers.
   C. It was a natural history museum.
   D. It was mostly a scholarly research institute.

17. Plato's sense of ''truth'' was:

   A. what was revealed by God.
   B. limited to mathematical proofs.
   C. underlying principles in any field.
   D. what was agreed to by consensus.

18. Eratosthenes was able to measure the angle of the sun at two distant places on the earth's surface *simultaneously* by:

   A. measuring at one place at midday on midsummer's day a year after measuring at the other place at the same time and date.
   B. having two teams measure angles at the same time and date.
   C. calculating the transit of the sun between measurements.
   D. calculating the movement (turning) of the earth between measurements.

19. One argument given that the "flight into Egypt" of Jesus Christ took place in Alexandria was:

A. Jesus Christ spoke Greek.
B. Jesus Christ knew the Greek version of the Bible.
C. Jesus Christ used the accentuation and punctuation of Alexandria.
D. Jesus Christ was against plagiarism.

20. What statement best fits Claudius Ptolemy?

A. He was an ancient astronomer.
B. He was an ancient astrologer.
C. He was both an astronomer and astrologer.
D. He was a historian.

21. A key difference between understanding and wisdom is:

A. wisdom is ancient; understanding is modern.
B. understanding can be accumulated across the generations; wisdom must be renewed in each generation.
C. understanding deals with things, whereas wisdom deals with people.
D. wisdom is subjective; understanding is objective.

22. The author's main point seems to be:

A. that the study of ethical truths is needed in today's religiously pluralistic world.
B. that we should all have the wisdom to adopt one religion or another.
C. that religious beliefs and ethical reasoning will always be at odds.
D. that people need both morality and ethics today.

23. From a historical point of view, this passage provides the reader with:

A. the names of important figures who lived in Alexandria.
B. a running commentary of the 1000 years during which Alexandria was the world's center of learning.
C. statements made by the great philosophers Aristotle and Plato regarding the teaching of wisdom to new generations.

D. documentation regarding the destruction of the library of Alexandria by Omar I in 642 A.D.

24. One of the great schools in Alexandria was in the disciplines of mathematics. It was founded by:

A. Euclid.   C. Aristotle.
B. Omar I.   D. Eratosthenes.

Passage IV (Questions 25–30)

In school-related and teacher-related cases, the charge of negligence is most often claimed by the plaintiff. As M. C. Nolte has said, "No person or school district can be held to account in damages where negligence is lacking."

A teacher is negligent either if he fails to carry out a duty owed a student, or if he unreasonably carries out a duty owed a student, and that specific omission or unreasonable act is established as the proximate cause of an injury suffered by that student. In actions brought against teachers, the first factor that must be established in proving that the teacher was negligent involves the identification and establishment by the plaintiff student of the legal duty or duties owed him by the defendant teacher.

Over the years, primarily through litigation, the duties of a teacher have been summarized in the following three categories: (1) proper instruction, (2) proper supervision, and (3) proper maintenance and upkeep of all equipment and supplies used by students. All three duties have been and still are fertile grounds for negligence suits against teachers.

The first and most vital of the teacher duties is the duty of instruction. There are two basic meanings for the term instruction. First, teachers owe students proper instruction that will result in the student's mastery of certain processes and basic skills. In recent years, there have been suits against public school systems and public school teachers claiming that they have breached this duty of instruction, with damaging results to the students. For example, in *Doe v. San Francisco Unified School District* the plaintiffs claimed that their son was never taught to read, and as a direct result of that inability the young man cannot obtain a job. A recent New York suit brought by parents whose son made little progress in a public school special education program due to lack of prop-

Adapted from Dr. Richard S. Vacca, "Teacher Malpractice." In *University of Richmond Law Review*, Vol. 8, no. 3 (Spring 1974).

er instruction offers another example of such litigation.

There is a second meaning, however, that has been given to the duty of instruction. Students should not be subjected to an activity in school without first receiving complete instructions from the teacher on how to perform that activity. Included in the instructions given by the teacher should be an explanation of the basic procedures involved, some suggestions on conduct while performing the assignment, and the identification and clarification of any risks that might be involved. Shop teachers, gym teachers, and science teachers seem to be more aware of this "need for instruction" than are regular classroom teachers; yet, all teachers are exposed to the same liabilities.

In cases like *Damgaard v. Oakland, Brigham Young University v. Lillywhite, Keesee v. Board of Education,* and *Crabbe v. County School Board,* the courts have consistently maintained that students should not be allowed to attempt an activity in school without first receiving proper instructions from the teacher, especially when the activity is potentially harmful and dangerous.

In deciding these cases the courts have offered several important behavioral guidelines for teachers, guidelines that, if followed, should help prevent teachers from being found negligent. Certain of these guidelines are as follows: Before allowing students to attempt tasks (1) consider the degree of difficulty involved in the activity, (2) consider the age, level of maturity, and past experience of the student, and (3) be certain to give careful instructions on how to perform the activity and identify and clarify any inherent dangers associated with the activity.

Numerous negligence actions have also been instituted against teachers claiming violation of a second teacher duty, the duty of supervision. In such suits the teacher's absence from the classroom when a student was injured is often claimed as the proximate cause of the resulting student injury. Another allegation frequently made by injured students is that although the teacher was present in the room, he failed to supervise the children closely enough while they were engaged in a potentially dangerous exercise, experiment, or procedure, and that the teacher's failure to provide close supervision was the proximate cause of the student's injury.

There is no uniform standard provided in case law to measure adequate, necessary, or proper supervision of students. What is adequate, necessary, or proper supervision is situational—it depends on a number of factors. Such factors as the age of the student, his experience, his judgment, his physical condition, and the difficulty of the task or activity must each be considered separately in determining the adequacy of teacher supervision.

25. Which of the statement(s) is/are *supported by* the passage?

   A. When filing a suit for negligence, the plaintiff should determine what the duties of the defendant were.
   B. Students have the right to be taught with the result being a certain mastery of subject matter.
   C. Instructors must maintain equipment.
   D. All of the above statements.

26. The duties of an instructor can be summarized as:

   A. effective teaching.
   B. proper guidance.
   C. upkeep of supplies.
   D. all of the above statements.

27. Under the category of instruction, which statements are *supported by* the passage?
   I. A teacher is responsible for progress of the student in the subject matter.
   II. Special education programs are subject to greater scrutiny.
   III. Risks must be clearly identified.
   IV. Explanations of procedures must be very detailed and explicit.

   A. I, II, and III   C. II and IV
   B. I and III   D. I, II, III, and IV

28. Of the following instructors, which have had a greater awareness in the area of giving directions?

   A. mathematics, science, and English
   B. gymnasium, biology, and history
   C. chemistry, gymnasium, and art
   D. shop, gymnasium, and science

29. In deciding cases, which factors have the courts considered?
   I. the difficulty of the task
   II. the maturity and experience of the student
   III. the risks associated with activities
   IV. the talents of students and teachers

   A. I, II, and III   C. II and IV
   B. I and III   D. I, II, III, and IV

30. When looking for a standard evaluating adequate, necessary, or proper supervision of students, which of the following might be considered?

    I.   judgment of the student
   II. chronological age of the student
  III. physical condition of the student
  IV. complexity of the task

  A. I, II, and III   **C.** I, II, III, and IV
  B. IV only   **D.** none of the
                              above

Passage V (Questions 31–37)

The process involved in the recovery from either chronic alcohol or substance abuse is a long one, mainly a lifetime pursuit. AA teaches that an alcoholic can never drink again, and it is generally held that relapse occurs more often when someone stops going to "meetings." Although empirical observations such as these have caused a considerable amount of doubt in the past, a measure of light is now being shed on the situation.

For example, some of the answers to the puzzle of the recovery process are suggested in two articles published in the first issue of the *Informer* by O'Brien and Rosecrans. They focus primarily on the environmental contingencies that cause drug dependent individuals problems when trying to stop using a specific chemical. Thus, the drug dependent individual is faced with many problems outside of his or her own internal need to feel good. For example, drug effects such as their self-administration, and the withdrawal syndrome following chronic use, can be elicited by external stimuli previously associated with previous drug use. A heroin-dependent individual in recovery may experience severe withdrawal symptoms if he or she enters a bar or restaurant previously associated with heroin withdrawal. Furthermore, an alcoholic when not under the influence of alcohol may have difficulty finding his or her car when parked during an alcoholic bout, but can remember where it is when drinking is resumed. This latter phenomena is better known as drug-induced state dependent learning, a pharmacological effect well documented in the human literature.

Thus, when one considers what a drug can do to an individual internally, and in conjunction with his or her environment, one wonders how anyone could become drug-free under the burden of such effects. However, it does happen many times over regardless of the odds. Thus, is recovery a magical phenomena, or is it scientifically based? The answer is not simple. One experiment conducted in rats may help us appreciate what might be going on during the recovery process. In this study, *Esposito et al* (Science *224:* 306-309 (1984) at the National Institute of Mental Health were evaluating how electrical stimulation (like ECS) affects energy metabolism in rat brain. Two groups of rats were studied; one group was allowed to stimulate itself by pressing a lever (self-stimulation), the other group was stimulated with same parameters, but the stimulation was elicited by the experimenter. The second group, thus, had no part in the electrostimulation of their brains. Interestingly, even though both groups of rats received the same level of stimulation, the brain area distribution pattern of increases in energy metabolism were quite different and contingent upon whether rat or experimenter turned on the stimulator.

This experiment is important, not because it provided a specific set of data, but because it demonstrated that a specific change in brain energy metabolism was controlled by each individual rat. The effect on energy metabolism was quite different when elicited by the experimenter. This simple experiment suggests that each individual, to recover from drug dependency, must operate on him or herself. This concept may have importance for two other reasons. First, treatment works only when the individual decides to take on recovery. Although this may appear to be a logical statement, many good professionals, including some in the areas of medical and mental health, do not appear to appreciate the difference between treatment and recovery. Secondly, during the recovery process, the individual is basically altering his or her behavioral conditioning and neurochemistry, which will allow the process to go forward. This can be done by extinguishing or altering the stimulus properties of the drugs that the individual is dependent on. "Don't drink and go to meetings." In scientific terms, the reinforcing effects of drugs are extinguished by not using them, and the stimulus properties are altered by joining forces with people who have also changed their environments. In addition, the social reinforcement and support in AA is also important to recovery because one is substituting alcohol or drugs with people, a much finer euphoriant. Therefore, success in recovery may not be as magical as was once thought, and may have a very precise and orderly basis. The awareness and knowledge of this scientific base can be helpful to both client and therapist.

Adapted from John A. Rosecrans, *Drug Dependence Outline*, MCV/VCU, 1990.

31. An appropriate title for this passage could be:

A. Withdrawal Syndrome.
B. Behavorial Conditioning and Withdrawal.
C. The Recovery Process.
D. Environmental Contingencies and Drug Use.

32. Recovery from drug addition:

A. involves a lifelong process.
B. is modulated by environmental factors.
C. can be associated with withdrawal symptoms.
D. includes all of the above.

33. According to the author:

A. certain tasks can be better learned while under the influence of psychoactive drugs.
B. certain tasks are easily performed while under the influence of drugs.
C. certain tasks my be difficult if not under the influence.
D. learning and performing of tasks are not drastically affected by drug use.

34. Which statement(s) is/are *supported* by the passage?

A. Neurochemical mechanisms play a role in drug addiction and recovery.
B. Environmental conditions may have drastic effects on an individual.
C. The individual is a key determinator.
D. All of the above.

35. According to the passage:

A. the addiction process is well understood.
B. the recovery process is well understood.
C. recovery is the reverse of addiction and depends solely on substitution of compounds.
D. none of the above statements is supported.

36. Most health professionals:

A. agree on the treatment plans of withdrawal and recovery.
B. appreciate that treatment and recovery are at times different.

C. are comfortable with the fact that neurochemical mechanisms are determining factors.
D. feel that AA does the best job in curing alcoholics.

37. The passage implies that the solutions to the drug addition and recovery are found:

A. in the individual.
B. in experimental models.
C. in organizations.
D. in environmental factors.

Passage VI (Questions 38–44)

Physicians like Hippocrates, Thomas Browne, and John Gregory emphasized that physicians must do the "right thing" for their patients, and most physicians take this to mean curing illness and preventing death. Gregory refreshingly reminds us that physicians are not always perfect. "I may reckon among the moral duties incumbent on a physician, that candor, which makes him open to conviction, and ready to acknowledge and rectify his mistakes. An obstinate adherence to an unsuccessful method of treating a disease, is based on a high degree of self-conceit, and a belief of the infallibity of a system." Erik Erikson takes the Golden Rule as his "baseline ... for wise and proper conduct" and points out that even though systematic ethicists may believe the concept too simple, the rule has "marked a mysterious meeting ground between ancient peoples surrounded by oceans and eras and is a theme hidden in the most memorable sayings of many thinkers." The Talmudic version of the Golden Rule, "What is hateful to yourself, do not to your fellow man" is similar to the Christian "Love thy neighbor as thyself." The Golden Rule is not a sufficient ethical principle, however, because it conceptualizes the idea that what is good for the physician is good for the patient. It expresses *beneficence,* which means that the physician, because of specialized knowledge and motivation, knows what is best for each patient.

The principle of beneficence, however, must be tempered by the countervailing idea of *autonomy.* The idea of human rights is a relatively recent development in social evolution. When physicians and priests were one and the same, the principle of beneficence was taken for granted. Patients were expected

Adapted from Dr. Stephen M. Ayres, "Moral Reasoning and Medical Decision Making," MCV/VCU, 1990.

to do what they were told and "doctors orders" became an everyday expression. The ethical principle of autonomy echoes Rousseau, Washington, and Jefferson in emphasizing the patient's primacy in making moral judgments about himself. The courts have generally held that constitutional rights permit an individual to determine what happens to himself and his property; many of these rights have been codified in what has been called a "Patient's Bill of Rights."

Rousseau pointed out that a social contract was necessary because of the inherent inequality among human beings. Some are wise, whereas others are dull, some are strong, whereas others are weak. This inequality is particularly striking in the patient-physician relationship. Physicians have wide knowledge and experience, whereas the patient may understand his own needs and values but has little information about his clinical state. Only detailed conversations with patients and their families can narrow this gap in such a way that people can make truly autonomous judgments about their own care.

Physicians frequently appear to ignore the required balance between the principles of beneficence and autonomy. A physician recommends radical mastectomy for breast cancer. No options are provided because the physician believes he knows best. The patient asks for a second opinion and the physician refuses saying "I cannot take care of you unless I can make all important decisions." Here is presumed beneficence gone amok. A moment later the patient refuses all surgery and the physician says kindly, "it's your life and you are free to do anything you like." Here the physician is ignoring the obvious worried state of the patient and threatening abandonment if the patient does not obey.

Aside from the physician's obvious arrogance and insensitivity, the key question must be: Is the patient completely autonomous when she refuses all treatment and walks out of the doctor's office? She has been told that she has cancer and must have what she believes to be a destructive surgical procedure. Fear of disfigurement and death have produced uncontrollable anxiety that causes her to attempt escape from the situation. True beneficence in this situation demands that the physican seek out the patient, and her family, and make certain that repeated efforts are made to present the true gravity of the situation. Beneficence does not mean the quick delivery of a series of commands but implies shared responsibility, patient education, and understanding, and gentle persuasion where necessary. *Indeed, correctly interpreting the proper balance between these two moral principles in any given situation could be considered one of the key responsibilities of the practice of medicine.*

The beneficence/autonomy concept must be related to the burden/benefit relationship of any proposed action. The balance between the risks or burden of continued treatment relative to any anticipated benefits must be carefully considered. Sometimes life itself, or the treatment proposed to sustain life, is so burdensome that the patient claims the right to allow the dying process to proceed. Granting seriously ill patients, or their families, the right to refuse life-lengthening treatment is an important human issue that is central to professional practice. In may respects, the judicial system is ahead of most physicians in understanding the issues under discussion. Artificial feeding, for example, a technique that many would consider to be part of the basic humane care required for all patients may also become burdensome in certain situations where any benefits from such intervention is minimal.

Obviously, the accuracy of a group of physicians to predict that meaningful life is no longer possible for the individual is central to any such decision. Such a need raises the issue of who can determine what is "meaningful life" and how can physicians best learn how to decide when the burden outweighs the benefit of any course of action.

38. Which of the following statement(s) is/are *supported by* the passage?

   A. The Golden Rule is not a sufficient ethical statement.
   B. Most physicians emphasize curing illness and preventing death.
   C. The Golden Rule views the physician as knowing what is best for the patient.
   D. All of the above.

39. Which of the following would probably have been chosen by the author as a title for the passage?

   A. The Development of the Medical Decision Making Process
   B. Physician Reasoning and Autonomy
   C. The Practice of the Golden Rule
   D. Moral Reasoning and Medical Decision Making

40. Regarding human rights, which statement(s) is/are NOT *supported by* the passage?

   A. Hippocrates lived before that principle was established.

B. Physicians must attempt to defeat the disease first and then explain their protocol.

C. The courts generally have backed the physician as to knowing what is best for the patient.

D. All of the above.

41. Which of the following statement(s) is/are *supported by* the passage?

    I. Patients are perfectly capable of making autonomous judgments.

    II. Beneficence implies understanding.

    III. Rousseau believed that people are quite similar.

    IV. Beneficence and autonomy go hand in hand to achieve good medical practice.

    A. I, II, and III   **C.** II and IV
    B. I and III   **D.** IV only

42. Which of the following statements is NOT *supported nor contradicted by* the information presented in the passage? Hippocrates:

    I. perceived medicine as a tripartite relationship between patient, disease, and doctor.

    II. believed that disease was determined to a great extent by the patient's environment and way of life.

    III. believed that there was nothing sacred about sickness and that each malady followed a distinct pattern (three stages).

    IV. thought of the physician as nature's helper who should reinforce the body's own defenses.

    A. I, II, and III   **C.** II and IV
    B. I and III   **D.** I, II, III, and IV

43. According to the passage, which of the following is/are correct?

    I. Life itself at times can be burdensome.

    II. Patient education is an essential element in true beneficence.

    III. The courts have a better grasp of the right to die concept than the physician.

    IV. Basic humane treatment must always be provided no matter what the benefit is.

    A. I, II, and III   **C.** II and IV
    B. I and III   **D.** I, II, III, and IV

44. The author of the passage argues for:

    I. education.

    II. balance.

    III. consultation.

    IV. patient rights.

    A. I, II, and III   **C.** II and IV
    B. I and III   **D.** I, II, III, and IV

Passage VII (Questions 45–51)

Another kind of editorial began in the April 1942 issue. It was the first to acknowledge America's entry into World War II. This informed youth how they could contribute to the war effort and attempted to inspire them to make such contributions. In an editorial "Little Things Can Help Win the War," the points were simple—stay healthy so you can work hard; assume minor responsibilities so adults can take major roles; save your pennies and dimes to buy Defense Stamps; and "most important of all," be confident. Confidence would provide "vision to see beyond today and its efforts and worries to the glorious day when we can all say, 'We, too, have fought a good fight and, all pulling together for the right cause, … we have won!' "

War effort editorials emphasized the need for collecting scrap metal and rubber, for maintaining fitness, and for growing "victory gardens."

To stress the need for staying fit, Hecht published the first guest editorial in *True Comics*. Colonel Theodore P. Bank, chief of the Athletic and Recreation Branch, Special Services Division of the War Department, wrote "The Importance of Physical Fitness Today." Bank mentioned time and effort being wasted because army recruits were unfit and work days were being lost in factories "because of sickness or injuries which are traceable directly to (young people's) lack of physical fitness."

On youth's involvement in food production, Hecht invited another guest writer, Wayne H. Darrow, director, U.S. Agricultural Labor Administration. His piece "You Can Help the Farmer Win the War," was carried on the first page of the August 1943 issue rather than on the inside front cover. Darrow wrote:

When the harvest is in this fall, everyone who has toughened his hands at farm work will be able to say that he has helped to win the war. Out on our farms this year there is a man's and a woman's job waiting for many thousand boys

From Dr. William E. Blake, Jr., "True Comics," VCU, 1990.

and girls. Our soldiers, sailors, and marines are counting on the farmers. Can the farmers count on you?

It could be thought that Hecht used editorials merely to sell magazines and to advance patriotism. He was indeed a skillful promoter, and he wanted the United States to win the war, but these aspects were less important than his major goal—a world of democracy, unity, and concord. He was an avid internationalist, a globalist.

In February 1943, in the midst of his war effort editorials, he wrote "It's Your World." The arguments were unusual, perhaps even risky for his own well-being, made as they were when the battle was at last shifting in favor of the Allies. This would not seem an appropriate moment to hint to children that the United States must bear some responsibility for the war. However, he attacked the retreat of the United States into isolationism following World War I. "So we celebrated our victory, crawled into our national shell and left the young democracies set up by the Versailles peace treaty to get along the best they could," he wrote. He continued the argument, "We hope and believe that never again will we be guilty of such failure to stand by. For one thing, we know now that withdrawing from our responsibilities after the last war was in a great measure responsible for World War II." He urged young people "to make this battle-scarred planet a safe and sane place to live in."

A similar article in January 1944 pointed out the rapid development of transportation and communication making the world smaller. "Learn to write, read, and speak another language—or two or three, if you can," he wrote. According to Hecht, advantages would be easier travel and more friendships in foreign countries. But also the linguist would be able to explain the principles of democracy.

In the following issue Hecht wrote another daring piece, which aroused hostility among some Americans. There was nothing subtle in the title, "An International Police Force." He maintained nations should not be free to act as they pleased. Nations should take their grievances to an international court and let judges decide. He advocated an international police force to enforce court decisions. "We can't have it both ways," he concluded. "We can't have lasting peace and at the same time insist upon all those national 'rights' which make the waging of wars inevitable."

March 1944 was the last issue of *True Comics* to carry an editorial. Paper had become scarce, and all comic magazines were forced to cut the number of pages. Features had to be discontinued and editorials seemed the most dispensable item.

Circulation figures for *True Comics* are available for each year of its publication, but it is impossible to know how widely young people were reading the editorials or what sort of impact they made.

The idea of a comic book with true stories was unique. Other publishers responded, turning out similar products, but *True Comics* stood alone in carrying editorials. These essays were clear witness to the broad, humanistic, and internationalist values and goals held by George J. Hecht; his determination to spread those ideals; and his confidence in the ability and willingness of American youth to read, to learn, and to do.

45. Which statement(s) is/are *supported by* the passage?
    I. The passage essentially is a history lesson.
    II. America's war effort is described.
    III. Youth and fitness are the main themes.
    IV. The fate of a comic book is described.

    A. I, II, and III   C. II and IV
    B. I and III   D. IV only

46. The publication was unique because it incorporated:

    A. true stories.
    B. color photographs.
    C. editorials.
    D. war stories.

47. The editorials stressed:

    A. recycling.
    B. patriotism.
    C. fitness.
    D. all of the above.

48. The publisher of this series could be considered a(an):

    A. communist.
    B. idealist.
    C. internationalist.
    D. socialist.

49. Which of the following is *supported by* the passage?

    A. The publisher was the first to portray America's entry into World War II in comic form.
    B. The publisher hoped to reach the young.
    C. The publisher himself wrote the editorial on fitness.
    D. Isolationism was proposed.

50. The feature of this publication was abandoned because:

A. the editor changed.
B. of competition.
C. a paper shortage occurred.
D. the war ended.

51. Which of the following is *contradicted by* the passage?

A. The editor believed that America's youth were willing to be responsible.
B. A linguist would serve democracy well.
C. The editor was somewhat of a free spirit.
D. A United Nations would prevent all future wars.

Passage VIII (Questions 52–58)

Herbert Hoover, engineer, self-made man, and great humanitarian hero of the First World War, went on to serve as food czar of the United States during its active war years, and returned to the international rescue business with the cessation of hostilities. As secretary of commerce during the prosperous 1920s, Hoover continued his commendable record of public service.

The 1930s, however, were less kind to his reputation. Elected president in 1928, he enjoyed a scant eight months in office before the collapse of the stock market created a catalyst for the onslaught of the Great Depression. The appearance of failure in combatting that economic and human tragedy, made worse by the Democrats' smear campaign, blighted his name. Despite his assertions that the depression had been beaten by the Summer of 1932, the voting public repudiated him in the presidential election of that year.

Out of office, he remained silent for a time and then took the offensive, first criticizing the New Deal and eventually even attacking President Franklin D. Roosevelt. An unsuccessful seeker of the Republican nomination in 1936 and 1940, Hoover struggled to make his voice heard as a critic of what he called unliberal policies. When war broke out in Europe in 1939, he assumed the dual role of passionate opponent of active United States involvement in the conflict and advocate of humanitarian relief to those caught behind enemy lines.

We gratefully acknowledge the help of Dr. Susan Esterbrook Kennedy, Professor of History and Geography, Virginia Commonwealth University, 1990.

Poland, Finland, Belgium, Holland, and Norway solicited Hoover's assistance almost immediately. He quickly established organizations to aid each of them with money, food, and other forms of nonmilitary support. But even in 1939, his efforts encountered obstacles, both real and propagandistic—in particular a nasty set of rumors about competition with the Red Cross. In 1940, the Hoover relief machine ran up against even more formidable opponents when Winston Churchill and Franklin Roosevelt assumed the posture that relief to these nations would lighten the burden that ought to fall upon their Nazi conquerors. Besides, said Churchill, the Germans would only steal whatever relief supplies were sent to those suffering under occupation.

For the first half of 1940, Hoover combined these relief efforts with a quiet campaign to get the Republican presidential nomination. Although he and his partisans would deny it in 1940 and later, Hoover engaged in a vigorous and carefully orchestrated program, directed toward bringing him a draft. But he would see himself as the victim of deliberate sabotage at the convention when the coveted nomination went to Wendell Willkie. Virtually ignored during the campaign, Hoover returned passionately to the cause of relief, offering the "Hoover Plan" for experimental feeding, which could be stopped instantly in the event of Nazi interference. But the official United States position remained negative. By the end of 1940, Hoover formed the National Committee on Food for the Small Democracies as a propaganda and lobbying organization to press for relief via the Hoover Plan.

Meanwhile, Hoover became increasingly alarmed at the growing danger that the United States might be drawn into an active role in the fighting. He continued to believe, as he had from the outbreak of hostilities, that Britain could not be defeated, that Germany could not win, and that a negotiated peace was possible. He concluded, therefore, that there was no need for American entry. But he distrusted Roosevelt's policies. Although Hoover's active opposition to war was nowhere near so vehement as it would become in 1941, that theme interweaves with his desire for office and his commitment to relief to present a highly complex scenario of his activities and motivations in 1940, and with it, a commentary on the state of the nation from the viewpoint of a still-influential citizen.

52. An appropriate title for this passage could be:

A. Herbert Hoover the statesman.
B. Dirty Politics.
C. Herbert Hoover the Humanitarian.
D. Herbert Hoover—Relief, Politics, and War.

53. Which of the following statements is NOT *supported nor contradicted by* the passage?

A. Hoover was a genius as an organizer.
B. Hoover was a humanitarian.
C. The Democrats ran an honest campaign in 1932.
D. Hoover felt that once being president was enough.

54. The passage pictures Roosevelt as:

A. a clean politician.
B. a humanitarian.
C. a self-made man.
D. not sympathetic to Hoover's efforts.

55. Which statement is *contradicted by* the passage?

A. Despite the ups and downs of his career, Hoover's name remained unblemished.
B. Hoover was part of the political scene for a long time.
C. Hoover did not have party support in his quest for reelection.
D. Other nations sought Hoover's help.

56. Which of the following is NOT *supported nor contradicted by* the passage?

A. The Hoover Plan was more appropriate.
B. The Marshall Plan was more appropriate.
C. The Berlin Airlift solved a severe problem.
D. All of the above.

57. Which of the following statements is *contradicted by* the passage?

A. Hoover competed with the Red Cross.
B. Churchill opposed Hoover's efforts.
C. Hoover opposed propaganda.
D. Hoover acted quickly when it came to relief.

58. Which statement applies to the passage as a whole?

A. Hoover is pictured as a committed individual.
B. The author is sympathetic and fair.
C. It is a quick overview of a long record of humanitarian service.
D. All of the above.

Passage IX (Questions 59–65)

Two ash samples received September 1989 and two ash samples received November 1989 were ignited to determine carbon content and then analyzed for mineral content. Data from the ash mineral analysis were used as input to the Bickelhaupt resistivity prediction model developed for the U.S.E.P.A. An additional computer run was performed to predict the resistivity of an ash that would result from burning 30% waste fuel containing 0.5% magnesium oxide along with the coal normally burned. The resistivity of the ash is an important factor in the performance of the air pollution control equipment used to control particulate emission from the combustion process.

The samples taken in September 1989 were taken from the hoppers of Units 15 and 16. The samples were taken while Unit 16 was having opacity problems to determine if resistivity problems related to ash chemistry were responsible for the performance problems. The analysis showed the ash mineral composition of the samples was virtually identical. The primary difference between the two ash samples was the loss on ignition, which was 23.33% for Unit 16 and 30.80% for Unit 15. The loss on ignition is presumed to be from unburned carbon.

With all of the carbon removed, the two samples are predicted to have approximately a 10^{11} ohm-cm resistivity at 450° F. This resistivity would lead to high sparking, and possible back corona in both units. Optimum resistivity for these units at their 450°F gas temperature is estimated to be about 7×10^9 ohm-cm. This resisitivy is lower than the 2×10^{10} ohm-cm, which is normally quoted as optimum for precipitators running at lower temperatures. The lower resistivity is required due to the lower dielectric strength of the flue gases at 450°. The lower dielectric strengths will promote back corona in ash layers sooner than units running the 200° to 250° F range.

The high resistivity predicted for the carbon free ash will change dramatically with the carbon levels indicated by the loss on ignition tests. Laboratory tests and field data from other ashes have shown large reductions in resistivity from similar carbon levels. The reductions are typically one to three orders of magnitude if the carbon is finely divided and well mixed with the ash. The benefits of the carbon are usually observed at higher gas temperatures, such as the 450° F$^+$ temperatures at which Units 15 and 16 are normally run. The higher unburned carbon levels on Unit 15 are believed to be responsible in part for the better performance of Unit 15 in September. A faulty spark sensing circuit on the automatic voltage con-

Adapted from a report by W. J. Borowy, VCU, 1990.

trollers for the outlet field of Unit 16 also was later found to have contributed to poor performance of the unit.

Ash samples from November 1989 were also analyzed. The higher sodium and iron content of the November ash samples resulted in an ash with a resistivity that was about five to six times less resistive than the September samples. ESP performance during this period of lower predicted resistivities was reported to be good.

Increases in ash magnesium oxide were estimated based on the following:

Fuel: 70% coal, 30% residue
Ash: 5.3%   0.5%

$(5.3 \times 70) + (0.5 \times .30)$ = total ash
   3.71   +   0.15   = 3.86% total ash.

On a percentage basis, the coal contributes 3.71/3.86 or 96.1% of the total ash, and the residue contributes 0.15/3.86 or 3.9% of the total ash. The 3.9 ash from residue was assumed to be mostly magnesium oxide. This was added to the sample with the highest magnesium oxide content to create the analysis for hypothetical Sample #5. The increase in magnesium oxide caused the predicted resistivity to increase about four times. The increase of resistivity will probably not cause operational problems with the favorable ash produced when the November samples were taken. However, low power levels and high opacity may be a problem if ash quality is similar to that encountered in September. If high resistivity problems occur when burning the high magnesium residue, injection of sodium sulfite (Na_2S) to increase the sodium oxide levels in the ash to 1.5% will lower resistivities to an acceptable level.

59. Data from the ash analysis was input into a computer model developed by:

A. U.S.D.A.
B. U.S.D.O.E.
C. U.S.D.O.T.
D. none of the above.

60. The primary difference between ash samples was:

A. one was from waste fuel and one was from coal.

B. the samples were collected at two different temperatures.
C. the loss on ignition.
D. none of the above.

61. What is the percent basis contribution of the coal to the total amount of ash produced?

A. 3.9 percent
B. 3.71 percent
C. 96.1 percent
D. 69.1 percent

62. A hypothetical sample #5 was created that increased the resistivity of the sample. What oxide was increased to create this sample?

A. sodium oxide
B. iron oxide
C. calcium oxide
D. magnesium oxide

63. What was the date of the first ash samples received?

A. September 1989
B. November 1987
C. November 1989
D. none of the above

64. Which of the following statement(s) is/are *supported by* the information in the passage?

I. Carbon content of the ash affects the electrical resistivity of the ash.
II. Magnesium oxide lowers the electrical resistivity of the ash.
III. Sodium oxide raises the electrical resistivity of the ash.

A. I only
B. II and III only
C. I and II only
D. I, II, and III

65. What is the probable reason this passage was written?

A. to discuss hazardous components of coal ash
B. to predict water treatment characteristics of a waste stream
C. to determine the impact of future fuel composition changes on electrical characteristics of fly ash
D. to calculate the composition of feed stock necessary in the production of resistors used in the electronics industry

PHYSICAL SCIENCES

10 PROBLEM SETS OF 5–10 QUESTIONS EACH
15 PROBLEMS FOLLOWED BY A SINGLE QUESTION
77 QUESTIONS
100 MINUTES

DIRECTIONS: The following questions or incomplete statements are in groups. Preceding each series of questions or statements is a paragraph or a short explanatory statement, a formula or set of formulas, or a definition. Read the written material and then answer the questions or complete the statements. Select the ONE BEST ANSWER for each question and indicate your selection by marking the corresponding letter of your choice on the Answer Form. Eliminate those alternatives you know to be incorrect and then select an answer from among the remaining alternatives. A periodic table is provided (see p 467). You may consult it whenever you wish to do so.

Passage I (Questions 66–71)

A human centrifuge is used to test and train pilots and astronauts to withstand the large "g-forces" experienced during flight. The centrifuge arm length is such that the subject moves in a large circle of radius 9 m. The maximum angular velocity is 4 radians/s. The subject normally faces inward toward the center of the circular path. ("eyeballs in").

During a test, the subject's respiratory and metabolic rate rise. The energy released per liter of oxygen consumed in human metabolism averages about 20,000 J/L.

66. What is the maximum linear (tangential) speed of the subject along the circular path at the maximum angular velocity of 4 radians/s?

    A. 18 m/s   C. 36 m/s
    B. 25 m/s   D. 226 m/s

67. A pilot of mass 82 kg (180 lbs) experiences 8 "g's" during one test for a period of 2 minutes. What is centripetal force, in newtons, acting on the pilot?

    A. 16 N   C. 960 N
    B. 660 N   D. 6400 N

68. In the earth frame of reference, what centrifugal force acts *on the pilot* during the test?

    A. The centrifugal force *on the pilot* is equal and opposite the centripetal force on the pilot.

    B. The centrifugal force *on the pilot* is 1 "g" larger than the centripetal force on the pilot.

    C. The centrifugal force *on the pilot* is 1 "g" smaller than the centripetal force on the pilot.

    D. There is *no* centrifugal force *on the pilot*.

69. The pilot's metabolic rate rises to 450 W and remains at that level during the 2 minute test period. What is the approximate number of liters of oxygen consumed by the pilot during the test period?

    A. 3 L   C. 6 L
    B. 4 L   D. 10 L

70. What force acts on the back of the pilot's seat?

    A. 0 N   C. 960 N
    B. 88 N   D. 6400 N

71. The pilot now faces outward ("eyeballs out"). What effect does this have on the centripetal force acting on the pilot?

    A. The centripetal force now points outward.

    B. The seat back now exerts an outward force.

    C. The centripetal force is replaced by the centrifugal force (now supplied by the pilot's seat harness).

    D. The centripetal force is unchanged (now supplied by the pilot's seat harness).

Passage II (Questions 72–77)

A periscope viewing system is to be used to observe the behavior of primates in a large environmentally controlled room on the upper floor of a large research facility. The periscope, like those used on submarines, is essentially a large, folded-path, low power telescope (using prisms to fold the light path). A sketch of the preliminary design appears below. Like all Newtonian telescopes, it uses a relatively long focal length objective lens to form a real image in front of the eyepiece lens (of shorter focal length). The observer looks though the eyepiece lens to see the final image, in the same manner that one would use a magnifying glass. The distance between the lenses is approximately equal to the sum of their focal lengths. The eyepiece, in this design, can be moved forward or back in order to focus on the primates as they move closer to or further away from the objective lens.

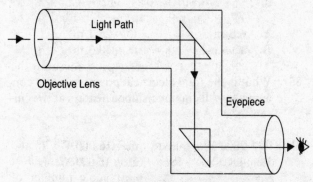

72. The total tube length of the three sections is to be 4 m. The objective lens available has a focal length of 3 m. What should the focal length of the eyepiece lens be?

  A. 0.75 m   C. 1.33 m
  B. 1 m   D. 7 m

73. A visitor seeing the sketch points out an important flaw that will require a design change. What is this flaw?

  A. The focal length of the eyepiece lens is too short.
  B. The images of the primates will be inverted.
  C. The objective lens should be a diverging lens.
  D. The prisms cannot be used in this way.

74. What will be the approximate magnification of this periscope?

  A. 0.67 ×   C. 3 ×
  B. 1 ×   D. 300 ×

75. The prisms (45-45-90° prisms) turn the light path through 90° by "total internal reflection" from the inside hypotenuse faces of the prisms when the incident angle is 45° as in the sketch. Can one use crown glass with an index of refraction of 1.52 for the prism?

  A. Yes, because the critical angle for crown glass is 47°.
  B. Yes, because the critical angle for crown glass is 41°.
  C. No, because the critical angle for crown glass is exactly 47°.
  D. No, because the critical angle for crown glass is 41°.

76. Describe the properties of the image that one sees with this preliminary design.

  A. real, inverted, magnified
  B. real, upright, magnified
  C. virtual, upright, same size as object
  D. virtual, inverted, magnified

77. The telescope is focused on a primate rather far away of the far side of the large habitat. As the primate moves rather close to the telescope, what must the observer do to see the primate clearly?

  A. No change, the image remains clear.
  B. Move the eyepiece away from the objective.
  C. Move the eyepiece closer to the objective.
  D. Use an inverting eyepiece because the image flips.

Passage III (Questions 78–82)

A large vertical cylindrical tank of water about 75 m tall is used by the U.S. Navy to train submariners in techniques used to safely escape sunken submarines in shallow waters. The tanks are used for physiological experiments also. Until very recently all submariners had to undergo a yearly physical test to show that they could escape from a depth of several hundred feet of water (without the use of any artificial breathing apparatus). The sailors enter an air lock and wait while the air pressure is increased until it equals the water pressure at the bottom of the tank. The bottom four feet of the air lock is filled with water. The door to the tank is then opened and the sailors take a final breath (of the high pressure air), swim out the door, and rise slowly to the surface. The trip to the surface takes several minutes. (During this time the swimmer exhales continuously.) The density of the water is 1000 kg/m^3.

78. If the water is incompressible, what pressure does the water exert at the bottom of the 75 m tall tank?

    A. 3.6×10^5 N/m^2 C. 72×10^5 N/m^2
    B. 7.35×10^5 N/m^2 D. 75×10^5 N/m^2

79. The answer to the preceding problem is the so-called gauge pressure. What is the absolute pressure at the bottom if the pressure of the atmosphere is 1.01×10^5 N/m^2?

    A. $4.6] 10^5$ N/m^2 C. 7.3×10^6 N/m^2
    B. 8.36×10^5 N/m^2 D. 7.6×10^6 N/m^2

80. A round glass view port of area 40 cm^2 is located halfway down at 36 m below the surface. What is the force on the view port in newtons?

    A. 1.4×10^7 N   C. 1.4×10^3
    B. 3.52×10^5 N   D. 2.3×10^3

81. If the sailor's total lung capacity is 6.3 liters and he takes in this volume of air at the pressure in the air lock; to what approximate volume, in liters, will the air expand as he rises to the surface (where the absolute pressure is 1 atmosphere)?

    A. 52 liters   C. 540 liters
    B. 67 liters   D. 670 liters

82. Because air contains 21% oxygen by volume, what is the partial pressure of oxygen in the lungs at the bottom of the 75 m escape tank?

    A. 2.12×10^4 N/m^2 C. 1.76×10^5 N/m^2
    B. 1.57×10^5 N/m^2 D. 1.01×10^6 N/m^2

Passage IV (Questions 83–87)

A soft drink bottling plant is building a large cylindrical tank with eight large electrical resistance heaters for the purpose of boiling city water in order to obtain distilled water for the soft drinks. The tank has a radius of 1.0 m. A 30 cm radius access hatch in the bottom of the tank is designed to withstand a maximum pressure of 19,600 N/m^2. The density of the water is 1000 kg/m^3. Each heater has a resistance of 10 ohms and normally draws a current of 20 amperes. A motor driven paddle stirs the water so that it is at nearly the same temperature throughout while being heated. The water starts to boil when it reaches a temperature of 100°C, with the heater current at 20 amperes.

83. What is the depth of the water in the tank if the maximum pressure on the bottom is 19,600 N/m^2?

    A. 2.0 m   C. 4.1 m
    B. 4.0 m   D. 8.2 m

84. What is the volume of the water in the tank in m^3?

    A. 6.3 m^3 C. 25.1 m^3
    B. 12.6 m^3 D. 50.3 m^3

85. What is the total electrical power in watts consumed by all eight resistance heaters at the current of 20 A?

    A. 2000 W   C. 16,000 W
    B. 4000 W   D. 32,000 W

86. The heater current is increased to 25 amperes. What is the voltage drop across each heater at 25 amperes?

    A. 250 V   C. 2500 V
    B. 600 V   D. 6250 V

87. At the higher heater current of 25 amperes, what is the temperature of the boiling water?

    A. 100 °C   C. 250 °C
    B. 125 °C   D. 625 ° C

Questions 88–96 are independent of any passage and of each other.

88. A mass on the end of a spring vibrates in simple harmonic motion with a frequency of 2 Hz. An identical mass is now attached to the original mass. What is the new frequency of oscillation?

    A. 1.4 Hz   C. 2.8 Hz
    B. 2.0 Hz   D. 4.0 Hz

89. A 60 kg person whose two feet cover a total area of 500 cm^2 exerts a pressure on the floor. What is the magnitude of this pressure?

    A. 11,800 N/m^2 C. 30,000 N/m^2
    B. 15,000 N/m^2 D. 960,000 N/m^2

90. The speed of sound in air is about 340 m/s. A sound of frequency 3400 Hz has what wavelength?

    A. 0.1 m   C. 34 m
    B. 10 m   D. 1156 m

91. A radioactive isotope has a half-life of 8 hours. At the end of 24 hours, what percentage of the original isotope will remain?

    A. 6.25%   C. 12.5%
    B. 10%   D. 25%

92. The absolute pressure of a gas increases by 33% at constant volume. What happens to the absolute temperature of the gas?

    A. The temperature triples.
    B. The temperature increases by 33%.
    C. The temperature increases by 67%.
    D. The temperature decreases by 33%.

93. The objective lens of a microscope is marked at 40X. An examination of the eyepiece shows that it is marked 10X. What is the magnification of this microscope?

    A. 4×   C. 140×
    B. 50×   D. 400×

94. A heart defibrillator in a hospital emergency room is set on 400 watt-s by the physician. When discharged across the patient's chest how many joules of energy are produced?

    A. 0.25 joules   C. 100 joules
    B. 40 joules   D. 400 joules

95. The patient whose heart is fibrillating in the preceding problem touched a 120 V source. A current of 100 milliamperes passed through his body and triggered the dangerous ventricular fibrillations in his heart. What was the average resistance of his body in ohms?

    A. .08 ohms   C. 1.2 ohms
    B. 0.83 ohms   D. 1200 ohms

Passage V (Questions 96–105)

A set of laboratory experiments designed to physically involve the students is planned for a high school physics course. They are to verify Newton's laws of motion and the conservation laws for linear and angular momentum. A pair of low carts on which the student sits are fitted with two complete skateboard wheel sets each. A laser beam and photogate can measure the velocities of such large objects using a commercial computer timing system. The forces required are measured with calibrated spring scales. The experiments are performed in the gymnasium to make use of its large smooth floor area. The instructor has devised a pulley and falling mass system to provide the constant forces to accelerate the cart-student systems, but most of the time she has the students provide the accelerating forces by walking backward while keeping the force reading constant on a spring scale. The experience of providing a constant force while accelerating gives the pulling student a "feel" for the real meaning of acceleration.

96. A student practices until he can pull a classmate at constant speed to just overcome friction. This requires a force of 9 N when the mass of cart-student is 90 kg. The student then accelerates the cart-student by pulling with a constant force of 18 N. What is the measured acceleration?

    A. 0.1 m/s^2 C. 1.2 m/s^2
    B. 0.8 m/s^2 D. 4.2 m/s^2

97. Two students of different masses sit on carts close together. They push off from one another and their velocities are measured just after they separate. The 60 kg student-cart has a speed of 1.2 m/s. The other student-cart has an opposite speed of 0.8 m/s. What is the mass of the second student-cart?

    A. 40 kg   C. 110 kg
    B. 90 kg   D. 120 kg

98. A student-cart of mass 80 kg has an initial speed through a photogate of 2 m/s. The frictional forces bring the cart to rest after it travels 8 m. What is the average total friction force that acted over the 8 m distance?

    A. 10 N   C. 40 N
    B. 20 N   D. 60 N

99. A student stands on a rotating frictionless stand with two large weights in his hands. While holding his arms in close to his sides, another student starts him spinning with a rotational angular velocity of 0.3 rev/s. He then sticks his arms out straight at shoulder height and his angular velocity slows to 0.2 rev/s. What is the ratio of his moment of inertia about his vertical spin axis when his arms are extended to his moment of inertia when his arms are at his sides?

   A. 0.6   C. 1.5
   B. 0.8   D. 2.5

100. A student-cart has a mass of 80 kg and an initial speed of 2 m/s. Another student then drops a 20 kg bag of sand onto the lap of the student on the cart. What is the new velocity of the student-cart-bag?

   A. 0.9 m/s   C. 1.2 m/s
   B. 1.0 m/s   D. 1.6 m/s

101. Two students whose cart-student masses are 120 kg and 80 kg sit on the essentially frictionless carts. They hold the ends of a light rope and pull until the carts bump together. They meet at their common center-of-mass. If they start 2 m apart, how far from the starting point of the heavier 120 kg mass is the meeting point?

   A. 0.4 m   C. 1.2 m
   B. 0.8 m   D. 1.4 m

102. One student-cart of mass 80 kg has an initial speed of 4 m/s and collides with another 80 kg student-cart which is at rest. The two carts lock together (due to a coupling mechanism) and move off together. What is their common velocity?

   A. 0.5 m/s   C. 2 m/s
   B. 1 m/s   D. 2.5 m/s

103. A student-cart of mass 100 kg is accelerated at 0.8 m/s^2 by the falling mass system that supplies a horizontal force of 90 N to a cord attached to the front of the cart. What is the friction force opposing the motion?

   A. 3 N   C. 60 N
   B. 10 N   D. 90 N

104. The 90 N force that accelerates the cart at 0.8 m/s^2 in the above problem is supplied by the tension in a cord passing over a frictionless pulley system to a weight that falls vertically. What is the mass of the falling weight?

   A. 5 kg   C. 40 kg
   B. 10 kg   D. 100 kg

105. In another trial, an 80 kg student-cart is to be accelerated from rest over a 10 m distance. The students calculate that the net force (including the tension in the cord and the opposing friction force) accelerating the cart is 100 N. What is the speed of the 80 kg student-cart at the end of the 10 m distance?

   A. 2 m/s   C. 5 m/s
   B. 4.5 m/s   D. 10 m/s

Passage VI (Questions 106–110)

Water is a weakly ionized compound having a $K_a = 1.0 \times 10^{-14}$. In the absence of added H^+ or OH^- ions, the $[H^+] = [OH^-]$. (It is recognized, of course, that H^+ actually is present for the most part in hydrated form as H_3O^+.) The K_a of benzoic acid is 6.6×10^{-5}.

106. The pH of pure water is:

   A. 3.0   C. 7.0
   B. 5.0   D. 9.0

107. Addition of 0.0001 moles of benzoic acid to a beaker containing 1 liter of water will result in benzoic acid solution of pH:

   A. between 3 and 4.
   B. between 4 and 5.
   C. between 5 and 6.
   D. between 6 and 7.

108. The pOH in question 107 would be:

   A. between 4 and 5.
   B. between 5 and 6.
   C. between 6 and 7.
   D. greater than 7.

109. If 1×10^{-12} moles of benzoic acid are dissolved in one liter of water, the pH will be about:

A. 6. C. 8.
B. 7. D. 9.

110. If 5×10^{-13} moles of sodium hydroxide are dissolved in the above one liter aqueous solution of 1×10^{-12} moles of benzoic acid, the pH will be:

A. between 4 and 5.
B. between 5 and 6.
C. between 6 and 7.
D. between 7 and 8.

Passage VII (Questions 111–115)

A solution of $AgNO_3$ (1×10^{-6} molar) is prepared. To this is added K_2CrO_4 until precipitation of Ag_2CrO_4 begins. The K_{sp} of Ag_2CrO_4 is 9×10^{-12}.

111. The precipitate begins at a K_2CrO_4 concentration of about:

A. 1×10^{-6}. C. 1×10^{-1}.
B. 1×10^{-3}. D. 1×10^{1}.

112. Addition of NaCl will bring about:

A. additional precipitation of Ag_2CrO_4.
B. a reaction that will dissolve the Ag_2CrO_4 precipitate.
C. precipitation of AgCl only if its K_{sp} is exceeded.
D. A and C.

113. Increasing the temperature will usually:

A. bring about more complete precipitation.
B. change the K_{sp}.
C. change the formula of the precipitate.
D. not be easily accomplished until ongoing precipitation is complete.

114. If the K_{sp}'s of AgBr, AgCl, and AgI are respectively 7.7×10^{-13}, 1.56×10^{-10}, and 1.5×10^{-16}, the addition of the sodium salt of which of these halides would first bring about precipitation of an insoluble salt?

A. NaBr
B. NaCl

C. NaI
D. all about the same (within a factor of 10)

115. If the sodium salts of the 3 halides in question 114 were added to a concentration that is one-half of that needed to bring about precipitation of that particular silver salt, the result would be:

A. precipitation of only the least soluble silver halide.
B. precipitation of part of each of the three silver halides.
C. precipitation of a portion of the two least soluble silver halides.
D. no precipitation.

Passage VIII (Questions 116–120)

Many metals react with oxygen to form oxides. Some of these oxides, such as Na_2O, CaO, and SrO, react with water to form basic solutions. (These oxides are called basic oxides or basic anhydrides.)

Many nonmetals can react with oxygen to form oxides as well. These nonmetal oxides, however, react with water to form acidic solutions. Thus they are called acid anhydrides.

116. Phosphorus would be expected to react with oxygen to form an oxide that will:

A. react with water to form an acidic solution.
B. react with water to form a basic solution.
C. react with water to form a neutral solution.
D. not react with water.

117. Nitrogen will react with oxygen to form an oxide (N_2O_5) that will:

A. react with water to form an acidic solution.
B. react with water to form a basic solution.
C. react with water to form a neutral solution.
D. not react with water.

118. One mole of Ca will react with oxygen to form an oxide that will react with water to form:

A. one mole of acid in solution.

B. one mole of base in solution.

C. two moles of acid in solution.

D. two moles of base in solution.

119. The solution in the question would require _____ for neutralization.

A. one mole of HCl

B. one mole of NaOH

C. two moles of HCl

D. two moles of NaOH

120. Burning of coal (without use of sufficient scrubbers) in the production of electricity is believed by many to be a major cause of "acid rain." If so, this is most likely because of the production of:

A. oxides of sulfur.

B. carbon dioxide.

C. carbon monoxide.

D. sodium oxide.

Passage IX (Questions 121–125)

Colligative properties of solutions are those properties that depend on the concentration of molecules or ions in solution rather than on their identities.

121. The freezing point of 1000g of water would be lowered most by the addition of one mole of:

A. ethylene glycol.

B. sodium chloride.

C. Na_2SO_4.

D. ethyl alcohol.

122. Calculations of freezing point depression resulting from solutes are based on:

A. molarity.

B. molality.

C. mole fraction.

D. A and B.

123. Colligative properties include:

A. boiling point elevation.

B. freezing point depression.

C. osmotic pressure.

D. more than one of the above.

124. It is noted that the addition of 46g of a solute to 1000g of water will lower the freezing point of water to $-2°C$. It could be predicted that the addition of 92g of the same solute to an identical 1000g of water in another container will:

A. lower the freezing point to $-4°C$.

B. lower the freezing point to $-8°C$.

C. produce a freezing point of $0°C$.

D. produce a freezing point of $+2°C$.

125. Several beakers are prepared, containing 1000g of the same solvent in each. Five grams of nonionizing solutes are added, one solute to each beaker. The greatest effect on boiling point will be noticed with the solute with the:

A. highest molecular weight.

B. highest melting point.

C. lowest molecular weight.

D. lowest melting point.

Passage X (Questions 126–135)

In a neutral atom, the number of orbital electrons is equal to the number of protons in the nucleus (atomic number). Orbital electron configurations may be shown in shorthand form and may be used to predict reactivity and valence. Krypton, for example, may be shown as $1s^22s^22p^63s^23p^63d^{10}4s^24p^6$. Neon is $1s^22s^22p^6$.

126. A neutral atom of the element $1s^22s^22p^63s^1$ would be expected to:

A. readily lose an electron to become an ion with a charge of $+1$.

B. readily lose two electrons to become an ion with a charge of $+2$.

C. readily gain three electrons to become an ion with a charge of -3.

D. be an unreactive (noble) element.

127. The above element has an atomic number of:

A. 8.   C. 18.

B. 11.   D. 19.

128. A neutral atom of the element $1s^22s^22p^63s^23p^63d^{10}4s^24p^5$ would be expected to react by:

A. losing one electron.

B. losing two electrons.

C. gaining one electron.

D. gaining three electrons.

129. An atom of atomic number 9, having an electron configuration of $1s^2 2s^2 2p^6$, would be:

   A. a neutral atom.
   B. an ion with a charge of $+1$.
   C. a noble element.
   D. an ion with a charge of -1.

130. An atom of atomic number 11, having an electronic configuration of $1s^2 2s^2 2p^6 3p^1$, would be:

   A. a neutral atom at ground state.
   B. an ion with a charge of $+1$.
   C. a neutral atom at an excited state.
   D. an ion with a charge of -1.

131. Noble elements include all of the following EXCEPT:

   A. helium.   C. neon.
   B. argon.   D. scandium.

132. The number of quantum numbers possessed by each orbital electron is:

   A. one.   C. three.
   B. two.   D. four.

133. The possible number of values of magnetic quantum number is:

   A. one.   C. three.
   B. two.   D. four.

134. The possible number of values of spin quantum numbers is:

   A. one.   C. three.
   B. two.   D. four.

135. In a particular atom, the number of electrons that possess all four quantum numbers identical to those of another electron is:

   A. zero.   C. two.
   B. one.   D. three.

Questions 136–142 are independent of any passage and of each other.

136. If one wished to remove substantially all of the chloride ions from an aqueous solution, this could be done by the addition of an aqueous solution of:

   A. KNO_3.   C. $AgNO_3$.
   B. Na_2SO_4.   D. starch.

137. If it is known that H_2S is a weak acid that ionizes to form $2H^+$ and S^{2-}, lowering the pH of a solution of H_2S by adding HCl should:

   A. raise the S^{2-} concentration.
   B. lower the S^{2-} concentration.
   C. have no effect on S^{2-} concentration.
   D. not be possible.

138. Which of the following aqueous solutions will have the lowest freezing point?

   A. 1 M NaCl.   C. 1.5 M glucose.
   B. 0.3 M Na_2SO_4. D. H_2O.

139. Consider this reaction: $Fe^{2+} \rightleftarrows Fe^{3+} + e^-$. Which of the following is correct?

   A. The reaction toward the right is an oxidation.
   B. The reaction toward the right is a reduction.
   C. The reaction toward the left is a reduction.
   D. A and C are correct.

140. The hydronium ion is:

   A. a protonated water molecule.
   B. formed by removal of H^- from a water molecule.
   C. an ion with the formula of H_2O^+.
   D. an uranium byproduct.

141. How many milliliters of $0.50N$ NaOH are required to neutralize 50 ml of $0.25N$ HCl?

   A. 25   C. 0.25
   B. 50   D. 2.5

142. A zwitterion is a molecule containing:

   A. both cationic and anionic functions.
   B. more than one cationic or anionic function.
   C. polar and nonpolar groups.
   D. a Z^+ charge.

WRITING SAMPLE

2 ESSAYS—TOPICS
60 MINUTES (30 MINUTES/TOPIC)

DIRECTIONS: Your response must be a unified, organized essay; it should contain fully developed, logically constructed paragraphs. Remember quality is more important than length. Before you begin writing, make sure you have read the item carefully and understand what is being asked. Write as legibly as possible. Because your essays will be scored as first-draft compositions, you may cross out and make corrections on your response booklet as necessary. It is not necessary to recopy your essay.

Part 1

Consider this statement:

Probably all laws are useless; for good men do not want laws at all, and bad men are made no better by them.

Demonax

Write a unified essay in which you perform these tasks. Explain the meaning of the above quote. Give specific examples of a time when good men would want laws and when bad men would be made better by them. Discuss the purpose of a set of imposed laws, what makes them useful or useless in serving this purpose.

Part 2

Consider this statement:

And thus your freedom when it loses its fetters becomes itself the fetter of a greater freedom.

Kahlil Gibran

Write a unified essay in which you complete the following tasks. Explain what you think the above statement means. Describe a specific situation in which freedom that has lost its fetters does not become the fetter of a greater freedom. Discuss the manner in which one type of freedom might put a restraint or a confinement on another type of freedom.

BIOLOGICAL SCIENCES

10 PROBLEM SETS OF 5–10 QUESTIONS EACH
15 PROBLEMS FOLLOWED BY A SINGLE QUESTION
77 QUESTIONS
100 MINUTES

DIRECTIONS: The following questions or incomplete statements are in groups. Preceding each series of questions or statements is a paragraph or a short explanatory statement, a formula or set of formulas, or a definition. Read the written material and then answer the questions or complete the statements. Select the ONE BEST ANSWER for each question and indicate your selection by marking the corresponding letter of your choice on the Answer Form. Eliminate those alternatives you know to be incorrect and then select an answer from among the remaining alternatives.

Passage I (Questions 143–151)

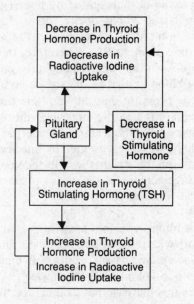

The pituitary gland is responsible for the secretion of thyroid stimulating hormone (TSH), which elicits an increased production of thyroid hormone from the gland; this thyroid hormone then may inhibit the pituitary via a negative feedback. Under hyperthyroid conditions, the following tests would give elevated values:

1. Basal metabolic rate (BMR)
2. Protein bound iodine (PBI)
3. Radioactive iodine uptake (RAI)

143. When TSH secretion falls, the secretion by the thyroid of thyroid hormone:

A. stays the same.
B. increases.
C. decreases.
D. will feed back upon the pituitary.

144. According to the schema given, if a normal individual is given an injection of TSH, his/her thyroid hormone production will first

A. show no noticeable change.
B. increase.
C. decrease.
D. lead to a decrease in pituitary TSH output.

Use the information in the flow chart and paragraph above, and in the following graphs, to answer questions 145–147.

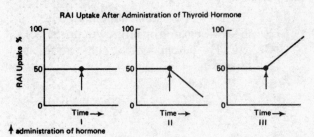

145. In which of the graphs is there evidence of thyroid malfunction?

A. I   C. I and III
B. I and II   D. III

146. Which graph(s) probably represent(s) the case of a typical hyperthyroid person?

A. II   C. I and III
B. I   D. II and III

147. Which of the graphs lead(s) you to believe that there is a breakdown in the normal thyroid-pituitary functional relationship?

A. I and III   C. II
B. III   D. II and III

148. A lack of iodine in the diet usually is associated with which disorder?

    A. acromegaly   C. rickets
    B. goiter   D. skin rash

149. Thyroid stimulating hormone (TSH) is produced by which of the following?

    A. acidophils (alpha cells)
    B. basophils (beta cells)
    C. delta cells
    D. chromophobes

150. Which of the following statements concerning the thyroid are correct?

    A. The gland is derived from the pharynx (foramen cecum of the tongue).
    B. Colloid is located extracellularly.
    C. T_3-triiodothyronine and T_4 thyroxine are the active principles.
    D. All of the above.

151. Hypersecretion of which hormone will result in acromegaly (giantism)?

    A. TSH—thyroid stimulating hormone
    B. STH—somatotropin (growth hormone)
    C. ACTH—adrenocorticotrophic hormone
    D. thyroxin

Passage II (Questions 152–156)

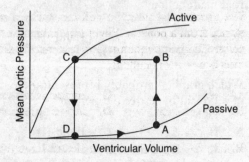

As the left ventricle of the heart contracts, it generates a pressure, which when more than that in the aorta causes the ejection of a volume of blood. The action of the ventricle can be represented as the relationship between the volume of blood in the ventricle and the intraventricular pressure. The relationship between ventricular pressure and volume is known as the Frank-Starling law of the heart and is shown above.

The lower curve represents the pressure volume relationship when the heart is being passively filled with blood during diastole (i.e., at rest). The upper curve represents the pressure-volume relationship as a result of contraction (i.e., systole). The volume at Point A is known as the end diastolic volume which is the volume of blood in the ventricle immediately preceding contraction. During systole, the ventricle contracts, but no blood is ejected until the pressure in the ventricle exceeds the pressure in the aorta. This phase of the cardiac cycle is known as isovolumetric contraction and is represented by line segment AB. When the aortic valve opens (point 3), blood is ejected without further increase in the ventricular pressure (line segment BC). Therefore, this phase of contraction is isotonic and results in the ejection of a volume of blood known as the stroke volume.

When the pressure that the ventricle can generate exactly equals the aortic pressure, the ejection of blood ceases, and the ventricle undergoes isovolumetric relaxation as represented by line segment CD. The blood from the atrium then fills the ventricle, and the pressure increase is the result of passive resistance of the ventricle (curve DA).

152. Assuming a constant mean aortic pressure, patients with renal failure may have an increased blood volume which results in an increased end diastolic volume in the ventricle. What effect does this increase have on cardiac function?

    I.   ventricular work remains constant
    II. stroke volume increases
    III. end systolic volume increases
    IV. ventricular work increases

    A. I, II, and III only   C. II and IV only
    B. I and III only   D. IV only

153. Patients with hypertension have a higher mean aortic pressure. If end diastolic volume stays constant:

    I.   stroke volume increases.
    II. ventricular work increases.
    III. end systolic volume decreases.
    IV. ventricular work may or may not increase.

    A. I, II, and III only   C. II and IV only
    B. I and III only   D. IV only

154. Patients with heart failure have an active pressure curve (i.e., upper curve) which is shifted downward and to the right as compared with that of normal. Assuming the end diastolic volume and the mean aortic pressure remain constant and the ventricle is capable of ejecting blood:

   I.   stroke volume decreases.
   II. end systolic volume increases.
  III. ventricular work decreases.
  IV. end systolic volume decreases.

A. I, II, and III only **C.** II and IV only
B. I and III only   **D.** IV only

155. With time, the blood volume of patients with heart failure tends to increase resulting in an increased end diastolic volume with a continued downward shift in the active pressure curve (i.e., upper curve). The increase in the end diastolic volume, as compared with the case of a failing ventricle without compensation referred to in the preceding question, will result in:

   I.   a stroke volume which may or may not increase.
   II. an increase in cardiac work.
  III. a decrease in end systolic volume.
  IV. an increase in stroke volume.

A. I, II, and III only **C.** II and IV only
B. I and III only   **D.** IV only

156. With a constant mean aortic pressure and as compared to normal, a compensated failure will show:

   I.   an increase in stroke volume.
   II. a stroke volume which may or may not decrease.
  III. a decrease in cardiac work.
  IV. an increase in end systolic volume.

A. I, II, and III only **C.** II and IV only
B. I and III only   **D.** IV only

Passage III (Questions 157–163)

In a laboratory experiment, red blood cells were placed into 0.5 M solutions and the appearance of the solutions was observed two hours later with the naked eye.

Solution	Cells
0.5 M glucose	no change
0.5 M sucrose	no change
0.5 M urea	hemolysis of RBCs
0.5 M glycerol	hemolysis of RBCs

157. How can the solutions of urea and glycerol be described with respect to the red blood cells?

A. isotonic   **C.** hypertonic
B. hypotonic   **D.** none of the above

158. The reason for these results is that:

   I.   the number of particles in the urea and glycerol solutions is greater than that in the glucose and sucrose solutions.
   II. glucose and sucrose form coatings around the red blood cells, which prevent their breaking.
  III. glucose and sucrose enter the cells but are immediately metabolized, therefore water does not enter the cells.
  IV. urea and glycerol can enter the cell, water follows them into the cell because it is then in greater concentration outside.

A. I and II only **C.** III and IV only
B. I and III only **D.** IV only

159. The property of the cell membrane that allows for this phenomenon to be demonstrated is called:

A. diffusion.   **C.** impermeability.
B. osmosis.   **D.** semipermeability.

160. The process by which a cell can move a substance from a point of lower concentration to a point of higher concentration (against the diffusion gradient) is called:

A. osmosis.   **C.** turgor pressure.
B. plasmolysis. **D.** active transport.

161. Which of the following structures are NOT considered modifications of the cell membrane?

A. basement membrane
B. terminal bars
C. desmosomes
D. intercalated discs

162. The plasma membrane of animal cells:

    A. is usually rigid.
    B. has selective channels made of proteins.
    C. is too thin to be seen by the use of any microscope.
    D. is composed only of proteins and carbohydrates.

163. Dialysis (as is used for the treatment of chronic kidney ailments) differs from the process of osmosis in the respect that:

    A. both solvent and solute pass through the membrane.
    B. solute selectively passes through the membrane only.
    C. solvent selectively passes through the membrane only.
    D. gases are the only substances that pass the membrane and blood is cleansed.

Passage IV (Questions 164–168)

The diagram below represents three generations of a human family, some of whose members have a non-lethal birth defect. The defect is caused by a single gene for which new mutations are very rare. The individuals with birth defects are represented by solid black symbols, whereas the individuals who have a normal phenotype are represented by open symbols. Males are represented by squares and females are represented by circles.

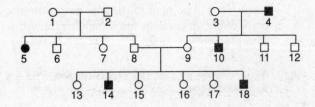

164. The defect is most likely caused by:

    A. an autosomal gene for which the defective allele is recessive to the normal allele.
    B. an X-linked gene for which the defective allele is recessive to the normal allele.
    C. an autosomal gene for which the defective allele is dominant to the normal allele.
    D. an X-linked gene for which the defective allele is dominant to the normal allele.

165. The genotype of individual number 1 in the family:

    A. is most likely to contain only normal alleles.
    B. is most likely to contain only defective alleles.
    C. is most likely to contain both normal and defective alleles.
    D. cannot be determined from the pedigree.

166. The genotype of individual number 4 in the family:

    A. is most likely to contain only normal alleles.
    B. is most likely to contain only defective alleles.
    C. is most likely to contain both normal and defective alleles.
    D. cannot be determined from the pedigree.

167. The genotype of individual number 7 in the family:

    A. is most likely to contain only normal alleles.
    B. is most likely to contain only defective alleles.
    C. is most likely to contain both normal and defective alleles.
    D. cannot be determined from the pedigree.

168. The genotype of individual number 8 in the family:

    A. is most likely to contain only normal alleles.
    B. is most likely to contain only defective alleles.
    C. is most likely to contain both normal and defective alleles.
    D. cannot be determined from the pedigree.

Passage V (Questions 169–178)

Blood is the fluid that circulates around in blood vessels to provide for gas exchange, waste removal, and nutrient procurement by the cells of the body.

Blood is composed of various types of cells and cell fragments (referred to as formed elements) and a fluid called plasma. The formed elements include erythrocytes or RBCs (red blood corpuscles), various types of leucocytes or WBCs (white blood cells), and thrombocytes or platelets.

In a clinical setting a number of tests are conducted on blood. One of these is to determine the packed cell volume or *hematocrit* (which is defined as the volume of formed elements relative to the total volume of blood). In order to determine an individual's hematocrit, 10 milliliters of blood are collected and placed in a heparinized centrifuge tube. Heparin is used to prevent clotting. The tube is spun for 15–20 minutes at 2500 rpm to sediment all the formed elements. The tube is then examined to determine the volume (in milliliters) of the packed formed elements. On the average, blood consists of approximately 45% formed elements and approximately 55% plasma; in other words, each 10 ml of blood will contain 4.5 ml of formed elements. The average "normal" packed cell volume or hematocrit is therefore 45% (i.e., 4.5 ml is 45% of 10 ml). Most of the sedimented formed elements are RBCs. A small region of WBCs and platelets will be located at the top of the region of formed elements; this layer is often referred to as the "buffy" coat.

A patient was seen by a physician who ordered a hematocrit as part of the patient's lab workup. Ten milliliters of blood were collected and treated as previously described. The diagram below shows the hematocrit tube at the end of centrifugation.

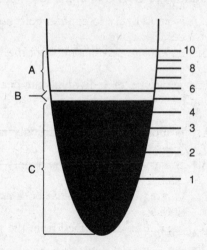

169. Region A consists of:

   A. fibrin clot material.
   B. plasma.
   C. serum.
   D. WBCs.

170. Region B consists predominately of:

   A. fibrin clot material.
   B. plasma.
   C. RBCs.
   D. WBCs.

171. The lower 5.5 ml consists predominantly of:

   A. fibrin clot material.
   B. platelets.
   C. RBCs.
   D. WBCs.

172. The hematocrit of this patient is:

   A. 45%.   C. 4.5 ml.
   B. 55%.   D. 5.5 ml.

173. The hematocrit of this patient is:

   A. normal.
   B. above normal.
   C. lower than normal.
   D. cannot be determined from the information given.

174. The components of the blood responsible for binding and carrying oxygen would be located in:

   A. region A.   C. region C.
   B. region B.   D. regions A and C.

175. The cellular components of the blood responsible for fighting infections would be located in:

   A. region A.   C. region C.
   B. region B.   D. regions B and C.

176. The components of the blood responsible for blood clotting would be located in:

   A. region A.   C. region C.
   B. region B.   D. regions B and C.

177. The major component found in region A would be:

   A. water.   C. sodium chloride.
   B. hemoglobin.   D. glucose.

178. The hematocrit of the patient, as compared to the normal value, suggests that the patient:

    A. lives at a high altitude.
    B. has sickle cell anemia.
    C. has pernicious anemia.
    D. has recently undergone excessive X ray treatment.

Passage VI (Questions 179–183)

A muscle fiber is a single muscle cell. Each fiber is composed of numerous cylindrical fibrils running the entire length of the fiber. The fibril exhibits light and dark bands—the I and A bands respectively. The I band is bisected by the M line. There is a somewhat lighter band within the A band that is called the H band. These striations are produced by the arrangement within the fibril of myofilaments; myosin is the thick myofilament, whereas actin is considered the thin myofilament.

179. A sarcomere is the area between:

    A. two A bands.   **C.** two I bands.
    B. two H bands.   **D.** two Z bands.

180. During contraction the lengths of the thick and thin myofilaments:

    A. increase.
    B. decrease.
    C. remain the same.
    D. first increase, then decrease.

181. If we could imagine observing a muscle contraction under a light microscope, we would see the narrowing of the:

    A. H and I bands.   **C.** Z bands.
    B. A bands.   **D.** H bands only.

182. If the muscle were deprived of ATP, which of the following would NOT be affected?

    A. the sodium pump of the muscle membrane
    B. the calcium pump of the sarcoplasmic reticulum
    C. the length of the myosin filaments
    D. the velocity of shortening

183. What is the internal activator substance that is released during excitation—contraction coupling?

    A. ATP   **C.** Ca^{2+}
    B. Mg^{2+} **D.** H^+

Passage VII (Questions 184–189)

During the inflammatory reaction, immune and paraimmune system cells circulating in microvessels adhere to the endothelium of these vessels in areas of tissue injury. The adherent cells then migrate across the endothelium into the injured tissue. The adherence of the cells to the endothelium is stimulated by cytokines such as tumor necrosis factor, TNF. The immune and paraimmune system cells may adhere to endothelial cells through binding of CD-18 molecules on the surfaces of the immune and paraimmune system cells to GMP-140 glycoproteins on the surfaces of endothelial cells. A series of experiments to evaluate these hypotheses is shown in figures 1–3. Figure 1 reports the binding of neutrophils, monocytes, and lymphocytes to plastic dishes coated with varying amounts of GMP-140. Figure 2 shows neutrophil adhesion to plastic dishes under varying conditions. Figure 3 shows neutrophil adhesion to cultured layers of vascular endothelial cells in the presence of varying concentrations of GMP-140 in the test solution.

Figure 1

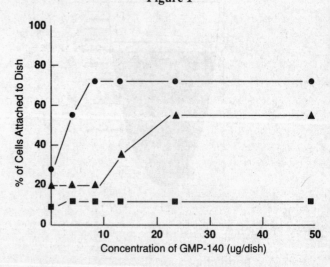

Adherence of neutrophils (▲), monocytes (●), and lymphocytes (■) to plastic dishes that had been coated with varying amounts of GMP-140.

Figure 2

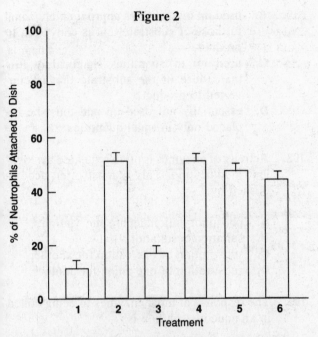

Effects of pretreatment of plastic dishes or neutrophils on the attachment of neutrophils to plastic dishes.
1—neither cells nor dish were pretreated
2—dish coated with GMP-140; no treatment of cells
3—dish coated with GMP-140 then treated with rabbit antibodies which bind to GMP-140
4—dish coated with GMP-140 then treated with rabbit antibodies which do not bind to GMP-140
5—dish coated with GMP-140; cells treated with antibodies which bind to CD-18
6—dish coated with GMP-140; cells treated with antibodies which do not bind to CD-18

Figure 3

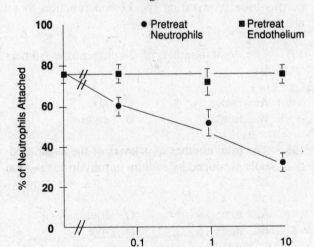

Effect of GMP-140 pretreatment on the binding of neutrophils to cultured endothelial cells.
Prior to the assay, aliquots of either neutrophils or endothelial cells were incubated with GMP-140 and subsequently washed by centrifugation. For the assay, pretreated neutrophils were mixed with untreated endothelial cells (●) or untreated neutrophils were mixed with treated endothelial cells (■).

184. As the concentration of GMP-140 used to coat plastic dishes was increased:

    A. the number of neutrophils attaching to the plastic tended to increase.
    B. the number of neutrophils attaching to the plastic tended to decrease.
    C. the tightness of binding of neutrophils to the plastic tended to increase.
    D. the tightness of binding of neutrophils to the plastic tended to decrease.

185. Plastic dishes that were not coated with GMP-140:

    A. did not bind monocytes.
    B. allowed attachment of about ¼ of the monocytes.
    C. allowed attachment of about ½ of the monocytes.
    D. allowed attachment of most of the monocytes.

186. Coating of plastic dishes with GMP-140:

    A. caused the largest increase in binding of neutrophils.
    B. caused the largest increase in the binding of lymphocytes.
    C. caused the largest increase in the binding of monocytes.
    D. caused approximately equal increases in binding of all cells.

187. The data presented:

    A. strongly support the hypothesis that neutrophils bind to GMP-140 on the surface of endothelial cells.
    B. strongly support the hypothesis that neutrophils use GMP-140 on the neutrophil surface to attach to endothelial cells.
    C. strongly refute the hypothesis that neutrophils bind to GMP-140 on the surface of endothelial cells.
    D. strongly refute the hypothesis that neutrophils use GMP-140 on the neutrophil surface to attach to endothelial cells.

188. The data presented:

A. strongly support the hypothesis that neutrophils bind to CD-18 on the surface of endothelial cells.

B. strongly support the hypothesis that neutrophils use CD-18 on the neutrophil surface to attach to endothelial cells.

C. strongly refute the hypothesis that neutrophils bind to CD-18 on the surface of endothelial cells.

D. strongly refute the hypothesis that neutrophils use CD-18 on the neutrophil surface to attach to endothelial cells.

189. Based on the data and information presented, a human patient who had a genetic defect that prevented synthesis of GMP-140 would probably be most severely impaired in:

A. phagocytosis of bacteria.

B. killing of virus-infected cells by natural killer cells.

C. cell-mediated immune responses to most targets.

D. humoral immune responses to most targets.

Passage VIII (Questions 190–194)

Enzymes have often been referred to as biological catalysts. They have many properties in common with other catalysts.

190. Enzymes are generally:

A. carbohydrates. C. lipids.
B. proteins. D. nucleic acids.

191. Enzymes function in reactions by:

A. increasing the net energy yield.

B. raising the energy level of the products.

C. decreasing the energy of activation.

D. changing the thermodynamic nature of a reaction, thus making a reaction thermodynamically favorable when it would not otherwise be so.

192. The nature of enzymes requires that the enzyme is:

A. used up in quantities greater than those of substrate that is converted to product.

B. used up in quantities approximately equal to those of substrate that is converted to product.

C. used up in quantities significantly less than those of the substrate that is converted to product.

D. essentially not used up and must be replaced only in small quantities.

193. Activity of enzymes is often regulated by covalent modification. This is most often accomplished by:

A. phosphorylation/dephosphorylation.
B. sulfation/desulfation.
C. substitution of one cation for another.
D. substitution of one anion for another.

194. The response of most enzymes to being boiled in an aqueous solution is:

A. substantially increased activity.
B. substantially decreased activity.
C. an increase of about 1 unit in isoelectric point.
D. no noticeable change is detected.

Passage IX (Questions 195–199)

All of the possible ketopentose sugar isomers have been synthesized in a research project. The ketopentose isomers have then been reduced with sodium borohydride, converting the ketone function to an alcohol.

195. The total number of 2-ketopentose isomers is:

A. two. C. six.
B. four. D. eight.

196. The total number of isomers of the sugar alcohols produced by sodium borohydride reaction is:

A. two. C. four.
B. three. D. five.

197. If all the sugar alcohols in the previous question were selectively oxidized so that the number 3 hydroxyl was converted to a ketone, there would be _____ chiral center(s) in each molecule.

A. one. C. three.
B. two. D. four.

198. The pentose(s) found in RNA usually consists of:

A. deoxyribose.   C. various pentoses.
B. ribose.   D. glucose.

199. If the sugar alcohols in question 196 were oxidized to convert carbon numbers 1 and 5 to carboxyls, the number of chiral centers would be:

A. none.   C. two.
B. one.   D. three.

Passage X (Questions 200–204)

The synthesis of proteins and nucleic acids is seen as being directed by a series of coded messages. The messages must be sent, received, and decoded.

200. The primary source or repository of information concerning synthesis of nucleic acids and proteins is considered to be:

A. protein.   C. RNA.
B. DNA.   D. peptides.

201. In the polymer that directs protein biosynthesis, there is a requirement of _____ unit(s) (or monomers) to code for each amino acid.

A. one   C. three
B. two   D. four

202. In a chromosome of higher animals there is(are) _____ strand(s) of DNA.

A. one   C. three
B. two   D. four

203. If 100 somatic cells of higher animals are allowed to divide once in ^2H_2O (water containing only deuterium), _____ of the cells will have only DNA containing deuterium.

A. none   C. one half
B. one fourth   D. all

204. Ultimately, synthesis of protein requires:

A. DNA.   C. protein.
B. RNA.   D. all of the above.

DIRECTIONS: Read each passage carefully, study each table, chart or formula, then answer the question following it. Eliminate those choices that you think to be incorrect and mark the letter of your choice on the answer sheet.

Maloney sarcoma tumors were implanted in Brown Norway (BN), Lewis (Le), and Lewis-Brown Norway (LBN) rats. Studies were then done to determine the types and amounts of host serum antibodies produced against the protein components of the virus contained in the tumor cells. The following data are from one such experiment.

ANTIPROTEIN 30 ACTIVITY IN SERA OF TUMOR BEARING BN, Le, AND LBN RATS

Host	AgB Phenotype	Mg Equivalent Day 25 Post Implant	Anti-p30 Antibody Day 31 Post Implant
BN	3/3	3.5 ± 0.8	5.3 ± 1.7
LBN	1/3	2.4 ± 0.4	4.5 ± 1.4
Le	1/1	0.4 ± 0.1	0.4 ± 0.2

205. The following statements are related to the information presented. Select the statement *supported by* the information given.

A. Brown Norway rats produced more anti-p30 antibody at both 25 and 31 days than the other two hosts.
B. On the basis of this information, Brown Norway rats are more resistant to cancer than either LBN or Le rats.
C. All three hosts produced more anti-p30 antibody at 31 days than they did at 25 days.
D. An AgB phenotype containing threes seems to be related to lower anti-p30 production.

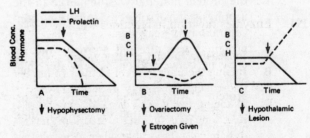

The graphs represent experimental results obtained when the pituitary gland was removed (A), the ovaries were removed (B) and lesions were placed in the hypothalamus (C), that part of the brain most closely related to the pituitary gland. The hormones LH and prolactin were measured in blood by radioimmunoassay.

206. It can be concluded from these results that:

    A. prolactin is produced by the ovaries.
    B. LH release stimulates prolactin release.
    C. ovarian hormones inhibit LH release, but not prolactin release.
    D. presence of the ovaries inhibits removal of LH from the blood.

The urophysis of teleosts secretes a neurohormone directly into the blood circulatory system. This secretory apparatus is believed functional in osmoregulation in fishes from marine and freshwater habitats. Fifteen blueback herring (*Pseudoharengus aestivalis*) were maintained in a marine aquarium at temperatures of 40°–45°. The fish were subjected to increasing salt concentration to a final concentration equal to twice that of seawater. At each concentration four of twelve urophyses were dissected and extracted, and electrophoresis on polyacrylamide gels were performed. Two specific bands of protein were identified as being specific to the urophysis. The amount of protein was determined by microdensitometry. The results are shown in the graph.

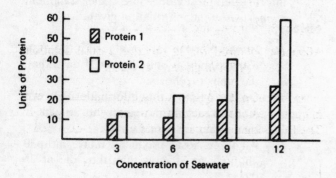

207. The experiment indicates that:

    A. the protein material was unaltered in the urophysis of fish subjected to varying concentrations of seawater.
    B. protein 1 was affected more by the increasing concentration of seawater than protein 2.
    C. protein 2 was affected more by the increasing concentration of seawater than protein 1.
    D. the data could not be analyzed.

An investigator had been studying the interrelationship (cooperation) of various cell types in tissue culture in the immune response to an antigen. The experiments conducted attempted to determine if spleen and mast cells were required for the production of antibody against a pollen. Various donor cells (spleen and mast cells) were injected into recipient rabbits whose immune system had been rendered nonresponsive by whole body X-irradiation. Antibody levels were determined in the serum of the recipients.

Experimental Groups		Antibody Level
A.	Spleen and pollen	0
B.	Spleen	0
C.	Mast cells and pollen	0
D.	Mast cells	0
E.	Spleen and mast cells and pollen	++
F.	Bone marrow and pollen	++
G.	Thymocytes and pollen	++

208. The following statements are related to the information presented above. Select the statement *not supported by* the information given.

    A. In the system under investigation, spleen and mast cells together are required for antibody production.
    B. Spleen cells are probably found in the thymus.
    C. Spleen cells or mast cells are essential to the antibody production against pollen.
    D. In the intact animal, the mast cells would probably be important as a source of antibody.

Four groups of rats were maintained under identical conditions. Three of the groups received drugs in their drinking water over a period of five weeks. The day before autopsy each rat received one microcurie of ^{131}I. At autopsy the thyroid glands from each group were pooled and weighed. Iodinated intermediates were isolated and their radioactivity determined. Remember iodide is trapped, oxidized, proteinated, and stored as part of the thyroid hormone.

^{131}I CONTENT
(counts/min./100 mg Thyroid Tissue)

Groups	Drug	Iodine Ion	Monoiodo-tyrosine	Trilodo-thyronine	Thyroxine	Av. Thyroid Wt. mg/100 g body wt.
1	None	6,120	10,140	7,520	35,990	14
2	A	55	46	13	62	76
3	B	40,976	10	9	14	88
4	C	1,592	2,025	1,970	8,985	4

209. Which group was treated with thyroxine, an inhibitor of the production of thyroid stimulating hormone by the pituitary gland?

A. Group 2   C. Group 4
B. Group 3   D. none of the above

After growing turkey red wheat for two years on a dry land farm, John Calendar had accumulated enough capital to move his family to a more fertile area. The first crops he planted on the new 1000-acre farm did well. The bar graphs below indicate his production of wheat and corn over the last five years. Bushels are plotted on the abscissa, and the numbers of acres planted in both crops are shown in parentheses.

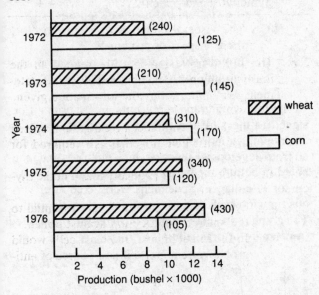

210. What was the average yearly proportion of wheat production to corn production?

A. 3/2   C. 10/9
B. 7/8   D. 5/7

Three greenhouses were constructed to examine different light cycles and their effects on the growth of several plants.

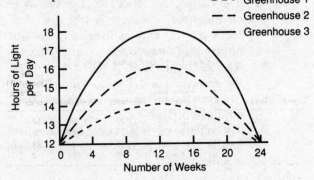

211. Plant X requires 15 hours of light per day for at least three weeks to exhibit a red coloration in its leaves. It may exhibit this highly desired feature in:

A. greenhouse 1.
B. greenhouse 1 and 2.
C. greenhouse 2 and 3.
D. all of the above.

One hundred ml of blood was drawn from a healthy male donor. Following centrifugation (4°C) and removal of the "buffy coat" by aspiration, hemoglobin was extracted from the pelleted red blood cells. The extracted hemoglobin was then divided into equal aliquots and these were treated as follows:

Aliquot 1: Analyzed on the day of extraction by polyacrylamide gel electrophoresis, followed by densitometer scanning of the stained gel

Aliquot 2: Stored for 30 days at room temperature

Aliquot 3: Stored for 30 days at 4°C

Aliquot 4: Stored for 30 days as a 50% solution (V/V) in glycerol at −20°C

At the end of the 30-day storage period, each of the aliquots was analyzed in the same way as aliquot 1. The following densitometer tracings were obtained:

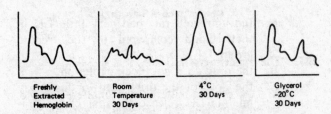

212. From these data it is clear that:

A. none of the storage conditions were able to maintain hemoglobin in an absolutely unchanged state.
B. hemoglobin peptides are strongly affected by heating.
C. hemoglobin contains peroxidase activity.
D. hemoglobin coupled with oxygen has a longer shelf life than hemoglobin coupled with CO_2.

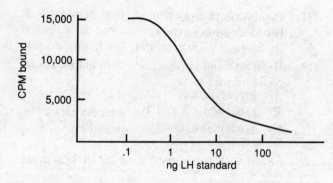

Blood samples from 10 female rats were withdrawn at 5 PM on the day of proestrus, when LH levels in the blood should be high if ovulation were to occur that night. The blood was assayed by double-antibody radioimmunoassay for LH. An antibody specific for LH is allowed to bind with the LH in the sample, then is partially displaced by radio-labeled LH whose binding to the limited amount of anti-LH is inversely proportional to the amount of unlabeled LH present (see standard curve). The antigen-antibody complex is precipitated with an antibody to the anti-LH, and the number of counts per minute bound in the precipitate is determined after the supernatant containing the unbound labeled LH has been poured off. The blood samples from 5 untreated rats (which ovulated) had cpm of 4000, 3000, 5000, 4000 and 3000, whereas those from 5 drug-treated animals had 5000, 13,000, 15,000, 3,000, 13,000.

213. It can be concluded from this study that:

A. the untreated rats had very little LH in their blood compared to the treated group.
B. the drug does not block ovulation.
C. the dose of the drug used in this study inhibits LH release in most of the animals.
D. ovulation occurred in three out of five of the treated rats.

Selective protein transport from the maternal circulation to the rat fetus is thought to occur via the visceral yolk sac. The maternal proteins are transferred to the yolk sac cavity and then must pass through the visceral endoderm, the visceral basement membrane (VBM), and the vitelline capillary endothelium to reach the fetal blood. Proteins X, Y, and Z were injected into a pregnant rat on day 12 of gestation and then were localized in the layers of the visceral yolk sac at 2 minutes, 6 hours, and 12 hours following injection. The results below demonstrate where each protein was localized at the three postinjection intervals.

Protein	Visceral Endoderm	VBM	Vitelline Endothelium	Fetal Blood
X	2 min.	6 hrs.	12 hrs.	—
Y	2 min., 6 hrs., & 12 hrs.	—	—	—
Z	2 min.	6 hrs.	12 hrs.	12 hrs

214. Based on the information given, select the statement *not supported by* the information given above.

A. All three proteins were absorbed at the same rate by the visceral endoderm.
B. The transport of protein X is blocked by the visceral basement membrane.
C. The visceral endoderm appears to block the transport of protein Y.
D. Protein X appears to be transported through the visceral endoderm.

The following graph represents an experiment designed to measure the rate of collagen synthesis in developing chondrocytes. Chondrocytes were isolated from developing sterna of chick embryos and incubated in culture media containing proline–^{3}H, a precursor of collagen. Specimens were fixed after various time intervals and prepared for autoradiography. The graph represents number of silver grains counted (μm/square of organelle).

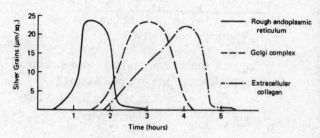

215. The following statements are related to the information presented. Select the statement *supported by* the information given.

A. The radioactive label found in the rough endoplasmic reticulum is transferred directly into the extracellular collagen without passing through the Golgi complex.
B. Radioactive isotope is incorporated into the extracellular collagen within 2 hours.
C. Collagen is a highly stable molecule and is not degraded.
D. The amount of rough endoplasmic reticulum in the cell increases during collagen synthesis.

216. Amino acids found in higher animals are usually:

A. optically inactive.
B. of the L-series.
C. of the D-series.
D. a racemic mixture.

217. Carbohydrates found in higher animals (such as glucose, fructose, and galactose) are usually:

A. optically inactive.
B. of the L-series.

C. of the D-series.
D. a racemic mixture.

218. D-glucose and L-galactose, both aldohexoses, could be said to be:

A. epimers.
B. diastereomers.
C. enantiomers.
D. A and B.

219. Foods with the highest number of kcal/g are the:

A. carbohydrates.
B. proteins.
C. fats.
D. nucleic acids.

Model Examination C Answer Key

Verbal Reasoning

1.	D	14.	C	27.	B	40.	D	53.	A
2.	D	15.	B	28.	D	41.	C	54.	D
3.	D	16.	D	29.	A	42.	D	55.	A
4.	A	17.	C	30.	C	43.	A	56.	D
5.	D	18.	A	31.	C	44.	D	57.	A
6.	D	19.	B	32.	D	45.	D	58.	D
7.	A	20.	C	33.	C	46.	C	59.	D
8.	D	21.	B	34.	D	47.	D	60.	C
9.	B	22.	A	35.	D	48.	C	61.	C
10.	D	23.	B	36.	C	49.	B	62.	D
11.	C	24.	A	37.	D	50.	C	63.	A
12.	B	25.	D	38.	D	51.	D	64.	A
13.	C	26.	D	39.	D	52.	D	65.	C

Physical Sciences

66.	C	82.	C	98.	B	113.	B	128.	C
67.	D	83.	A	99.	C	114.	C	129.	D
68.	D	84.	A	100.	D	115.	D	130.	C
69.	A	85.	D	101.	B	116.	A	131.	D
70.	D	86.	A	102.	C	117.	A	132.	D
71.	D	87.	A	103.	B	118.	B	133.	C
72.	B	88.	A	104.	B	119.	C	134.	B
73.	B	89.	A	105.	C	120.	A	135.	A
74.	C	90.	A	106.	C	121.	C	136.	C
75.	B	91.	C	107.	B	122.	B	137.	B
76.	D	92.	B	108.	D	123.	D	138.	A
77.	B	93.	D	109.	B	124.	A	139.	D
78.	B	94.	D	110.	A	125.	C	140.	A
79.	B	95.	D	111.	D	126.	A	141.	A
80.	C	96.	A	112.	C	127.	B	142.	A
81.	A	97.	B						

Biological Sciences

143.	C	159.	D	175.	B	190.	B	205.	A
144.	B	160.	D	176.	B	191.	C	206.	C
145.	C	161.	A	177.	A	192.	D	207.	C
146.	B	162.	B	178.	A	193.	A	208.	D
147.	A	163.	A	179.	D	194.	B	209.	C
148.	B	164.	A	180.	C	195.	B	210.	B
149.	B	165.	C	181.	A	196.	B	211.	C
150.	D	166.	B	182.	C	197.	B	212.	A
151.	B	167.	C	183.	C	198.	B	213.	C
152.	C	168.	C	184.	A	199.	C	214.	B
153.	D	169.	B	185.	B	200.	B	215.	B
154.	A	170.	D	186.	C	201.	C	216.	B
155.	C	171.	C	187.	A	202.	B	217.	C
156.	C	172.	B	188.	D	203.	A	218.	B
157.	B	173.	B	189.	A	204.	D	219.	C
158.	D	174.	C						

Explanation of Answers for Model Examination C

VERBAL REASONING

1. **D.** At the beginning of paragraph two the point is made that questions remain concerning custody and storage of data. The article starts with the question who owns scientific data, which clearly eliminates **A.** The passage points out that the federal government expects an institution to claim ownership of data if it resulted from federally sponsored programs. The article does not specify as to the investigator's responsibility to preserve data.

2. **D.** The passage makes the argument that it is truly necessary to establish ownership of data. A point is made that in industry, the ownership of data is well established and formalized in employment contracts. The author indicates that the period data must be stored is unspecified, and that it is not a universal practice of universities to claim ownership of scientific data.

3. **D.** Statement **A** is refuted in paragraph two; the author questions the mode and method and state of preservation. Paragraph two, clearly does not give us an answer as to the cost factor and as to who bears the burden. There is no general agreement as to when data preservation and protection should start. **D** is supported by the passage in paragraph two, and it is pointed out that many issues remain unsolved in the custody battle over data.

4. **A.** Paragraph one indicates that in industry, data stays with the employer, whereas institutions lack clear policies. It is argued that no established lines of command exist in many cases as to who owns the data when the team approach (paragraph three) is used. At the end of paragraph one, it is pointed out that federal agencies do not provide for the transfer of ownership of scientific data with ownership rights.

5. **D.** Paragraph three states at the beginning that there are differences between discovery and verification of claims. The author points out in the same paragraph that the need for formal written arrangements exists when it comes to data, and that public policymakers need to establish definitions and definitive guidelines. The author not only asks institutions to assume a leadership role, but assigns this responsibility to them.

6. **D.** None of the issues cited in the question is discussed in the passage.

7. **A.** In the middle of the first paragraph, it is made clear that no great consistency exists as far as policy is concerned regarding the ownership of data of trainees.

8. **D.** Paragraphs one and two could be entitled acute pharmacological experience, whereas paragraph three deals with drug effects as a prelude to dependency. Paragraph four discussed learning aspects, and paragraphs five and six deal with neurochemical aspects.

9. **B.** Paragraph one makes it perfectly clear that the dependence process starts with the initial exposure. It is also emphasized that after taking a drug an individual may feel pleasure (or less pain), but that the word pleasurable has many meanings and may not be related to "feeling good."

10. **D.** Paragraph one emphasizes that people take psychoactive drugs for many reasons that essentially meet their own individual needs, whether it be feeling good, peer pressure, or whatever.

11. **C.** Paragraphs two and five make the statement that most drugs produce their effects via an alteration of brain neurochemistry, which can lead to other more long-term problems. Alteration of the mind is not specific, and drugs do not act in a very predictable way.

12. **B.** Paragraph three discusses the phenomenon of conditioned stimulus and points out that

the use of a drug can come under environmental control. Although the role of ritual is mentioned, it certainly is not the order of the day. Placebo does not routinely replace the chemical substance. No mention is made anywhere in the passage as to side effects.

13. **C.** Paragraph four deals with learned behaviors. There is no implication that learning or performing of tasks is enhanced by the consumption of psychoactive drugs. The point is made that there is the development of behavioral tolerance and that persons learn to adapt to the drug state to a degree. The example is given of an individual having difficulty finding the liquor store when sober. No credence is given in the passage to the statement that behavioral tolerance lessens the effects of drug affliction.

14. **C.** Paragraph two emphasizes that chronic drug use will introduce variables that may take over drug taking behavior, and that individuals will lose ability to control this behavior. The last paragraph mentions that chemotherapy is a modality in use, but no cure is implied. The passage as a whole focuses on the neurochemical imbalance elicited by drug use; paragraph five states that drugs have profound effects on specific neurotransmitter systems.

15. **B.** Although the reader may reach similar conclusions as those presented in statements **A** and **C**, the only statement that is specifically made by the author is statement **B**. Paragraph two states that drugs do not always serve as primary reinforcers of behavior, but have important secondary reinforcing qualities.

16. **D.** Paragraph one indicates that at Alexandria teaching was limited to only what was necessary to train researchers for the next generation. The focus was on improving understanding so that each generation could inherit a more advanced civilization.

17. **C.** Paragraph two makes it clear that Plato marveled at the underlying principles of mathematics and tried to find underlying principles or "truths" in other fields of study.

18. **A.** Paragraph three deals with the second librarian Eratosthenes who measured the size of the earth; he measured the angle of the sun (six degrees) at midday on mid-summer's day at Alexandria because he knew from previous trips to Syrene (near today's Aswan Dam) that the sun shone to the bottom of its wells (zero degrees) on that very day and time each year. He only had to measure the distance between these two places to calculate the circumference of the earth.

19. **B.** Paragraph four indicates that Aristophanes the third librarian commissioned 70 scholars to translate the Bible into Greek and that this translation, which became known as the *Septuagint*, was used by Jesus Christ. The point is also made that evidence suggests that the "flight into Egypt" took place in Alexandria.

20. **C.** Paragraph seven tells us that Ptolemy wrote 13 books on astronomy, and that in his books on astrology he summarized the beliefs of the Greeks, Egyptians, and Persians and gave us the horoscope and Zodiac signs used today.

21. **B.** Paragraph nine makes the argument that whereas understanding could be accumulated in libraries and transmitted by books from generation to generation, wisdom has to be reinspired again and again by individuals in each generation.

22. **A.** The last paragraph indicates that during periods of ebbing or pluralistic religious beliefs (like today), ethics become necessary to form a behavioral consensus, to "hold these truths."

23. **B.** Paragraph one describes the great library and museum of Alexandria. The remaining paragraphs discuss the great figures who played a role in making Alexandria the center of higher learning for almost a thousand years.

24. **A.** The school of mathematics was founded by Euclid around 300 B.C.

25. **D.** Paragraphs two, three, and four address the issues cited in statements **A, B,** and **C**.

26. **D.** Paragraph three summarized the duties of a teacher as proper instruction, supervision, and maintenance of all supplies.

27. **B.** Statements I and III are correct. Paragraph four indicates that teachers owe students proper instruction that will result in the student's mastery of certain processes and basic skills. Paragraph five makes the point that risks must be identified and clarified.

28. **D.** Paragraph five states that shop, gym, and science teachers have been more aware than regular teachers of the need for specific guidance and instruction.

29. **A.** Paragraph seven cites that the courts have offered several behavioral guidelines; statements I, II, and III are summaries of them.

30. **C.** The last paragraph indicates that all four choices are appropriate and supported by the passage.

31. **C.** A thorough reading of the passage will leave the reader with only one major theme. The writer has clearly focused on the recovery process and its many facets.

32. **D.** Paragraph one indicates that a long-term proposition is encountered in the recovery from addiction. It is a lifetime pursuit and, as AA points out, relapse frequently occurs when people stop attending meetings. Drug use as recovery depends on many factors, and the environment plays a major role in both. As is common with many compounds taken for a long period, (psychoactive drugs or steroids administered under supervision) stoppage usually results in withdrawal symptoms.

33. **C.** Under no circumstances is the point made that drug use enhances learning or the performing of tasks. Psychoactive drugs are definitely detrimental to all aspects of an individual's functioning. The point is made that there is a drug-induced state dependent learning and the example is that a person sober might have a problem finding the car, but when under the influence the person "may" remember where it is.

34. **D.** Every statement is substantiated by the passage. Drugs or electrical stimulation produce their effects via an alteration of the brain's neurochemistry. The environment, it is pointed out in paragraph two, plays a key role in the addiction and recovery process. Paragraph four emphasizes that the individual determines to a great extent his/her own fate.

35. **D.** Neither addiction or recovery are simple or well understood processes. Recovery, as paragraph four indicates, involves commitment on the part of the user to stop using the drug and to reinforce his actions by changing and utilizing environmental and social phenomena to help him in the lifelong process.

36. **C.** The passage does not address treatment of drug addiction. Paragraph four does point out that many good professionals do not appear to appreciate the difference between treatment and recovery. No indication is given that AA is the appropriate avenue to cure alcoholics. Paragraphs three and four should leave no doubt in the reader's mind that neurochemical aspects are determining factors in addiction, treatment, and eventual recovery.

37. **D.** Individual variations and commitment are emphasized. Animal experiments are essential. Organizations like AA, as is pointed out in paragraph four, help in the substitution of the drug with people and provide social reinforcement. Throughout the passage environmental aspects are highlighted.

38. **D.** The passage in paragraph one emphasizes that the Golden Rule is not a sufficient ethical principal because it fosters the idea that what is good for the physician is good for the patient. Paragraph one also emphasizes that physicians must do the "right thing" and indicates that most feel that this means curing illness and postponing death. Gregory does point out that physicians are not perfect and should acknowledge and rectify their mistakes.

39. **D.** Although the passage touches upon medical decision making, reasoning and autonomy of the patient, the application and interpretation of the Golden Rule, the central theme is philosophical and the best and most encompassing title would be "Moral Reasoning and Medical Decision Making."

40. **D.** None of the statements posed are supported by the passage. The passage points out that Hippocrates preached the Golden Rule and that certainly is part of the principal of human rights. A very strong argument is made in paragraphs four and five in favor of the physician explaining in an appropriate, understanding, sensitive, compassionate, and thorough manner the disease process to the patient and reaching a mutual consensus in order to delin-

iate an appropriate course of action suitable for the individual, the family, and accepted medical practice. Paragraph two makes it quite clear that the courts generally have held that the constitutional rights permit an individual to decide what happens to himself, and these rights have been called the "Patient's Bill of Rights."

41. **C.** Throughout the passage it is stressed that a give and take attitude must exist in the decision making process, and paragraph three points out that Rousseau advocated a social contract because human beings are different. Paragraph four leaves no doubt that beneficence and autonomy must be weighed and applied to reach a decision.

42. **D.** Although every statement is correct and was espoused by Hippocrates, the passage does, however, not deal with them and so it neither contradicts nor supports the information presented in the question.

43. **A.** Paragraph six emphasizes that burden/benefit aspects of treatment must be weighed. Sometimes life itself, or the treatment proposed to sustain life, is so problematical that patients opt for the right to die. It was previously pointed out that education of the patient is essential for proper medical practice. Paragraph six makes the point that the courts understand the concept of the right to die better than most physicians. The paragraph gives the example of artificial feeding, which may become so problematical in the respect that any benefit from the intervention is minimal.

44. **D.** There should be no doubt in the reader's mind that the passage argues strongly for education, a balance in the decision making process, consultation between physician and patient, and among physicians, and above all that patients' rights should never be negated.

45. **D.** The last paragraph makes it perfectly clear that the history of a comic book (*True Comics*) is detailed.

46. **C.** The last paragraph points out that the idea of a comic book with true stories was unique, but *True Comics* stood alone in the respect that it carried editorials.

47. **D.** A thorough reading leads the reader to conclude that besides selling magazines, the publisher preached recycling, patriotism, and fitness.

48. **C.** Paragraph three ends with the statement that the publisher was an avid internationalist, a globalist.

49. **B.** Paragraph one clearly indicates that it was an editorial in the comic book that was the first acknowledgment of America's entry into World War II. The editor was interested in reaching the young and making them aware how they could contribute to the national effort.

50. **C.** Paragraph eight mentions that paper had become scarce and all comic books were forced to cut the number of pages, and editorials seemed dispensable.

51. **D.** The last paragraph makes it perfectly clear that Mr. Hecht had confidence in the ability and willingness of American youth. It is pointed out in paragraph six that a linguist would be able to explain the principles of democracy. The whole passage deals with the ideas and ideals of a strong willed and daring individual; the first sentence of paragraph seven should be convincing. Although the editor talks about international courts and forces, he does not propose the notion that such cooperation would prevent all future wars.

52. **D.** Of the four titles listed "Herbert Hoover—Relief, Politics, and War" is the most appropriate one. Herbert Hoover was the food czar of the United States during World War I and thereafter helped with international relief efforts. He became president in 1928 and after his loss to Roosevelt in 1932 continued a role in the political arena. He was afraid that the United States would enter World War II and hoped for a negotiated peace.

53. **A.** Although it is true that Hoover had many contacts and was a brilliant organizer, our passage really does not focus on this issue at all. Paragraph one pictures Hoover as a humanitarian and paragraph two mentions that the Democrats ran a smear campaign. Hoover as is mentioned in many places in the passage actively sought the presidency continuously.

54. **D.** Roosevelt ran a smear campaign against Hoover (paragraph two). No mention of humanitarianism and of being self-made is made in the passage. It is, however, clear from paragraph four that Roosevelt opposed the relief efforts.

55. **A.** Paragraph two mentions that Hoover's name was blighted by the 1932 campaign. Hoover was influential from World War I until his death. Paragraphs three and five detail the convention defeats, and four indicates that Poland, Finland, Holland, Belgium, and Norway solicited his help.

56. **D.** All three statements made are not addressed by the passage.

57. **A.** Paragraph four mentions that a nasty set of rumors hinted that Hoover's relief efforts competed with the Red Cross; in this paragraph both Roosevelt's and Churchill's oppositions are mentioned. The National Committee on Food for the Small Democracies was a propaganda organization. Paragraph four points out that Hoover acted quickly to aid with money, food, and other such supplies.

58. **D.** There can be no doubt in the reader's mind that Hoover was service oriented, had a long record, and was committed. No sides were taken by the author, and in that respect a fair and sympathetic job was done.

59. **D.** The opening paragraph states the computer model was developed by the U.S.E.P.A.

60. **C.** Paragraph two states that the primary difference ... was the loss on ignition.

61. **C.** Paragraph six states that the coal contributed 3.71/3.86 or 96.1% of the total ash.

62. **D.** Magnesium oxide was added in the hypothetical sample to increase resistivity as indicated in paragraph six.

63. **A.** Paragraph one states that two ash samples were received September 1989 and two ash samples were received November 1989.

64. **A.** Paragraph six indicates that magnesium oxide increased resistivity, whereas sodium oxide lowers resistivity.

65. **C.** The laboratory work and the computer modeling work was done to predict the effects of a change in chemical composition of a waste fuel on the electrical resistance of the ash produced.

PHYSICAL SCIENCES

66. **C.** The tangential (linear) velocity of an object moving around a circular path (velocity tangent to the circle) is proportional to the angular velocity.

   $v = r w$, where r is the radius (9 m in this case) and w is the angular velocity (which must be in radians/s for use in this formula).

67. **D.** A "g" force is equal to the actual weight, mg, of a person or object, so:

   $8 \text{"g's"} = 8(82 \text{ kg})(9.8 \text{ m/s}^2 = 6429 \text{ N}.$

68. **D.** The centrifugal force is the "equal and opposite force" of Newton's third law and thus does NOT act *on* the *pilot*. It is the force that the pilot exerts *on* the *back of his seat*.

69. **A.** Power in watts is the rate of energy use, thus the energy, $E = P \times t$ or $E = 450$ watts $\times$ 120 seconds $= 54,000$ joules and liters of O_2 consumed $= 54,000 \text{ J}/(20,000 \text{ J/L}) = 2.7 \text{ L}.$

70. **D.** According to Newton's third law, the pilot exerts a force of 8 "g's" on his seat back. Notice that this *is* the centrifugal force and it *is* a real outward force on the seat back. (The pilot, in his rotating "frame of reference," feels as if a large outward force is pushing him into the seat back. This force is a "fictitious" force because the only real force acting on him is the inward centripetal force.)

71. **D.** The necessary inward-pointing centripetal force is unchanged. Nothing has changed except the device that supplies the centripetal force.

72. **B.** It is given in the passage that the telescope length is approximately equal to the sum of the focal lengths. If the total length is 4 m, then the value of f_e is 4 m $- f_o = 1$ m.

73. **B.** The objective lens forms a real, inverted image. The eyepiece acts in the same way that a magnifying glass does. The observer looks through the eyepiece and sees a final, virtual image that has the same orientation as the first image (that is, the final image is still inverted). This can be corrected by inserting a third lens, known as an erecting lens, between the objective and eyepiece.

74. **C.** The magnification of a simple Newtonian telescope is the ratio of the objective focal length to the eyepiece focal length:

$$M = f_o/f_e = 3/1 = 3 \times.$$

75. **B.** This question requires an understanding of total internal reflection. The critical angle is the incident angle for which Snell's law of refraction predicts a refracted angle of 90°, for light rays traveling from a medium of larger index of refraction toward a medium of lower index of refraction. Here the light ray is incident inside the glass prism toward air of index, $n_{air} = 1$. Using Snell's law:

$n_{glass} \sin \emptyset_c = n_{air} \sin 90°$, and because $n_{glass} = 1.52$; $\sin \emptyset_c = 1/1.52$ and $\emptyset_c = 41°$.

76. **D.** The objective lens is a projection lens, producing an inverted real image. The first image lies within the focal length of the eyepiece, which therefore acts as a magnifying glass, forming a virtual, enlarged image. The eyepiece does not invert the image.

77. **B.** As the object (primate) moves closer to the objective, the real image formed by the objective is further away from the objective, i.e., closer to the original position of the eyepiece. To see the image clearly, the eyepiece must be moved "back" away from the objective in order to focus the second (virtual) image clearly. (It is the eyepiece that is adjustable in telescopes and binoculars.) This is similar to holding this printed page too close to your eyes to see clearly. If you hold the page still and move your head away you will be able to see the print clearly.

78. **B.** The pressure is due to the weight of a column of fluid 75 m tall. $P = dgy$; where $d =$ density of the liquid, and y is the depth below the surface; g is the acceleration of gravity, 9.8 m/s².

79. **B.** The gauge pressure is the pressure over and above the atmospheric pressure. (The gauge pressure is that read by an automobile tire gauge, for example.) Thus the absolute pressure = 1 atm + gauge pressure.

80. **C.** Because pressure = force/unit area, the force is $F = PA$, where A is the area in square meters of the view port. ($A = 40$ cm² $= 40 \times 10^{-4}$ m²). The pressure is the gauge pressure, dgy, at $y = 36$ m.

81. **A.** Treating the air as an ideal gas, we see that $P_1V_1 = P_2V_2$, or $V_2 = P_1V_1/P_2$. Notice that we must use the absolute pressures in this expression. Then $P_1 = 8.36 \times 10^5$ N/m² and $P_2 = 1.01 \times 10^5$ N/m².

82. **C.** The partial pressure is the same fraction (0.21) of the total absolute pressure of 8.36×10^5 N/m² as the fraction of oxygen by volume in ordinary air.

83. **A.** The hydrostatic pressure due to the weight of a fluid increases linearly with depth and depends on the density of the fluid. $P = dgh$, where d is the density and h the depth from the fluid surface. Then $h = P/dg = 19600/(1000 \times 9.8) = 2.0$ m.

84. **A.** This is a straightforward geometry problem. The volume of the water in the cylindrical tank equals the product of the horizontal cross-sectional area times the height of the water. ($V = Ah$) The area is that of a circle, $A = \pi r^2$, hence $V = \pi (1 \text{ m})^2 (2 \text{ m}) = 6.3$ m³.

85. **D.** The questions requires a knowledge of the electrical power consumed by a resistance R. $P = IV = I^2R$. Each resistor with the same current of 20 amperes consumes 4000 watts so the eight resistors consume 32,000 watts.

86. **A.** This problem is solved by the use of Ohm's law, $V = IR = (25 \text{ A}) (10 \text{ ohms}) = 250$ V.

87. **A.** The boiling of the water involves a change of state from the liquid to the vapor state. Like most substances that form crystalline solids, the melting point and boiling point temperatures of water occur at precise temperatures. The "latent heat of vaporization" concept illustrates the fact that the energy supplied to the water at its boiling point temperature (100°C at

1 atmosphere) goes entirely into the change of state. The added energy at the higher current of 25 amperes causes a faster change of state (faster boiling) but *does not* increase the boiling point temperature).

88. **A.** This question requires a knowledge of the formulas dealing with simple harmonic motion. The frequency of oscillation of a mass, m, on the end of a spring of spring constant, k, is given by:

$f = \frac{1}{2\pi}\sqrt{\frac{k}{m}}$. If one now takes the ratio of the new frequency (f_2) to the old frequency (f_1), using the appropriate masses $(m$ and $2m)$, the constants and the unknown spring constant may be cancelled, leaving:

$$\frac{f_2}{f_1} = \sqrt{\frac{m_1}{m_2}}$$

so $f_2 = 2\text{Hz}\sqrt{\frac{1}{2}} = 1.4$ Hz.

89. **A.** Pressure = force/unit area. The force is the person's weight, mg. The area must be converted to SI units of m^2. Thus;

$$P = \frac{60 \text{ kg} \times 9.8 \text{ m/s}^2}{500 \text{ cm}^2 \times 10^{-4} \text{ m}^2/\text{cm}^2} = 11,800 \text{ N/m}^2.$$

90. **A.** The question deals with the basic relation for the velocity of *any* wave (sound waves, water waves, light waves).

velocity = frequency × wavelength.

$$\text{wavelength} = \frac{340 \text{ m/s}}{3400 \text{ Hz}} = 0.1 \text{ m}.$$

91. **C.** The half-life is the time required for the quantity of a substance to decrease by a factor of 1/2. At the end of each half-life, 1/2 of the quantity that existed at the beginning of that particular half-life remains. Because 24 hours corresponds to three half-lives for this isotope, the fraction remaining is given by:

$1/2 \times 1/2 \times 1/2 = 1/8$ or 12.5%.

92. **B.** This question requires knowledge of the ideal gas law formula:

$$P_1 V_1/T_1 = P_2 V_2/T_2.$$

In this problem, because the volume is con-

stant, $V_1 = V_2$, the pressure is directly proportional to the absolute temperature. The temperature increases by exactly the same factor as the increase in pressure of 33%.

93. **D.** The magnification of a microscope is given by the product of the magnifications of objective and eyepiece. $M = M_o M_e$.

94. **D.** The metric power unit is the watt defined as 1 watt = 1 joule/s. (Power is the time rate of doing work.) Therefore 1 joule = 1 watt-s and 400 watt-s is equal to 400 joules.

95. **D.** This question requires only a knowledge of the simple form of Ohm's law, $V = IR$. One must convert the current to amperes. (100 mA = 0.1 A.) The resistance is thus $120V/0.1A = 1200$ ohms.

96. **A.** Newton's second law states that the net force equals the product of mass and acceleration: $F_{net} = ma$. In this case the net force is the difference between the applied force (18 N) and the force of friction (9 N): $F_{net} = F_a - F_f = 18 - 9 = (90)a$.

97. **B.** The total momentum of the two-cart system is zero before the students push off, and remains zero after they separate. Then: $0 = m_1 v_1 + m_2 v_2$. Thus, $v_2 = (60 \text{ kg})(1.2 \text{ m/s})/(0.8 \text{ m/s})$.

98. **B.** The initial kinetic energy is used up in doing work against the frictional force as the student-cart is brought to rest. Using the conservation of energy principle: $F_f x = 1/2 \, mv^2$, where $x = 8$ m. Then: $F_f = 20$ N.

99. **C.** We know that the total angular momentum of the student is conserved (constant). Because he is capable of changing his moment of inertia about the vertical axis of spin by extending his arms or pulling them in, we can find the ratio of the moments of inertia by using the conservation law in the form: $I_1 \, \Omega_1 = I_2 \, \Omega_2$. Then: $I_2/I_1 = \Omega_1/\Omega_2 = 1.5$.

100. **D.** Linear momentum is conserved in this problem. The addition of mass causes a decrease in the velocity as given by: $m_1 v_1 = (m_1 + m_{sand})V_2$. $V_2 = 1.6$ m/s.

101. **B.** The center-of-mass will not move because the forces exerted by pulling on the rope are internal forces to the two-cart system. It is nearer the larger mass, and is found by using the formula for the cm: $X_{cm} = (m_1x_1 + m_2x_2)/(m_1 + m_2)$. We are allowed to place the origin of the coordinate system anywhere we choose. Placing the origin at the original position of the larger mass, $x_1 = 0$ and $x_2 = 2$ m. $X_{cm} = (0 + (80)(2))/(200$ kg$) = 0.8$ m.

102. **C.** Conservation of momentum applies to this completely inelastic collision as follows: $m_1v_1 = (m_1 + m_2)V$. Then $V = (80$ kg$)(4$ m/s$)/(80 + 80) = 2$ m/s.

103. **B.** The net force accelerates the 100 kg mass according to Newton's third law. The net force here is the difference between the applied 90 N force and the opposing friction force. $F_{net} = 90 - f = ma = 100$kg $\times 0.8$ m/s^2. Solving for f we find that $f = 10$ N.

104. **B.** The falling weight can be isolated so that we can apply Newton's third law to it alone. The weight force due to the mass acts downward and the 90 N tension upward. The third law then shows that: $mg - 90 = ma$, which we solve for the unknown mass, m. $m(g-a) = 90$ N. $m(9.8-0.8) = 90$. Then $m = 10$ kg.

105. **C.** The work done in accelerating the cart is equal to the gain in kinetic energy: $F_{net}x = 1/2\ mv^2$, or $(100$ N$)(10$ m$) = (1/2)\ 80v^2$ and then $v = 5$ m/s.

106. **C.** Both $[H^+]$ and $[OH^-] = 1.0 \times 10^{-7}$. The pH = 7.0.

107. **B.** $K_a = \dfrac{[H^+][B^-]}{[HB]} = 6.6 \times 10^{-5} = \dfrac{[H^+]^2}{0.0001}$
$[H^+]^2 = 6.6 \times 10^{-9} = 66 \times 10^{-10}$

Because the square root of 66 is about 8, $[H^+] = 8 \times 10^{-5}$ or between 1×10^{-4} and 1×10^{-5}
pH $= -\log [H^+]$ and is between 4 and 5. Although water itself contributes $[H^+] = 1 \times 10^{-7}$, this is negligibly small in comparison to the H^+ from benzoic acid. Thus, in this example, the H^+ from water may be neglected.

108. **D.** pH + pOH = 14
Although in pure water pH = pOH, that is not the case here. Because pH is between 4 and 5, however, this pOH will be between 9 and 10.

109. **B.** $K_a = \dfrac{[H^+]^2}{1 \times 10^{-12}} = 6.6 \times 10^{-5}$

$[H^+]^2 = 6.6 \times 10^{-17} = 66 \times 10^{-18}$
$[H^+] =$ about 8×10^{-9} or 0.08×10^{-7}.

This is very small compared to the $[H^+]$ of 1.0×10^{-7} supplied by ionization of water. Thus the pH approximates 7.

110. **A.** Henderson-Hasselbalch formula

$$pH = pK_a + \log \frac{[salt]}{[acid]}$$

When the concentrations of salt and acid are equal, pH = pK_a. By inspection of $K_a = 6.6 \times 10^{-5}$, its negative log would be between 4 and 5. Thus the pK_a and the resulting pH are between 4 and 5.

111. **D.** $K_{sp} = 9 \times 10^{-12} = [Ag^+]^2 [CrO_4^=]$
$= (1 \times 10^{-6})^2 [CrO_4^=] = 9 \times 10^{-12}$
$[CrO_4^=] = 9$ or approximately 1×10^1

112. **C.** Addition of Cl^- ions will bring about precipitation of AgCl when its K_{sp} is exceeded.

113. **B.** The K_{sp} is given for a particular temperature and will change with temperature. It may speed the reaction but will not likely bring about more complete precipitation.

114. **C.** The K_{sp} with the smallest number represents the one with the lowest solubility.

115. **D.** The K_{sp}'s are independent of each other. If the K_{sp} of one is not reached, no precipitation will occur.

116. **A.** Phosphorus, a nonmetal, will react with oxygen to form an oxide. This oxide will react with water to form an acidic solution.

117. **A.** Nitrogen, a nonmetal, will react with oxygen to form an oxide. This oxide will react with water to form an acidic solution.

118. **B.** One mole of Ca will form one mole of CaO by oxidation. This will form one mole of $Ca(OH)_2$ by reaction with water.

119. **C.** One mole of $Ca(OH)_2$ will require two moles of HCl for neutralization.

120. **A.** Oxides of sulfur are produced during burning of coal. These acid anhydrides react with water to form acids. Carbon dioxide can react

with water to form the weak acid, carbonic acid. There is already a substantial amount of carbon dioxide in the atmosphere. Although carbon dioxide above the earth may contribute to other problems, it has not been suggested to contribute to acid rain.

121. **C.** One mole of each would exert the same effect, but only if they are not ionized. NaCl produces 2 ions per molecule, and Na_2SO_4 produces 3 ions per molecule. Colligative properties depend on the number of particles.

122. **B.** Molality (moles of solute per 1000g of solvent) is used in calculations of colligative properties. Further calculations are required if there is ionization.

123. **D.** All of these are colligative properties.

124. **A.** Without knowing the identity of the solute, we know that twice the amount will lower the freezing point twice as much.

125. **C.** If the weight is the same, the non-ionizing solute with the lowest molecular weight will have the largest number of dissolved molecules.

126. **A.** Loss of a single electron in the 3s orbital leaves the stable electronic configuration of the noble gas, neon.

127. **B.** In a neutral atom, the number of electrons in orbitals equals the number of protons in the nucleus. The latter defines the atomic number.

128. **C.** Gain of an additional electron would give the stable electronic configuration of the noble element, krypton.

129. **D.** Note that the number of electrons exceeds the atomic number (and the number of protons) by one. Thus, this would be an ion with a charge of −1.

130. **C.** The fact that the number of electrons is equal to the atomic number indicates that this is a neutral atom. The fact that the outermost electron is in the 3p orbital rather than the expected 3s orbital indicates that the atom is in an excited state.

131. **D.** Noble elements include helium, neon, argon, krypton, xenon, and radon.

132. **D.** Each orbital electron possesses four quantum numbers—principal, angular momentum, magnetic, and spin.

133. **C.** Possible values of magnetic quantum number are −1, 0, and +1.

134. **B.** Possible values of spin quantum number are $+\frac{1}{2}$ and $-\frac{1}{2}$.

135. **A.** No two electrons in an atom possess all four identical quantum numbers.

136. **C.** Silver ions will react with chloride ions and precipitate as AgCl.

137. **B.** $H_2S \rightleftarrows 2H^+ + S^{2-}$. By the common ion effect, lowering the pH (increasing the H^+ concentration) will lower the S^{2-} concentration by displacing the reaction to the left.
$K_i = \dfrac{[H^+]^2[S^{2-}]}{[H_2S]}$.
If $[H^+]$ increases, $[S^{2-}]$ must decrease.

138. **A.** Freezing point depression in water depends only on the number of solute particles per unit volume
$1\ M$ NaCl $= 2 \times 1 \times 6.02 \times 10^{23}$ particles per liter
$0.3\ M\ Na_2SO_4 = 3 \times .3 \times 6.02 \times 10^{23}$ particles per liter
$1.5\ M$ glucose $= 1 \times 1.5 \times 6.02 \times 10^{23}$ particles per liter
$0.5\ M\ BaSO_4 = 2 \times 0.5 \times 6.02 \times 10^{23}$ particles per liter
Dividing by 6.02×10^{23} we can see that the comparative figures are NaCl, 2; Na_2SO_4, 0.9; glucose, 1.5; and $BaSO_4$, 1.0. Thus, the NaCl solution has the greatest number of particles per unit volume (considering the ionization of NaCl, Na_2SO_4 and $BaSO_4$), and it will have the lowest freezing point.

139. **D.** A reaction in which electrons (e^-) are removed is termed an oxidation reaction; the adding of electrons to an atom or molecule is termed a reduction reaction.

140. **A.** The hydronium ion, H_3O^+, is a protonated water molecule. $2H_2O \rightleftarrows H_3O^+ + OH^-$

141. **A.** As long as the volume units are the same, $N_1V_1 = N_2V_2$

$$V_2 = \frac{N_1V_1}{N_2} = \frac{(50)(0.25)}{0.50} = 25 \text{ ml}$$

142. **A.** This is a definition of the zwitterion; an example is the amino acid, glycine.

WRITING SAMPLE

Part 1, Essay

One must point out that Demonax begins his assertion with "probably." The statement then takes on a more questioning or probing tone, as if he is asking for a contradiction. This tone colors an attitude that is already filled with a sort of shrugging resignation or apathy. Demonax clearly believes that laws do not serve their intended purpose. It seems that, to him, that purpose would be to change the nature of men who are not "good." He says, in effect, that good men do not need laws in order to be good and that bad men will remain bad with or without laws.

This is probably true. However, it is not clear that Demonax explored the possibility that laws might serve another purpose. Among some probable other things, laws serve as guidelines by which men can operate in social groups. Even a very good man might want to know on which side of the street he should drive. Laws might also be a deterrent to bad behaviors as well. A bad man who might steal the purse of an elderly blind woman might be deterred by the knowledge that the law calls for a prison sentence for so doing. The man is made no better by the law, but the life of the blind woman might be.

Laws are useful as a set of guidelines, rules, or agreements, accepted by a group of people who wish to live interdependently. They save time for people who otherwise would have to continuously be deciding upon the methods to use in everyday social interactions. More controversial, but also inevitable, is the fact that they also uphold a moral code that is agreed upon hopefully by the majority. Without any laws, we would, in fact, be less free to move about in more important endeavors because we would be constantly battling each other for time and space. Imagine an interstate highway with no traffic regulations, for example. Or imagine trying to maintain possession of one's home if there were no laws to say that it was your home between the time when you left for work and the time when you returned from work. As an effort to change the nature of a human being, laws are, indeed, probably useless. But, as an effort to change the nature of our social lives, they are clearly invaluable and mean the difference between living in civilization and living in chaos.

Part 1
Explanation of First Response: 5

The paper focuses on the statement and addresses each of the three writing tasks. In the first paragraph the writer begins the explanation of the statement by noting that it is qualified with the word "probably," an explanation that is completed with a paraphrase of the quotation. The second paragraph presents specific situations in which laws do, in fact, serve good purposes. The final paragraph balances the extremes, exploring those things about laws that make them useful for people living together in social situations, which is a pragmatic position, but arguing that laws probably do not change human beings.

This is a tightly reasoned essay that makes good use of concrete examples. The writing is clear, and the sentences are nicely paced. Paragraph two is potentially a strong one, with its example of the elderly woman's purse; but it would benefit from a bringing together of ideas at the end, a sentence to clinch the paragraph. With fuller development of this paragraph and a brief expansion of the idea in paragraph one that, to Demonax, laws do not serve their intended purpose, the essay would receive a 6 rather than a 5.

Part 2, Essay

With the thought of the concept of freedom comes naturally the question, from what? Freedom does not exist without the possibility, really the latent presence of restraint. What Gibran says is that an increase in one freedom would necessarily imply a restraint on another. This is because an increase in a man's freedom always means also an increase in his domain of responsibility. For example, as an infant, a person could be seen as either totally free or totally without freedom. An infant is totally free from responsibility and obligation, yet totally dependent on and restrained by his caretakers. What Gibran understands is that, the greater one's realm of existence and the broader one's scope of knowledge, the greater also is one's realm and scope of responsibility. As you commit an act, the act becomes a part of you, a fetter perhaps, and certainly a history or past to which you are then forever confined and from which you never will be free.

From this point of view, there are certainly no possible examples of a freedom that implies no restraints, for existence itself implies a certain restraint. Even a freedom to die would imply a restraint from the opportunity to live. The point is that one thing or act at a point in the realm of time and space forbids the existence of another at that point. With every act and thought then, we redefine our own existence; with definition comes restraint, and with restraint comes the inhibition of some freedom.

What Gibran is apparently trying to do is to point beyond an immediate goal of freedom to the new existence beyond it. For example, once a person is free of the yoke of his parents and family, that freedom puts a new and greater yoke, that of responsibility on his shoulders throughout the remainder of his life. Gibran is not arguing against freedom, however, but is suggesting a more mature, wiser view of freedom than that of freedom as an end in itself. As one's vision expands, one will have greater and greater freedoms. But with that vision will also come knowledge and with knowledge will come responsibility. And so, as we seek to broaden our scope of existence, we also seek to make our burden a bit heavier. And this becomes a good thing.

Part 2
Explanation of Second Response: 4

The paper addresses all three objectives, and it does an especially nice job with one and three. Paragraph one focuses sharply on the explanation of the quotation. This is perhaps the most difficult of the tasks for this quotation because of its seeming paradox. The paragraph also provides the example of the infant, who could be considered either totally free or totally without freedom. Paragraph two does not confront the second task as directly as does paragraph one. Though there is a clear attempt here to explore the possibility of a freedom that would not imply a burden or an obstacle to a greater freedom, the paragraph stops short of providing a specific situation that illustrates the point. If there were a more direct confrontation of the second task, this essay would receive a higher rating. Paragraph three reconciles the extremes and examines the implications of the statement.

The writing in this paper is clear and well controlled. Each of the paragraphs is organized around a topic that gives unity to the paper. Its sentences are varied and flow nicely from one to the next. The weakest aspect of the paper is that it lacks concrete details to illustrate its points from the beginning of paragraph two to the end. With the addition of such details and with a direct confrontation of the task in paragraph two, its rating would move to 5 or 6.

BIOLOGICAL SCIENCES

143. **C.** Thyroid stimulating hormone (TSH) produced by the pituitary gland stimulates the thyroid gland to produce its hormones T_3 (triiodothyronine) and T_4 (tetraiodothyronine or thyroxine). TSH modulates the iodide trapping mechanisms; hypersecretion results in goiter and exophthalmos, whereas hyposecretion leads to diminished thyroid function and lethargy.

144. **B.** See explanation for question 143.

145. **C.** When thyroxin is administered, one would expect that the iodide uptake would decrease; in graph I it stayed level, whereas in graph III an increase of uptake is exhibited. Both experimental conditions indicate some evidence of thyroid malfunction.

146. **B.** A hyperthyroid individual would not be expected to show additional uptake because the gland already is working at an elevated level. When thyroid hormone was administered as in our experiments, normally the uptake should have decreased; it stayed the same however.

147. **A.** When thyroxin is administered, TSH production diminishes and RAI uptake should drop. This did not occur in graph I while graph II demonstrates the expected normal. Graph III shows an increase in uptake indicating that the pituitary is not responding to the negative inhibitory feedback that thyroxin elicits; TSH production should decrease at the time of thyroxine administration.

148. **B.** Acromegaly is a result of pituitary oversecretion of growth hormone. Lack of iodine will result in goiter development of the thyroid gland. Rickets is due to vitamin D deficiency. A skin rash is not a specific lesion that can be associated with only one specific cause as the others listed.

149. **B.** Acidophils produce somatotropic hormone (STH) and luteotropic hormone (LTH) or prolactin. Beta cells produce thyroid stimulating hormone (TSH), adrenocorticotropic hormone (ACTH), and melanocyte stimulating hormone (MSH). Delta cells produce luteinizing hormone (LH) (called interstitial cell stimulating hormone in the male), and follicle stimulating hormone (FSH). Chromophobes are considered resting cells.

150. **D.** All statements are correct. The thyroid originates from the foramen cecum region of the tongue. Its structural unit is the follicle, a unit of epithelial cells that surround a colloid space. Colloid is located extracellularly and contains thyroglobulin. T_3 and T_4 are the active thyroid principles and are released into the bloodstream and carried on proteins to the tissues.

151. **B.** Acromegaly and (or) giantism is due to over-activity of the alpha cells of the pituitary, which secrete growth hormone. If a person is affected before puberty, he or she will develop into a fairly well-proportioned giant. After maturity, an increase in the size of the hands and feet and massive development of the bones comprising the face are consequences. In the adult, strictly speaking, the term acromegaly must be applied to this condition.

152. **C.**

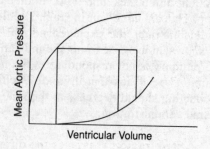

If aortic pressure is unchanged and end diastolic volume increases, the stroke volume or the difference between end diastolic volume and end systolic volume is larger. Ventricular work is equal to:

Work = Pressure • Stroke Volume = Force/ Area • Volume = Force • Length

or the area under the curve. The kinetic energy of the ejected blood can be ignored because it represents ≈5% of the total energy and stays constant under most conditions. The area subtended by the pressure-volume loop increases as does the work in this case. Because the contractility of the heart represented by the upper curve remains constant, the end systolic volume also remains constant.

153. **D.**

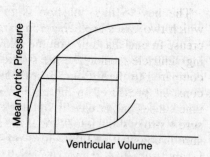

Whereas the pressure to eject blood must increase, the volume of blood the ventricle ejects is less. Therefore, the ventricular work depends on the exact nature of the two curves. Because the ventricle cannot maintain the required pressure at low volumes, the total volume of blood ejected is less and the end systolic volume is increased.

154. **A.**

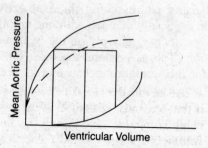

In this case, the ventricle is incapable of generating the same pressure at low volumes. Therefore, the volume of blood ejected is less (i.e., the stroke volume is smaller), and the end systolic volume is correspondingly larger. Note that this question is a play on words. If the stroke volume decreases with a constant end diastolic volume, the volume left in the ventricle after contraction will be more. The ventricular work is reduced because the pressure remains constant while the volume of blood ejected falls so that the product of the two decreases.

155. **C.**

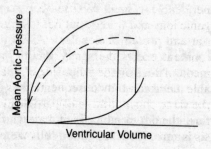

The key to this question is to remember which two cases are being compared. The increase in end diastolic volume allows the failing ventricle to increase the stroke volume as compared to the uncompensated case. With a constant pressure, an increase in stroke volume causes an increase in the work (i.e., pressure ● stroke volume). Because the aortic pressure is constant and the active pressure curve is unchanged in the two cases, the volume remaining in the ventricle at the point at which the ventricle stops ejecting blood will remain constant.

156. **C.**

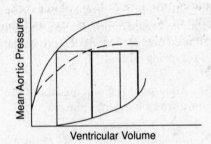

The key to this question, as in question 155, is that one must remember what conditions are being compared. Increasing the end diastolic volume sufficiently could theoretically allow a failing ventricle to eject a larger stroke volume than is the case in normals. However, the compensation for a failing ventricle usually is not sufficient for this to occur under physiological conditions. Because the stroke volume is indeterminate relative to the normal condition, the ventricular work is also indeterminate given a constant mean aortic pressure. Because by definition a failing ventricle cannot maintain the same pressure at low volumes, the end systolic volume must increase in comparison to that of normal.

157. **B.** The definitions of isotonic, hypotonic, and hypertonic need to be recalled. Remember that the structure placed in a medium is surrounded by a semipermeable membrane; the structure is permeable to small particles (e.g., certain inorganic ions and water), but not to large particles (fat and protein molecules). An isotonic environment exerts the same osmotic pull as the medium does on the other side of a semipermeable membrane. It consequently has to possess the same concentration of particles and, therefore, the net gain or loss of water during osmosis is zero. If the red blood cells were placed in a hypotonic solution, hemolysis would occur because a hypotonic solution would exert a lesser osmotic pull than the medium on the other side of a semipermeable membrane (the inside of the RBC); the medium would possess a smaller concentration of particles and consequently would lose water during osmosis. In our case, the red blood cells were hypertonic in relation to the medium and exerted a larger osmotic pull than the medium on the other side of the semipermeable membrane because it possessed a greater concentration of particles and consequently accumulated water during osmosis.

158. **D.** In this experiment, urea and glycerol did enter the red blood cell and water consequently followed because it was in greater quantity outside and tried to establish an equilibrium.

159. **D.** Cell membranes are described as semipermeable because they allow some materials to pass while they block others. All materials that pass membranes must be either a liquid or dissolved in a liquid. Molecules also must be fairly simple, but molecular size is not the limiting factor because amino acids pass less readily than do many smaller molecules. Osmosis is the passage of liquids through a membrane; usually water through the semipermeable membrane. Diffusion is the passage of molecules from a more concentrated environment to a less concentrated region; equalization is usually the end result.

160. **D.** Active transport involves the diffusion of molecules against a gradient; this is an energy consuming phenomenon. The process of moving substances from an area of lower concentration to where they are in a higher concentration is selective, and requires respiration. Osmosis and diffusion are described in the explanation for question 159. Turgor pressure involves the passage of water into a cell at a faster rate than it can leave; the cell becomes plump and filled (turgid). At times the force results in bursting the structures. Plasmolysis is defined as a shrinking of protoplasm due to the loss of water from a cell.

161. **A.** Layers of material (probably mucopolysaccharide) secreted by the cell are found on the surface of the cell. The most prominent layer is the basement membrane, or basal lamina. These structures are boundaries and must be

traversed by material entering and leaving the cell. Cells must be held together; adjacent cell membranes interdigitate and intercellular cement is utilized. A desmosome is a specialized area of connection between adjacent cellular membranes (macula adherens). A terminal bar is a dense area surrounding the apical cellular surface. It includes the tight junction (zona/occludens) and the loose junction (zona adherens). In cardiac muscle, several cardiac muscle cells join end to end at a specialized junctional zone known as an intercalated disc.

162. **B.** Some of the proteins embedded in the lipid layers of membranes are shaped to form channels with "gates," which open only to certain materials or under certain conditions.

163. **A.** Osmosis is a process in which solvent passes from an area of lower solute concentration to an area of higher solute concentration. In dialysis solvent and solute both pass through the membrane.

164. **A.** The defect cannot be dominant because individual 5 was produced by two normal parents who would have no defective alleles if the defect is dominant (either autosomal or X-linked). The defect is unlikely to be X-linked recessive because unless a new mutation occurred, individual 5 should have received a normal allele for the gene on her X from her father (individual 2) and therefore could not express a recessive X-linked defect. Therefore the most likely possibility (using the assumptions of a single controlling gene and very rare mutations) would be an autosomal gene for which the defective allele is recessive to the normal allele.

165. **C.** Unless a new mutation occurred, individual 1 would have to have one normal allele (which produced the normal phenotype) and one defective allele (which was contributed to individual 5 along with a defective allele from individual 2) to produce individual 5's defective phenotype.

166. **B.** Individual 4 would have to contain two defective alleles to produce the defective phenotype.

167. **C.** Individual 7 would have to contain at least one normal allele to produce her normal phenotype. Her other allele cannot be determined

with certainty from the data given. Because her parents are probably both heterozygotes (see above), she has a ⅓ probability of having two normal alleles and a ⅔ probability of having one normal and one abnormal allele.

i.e., $Nn \times Nn$
¼ NN : ⅔ Nn : ¼ nn

defective phenotype
⅔ of normal phenotype
⅓ of normal phenotype

Therefore she is most likely to contain one normal and one defective allele.

168. **C.** Individual 8 would have to contain one normal allele (to produce his normal phenotype) and one abnormal allele (because he contributed one of the two defective alleles in each of offspring 14 and 18).

169. **B.** The upper region consists of the fluid portion of the blood, the plasma.

170. **D.** The thin "buffy" layer is the white blood cells and platelets.

171. **C.** After centrifugation, the packed volume of formed elements was 5.5 ml. As stated previously, most of the formed elements are RBCs.

172. **B.** After centrifugation, the volume of packed formed elements of the patient was 5.5 ml. Because hematocrit is defined as the relative volume of formed elements, the hematocrit of this patient is 55% (i.e., 5.5 ml out of 10 ml, or 55% of the total blood volume, was occupied by formed elements).

173. **B.** The hematocrit of this patient, 55%, is higher than the normal average value of 45%.

174. **C.** Region C consists of RBCs. These cells contain hemoglobin, which binds and carries oxygen.

175. **B.** Region B, the "buffy" coat, consists of WBCs and platelets. The WBCs consist of a number of cell types, some of which are responsible for fighting infections.

176. **B.** Region B, the "buffy" coat, consists of WBCs and platelets. The platelets are responsible for triggering the cascade of events that results in the formation of blood clots.

177. **A.** The major component of blood plasma is water.

178. **A.** Because the patient's hematocrit is higher than the normal value, the patient has more formed elements, largely RBCs, than a normal individual. Because RBCs are responsible for binding and carrying oxygen, a higher hematocrit might suggest that the individual has a higher physiological demand for oxygen. Such a condition is seen in individuals living at high altitudes where the oxygen concentration of the air is lower (compared to the oxygen concentration of air at sea level).

179. **D.** A sarcomere, the area between two Z bands, is the functional unit of muscle; it is the region between two Z lines and consists of an A band and half of two abutting I bands.

180. **C.** According to the sliding filament theory (Huxley) the sarcomere response to excitation involves the sliding of thin and thick myofilaments past one another making and breaking chemical bonds with each other as they go. Neither the thick nor thin myofilaments change in length.

181. **A.** If we observed this contraction under the light microscope, we would see the narrowing of the H and I bands during contraction while the width of the A band would remain constant.

182. **C.** The immediate energy source for contraction is ATP which can be hydrolyzed by actomyosin to give ADP, P_1, and the energy which is in some way associated with cross-bridge motion. The ultimate source of this ATP is the ATP produced by the intermediary metabolisms of carbohydrates and lipids. As mentioned in previous answers the length of the myosin filaments would NOT be affected by ATP.

183. **C.** Calcium ions released following an action potential in the fiber membrane and T-tubules bind with troponin. Calcium-troponin binding removes the inhibition of actomyosin formation. The sarcoplasmic reticulum concentrates calcium ions (Ca^{2+}) within its lumen, but depolarization of the T-tubule membrane induces the nearly terminal cisternae of the sarcoplasmic reticulum to release this Ca^{2+} into the sarcoplasm among the myofilaments. The Ca^{2+} becomes associated with the troponin of the thin myofilament, bringing about contraction.

184. **A.** As shown in Figure 1, the percent of neutrophils bound increased from about 20% to about 50% as GMP-140 concentration increased. Tightness of binding, (C) and (D), was not measured, although it could contribute to the increased number of attached cells.

185. **B.** Figure 1 indicates that about ¼ of monocytes attached at a GMP-140 concentration of zero.

186. **C.** According to Figure 1, coating with GMP-140 caused little change in lymphocyte attachment, increased neutrophil attachment from about 20% up to about 50%, and increased monocyte attachment from 25% to about 75%.

187. **A.** Because GMP-140 coating of dishes increased neutrophil attachment (Figure 1), the neutrophils clearly attach to GMP-140. Pretreatment of neutrophils with GMP-140 (Figure 3) decreased attachment of the neutrophils to cultured endothelial cells, indicating that the GMP-140 binding sites on neutrophils are involved in endothelial attachment.

188. **D.** Treatment of neutrophils with antibody against CD-18 had no effect on attachment of neutrophils to GMP-140-coated dishes, so CD-18 on neutrophils is apparently not involved.

189. **A.** Neutrophils and macrophages (derived from monocytes) are most important in phagocytosis and if these cells could not easily leave vessels in inflammation sites, phagocytosis of bacteria should be impaired. Lymphocytes would not be affected because they do not appear to depend on GMP-140, so natural killer activity (due to large granular lymphocytes), cell-mediated responses (using helper T lymphocytes and cytotoxic T lymphocytes), and humoral responses (using helper T lymphocytes and B lymphocytes) should not be heavily affected. Some reduction in cell-mediated and humoral responses could occur due to reduction in macrophages available to serve as antigen-presenting cells and/or cytokine sources.

190. **B.** Enzymes are generally protein in nature, thus largely polymers of amino acids. Some other material may be present as well. The recent recognition of a small number of nucleic acids (ribozymes) that act on enzymes does not invalidate the question.

191. **C.** Enzymes function in reactions by decreasing the energy of activation. The net energy yield (positive or negative) is not affected, and a thermodynamically unfavorable reaction will not proceed simply by addition of an enzyme.

192. **D.** Enzymes are considered not to be used up in reactions. Incidental loss or destruction of enzyme does require replacement however.

193. **A.** Covalent modification would not include changes of ions. Phosphorylation/dephosphorylation is often used as a means of regulation of activity of various enzymes. Sulfation/desulfation is seldom if ever employed.

194. **B.** The response of most enzymes to being boiled in aqueous solution is substantially decreased activity as a result of enzyme denaturation. (Remember that enzymes are proteins in general.) More moderate increase in temperature increases the activity of an enzyme.

195. **B.** The number of possible isomers is four. Note that positions 3 and 4 are chiral and thus may have the hydroxyl group on either side. Thus $2 \times 2 = 4$.

196. **B.** Although there appear at first glance to be three chiral centers, this is not so; the number 3 carbon is *not* attached to four nonidentical groups. Thus only four isomers appear to be possible, but it can be seen that two of these are identical and thus there are two optically active isomers and one optically inactive isomer.

197. **B.** There are two chiral centers.

198. **B.** Ribose is found in RNA, contributing to the name, ribonucleic acid. Deoxyribose is found in DNA.

199. **C.** As seen in the explanation for question 196, there are only two chiral centers (carbons 2 and 4).

200. **B.** DNA is the primary source of information. It is usually considered that DNA directs the synthesis of RNA and that RNA directs the synthesis of protein. DNA also directs its own replication. In some cases (for example the retroviruses), RNA can direct the synthesis of DNA.

201. **C.** RNA directs the synthesis of protein (see above) and three nucleotide bases are required to code for each amino acid.

202. **B.** Paired strands of DNA are found in the chromosomes of higher animals.

203. **A.** None of the cells will have only DNA containing deuterium. Each cell will have two strands of DNA for each chromosome, and one strand of each pair will contain deuterium.

204. **D.** As stated above, DNA is required to code for RNA and RNA is required to code for protein. The enzymes that actually carry out the biosynthesis are protein. (It might be argued that DNA is not required, but *ultimately* DNA is required for RNA synthesis.)

205. **A.** This study investigated the response of antibody produced by a host against the protein of the virus inducing tumor. Statements **C** and **D** are contradicted by the evidence. There is no information to either confirm or deny statement **B**, however, it is clear that Brown Norway rats produced antibody at both time periods and, therefore, statement **A** is supported by the data presented.

206. **C.** From the experimental data, one can conclude that prolactin and LH are both produced by the pituitary, that the hypothalamus stimulates LH release, but inhibits prolactin release, and that ovarian hormones inhibit LH release, but not prolactin release. Lactogenic hormone or luteotrophic hormone (LTH) or prolactin is secreted by the acidophils (alpha cells) of the pituitary. This hormone: (1) promotes growth of the breast, which has been stimulated already by estrogen and progesterone; (2) promotes and maintains lactation; (3) helps in maintenance of the corpus luteum; and (4) promotes maternal instinct.

207. **C.** The experiment was performed to determine the effect of salinity concentrations on the secretory proteins of the urophysis. The data shows that protein 2 was affected more (twice) by the increasing concentration of seawater than protein 1.

208. **D.** Careful analysis of the data shows that in the system under investigation, spleen cells and mast cells together are required for antibody production, that spleen cells are probably found in the thymus and that X-irradiation is an important tool in immunological work. Statement **C**, implying that spleen cells or mast cells are essential to the antibody production against pollen is contradicted by the data because bone marrow and pollen and thymocytes and pollen show a response. Statement **D** is not supported nor contradicted by the experiment, even though mast cells are known to produce histamine and their activity is controlled by certain nasal sprays limiting their effects after exposure to certain substances.

209. **C.** Beta cells of the pituitary produce thyroid stimulating hormone, which stimulates the thyroid to produce its hormones T_3 (triiodothyronine) and T_4 (tetraiodothyronine or thyroxin). Iodides consumed in food and water are absorbed and carried to the iodide pool in the extracellular fluid via the circulatory system. Five events are involved in hormone production: (1). trapping iodide; (2). oxidation of iodide to organic iodine; (3). synthesis of hormone; (4). storage as the thyroglobulin moiety; and (5). release of the active principle into the circulation. TSH greatly influences the trapping mechanism; thiocyanates block trapping, whereas thiouracil blocks the oxidation and synthetic steps. The data shows that Group 4 received thyroxine, which inhibited TSH production, whereas Group 2 was treated with thiocyanate, which affected the iodine pump. Group 3 received propylthiouracil, an inhibitor of iodine oxidation; in Group 2 iodine is not taken up and no radioactivity can be measured.

210. **B.** The five-year total of wheat was 49; for corn it was 56. The ratio is thus 7⁄8.

211. **C.** Scanning of the graphs comparing the number of daylight hours clearly shows that only in greenhouses 2 and 3 are there provided 15 hours of light per day for several weeks, which is necessary for Plant X. If the question would have been that Plant Y will only bear fruit when the period of darkness is 8 hours or less, it could not have born fruit in greenhouse 1. However, if Plant Z will only form flowers and seeds when exposed to days of no more than 15 hours in length, it certainly could not have been native in areas simulated by greenhouses 2 and 3.

212. **A.** Blood is composed of cells and plasma. Plasma constitutes about 55% of blood volume, and cellular elements about 45%. The normal red blood cell hematocrit is about 36–45%. Hemoglobin, a complex molecule of iron and protein, is a key element of the RBC; the RBC carries oxygen from the lungs to the tissues and transports carbon dioxide from the tissues to the lungs. In the breakdown of hemoglobin, bilirubin is excreted and iron is retained. The purpose of the experiment was to test the effect of different storage conditions on hemoglobin composition as revealed by gel electrophoresis. Although none of the storage conditions were able to maintain hemoglobin in an absolutely unchanged state, storage at −20°C in glycerol allowed the least change from the fresh configuration.

213. **C.** The suppressed plasma levels of FSH and LH during the follicular phase of the menstrual cycle are due to the negative inhibitory effects of estrogen being secreted from developing follicles. The small, abrupt rise in plasma estrogen is believed to trigger the ovulatory LH surge (by suspension of negative or positive feedback). During the luteal phase, estrogen and progesterone again establish the negative-feedback suppression and luteal failure occurs on day 26. The higher levels of bound LH in the treated animals indicate that these animals had lower LH levels; the drug seems to inhibit LH release.

214. **B.** Examination of the data shows that all three proteins were absorbed at the same rate (2 minutes) by the visceral endoderm; the visceral endoderm appeared to block the transport of protein Y, whereas protein X appeared to be transported through it. The statement that the visceral basement membrane blocked the transport of protein X is not supported by the data because it is found at the next level, namely, the vitelline endothelium. The vitelline endothelium does, however, block protein X from entering the fetal blood.

215. **B.** The fiber components of connective tissue add strength and support. They are collagenous, elastic and reticular in nature; collagen fibers are the most numerous fiber type. The graphs show that labeled proline starts to appear in the collagen in under 2 hours, so **B** was supported by the evidence. Statements **A** and **C** were contradicted by the information given, and **D** is neither supported nor contradicted.

216. **B.** Glycine has no chiral center, but other amino acids in higher animals are ordinarily of the L-series.

217. **C.** Carbohydrate monosaccharides found in higher animals are generally of the D-series.

218. **B.** Epimers differ in configuration at only one carbon. Enantiomers are nonsuperimposable mirror images. Diastereomers are nonsuperimposable nonmirror images.

219. **C.** The number of kcal/g for the classes of food material are: carbohydrates, 4; proteins, 4; and fats, 9. The nucleic acids are not considered as a class of food.

The MCAT
Model Examination D

ANSWER SHEET

DIRECTIONS: After locating the number of the question to which you are responding, fill in the circle containing the letter of the answer you have selected. Use pencil (not a ballpoint pen) to completely blacken the circle.

VERBAL REASONING

1. Ⓐ Ⓑ Ⓒ Ⓓ
2. Ⓐ Ⓑ Ⓒ Ⓓ
3. Ⓐ Ⓑ Ⓒ Ⓓ
4. Ⓐ Ⓑ Ⓒ Ⓓ
5. Ⓐ Ⓑ Ⓒ Ⓓ
6. Ⓐ Ⓑ Ⓒ Ⓓ
7. Ⓐ Ⓑ Ⓒ Ⓓ
8. Ⓐ Ⓑ Ⓒ Ⓓ
9. Ⓐ Ⓑ Ⓒ Ⓓ
10. Ⓐ Ⓑ Ⓒ Ⓓ
11. Ⓐ Ⓑ Ⓒ Ⓓ
12. Ⓐ Ⓑ Ⓒ Ⓓ
13. Ⓐ Ⓑ Ⓒ Ⓓ
14. Ⓐ Ⓑ Ⓒ Ⓓ
15. Ⓐ Ⓑ Ⓒ Ⓓ
16. Ⓐ Ⓑ Ⓒ Ⓓ
17. Ⓐ Ⓑ Ⓒ Ⓓ
18. Ⓐ Ⓑ Ⓒ Ⓓ
19. Ⓐ Ⓑ Ⓒ Ⓓ
20. Ⓐ Ⓑ Ⓒ Ⓓ
21. Ⓐ Ⓑ Ⓒ Ⓓ
22. Ⓐ Ⓑ Ⓒ Ⓓ
23. Ⓐ Ⓑ Ⓒ Ⓓ
24. Ⓐ Ⓑ Ⓒ Ⓓ
25. Ⓐ Ⓑ Ⓒ Ⓓ
26. Ⓐ Ⓑ Ⓒ Ⓓ
27. Ⓐ Ⓑ Ⓒ Ⓓ
28. Ⓐ Ⓑ Ⓒ Ⓓ
29. Ⓐ Ⓑ Ⓒ Ⓓ
30. Ⓐ Ⓑ Ⓒ Ⓓ

31. Ⓐ Ⓑ Ⓒ Ⓓ
32. Ⓐ Ⓑ Ⓒ Ⓓ
33. Ⓐ Ⓑ Ⓒ Ⓓ
34. Ⓐ Ⓑ Ⓒ Ⓓ
35. Ⓐ Ⓑ Ⓒ Ⓓ
36. Ⓐ Ⓑ Ⓒ Ⓓ
37. Ⓐ Ⓑ Ⓒ Ⓓ
38. Ⓐ Ⓑ Ⓒ Ⓓ
39. Ⓐ Ⓑ Ⓒ Ⓓ
40. Ⓐ Ⓑ Ⓒ Ⓓ
41. Ⓐ Ⓑ Ⓒ Ⓓ
42. Ⓐ Ⓑ Ⓒ Ⓓ
43. Ⓐ Ⓑ Ⓒ Ⓓ
44. Ⓐ Ⓑ Ⓒ Ⓓ
45. Ⓐ Ⓑ Ⓒ Ⓓ
46. Ⓐ Ⓑ Ⓒ Ⓓ
47. Ⓐ Ⓑ Ⓒ Ⓓ
48. Ⓐ Ⓑ Ⓒ Ⓓ
49. Ⓐ Ⓑ Ⓒ Ⓓ
50. Ⓐ Ⓑ Ⓒ Ⓓ
51. Ⓐ Ⓑ Ⓒ Ⓓ
52. Ⓐ Ⓑ Ⓒ Ⓓ
53. Ⓐ Ⓑ Ⓒ Ⓓ
54. Ⓐ Ⓑ Ⓒ Ⓓ
55. Ⓐ Ⓑ Ⓒ Ⓓ
56. Ⓐ Ⓑ Ⓒ Ⓓ
57. Ⓐ Ⓑ Ⓒ Ⓓ
58. Ⓐ Ⓑ Ⓒ Ⓓ
59. Ⓐ Ⓑ Ⓒ Ⓓ
60. Ⓐ Ⓑ Ⓒ Ⓓ

61. Ⓐ Ⓑ Ⓒ Ⓓ
62. Ⓐ Ⓑ Ⓒ Ⓓ
63. Ⓐ Ⓑ Ⓒ Ⓓ
64. Ⓐ Ⓑ Ⓒ Ⓓ
65. Ⓐ Ⓑ Ⓒ Ⓓ

PHYSICAL SCIENCES

66. Ⓐ Ⓑ Ⓒ Ⓓ
67. Ⓐ Ⓑ Ⓒ Ⓓ
68. Ⓐ Ⓑ Ⓒ Ⓓ
69. Ⓐ Ⓑ Ⓒ Ⓓ
70. Ⓐ Ⓑ Ⓒ Ⓓ
71. Ⓐ Ⓑ Ⓒ Ⓓ
72. Ⓐ Ⓑ Ⓒ Ⓓ
73. Ⓐ Ⓑ Ⓒ Ⓓ
74. Ⓐ Ⓑ Ⓒ Ⓓ
75. Ⓐ Ⓑ Ⓒ Ⓓ
76. Ⓐ Ⓑ Ⓒ Ⓓ
77. Ⓐ Ⓑ Ⓒ Ⓓ
78. Ⓐ Ⓑ Ⓒ Ⓓ
79. Ⓐ Ⓑ Ⓒ Ⓓ
80. Ⓐ Ⓑ Ⓒ Ⓓ
81. Ⓐ Ⓑ Ⓒ Ⓓ
82. Ⓐ Ⓑ Ⓒ Ⓓ
83. Ⓐ Ⓑ Ⓒ Ⓓ
84. Ⓐ Ⓑ Ⓒ Ⓓ
85. Ⓐ Ⓑ Ⓒ Ⓓ
86. Ⓐ Ⓑ Ⓒ Ⓓ
87. Ⓐ Ⓑ Ⓒ Ⓓ
88. Ⓐ Ⓑ Ⓒ Ⓓ

89. Ⓐ Ⓑ Ⓒ Ⓓ
90. Ⓐ Ⓑ Ⓒ Ⓓ
91. Ⓐ Ⓑ Ⓒ Ⓓ
92. Ⓐ Ⓑ Ⓒ Ⓓ
93. Ⓐ Ⓑ Ⓒ Ⓓ
94. Ⓐ Ⓑ Ⓒ Ⓓ
95. Ⓐ Ⓑ Ⓒ Ⓓ
96. Ⓐ Ⓑ Ⓒ Ⓓ
97. Ⓐ Ⓑ Ⓒ Ⓓ
98. Ⓐ Ⓑ Ⓒ Ⓓ
99. Ⓐ Ⓑ Ⓒ Ⓓ
100. Ⓐ Ⓑ Ⓒ Ⓓ
101. Ⓐ Ⓑ Ⓒ Ⓓ
102. Ⓐ Ⓑ Ⓒ Ⓓ
103. Ⓐ Ⓑ Ⓒ Ⓓ
104. Ⓐ Ⓑ Ⓒ Ⓓ
105. Ⓐ Ⓑ Ⓒ Ⓓ
106. Ⓐ Ⓑ Ⓒ Ⓓ
107. Ⓐ Ⓑ Ⓒ Ⓓ
108. Ⓐ Ⓑ Ⓒ Ⓓ
109. Ⓐ Ⓑ Ⓒ Ⓓ
110. Ⓐ Ⓑ Ⓒ Ⓓ
111. Ⓐ Ⓑ Ⓒ Ⓓ
112. Ⓐ Ⓑ Ⓒ Ⓓ
113. Ⓐ Ⓑ Ⓒ Ⓓ
114. Ⓐ Ⓑ Ⓒ Ⓓ
115. Ⓐ Ⓑ Ⓒ Ⓓ
116. Ⓐ Ⓑ Ⓒ Ⓓ
117. Ⓐ Ⓑ Ⓒ Ⓓ
118. Ⓐ Ⓑ Ⓒ Ⓓ

119. Ⓐ Ⓑ Ⓒ Ⓓ
120. Ⓐ Ⓑ Ⓒ Ⓓ
121. Ⓐ Ⓑ Ⓒ Ⓓ
122. Ⓐ Ⓑ Ⓒ Ⓓ
123. Ⓐ Ⓑ Ⓒ Ⓓ
124. Ⓐ Ⓑ Ⓒ Ⓓ
125. Ⓐ Ⓑ Ⓒ Ⓓ
126. Ⓐ Ⓑ Ⓒ Ⓓ
127. Ⓐ Ⓑ Ⓒ Ⓓ
128. Ⓐ Ⓑ Ⓒ Ⓓ
129. Ⓐ Ⓑ Ⓒ Ⓓ
130. Ⓐ Ⓑ Ⓒ Ⓓ
131. Ⓐ Ⓑ Ⓒ Ⓓ
132. Ⓐ Ⓑ Ⓒ Ⓓ
133. Ⓐ Ⓑ Ⓒ Ⓓ
134. Ⓐ Ⓑ Ⓒ Ⓓ
135. Ⓐ Ⓑ Ⓒ Ⓓ
136. Ⓐ Ⓑ Ⓒ Ⓓ
137. Ⓐ Ⓑ Ⓒ Ⓓ
138. Ⓐ Ⓑ Ⓒ Ⓓ
139. Ⓐ Ⓑ Ⓒ Ⓓ
140. Ⓐ Ⓑ Ⓒ Ⓓ
141. Ⓐ Ⓑ Ⓒ Ⓓ
142. Ⓐ Ⓑ Ⓒ Ⓓ

WRITING SAMPLE
Use separate ruled sheets of paper.

BIOLOGICAL SCIENCES

143. Ⓐ Ⓑ Ⓒ Ⓓ
144. Ⓐ Ⓑ Ⓒ Ⓓ
145. Ⓐ Ⓑ Ⓒ Ⓓ
146. Ⓐ Ⓑ Ⓒ Ⓓ
147. Ⓐ Ⓑ Ⓒ Ⓓ
148. Ⓐ Ⓑ Ⓒ Ⓓ
149. Ⓐ Ⓑ Ⓒ Ⓓ
150. Ⓐ Ⓑ Ⓒ Ⓓ
151. Ⓐ Ⓑ Ⓒ Ⓓ
152. Ⓐ Ⓑ Ⓒ Ⓓ
153. Ⓐ Ⓑ Ⓒ Ⓓ
154. Ⓐ Ⓑ Ⓒ Ⓓ
155. Ⓐ Ⓑ Ⓒ Ⓓ
156. Ⓐ Ⓑ Ⓒ Ⓓ
157. Ⓐ Ⓑ Ⓒ Ⓓ
158. Ⓐ Ⓑ Ⓒ Ⓓ
159. Ⓐ Ⓑ Ⓒ Ⓓ
160. Ⓐ Ⓑ Ⓒ Ⓓ
161. Ⓐ Ⓑ Ⓒ Ⓓ
162. Ⓐ Ⓑ Ⓒ Ⓓ
163. Ⓐ Ⓑ Ⓒ Ⓓ
164. Ⓐ Ⓑ Ⓒ Ⓓ
165. Ⓐ Ⓑ Ⓒ Ⓓ
166. Ⓐ Ⓑ Ⓒ Ⓓ
167. Ⓐ Ⓑ Ⓒ Ⓓ

168. Ⓐ Ⓑ Ⓒ Ⓓ
169. Ⓐ Ⓑ Ⓒ Ⓓ
170. Ⓐ Ⓑ Ⓒ Ⓓ
171. Ⓐ Ⓑ Ⓒ Ⓓ
172. Ⓐ Ⓑ Ⓒ Ⓓ
173. Ⓐ Ⓑ Ⓒ Ⓓ
174. Ⓐ Ⓑ Ⓒ Ⓓ
175. Ⓐ Ⓑ Ⓒ Ⓓ
176. Ⓐ Ⓑ Ⓒ Ⓓ
177. Ⓐ Ⓑ Ⓒ Ⓓ
178. Ⓐ Ⓑ Ⓒ Ⓓ
179. Ⓐ Ⓑ Ⓒ Ⓓ
180. Ⓐ Ⓑ Ⓒ Ⓓ
181. Ⓐ Ⓑ Ⓒ Ⓓ
182. Ⓐ Ⓑ Ⓒ Ⓓ
183. Ⓐ Ⓑ Ⓒ Ⓓ
184. Ⓐ Ⓑ Ⓒ Ⓓ
185. Ⓐ Ⓑ Ⓒ Ⓓ
186. Ⓐ Ⓑ Ⓒ Ⓓ
187. Ⓐ Ⓑ Ⓒ Ⓓ
188. Ⓐ Ⓑ Ⓒ Ⓓ
189. Ⓐ Ⓑ Ⓒ Ⓓ
190. Ⓐ Ⓑ Ⓒ Ⓓ
191. Ⓐ Ⓑ Ⓒ Ⓓ
192. Ⓐ Ⓑ Ⓒ Ⓓ
193. Ⓐ Ⓑ Ⓒ Ⓓ

194. Ⓐ Ⓑ Ⓒ Ⓓ
195. Ⓐ Ⓑ Ⓒ Ⓓ
196. Ⓐ Ⓑ Ⓒ Ⓓ
197. Ⓐ Ⓑ Ⓒ Ⓓ
198. Ⓐ Ⓑ Ⓒ Ⓓ
199. Ⓐ Ⓑ Ⓒ Ⓓ
200. Ⓐ Ⓑ Ⓒ Ⓓ
201. Ⓐ Ⓑ Ⓒ Ⓓ
202. Ⓐ Ⓑ Ⓒ Ⓓ
203. Ⓐ Ⓑ Ⓒ Ⓓ
204. Ⓐ Ⓑ Ⓒ Ⓓ
205. Ⓐ Ⓑ Ⓒ Ⓓ
206. Ⓐ Ⓑ Ⓒ Ⓓ
207. Ⓐ Ⓑ Ⓒ Ⓓ
208. Ⓐ Ⓑ Ⓒ Ⓓ
209. Ⓐ Ⓑ Ⓒ Ⓓ
210. Ⓐ Ⓑ Ⓒ Ⓓ
211. Ⓐ Ⓑ Ⓒ Ⓓ
212. Ⓐ Ⓑ Ⓒ Ⓓ
213. Ⓐ Ⓑ Ⓒ Ⓓ
214. Ⓐ Ⓑ Ⓒ Ⓓ
215. Ⓐ Ⓑ Ⓒ Ⓓ
216. Ⓐ Ⓑ Ⓒ Ⓓ
217. Ⓐ Ⓑ Ⓒ Ⓓ
218. Ⓐ Ⓑ Ⓒ Ⓓ
219. Ⓐ Ⓑ Ⓒ Ⓓ

Model Examination D

VERBAL REASONING

9 PASSAGES
65 QUESTIONS
85 MINUTES

DIRECTIONS: The questions are based on the accompanying passages. Read each passage carefully, then answer the following questions. Consider only the material within the passage. For each question, select the *ONE BEST ANSWER* and indicate your selection by marking the corresponding letter on the Answer Form.

Passage I (Questions 1–7)

Until the 1960s, the federal government's role in special education was limited. It supported programs for exceptional children by (1) supplying matching funds to state and local agencies; (2) granting funds for research in all areas of exceptionality; (3) disseminating information; (4) providing consultative services to state and local groups; and (5) distributing fellowships for the training of professionals in all areas related to special education (Kirk, 1962). It has been observed that "the best index of maturity in a society is the attention it pays to its handicapped, its poor, its abandoned" (Jordan, 1962, p. 9). In that sense, 1965 was the coming of age in America. P.L. 89–10, the Elementary and Secondary Education Act (ESEA) of 1965, made funds available to public schools for programs for children from low-income families. Congress used the term *educationally disadvantaged,* which was defined to include exceptional children. Later in 1965, P.L. 89–313 amended Title I of the ESEA to provide more direct aid for the education of exceptional children in state-operated or state-supported institutions.

The following year, P.L. 89–750, the ESEA Amendments of 1966, authorized significant sums of money for the "initiation, expansion, and improvement of programs and projects for the education of the handicapped" (Meisgeier and King, 1970, p. 294). The provisions of the amendments were directed to children from ages three to twenty-one.

P.L. 89–750 also required the Commissioner of Education to establish within the Office of Education two bodies related to the problems of exceptional children. One was the Bureau of Education for the

Adapted from T. E. McGovern, D. A. Draper, and R. S. Vacca, "Introduction: Legislation and Litigation." In N. H. Fallen and T. E. McGovern, *Young Children with Special Needs.* Columbus, Ohio: Charles E. Merrill Co., 1978.

Handicapped, which was responsible for administering programs and projects relating to the needs of exceptional persons. The other group to be organized was the National Advisory Committee on Handicapped Children, which was to serve in an advisory capacity to the Commissioner.

P.L. 90–247, the ESEA Amendments of 1967, demonstrated the federal government's increased involvement in special education. It made provisions for a variety of services for the handicapped, including regional resource centers and centers and services for deaf-blind children. The establishment of centers for deaf-blind children met a critical need in the field of education since a rubella epidemic in the early 1960s had resulted in the birth of thousands of children with multiple handicaps.

Entitled the Handicapped Children's Early Education Assistance Act of 1968, P.L. 90–538 authorized experimental preschool programs for the handicapped. It was hoped that the three years of operation authorized by the Act would demonstrate conclusively that disabilities would be alleviated or corrected in 50% or more of the exceptional children if medical and special educational services were provided during the formative years (Minskoff, 1970).

One piece of federal legislation related to the handicapped was passed in 1970. It was P.L. 91–230, the Elementary and Secondary Education Assistance Programs Extension. Under Title VI, the Education of the Handicapped Act was created, which encompassed all Office of Education programs established to meet special educational needs. Among the authorizations were special programs for children with specific learning disabilities.

The most recent and most significant piece of legislation for the cause of exceptional children in general, and of young, special children in particular, is

P.L. 94–142, the Education for All Handicapped Children Act, enacted in November 1975. The scope of this act, by virtue of its comprehensive requirements, reaches far beyond any past legislation to meet the needs of exceptional children. Some of the major mandates of the new law are:

1. A free public education for all handicapped children between the ages of three and eighteen by September 1978, and for all those between the ages of three and twenty-one by September 1980. Exceptions are allowed in states where school attendance laws do not include children in the three to five and eighteen to twenty-one ranges.

2. An *individualized educational plan* must be written for each handicapped child. Such a program must be developed through the joint efforts of a qualified school official, the child's teacher, the parent or guardian, and whenever possible, the child.

3. The handicapped and nonhandicapped child must be educated together to the maximum extent appropriate. Special classes and separate schools are possible only when the nature or severity of the handicap is such that education in regular classes cannot be achieved satisfactorily.

4. All tests and other evaluation instruments and their implementation must not be racially or culturally discriminatory.

5. All policies, programs, and procedures for educating handicapped children must have prior public notice and prior parent involvement and consultation.

6. All rights and guarantees of this new law apply to handicapped children in private as well as public schools.

7. All state-level agencies currently responsible for special education will have jurisdiction over all educational programs for handicapped children offered within a given state.

8. Each governor will appoint an *advisory panel* to advise and assist in the overall implementation of the law's requirements (Goodman, 1976).

With the first requirement, early childhood–special education becomes a legal mandate. The downward extension of special education services to the preschool years will have a significant impact on the development of young, handicapped children. Early identification, appropriate placement, and special programming will greatly increase the probability of the special child's achieving his full potential.

1. The main object of this passage is to:

   A. list the laws that relate to special education.
   B. highlight the increasing role of the federal government in the area of special education.
   C. point out that early childhood special education is a legal mandate.
   D. inform the public about the rights of handicapped children.

2. Which of the following statements does NOT describe a manner in which the federal government supported programs for exceptional children before the 1960s?

   A. matching state and local funds and supplying research grants
   B. providing a free public education for all handicapped children
   C. disseminating information and providing consultative services
   D. distributing fellowships to train professionals in all areas of special education

3. The Education of the Handicapped Act encompassed all Office of Education programs established to meet special needs. Under which of the following public laws was this act created?

   A. P.L. 90–247, the ESEA Amendments of 1967
   B. P.L. 90–538, the Handicapped Children's Early Education Assistance Act of 1968
   C. P.L. 91–230, the Elementary and Secondary Education Assistance Programs Extension of 1970
   D. P.L. 94–142, the Education for All Handicapped Children Act of 1975

4. According to the descriptions given in this passage, handicapped children include:

   A. those who are physically handicapped.
   B. those who are mentally handicapped.
   C. those who are emotionally handicapped.
   D. none of the above.

5. P.L. 94–142, the Education for All Handicapped Children Act, is the most significant piece of legislation for the cause of exceptional

children. This act provides handicapped children with:

A. a free public education.
B. an individualized educational plan.
C. education with regular children as much as possible.
D. all of the above.

6. According to the passage, a significant effect of the free public education mandate of P.L. 94–142 is:

A. the downward extension of special education services to preschool children.
B. the increased number of regulations placed on local school systems.
C. the opportunity provided for each handicapped child to achieve his/her full academic potential.
D. the need to set up advisory panels to advise and assist school districts in carrying out the law.

7. Mrs. Smith, Anthony's third-grade teacher, is worried because the child is having severe difficulty in math, despite all the extra attempts that have been made to help him. Mrs. Smith has discussed this lack of progress with Anthony's parents several times.

Which of the following scenarios supports mandate 5 of P.L. 94–142?

A. Mrs. Smith discusses the situation with her principal. The principal has a conference with the parents and suggests that evaluation for possible special education placement may be appropriate.
B. Mrs. Smith is convinced that Anthony has a learning disability. She asks the school counselor to administer a series of achievement tests.
C. A complete evaluation is conducted on Anthony. The principal informs his parents that he qualifies for help through the school's special education department.
D. Mrs. Smith is very fond of Anthony and wants him to succeed. She persuades the school's learning disabilities teacher to work one-on-one with him during math period.

Passage II (Questions 8–15)

To establish a prima facie case of sex discrimination in compensation, an employee must present data that compare her salary to that of male coworkers doing the same job under the same circumstances. The standard or test that has emerged from case law is called the equal pay for equal work standard. Not to be confused with the idea that one must hold a job identical to that of someone else, the standard is built on a concept that evaluates jobs within a context of substantial equivalency. The issue to probe thus becomes: Is complainant's job equal in effort and responsibility to that of a male counterpart? A corollary question also is asked. Do the two incumbents in these jobs (the male and the female) possess comparable skills?

On March 11, 1974, the Secretary of Labor took action against Columbia University and its president, seeking to enjoin the University from discriminating against its female custodial workers (classified as light cleaners). Alleging a violation of the Equal Pay Act on the basis of sex, the evidence showed that female light cleaners were paid a lower hourly rate than male heavy cleaners. At trial, the court came to the conclusion that the jobs of light cleaners and heavy cleaners were different. And, because the job of heavy cleaners involved greater effort than that of light cleaners, the plantiff had failed to sustain the burden of establishing the idea of equal work within the meaning of the Act.

On appeal, the Second Circuit Court of Appeals focused its attention on the "equal effort" criteria in connection with the workers' primary duties. The Court stated:

> The concept of "effort" in the act is straightforward. It calls for a direct comparison of the amount of physical exertion required by the jobs; there is no factor added to compensate for physiological differences between men and women. Based on our careful review of the record before us we cannot say that the district court was clearly erroneous in making this direct comparison and in finding as a fact that heavy cleaning involves "greater effort."

The court also noted that the differences between the heavy cleaner and light cleaner jobs were known by the employees. Furthermore, no heavy cleaner job had ever been denied to a woman. In fact, in 1972, Columbia opened a heavy cleaner category to women, and seven light cleaners were accepted into

Adapted from Richard S. Vacca: "Sex Discrimination in Public School Employment." In S. B. Thomas, N. H. Cambron-McCabe, and M. M. McCarthy, Eds, *Education and the Law*. New York: Institute for School Law and Finance, 1983.

on-the-job training for that position. However, after seven weeks, four of the seven workers transferred back to light cleaning.

In conclusion, the circuit court held that based on the evidence of the understanding and experience of the individuals most closely involved, together with the undisputed fact that heavy cleaning called for greater effort, there was no valid claim of unequal pay for substantially equivalent work within the meaning of the Equal Pay Act.

A new and more controversial standard in sex discrimination cases involves the notion of comparable worth. Under the theory of comparable worth, one must look beyond the equal pay for equal work criterion. In such cases, the female plantiff argues the intrinsic worth, or the intrinsic difficulty of her job, as compared to other jobs in the same organization. Such an argument thus carries the complaint beyond the confines of an equal wage matter and places it under the broader umbrella protection of Title VII.

The judiciary has not yet endorsed the notion of comparable worth, but the Supreme Court has ruled that Title VII provides a remedy for sex discrimination in compensation beyond that covered by the Equal Pay Act. The matter arose in Washington County, Oregon, when four women guards in the female section of the county jail alleged that they were paid unequal wages for work substantially equal to that performed by male guards. In their complaint, the women guards charged that because of intentional discrimination, the county set the pay scale of female guards (but not male guards) "at a level lower than that warranted by its own survey of outside markets and the worth of the jobs."

After an adverse decision at trial, the female guards appealed to the Eighth Circuit Court of Appeals. The appellate court reversed the trial court and held that petitioners were not precluded from suing under Title VII, solely because their jobs were not substantially equal to higher-paying jobs held by male employees. The Supreme Court agreed and ruled in *County of Washington v. Gunther* that the wage differentials were based on intentional sex discrimination even though female guards did not actually perform work equal to that of male guards. Although not adopting the controversial concept of comparable worth, the Court left the door open for a comparable worth argument to be raised in future litigation.

It is significant to note that Justice Rehnquist for the four dissenters in *Gunther* strongly stated that this decision could spell the nullification of the Equal Pay Act if future plantiffs are allowed to substitute the comparable worth standard for that of the equal pay for equal work standard. He asserted that the majority's opinion must be read narrowly ("the opinion does not endorse the so-called 'comparable worth'

theory): though the Court does not indicate how a plaintiff might establish a prima facie case under Title VII, the Court does suggest that allegations of unequal pay for unequal, but comparable, work will not state a claim on which relief may be granted."

Others would argue that the Supreme Court's decision in *Gunther* establishes a possibility for plaintiffs in future cases to be given the opportunity to produce evidence showing a Title VII violation based on a comparable worth, rather than on an equal work basis. For example, female teachers might argue that over the years the historical pattern and practice in public school systems have inflated the value and salaries of certain jobs simply because they were held by men, while depressing the value and salaries of other jobs because they were held by women, even though each of the jobs is of comparable worth to the school system.

8. When one investigates an equal pay issue, attention must be given to:

  I. equal worth.
 II. equal effort.
III. equal length of employment.
 IV. equal responsibility.

A. I, II, and III   C. II and IV
B. I and III   D. I, II, III, and IV

9. Which of the following statement(s) is/are *supported by* the passage?

A. Identical jobs should receive equal reimbursement.
B. Substantial equivalency is at the bottom of the issue.
C. The question also to be asked is whether the concerned possess equal levels of education.
D. Effort, attitude, drive, and determination are important considerations in equal pay for equal work cases.

10. In sex discrimination cases the courts:

  I. have considered the fact that women bear children.
 II. have decided that maternity leave is a constitutional right.
III. have allowed the notion of physical and physiological differences.

IV. view the Equal Pay Act and the Title VII laws as equal in impact.

A. I, II, and III   C. II and IV
B. I and III   D. neither I, II, III, nor IV

11. The Columbia University case illustrates:

A. that on-the-job training is essential in avoiding problems.
B. the haphazard approach used by the Department of Labor in filing suit.
C. that employees are not always aware of differences in their jobs.
D. the well-defined limits of the Equal Pay Act in regard to the equal effort interpretation.

12. Which of the following statement(s) is/are *supported by* the passage?

I. Comparable worth is a complex issue.
II. In comparable worth issues one must probe well beyond the equal pay for equal work issues.
III. The Supreme Court considers Title VII as a remedy for sex discrimination.
IV. The judiciary has endorsed Title VII.

A. I, II, and III   C. II and IV
B. I and III   D. I, II, III, and IV

13. In the Oregon case:

I. the first trial ended with a ruling for the county.
II. the first trial resulted in no definitive decision.
III. the appellate court did not preclude a suit based on job unequality.
IV. the Supreme Court adopted the concept of comparable worth.

A. I, II, and III   C. II and IV
B. I and III   D. I, II, III, and IV

14. Which of the following is/are *supported by* the passage?

I. There were four dissenters to the Supreme Court decision.
II. Concern was voiced about the future effectiveness of the Equal Pay Act.

III. It is anticipated that litigation might substitute the principle of comparable worth for the argument equal pay and equal work.
IV. The majority opinion clearly defined the limits of the decision in the *County of Washington v. Gunther* case.

A. I, II, and III   C. IV only
B. I and III   D. I, II, III, and IV

15. The main theme of this passage can be considered to be:

A. Equal Pay Act v. Title VII.
B. comparable worth.
C. sex discrimination.
D. judiciary policy making.

Passage III (Questions 16–24)

There have been two controversies over Eoanthopus, and it is the first of them that has the incongruous mandible for its theme. The question at issue was whether this specimen represents a single creature or two different ones. Scientists made reconstructions reconciling jaw and skull; however, one group described the jaw as an ape's separately from the skull that was assigned to Homo sapiens. The finder's argument ran as follows: All of the remains were found very close together. The lower jaw and brain case were both of a similar brown color and apparently in the same state of fossilization. The jaw, even though ape-like, did have human features, particularly in the teeth. The molar teeth had apparently been worn to a flatness never seen in apes, and only expected if the jaw had belonged to a type of human being. The roots of the teeth seen radiologically also resembled human teeth. The appearance of this ape-like man at the beginning of the Ice Age was just what many authorities expected to find. Shortly thereafter, a canine tooth, ape-like, but worn in a way never found in modern apes, was found. This was strong support for the missing link interpretation and man's ape-like ancestry. Questions remained concerning how anatomically the jaw could have worked as part of a human skull, and the wear of the teeth.

Three years later, about two miles away from the first site, pieces of a thick braincase and a molar tooth (both similar to the first find) were unearthed. The

From H. R. Seibel, "The Piltdown Hoax," *Bioscope*, 1962.

climate was ripe for the view that the human ancestor would show a combination of ape and man. However, as more human fossils were found in other parts of the world, this particular specimen differed from all in regard to skull characteristics. Their braincases were far more ape-like and their jaws less so, and a consistent line of evolution was found. Restorations of the cranium resulted in the revisions of brain volume, but in the end the controversial specimen had a brain of modern size to go with its modern skull.

If the remains were old, they could be accepted even though odd and isolated. When the fluorine method was applied, it was found that neither jawbone nor braincase contained more than small traces of fluorine meaning that the specimen did not date before the Ice Age. The specimen was now believed to be 50,000 and not 500,000 years old, making it an evolutionary absurdity with no known ancestor or descendants. An explanation was to suppose that a piece of modern ape jaw had been deliberately placed with an ancient braincase and both suitably stained. Another fluorine analysis placed the braincase as ancient, but the jaw and teeth in modern times. In fact, chemical analysis showed that the jaw and teeth contained the same amount of nitrogen and organic carbon as modern specimens, the calvarium, however, much less. Ruling out that the organic matter was not gelatin or glue with which the specimen had been impregnated as a means of hardening was accomplished with electron microscopy because the jaw showed preserved fibers of organic tissue and the calvarium lacked this feature. Besides this, it was established that the jaw had been colored artificially with iron to match the calvarium.

The first specimen was apparently made up by placement of an artificially abraded molar tooth of an orangutan with a piece of thick frontal bone; the last fragment found duplicated the thinnest part of the first skull. Chromium detected in the jaw indicates that a dichromate solution was used in an attempt to assist the oxidation of iron salts used to stain these specimens.

16. The skull was classified to belong to:

    I. a vertebrate.
    II. a mammal.
    III. a man.
    IV. an ape.

    A. I, II, and III   C. II and IV
    B. I and III   D. I, II, III, and IV

17. This passage was probably written by:

    A. a historian.   C. a sociologist.
    B. an anthropologist.   D. an archeologist.

18. From the passage one could surmise that flourine:

    A. was obtained from drinking water.
    B. was absorbed from the soil.
    C. becomes more concentrated.
    D. is a by-product of the decay process.

19. If the jawbone was modern, its fluorine content in relation to the braincase would have been:

    A. the same.
    B. more.
    C. less.
    D. not important in the solution.

20. The analysis of iron was used to establish:

    A. a color comparison.
    B. the organic matrix pattern.
    C. the age of the specimens.
    D. none of the above.

21. The piece of fossil found last was:

    A. not unusual in size.
    B. thick.
    C. thin.
    D. none of the above.

22. With age iron salts:

    A. are reduced.   C. deteriorate.
    B. are halogenated.   D. are oxidized.

23. Chromium:

    A. is naturally found in bones.
    B. is absorbed from the surrounding areas by a specimen.
    C. is used as a parameter in testing fossils.
    D. none of the above.

24. The passage mainly deals with:

    A. the development of experimental methods of studying fossils.
    B. the verification of the missing link.
    C. a valuable fossil find.
    D. a brilliantly devised falsification.

Passage IV (Questions 25–32)

End-user computing (EUC) is computing that is performed by the users for the users independently of the information systems (IS) department. It usually involves the use of personal computers and "off the shelf" shrink-wrapped PC software, such as popular favorites Lotus 1-2-3 or dBASE III+.

EUC is with us for three primary reasons: (1) computers, including PCs, are the tool for the job in an information-driven society; (2) the extended wait for IS application development services due to enormous backlogs is unacceptable; and (3) the phenomenal decrease in price of microcomputers has made them easily affordable.

All indicators point to a future where the PC is as commonplace an office fixture as the telephone is today. It has been estimated that within large companies, the ratio of PCs to white collar workers is about 1:2, but is expected to change to 1:1 in the early 1990s.

Advantages and disadvantages of EUC are numerous. Advantages include (1) users of EUC can help themselves by doing their own simple applications development and implementation, thereby freeing IS professionals to develop large, complex corporate systems; (2) users do not have to articulate system requirements to an analyst, thereby eliminating the possibility of flawed systems design due to poor communications; and (3) users will be much more likely to implement self-developed systems due to the high probability of user acceptance criteria being met.

Disadvantages include the distinct possibility of (1) hardware and software incompatibility; (2) data security problems; (3) difficulty of evaluating/purchasing the most cost effective EUC hardware and software; (4) data integrity problems resulting from data redundancy, and file sharing and file transmission errors; (5) further widening the rift between IS and users; (6) the complexity of successful management; and (7) systems developed without regard for IS-type standards and procedures and generally accepted data processing practices, resulting in poor matching of systems to organizational objectives, incorrect or incomplete systems, inefficient and/or ineffective systems, or poorly documented systems.

The implications for IS include (1) less involvement with small scale systems development projects; (2) permitting of access to a wide variety of users of corporate data, plus management of the micro-to-mainframe link and associated hardware and software; and (3) security issues concerning data protection from the standpoint of privacy as well as validity.

The management of EUC is a tremendous challenge to organizations. The current management structure most companies use is the information center, which is staffed by employees with the expertise to help users work effectively with their own application developments. There are two types of basic information center (IC) structures, the IBM Canada type and the distributed type. The IBM Canada type utilizes a staff of widely experienced employees who report to the same manager and work with users on start-to-finish developments. This can be advantageous because it provides a single-user interface, and because support representatives have stronger applications knowledge. However, they do not get exposed to as wide an area of corporate applications.

The second basic IC management structure, the distributed type, has specific functional areas, with each group reporting to a different manager. The areas are (1) manager; (2) consultant, the first person the user deals with, who helps the user pick the appropriate hardware and software; (3) the product specialist, who actually assists with development, and is assigned to projects using one of the software packages he or she is proficient in; and (4) technical support, which sets up and supports hardware and communications functions such as micro-to-mainframe links.

In addition to responsibilities listed above, other tasks of the IC include helping with evaluation and purchase of compatible hardware and software, helping to draft and enforce application development standards, and training. However, as mentioned earlier, IC management is no easy task. Many ICs are already experiencing the same backlogs as their IS counterparts. Not only is EUC demand growing rapidly, but constant technological change is occurring. The trend of the information center is toward "interactive-connectivity" of data, graphic, and voice processing equipment for all of the following (1) mainframes, minis, and PCs; (2) local and wide area networks; (3) individual terminals; (4) facsimile machines; (5) copiers; (6) telecommunication equipment; and (8) video transmission equipment and systems.

So, with all this growing importance to organizations, who controls the ICs; users or IS? The prevalent wisdom is to make the ICs separate but equal to IS, in order to give them the power and autonomy with which to properly function.

In order for the IC to be successfully implemented, the support of top management is imperative. They must be convinced that EUC will occur in a manner that is consistent with organizational objectives. IC strategic planning is therefore required, and should also be considered in company-wide planning. According to experts, PC adoption must be incorporated in an overall strategic plan because, otherwise, difficulties will appear down the road.

From Ben Owen, "Systems Performance Evaluation," MCV/VCU, 1990.

25. Based on the information in the passage, which of the following statements summarize(s) the author's purpose?

    I. defining EUC and its future direction
    II. describing advantages and disadvantages of EUC
    III. discussing implications of EUC on traditional corporate information systems departments and associated management strategies

    A. I only   C. I and II only
    B. II only   D. I, II, and III

26. Which of the following factors explain the tremendous growth of EUC?

    I. computers are the tool for the job in an information-driven society
    II. the unacceptable waiting period for development of applications by information systems due to backlogs
    III. the sharp drop in prices of microcomputers

    A. I only   C. I and II only
    B. II only   D. I, II, and III

27. According to the passage, by the early 1990s large companies will experience a:

    I. 500% increase in the ratio of all workers to computers.
    II. a 100% increase in the ratio of computers to white collar workers.
    III. growing disparity between educational level and computer-related jobs.

    A. I only   C. I and II only
    B. II only   D. I, II, and III

28. Which of the following statements was/were listed as advantages of EUC?

    I. End-users can develop their own simple applications without waiting for help and authorization of information systems.
    II. Potential communications problems are reduced, due to the elimination of expressing systems requirements to an analyst.
    III. Implementation of developed systems will be more likely to occur.

    A. I only   C. I and II only
    B. II only   D. I, II, and III

29. Which of the following statements was/were listed as disadvantages of EUC?
    I. potential compatibility problems between third and fourth generation computer languages
    II. the complexity of successful EUC management
    III. the inability of vendors to develop PC communications standards

    A. I only   C. I and II only
    B. II only   D. I, II, and III

30. The implications of EUC for information systems departments include:

    I. more involvement with small scale systems development projects.
    II. permitting corporate data access to a wide variety of users.
    III. development of "user-friendly" report writers for end-users.

    A. I only   C. I and II only
    B. II only   D. I, II, and III

31. Information centers have become the corporate answer for management of EUC. Which of the following best describes the desired organizational structuring of the IC?

    A. EUC placed under the auspices of the information systems department
    B. EUC placed under the auspices of the respective user areas
    C. EUC made an independent group
    D. EUC allowed to develop "laissez faire" to determine the optimum placement within the organization

32. Among the following issues, which is the most crucial to the success of EUC in an organization?

    A. hardware and software compatibility between microcomputers and mainframes
    B. reliable micro-to-mainframe communication links
    C. development of EUC standards and policies
    D. incorporation of EUC into company-wide strategic planning

Passage V (Questions 33–38)

"In this way you shall set the fiftieth year apart and proclaim freedom to all the inhabitants of the land." In this way the ancient writer of *Leviticus* had God speak through Moses for the purpose of commemorating the entrance of the people of Israel into the "Promised Land." This is not the oldest reference to the celebration of an "anniversary," but it does show that celebrating anniversaries is a very old practice, and it also illustrates the role of round numbers in such celebrations.

Thus, the institution's celebration of its one hundred fiftieth year of existence adheres to a very old tradition. We celebrate birthdays and wedding anniversaries annually, whereas we usually commemorate the formation of institutions, businesses, churches, nations and schools on the round-numbered years. (Even with birthdays and weddings we call special attention to the "big" years—tenth, twenty-fifth, fiftieth, and so on.) That we do so, may have something to do with the fact that our numbering is on the base ten system, and the round numbers are those that finish the pattern. Although that explains why we pick the round numbers for our large celebrations, it does not explain why we think it important to celebrate such occasions. A brief discussion of why we *do* observe anniversaries is also an argument for why we *should* do so.

Perhaps the most obvious reason for celebrating the birth of an institution or the commemoration of some dramatic event is our belief that there was a good in it worth perpetuating. Thus, John Adams said of the 1776 Resolution of Independence:

> I am apt to believe that it will be celebrated by succeeding generations as the great anniversary festival. It ought to be commemorated as the day of deliverance, by solemn acts of devotion to God Almighty. It ought to be solemnized with pomp and parade, with shows, games, sports, guns, bells, bonfires, and illuminations, from one end of this continent to the other, from this time forward for evermore.

Quite obviously, Adams believed that the launching of a free and independent nation was an act of such worth as to warrant regular celebration. It might be noted in passing that the inauguration of a new enterprise is always an act of hope. It is only at some future time, when folk have seen how an organization, institution, or nation has turned out—when growth and achievement became history—that there can be a confident celebration of the founding day.

From Dr. William E. Blake, Jr., VCU's Sesquicentennial Celebration, 1989.

But there is also an almost contradictory reason for anniversary celebrations. Instead of perpetuating ancient values they are often viewed as the occasion for a new beginning. As James Russell Lowell wrote, "New occasions teach new duties; time makes ancient good uncouth." So, anniversaries offer the opportunity to reflect on the path traveled, where a people are, where they wish to go next, and what's the best way to get there.

Anniversaries are also a time to honor the people who started the enterprise. Even if it is a romantic conception, we usually think of these pioneers as the hardier sort, whose lives and efforts are worthy of emulation.

Perhaps there is in anniversary celebrations something of an attempt to recapture or to *capture* the drama and emotion of the founding days. Nostalgia, even if it is variously felt, seems to be pleasant to the human spirit. Even if it is tinged with sadness, it is still treasured. Just call to mind (if you can) the lyrics of "Love's Old Sweet Song."

We must confess that part of the motivation for celebrating anniversaries is just plain, human pride. It doesn't matter whether one was among the founding party or joined the institution much later. If the organization has had a long, distinctive history, one may say, "I helped put that together" or "That eminent institution values me enough to make me a part of it." The power of human pride cannot be underestimated as the motor of an institutional machine.

And we cannot ignore the commercial motivation behind anniversary celebrations. It is not just business organizations that stress, "One Hundred and Fifty Years of Faithful Service to the Community." Organizations of all varieties—churches, clubs, social and humane societies, *and* schools—use anniversaries to emphasize their legitimacy, durability, and trustworthiness and use the occasion to appeal for continued—and expanded—patronage by the public. All of these motivations are *implicit* in a celebration. There is real value in making them *explicit*. To be consciously aware of *why* we're celebrating would make the occasion more meaningful and enjoyable.

33. Which of the following statements are *neither supported nor contradicted by* the passage?

   A. After 50 years, the Jews celebrated their leaving Egypt.
   B. God spoke to Moses to initiate the celebration.
   C. Most celebrations are joyous events.
   D. Celebrations are a part of civilizations.

34. Which of the following statements is/are *supported by* the passage?

    I. There is a logical reason for celebrating.

    II. Round-numbered year festivities are usually special.

    III. Our mathematical system depends on round numbers that enhance remembering events.

    IV. Independence Day should be observed for always.

    A. I, II, and III   **C.** II and IV
    B. I and III   **D.** IV only

35. The passage supports the notion(s):

    A. that Founding Day is an act of hope.
    B. that history will be the determining factor.
    C. that a celebration is a renewal.
    D. that all of the above are valid.

36. Which of the following statements is/are *supported by* the passage?

    A. Nostalgia is good for mankind.
    B. Pioneers are usually worthy of emulating.
    C. People need a time to reflect.
    D. All of the above are viewed positively by the author.

37. The author believes:

    A. that a sense of being a part of history is productive.
    B. entrepreneurship is part and parcel of a festival.
    C. justification for existence is a motive for anniversary celebrations.
    D. all of the above statements.

38. The passage could properly be titled:

    A. Our One Hundred Fiftieth-Year Celebration.
    B. Why We Celebrate.
    C. Founding Day.
    D. A History of Anniversary Celebrations.

Passage VI (Questions 39–44)

Myths and fairy tales are most often told and remembered as plots (who did what to whom and what happened). But they actually endure in our continuing imaginations because of the "character" of the characters involved. If you place Oedipus into Daedalus's story, or Narcissus into Odysseus's story, you won't have the same story. Cinderella wouldn't do what Red Riding Hood does, nor would Jack-in-the-Beanstalk do what Hansel does. The character doesn't merely *follow* a plot line—the plot happens *because* of the particular human weaknesses and strengths of the particular character.

Underlying all these characters, of course, are larger issues, such as greed and selfishness, pride, acceptance of fate, compassion, cleverness, and risk. But what distinguishes one character from another are the choices, actions, and consequences of those choices peculiar to the individual character. When a teenager (like Theseus) is faced with a dilemma of State (his country must pay human sacrifice tribute in the form of seven youths and seven maidens to a more powerful country), there are a number of choices or decisions he can make. He can ignore the whole problem (it's not his fault, after all); he can take personal responsibility for solving the problem, either because he wants to be a Big Hero or because (as son of the King) he must learn to face problems if he expects to inherit the throne; or he might simply be in a boastful or adventuresome mood when the idea crosses his mind. Once Theseus commits himself to the task (destroying the Minotaur, symbol of the opposing country's power), there are further choices: He can take all the credit but allow his underlings to do all the hard work; he can sacrifice himself on a seemingly impossible task (finding and destroying the Minotaur in its Labyrinth); or he can take advantage of a girl's love for him (agreeing to take Ariadne away with him if she gives him the secret of the Labyrinth). And once he's solved the primary problem of the Minotaur, there are even more choices: does he really want to take Ariadne back with him as he promised? Should he take time out to change the color of his ship's sails (as he promised his father) when he's being pursued by an angry enemy? Because he doesn't change the sails, he directly causes his father's suicide; because he chooses to leave Ariadne behind, he indirectly sets up an even more tragic chain of events in his own life that won't become apparent for a number of years. The series of choices and consequent actions that Theseus

Adapted from Sally V. Doud, "Essay Test Introduction," VCU, Spring 1990.

takes thus becomes the plot we know, only after we look back on it.

Young people still face seemingly impossible tasks today. These might involve the State (expose corruption, act on one's conscience, protest the military draft), or they might involve other people and relationships (whether to live up to an agreement made under different circumstances, such as an engagement, marriage, contract, job, project). People still have to decide whether to try and save a sinking ship, or whether to catch the first lifeboat; whether to admit a harsh truth or to avoid it (lie, exaggerate, use diplomacy, pass blame, run away). Can or should one be loyal to a person or way of life one no longer cares about? What are the risks and benefits of any decision? Does it still "pay" to be a hero, or do other occupations seem more lucrative? Is the difference between a hero and a fool merely success? Should you get involved with someone else's problem or shrug it off? Should you take a stance or merely cast your eyes to heaven and wait for divine intervention and fate? Also, it isn't always easy to separate personal ego or animal needs from more "noble" desires to bring about social or human justice, and often the two run along together for a considerable distance before they part ways. These are matters for contemporary characters in contemporary stories, but these are the same matters Theseus dealt with. We still have our Minotaurs, escape ships, labyrinths, tasks, Ariadnes, and Theseuses, though the forms are different each time. That's why myth and fairy tales (based on folktales or myths) are called Universal.

39. The most appropriate title for this essay would be:

    A. The Role of Fate in Contemporary Life.
    B. Red Riding Hood and Theseus: Two Versions of the Same Character.
    C. Universal Aspects of Everyday Experience.
    D. Myth is Dead.

40. According to the author of the passage:

    A. people today do not face impossible tasks as did the characters in the Greek myths.
    B. the outcomes of fairy tales and myths are rarely determined by choices the characters have made.

    C. myths and fairy tales are universal because the choices that are faced by characters in them are similar to the ones faced by people of all times.
    D. there are fewer choices for heroes today than there were for the heroes of Greek myths.

41. One might infer from this passage that:

    A. Theseus is responsible for the death of his father.
    B. one should not sacrifice himself to a seemingly impossible task.
    C. Theseus should not be blamed for the suicide of his father.
    D. in making decisions, individuals should wait for divine intervention.

42. According to the author of the passage:

    A. plots proceed as a pattern of cause and effect events.
    B. plots are always the same from one story to the next.
    C. plots are merely an accumulated series of events.
    D. plots are the most important part of any story.

43. The most important part of the passage is:

    A. that we not forget the story of Theseus and his adventures surrounding the Labyrinth.
    B. stories change, but the realm of human choices remains the same.
    C. universality deals with language.
    D. we are always punished for our misdoing.

44. According to the passage, the primary problem facing Theseus is:

    A. how he can reward Ariadne for giving him the secret of the Labyrinth.
    B. the killing of the Minotaur.
    C. the changing of his ship's sails so as to inform his father of his fate.
    D. how he will rid himself of guilt after he has killed the Minotaur.

Passage VII (Questions 45–50)

Caricature is a device satirists commonly use in their work. Why is it so common? Caricatures grab readers' or viewers' attention; moreover, they are funny. Caricatures distort reality and that distortion is often hilarious. An audience that will appreciate the caricature recognizes the incongruity between the real object and the satirist's portrayal of it. They also understand why the satirist is attacking this object. In effect, the appreciative audience says, "Of course, this is all out of proportion. But, you know, he's got a point there. This person (place, thing) really does have a weak spot." Meanwhile, as they muse on the message, they are reacting to the incongruities, the exaggeration, with anything from a wry smile to convulsive laughter.

What exactly is a caricature? I would define it as a pictorial (drawing, painting, sculpture, collage, mask, dramatization) or verbal (poem, essay, descriptive sketch in fiction or nonfiction) exaggeration of an object (person, place, thing, situation, organization). The distortion must be based on a fact about the object, for example, bushy eyebrows. The artist or writer just stretches that fact all out of shape; the politician's eyebrows are not *that* bushy. He plays with his object as if it were a glob of silly putty or bread dough. He kneads it, rolls it up, flattens it, stretches it out, shapes it any way to suit his fancy. He must not go so far as to make the object completely unrecognizable, but he has a lot of room to play with his object.

One thing that happens when an object becomes so pliable in the hands of an artist or writer is that the object instantly plummets in value. It becomes ridiculous, at least to some extent, and not as important as it had been. Often the satirist's purpose is to show that the object, because of people's vanity or hypocrisy, is considered more valuable than it really is. By doing a caricature of it, he deflates its value. Furthermore, the artist or writer shows that he has control over the object, at least temporarily. He is exerting his power by the way he portrays the object. It's as if he's saying, "Ah ha! You thought you were so important. But look at you now, the way *I*'ve made you. I'm calling the shots for now." Needless to say, the people being caricatured rarely think kindly about the creators of the satire—not only do the caricatures deflate their importance, but also the caricatures show that the people who are being satirized don't have control over their image.

It's important to note that one of the effects of caricature is to dehumanize the person being carica-

tured. This dehumanization is even there in the language of how we discuss satire: the word "object." As the audience, we often enjoy seeing a vaunted person being devalued by caricature and agree that the devaluation is often deserved. But does the means justify the end? Caricatures certainly work, and creators and audience have a lot of fun while criticizing the object. However, a side effect is that caricatures serve as one out of many ways we tend in our society to dehumanize each other. Rarely does the creator or the audience notice this; we're caught up in the laughter and disregard any objections to a caricature by saying, "It's just a joke. Don't you have a sense of humor? He (object of caricature) deserved it anyway." Yes, it's just a joke. But also, yes, it makes it easier for us to view people as objects to be manipulated, vilified, destroyed. Think back to the caricatures we did of the Japanese in World War II. It is much easier to work up enthusiasm for killing people when they are depicted as hideous monsters. Hitler readily used caricature to depict Jews as less-than-human animals.

Exaggeration, playing the extremes against each other, distortion—these are all elements of caricature. Caricatures are a quite effective means for satire—creators enjoy creating them, audiences respond eagerly to them, they make their point. However, they are not innocuous little creatures; they can be used to stereotype and dehumanize people. Also, as we use them casually day after day, we sometimes don't even notice anymore that they are caricatures. The cartoon character becomes the norm. Wiley the Coyote makes falling off cliffs, holding an exploding piece of dynamite, or being crushed with huge stones seem like normal, everyday events; he is just a little frazzled after each episode. Numbed day after day with caricatures, might we begin to think of life as a cartoon?

45. Which of the following statements about caricatures is NOT *supported by* the passage?

   A. Caricatures do not have to be pictures.
   B. People who are satirized often lose the public's respect.
   C. People who are satirized often deserve the ridicule.
   D. Caricatures can be based on falsehoods.

46. According to the passage, people laugh at caricatures because:

   A. bushy eyebrows and other such facial quirks are naturally funny.

B. we laugh at people who are vain and hypocritical.

C. we recognize the incongruities between the object and the caricature of it.

D. the people who create caricatures have a good sense of humor.

47. Which of the following statements best sums up the author's opinion of caricatures?

A. Caricatures are hilarious.

B. Caricatures reveal the hypocrisies of our society.

C. Caricatures have insidious effects.

D. People who do not appreciate caricatures have no sense of humor.

48. According to the passage, caricatures are effective forms of satire because:

I. ridicule devalues an object.

II. caricatures appeal to many kinds of audiences.

III. the satirist controls his object's public image.

A. I and II

B. II and III

C. I and III

D. I, II, and III

49. According to the passage, caricatures can be dangerous because:

A. people satiated with exaggeration may not recognize the norm.

B. a person who is satirized may not deserve the ridicule.

C. caricatures divert our attention from real problems.

D. caricatures give satirists too much power over society.

50. Of the following titles, which is most appropriate for the passage?

A. The Cruel Art of Caricature

B. Caricature and Understatement

C. Caricature: Exaggeration as a Satirist's Tool

D. Cartoon Art

Passage VIII (Questions 51–59)

On a physiological level, aggression is a neurochemical impulse, causing tension that necessitates a physical release. According to the evolutionist position, aggression as instinct can be traced from some of the earliest primitive animal forms from which we humans draw a common ancestor, and must therefore, by reason of evolution as well as observed behavioral patterns, be attributable to man. If conflict is the father of all things, it may be the activating force behind all human behavior (love as well as hate), and its ritual forms of appeasement and redirected activity provide a basis for culture.

In order that aggression be considered an element of man's genetic inheritance, some explanation must be offered for its existence in his past. Ethologists maintain that aggression in earliest man, as in all of the lower animals, had a distinct survival advantage, most commonly linked to the defense of territory. "What directly threatens the existence of an animal species," says Konrad Lorenz, "is never the 'eating enemy' but competition" within the species. In this sense, intraspecies aggression provides for the even distribution of a particular species over an inhabitable area; a form of population control as well as quality control. The stronger animal will control the more advantageous territory and subsequently corner the hardier breeding population. Man's traditional attachment to his land is seen as a modern refinement of his territoriality; most human conflicts can be traced back to dispute over land itself or to his sense of independence concerning his property.

According to Robert Ardrey, the defense of the territory holds animals together in breeding pairs or larger groups; but the most powerful defense is offered by the pair, thereby encourages bonding, to even further selective advantage. Territoriality is also psychological, providing the three basic animal needs: security, identity, and stimulation. The first two are self-explanatory; with the third we are more concerned, for stimulation—by other animals of one's kind—is accomplished through aggression. This may take the form of *inward antagonism,* bickering among one's closest neighbors, which serves no apparent purpose except perhaps sheer stimulation; yet this is considered responsible for socialization. The growth of population into congested cities instead of more evenly spacing out has even been interpreted in this context to be a reaction of man's aggressive needs rather than a practical understanding of cooperation.

Stimulation through aggression can also take the form of *outward antagonism,* the defense of a species

Adapted from Sally V. Doud, "Aggression and Human Nature," VCU, 1976.

group of its territory against outsiders; uniting its members in a common cause and often considered the basis for the human Nation.

Another important aspect of aggression, says Lorenz, is its role in securing the personal bond. "The danger in aggression is its spontaneity ..." therefore, "... aggression of animals toward their own kind is held in check by inhibiting mechanisms" such as ritualization of fighting, appeasement gestures, and redirected activity. As each relationship between two members of the species must be individually negotiated, this constitutes the beginnings of personality. Various forms of greeting as well as many human emotional expressions, such as laughter, are considered ceremonies of redirected activity or appeasement; Lorenz notes that everyone is aware of how laughter tends to create a bond.

Lionel Tiger provides an example of aggression's role in establishing order and custom within a human society: competition between several age groups of males (for females, for prestige) is often responsible for rigid initiatory tradition, along with other political measures prohibitive to one group while enhancing the chances of a second.

The human being who voluntarily places himself within the power of the law embodies the theory of inhibiting mechanisms. Members of the Cheyenne tribe who broke the law during a hunt willingly submitted to the authority of the Shield Soldiers, a gesture of ritual appeasement. In turn, the Shield Soldiers rendered only token punishment, and that on the property of the offenders, acknowledging the appeasement gesture by a redirected activity.

The theory of innate aggression carried to its ultimate climax presents us with the uncomforting image of man with "killer instincts." Although Ardrey points out that territoriality is defensive, that early man hunted because he was hungry, still others point to cannibalism as human acts of aggression as well as a cultural phenomenon.

The more dangerously aggressive the particular species is, the firmer is the bond necessary to prevent intraspecies destruction. Here is man's anomaly: he is devoid of the more elaborate safety devices to prevent the abuse of his killing power, because these devices were unnecessary in the harmless protohuman for whom quick and easy killing was impossible. The acquisition of weapons threw off the natural balance, for now he is capable of great destruction without the accompanying mechanics of inhibition; the Cain and Abel, the master of war, the deadly predator who kills for enjoyment.

"It is true," says Morton Hunt, "like other animals, we are impelled to action by hunger, fear, anger, sexual desires ... but are not directed by instinct to take specific actions in order to satisfy those desires. ... Man may be innately aggressive ... but he is not programmed ... the drive can be directed to many different ends." The apparatus with which we are equipped to speak is a product of our evolution, and the particular language is culturally transmitted.

The emphasis then is on interdependence of instinct and culture; no longer is man at the mere beck and call of his instincts, but capable of exercising control over them. His intelligence permits him the conscious choice of goals.

51. The passage suggests that:

    A. aggression has not yet been traced to earlier evolutionary forms than man.
    B. aggression is a neurochemical impulse.
    C. unlike hunger, aggression does not require release.
    D. aggression seeks direct expression or appeasement and therefore is not redirected into culture building activities.

52. According to Lorenz, the greatest threat to the survival of an animal species is:

    A. what he calls the "eating enemy."
    B. natural disaster.
    C. various forms of pollution.
    D. competition within the species.

53. The passage suggests that of the three basic animal needs, the one that is thought to account for bickering among one's closest neighbors is:

    A. identity.
    B. security.
    C. stimulation.
    D. structure.

54. The passage asserts that one of man's greatest anomalies is that:

    A. he instinctively pairs with or bonds to another human being, but that he cannot remain monogamous throughout his life cycle.
    B. he possesses the "killer instinct" but lacks the internal controls or safety devices that restrict this instinct.
    C. he has free access to weapons but lacks the "killer instinct" to take full advantage of them.
    D. man is territorial and nomadic at the same time.

55. Morton Hunt, who is quoted in the essay, asserts that:

A. man is innately aggressive, but he is not biologically programmed as to how to direct his aggression.
B. cultural transmission plays only a minor role in determining how aggression is channeled from generation to generation.
C. it is a mistake to think of man as innately aggressive.
D. the existence of anger in man differentiates him from other animals.

56. One might infer from this passage that:

A. the existence of aggression in lower animals is unimportant in the study of aggression in man.
B. aggression plays a very important role in determining the ways in which human beings interact in social groups.
C. humans are not territorial.
D. people live in cities because of innate cooperativeness.

57. The most appropriate title for this essay would be:

A. Lorenz On Aggression.
B. The "Killer Instinct" in Man.
C. Man as Pure Instinct.
D. Aggression as the Basis for Culture.

58. The growth of population into congested cities rather than an even spacing out has been interpreted in the context of Ardrey's ideas as:

A. a natural need in man to cooperate.
B. the herding instinct.
C. a need for sharing material goods.
D. a reaction of man's aggressive needs.

59. Members of the Cheyenne tribe who broke the law during a hunt:

A. rebelled against punishment, thus exhibiting aggression.
B. willingly submitted in a gesture of ritual appeasement.
C. insisted that their punishment be on their own land.
D. never broke the same law twice, thus suppressing aggression.

Passage IX (Questions 60–65)

Because the ability to write well is so crucial to success in school, educators are paying more attention to assessments of writing. States have begun requiring students to take minimum competency tests before graduation or before entering high school. Colleges want to limit admissions to students who have shown a certain level of competency in writing. Or they want to place students in an appropriate level of freshman English. How are all these decisions on proficiency, admissions, placement, and exemption made? Tests. Because decisions have to be made on large numbers of students, the tests are large scale assessments, tests that *everyone* in the group (school, state, nation) takes.

There are two major types of tests—direct assessments and indirect assessments. Direct assessments are tests that use readers to judge actual samples of students' writing, writing done in timed in-class sessions on a common topic. Indirect assessments are tests that use answers to multiple-choice questions to judge students' knowledge about certain aspects of writing, such as mechanics or grammar.

Statistics show that multiple-choice tests are very reliable, meaning that students' scores are consistent (if Johnny retakes the test, he is likely to receive about the same score), but how valid they are is speculative (validity refers to what extent a test actually tests what it purports to test). Because multiple-choice questions can test only reading and editing skills for the most part, the scores have meaning only about a student's knowledge of those areas tested. G. Conlan points out that multiple-choice questions have become more sophisticated recently in the types of knowledge tested and can test such things as principles of organization, logic, ability to shift parts of sentences, and sensitivity to idioms. But still it is someone else's text. Does ability to edit someone else's text necessarily mean ability to *create* texts of one's own?

If we want to measure writing skills, a test that requires a person to write would likely be a more valid test than one that doesn't. However, direct assessment is not proving to be a panacea either. A valid test must necessarily be reliable also; many of the problems with direct assessment testing have to do with reliability. If we change the wording of test topics, the testing conditions, or the readers scoring essays, scores can change dramatically.

Reliability problems are most conspicuous in the scoring process. Here is the main objection to direct assessment—different readers have different reactions to the same essay. How can we determine if an

Adapted from Rebecca Dale, "Direct-Indirect Assessment of Writing," Capitol Writing Project, VCU, Summer 1989.

essay has been scored accurately? Reader-response theory has pointed out that readers "recreate" a text when they read it, that interpretation depends on what readers bring to the experience of reading a text as well as what writers put into the text.

Administrators of these tests try to cope with this problem in several ways. One, they develop scoring guides that specify the criteria to be used in evaluating the student papers. Whether they use holistic scoring (scoring an essay as a whole), primary trait scoring (a type of holistic scoring focusing on certain traits found in the particular mode of discourse tested), or analytic scoring (scoring subcategories, such as content, organization, mechanics, and adding the scores up), they all specify in the scoring guides the characteristics of a paper for each score in the scoring range.

Secondly, test administrators train readers with "anchor" papers and trial grading runs. This is sometimes referred to as "calibrating the readers." Readers need to internalize the criteria in the scoring guide, and by comparing their judgments on an essay to an anchor paper whose score has been predetermined, they can get a feel for how lenient or rigorous the scoring should be. The trial grading runs, where each of the readers grades some sample essays, give additional calibration. After grading the samples, the readers discuss the scores they gave, along with their reasons for assigning those scores. The discussion of discrepancies brings up issues in how to apply the criteria and allow the group to reach greater consensus on what the various scores mean.

Thirdly, each essay is read by two readers, each unaware of the score the other reader has given it. If the scores differ by more than one point, a third reader reads the essay. White considers the practice of multiple readings essential:

Although there is a constant temptation to reduce the costs by reducing the second reading to samples or by eliminating second readings altogether, such an economy renders the reading unaccountable and unprofessional.

Scores do vary. "Most papers, if rescored by the same readers at the same reading, would probably receive different scores."

These measures in administering tests help increase reliability in scoring essays, but they do not solve the problem. Readers react to the topic and unintentionally may bring some bias to their grading. In cases where readers are aware of their own bias, they even may try to compensate for their bias and be too lenient in grading essays that offend them.

Another problem is reader drift. Readers who are reading hundreds of essays at a time may be more or less lenient at some times than at others. For example, a paper read right after a brilliant one is more likely to receive a lower score than if it's read after an average one. Barritt, Stock, and Clark have raised a provocative question in their study of how expertly trained readers of students' texts can disagree widely in scoring: They found that readers expected to find "average" student papers, and they could agree on scores for papers that met their expectations. But when they read papers that did not fit their expectations of an "average" student, their scores differed widely. S. Freedman had a similar finding in a comparison of student and professional writers: Evaluators gave student work fairly consistent scores, but in scoring the professional essays, "the raters disagreed violently with one another."

60. According to the passage, indirect assessments of writing have been criticized because:

A. scores are unreliable.
B. only reading and editing skills are tested.
C. the tests are biased.
D. evaluators cannot agree on the criteria for scoring.

61. Which of the following statements does the passage state or imply is/are true?

I. A reliable test is necessarily valid.
II. A valid test is necessarily reliable.
III. A test may be reliable, but not valid.
IV. A test may be valid, but not reliable.

A. I and II   C. II and III
B. III and IV   D. II only

62. Which of the following statements best sums up the importance of reader-response theory to the problems of evaluating essays on large-scale assessments?

A. Scoring guides are necessary to set the criteria by which essays are judged.
B. Evaluators are influenced by their own ideas.
C. Evaluators need to be calibrated.
D. Evaluators give inconsistent scores to professional essays.

63. According to the passage, administrators deal with the reliability problems in scoring direct assessments by all EXCEPT which of the following?

A. essays are scored by multiple readers.
B. evaluators must use specific criteria in judging essays.
C. holistic scoring, primary trait scoring, or analytic scoring is used.
D. evaluators are trained with "anchor papers."

64. According to the passage, which of the following affects the reliability of scores on essays?

A. Multiple readings mean that scores will likely differ.
B. Evaluators may not agree on which criteria are the most important.
C. An average paper read after an outstanding one may receive a lower score than if it's read after another average one.

D. Trial grading runs do not give sufficient calibration.

65. Which statement probably best sums up the author's evaluation of the ways to test writing in large-scale assessments?

A. Indirect assessments are better than direct assessments because of the reliability problems involved in direct assessments.
B. Direct assessments are better than indirect assessments because they test a student's ability to create a text.
C. Evaluators of essays in direct assessments need to be carefully trained.
D. Both indirect assessments and direct assessments have only limited value.

PHYSICAL SCIENCES

10 PROBLEM SETS OF 5–10 QUESTIONS EACH
15 PROBLEMS FOLLOWED BY A SINGLE QUESTION
77 QUESTIONS
100 MINUTES

DIRECTIONS: The following questions or incomplete statements are in groups. Preceding each series of questions or statements is a paragraph or a short explanatory statement, a formula or set of formulas, or a definition. Read the written material and then answer the questions or complete the statements. Select the ONE BEST ANSWER for each question and indicate your selection by marking the corresponding letter of your choice on the Answer Form. Eliminate those alternatives you know to be incorrect and then select an answer from among the remaining alternatives. A periodic table is provided (see p467). You may consult it whenever you wish to do so.

Passage I (Questions 66–70)

In a physics class, an experimental motion experiment is devised to allow the study of the motion of a number of objects under a variety of conditions. One part involves projecting identical steel or wooden balls at a variety of initial angles and speeds, starting at various heights above the floor. Equipment, such as protractors and photogate timers, is available so the angles and speeds are known. Rectangular metal blocks of various masses can be slid across horizontal surfaces and also down inclined planes. The surfaces vary from essentially frictionless to quite rough surfaces. The balls can be rolled down the inclined planes also. The masses of each object are measured in advance and the velocities can be measured at any point of the motion with the photogate timers.

66. One of the identical balls is dropped from the edge of a lab table 1.1 m high at the same instant another one is projected horizontally with an intial velocity of 2 m/s. If there is no air resistance, what are the times for the two balls, respectively, to strike the floor?

   A. 0.11 s, 0.11 s   C. 0.47 s, 0.95 s
   B. 0.47 s, 0.47 s   D. 1.2 s, 2.3 s

67. One ball is projected horizontally with an initial horizontal velocity of 10 m/s while a second is projected at an angle of 30° *above* the horizontal with the same initial speed. Both balls strike a vertical wall that is exactly 10 m away. How long does it take each ball, respectively, to hit the wall?

   A. 0.87 s, 1.5 s   C. 1 s, 1 s
   B. 1 s, 0.87 s   D. 1 s, 1.5 s

68. A rectangular block of mass 1 kg and one of mass 3 kg are projected across a rough surface with the same starting speed of 4 m/s. The coefficient of friction is 0.4. How far do the blocks slide, respectively?

   A. 2 m, 2 m
   B. 3 m, 2 m
   C. 4 m, 4 m
   D. 6 m, 2 m

69. One of the balls is released from rest at the top of an inclined plane 0.5 m high and rolls down without slipping. At the same instant a rectangular block is released and slides down a frictionless plane which is also 0.5 m high. Which of the two objects has the greater speed at the bottom of the inclines?

   A. The ball.
   B. The block.
   C. Both have the same speed.
   D. The question cannot be answered because there is not enough information given.

70. A wooden ball of mass 0.4 kg is dropped down a circular stairwell. It is observed to reach a terminal velocity of 35 m/s and continues falling at that speed. What is the force of air friction acting on the ball?

   A. 3.9 N
   B. 7.8 N
   C. 14 N
   D. 28 N

Passage II (Questions 71–76)

The students in an introductory physics class are nearly all in premedicine, so the instructor decides to have one lab session in which all the topics are related to the human body and its physiology. The students' blood pressures, temperatures, weights (masses), height, and so on can be measured. The instructor has obtained clinical equipment to test hearing, sight, pulmonary function, metabolic rates, and so on with reasonable accuracy.

71. The lab instructor weighs 205 pounds. If 1 kg weighs 2.2 pounds, what is the instructor's mass in kg. and his weight in newtons?

    A. 45.5 kg and 446 N
    B. 78 kg and 674 N
    C. 93.2 kg and 913 N
    D. 451 kg and 46 N

72. The average aortic pressure for a student is determined to be 100 mmHg. What is the gauge pressure in the foot artery, which is 1.35 m below the aorta? (The density of blood is 1050 kg/m^3.)

    A. 120 mmHg   C. 405 mmHg
    B. 205 mmHg   D. 660 mmHg

73. The metabolism for one of the women in the class requires about 2000 kcal per day. Given a food intake of 3200 kcal per day for a period of two weeks, what mass of fat corresponds to the excess food intake? The energy of oxidation for fats and oils is 9.5 kcal per gram.

    A. 440 g   C. 1240 g
    B. 860 g   D. 1700 g

74. It is known that in human metabolic processes, the ratio of energy released to oxygen consumed is about 20,000 joules/liter. A student with a basal metabolic rate of 95 W steps up and down repeatedly on a step for 10 minutes. The student's metabolic rate rises to an average of 630 W during the 10 minutes. What is the approximate number of liters of oxygen the student consumes during the exercise period?

    A. 9 L   C. 45 L
    B. 19 L   D. 134 L

75. A simple experiment in static equilibrium can determine the vertical position of a student's center-of-mass above the soles of the feet. The student lies on a board resting on two bathroom scales set on zero. The centers of the scales are 1.83 m apart. The head scale reads 90 pounds whereas the scale at his feet reads 100 pounds. What is the location of the center-of-mass above the soles of his feet?

    A. 0.60 m   C. 1.03 m
    B. 0.87 m   D. 1.23 m

76. A student wants to lose 1 pound of fat (0.4545 kg) by exercising as above. (1 kcal = 4186 joules.) The average rate of energy expended is 500 watts (above that required for ordinary metabolism). For how many hours will the student have to exercise continuously?

    A. 0.5 hours   C. 23.5 hours
    B. 10.0 hours   D. 455 hours

Passage III (Questions 77–81)

A set of experiments in the physics lab is designed to develop understanding of simple electrical circuit principles for direct current circuits. The student is given a variety of batteries, resistors, and DC meters; and is directed to wire series and parallel combinations of resistors and batteries making measurements of the currents and voltage drops using the ammeters and voltmeters. The student calculates expected current and voltage values using Ohm's law and Kirchhoff's circuit rules and then checks the results with the meters.

77. A student connects a 6-volt battery and a 12-volt battery in series and then connects this combination across a 10-ohm resistor. What is the current in the resistor?

    A. 0.8 A   C. 1.8 A
    B. 0.9 A   D. 3.6 A

78. Resistors of 4 ohms and 8 ohms are connected in series. A battery of 6 volts is connected across the series combination. How much power, in watts, is consumed in the 8-ohm resistor?

    A. 0.67 W   C. 12 W
    B. 2 W   D. 24 W

79. Two 4-ohm resistors are connected in series and this pair is connected in parallel with an 8-ohm resistor. A 12-volt battery is connected across the ends of this parallel set. What power, in watts, is consumed in the 8-ohm resistor in this case?

A. 0.9 W   C. 4.4 W
B. 2.0 W   D. 18 W

80. A 6-volt battery is connected across a 2-ohm resistor. What is the heat energy dissipated in the resistor in 5 minutes?

A. 430 joules   C. 4300 joules
B. 560 joules   D. 5400 joules

81. A 12-volt battery is connected across a 4-ohm resistor and the heat energy dissipated in the resistor in 10 minutes is used to heat 2 kg of water (which is thermally insulated so that no heat escapes). The initial temperature of the water is 20°C and the specific heat of the water is 4184 joule/kg-°C. What is the final temperature of the water at the end of the 10 minutes of heating?

A. 22.6 °C   C. 34.2 °C
B. 28.4 °C   D. 56.4 °C

Passage IV (Questions 82–87)

A set of introductory physics experiments is for the purpose of studying different types of wave motion in different aspects. The student can generate mechanical waves on strings, sound waves in different media, light waves, and water waves in ripple tanks. The plan is to show the similarities (and differences) between different kinds of waves, and to study the propagation of waves through differing materials.

82. A small loudspeaker sends a sound wave into a tube, which is closed on the other end, and a loud resonance is obtained at a frequency of 340 Hz. The tube is 25 cm long. It is known that the open end is an antinode of the standing wave and the closed end is a node. If the 340 Hz resonance is the lowest frequency resonance (the fundamental frequency), what is the speed of sound in the air?

A. 120 m/s   C. 340 m/s
B. 280 m/s   D. 680 m/s

83. The highest sound frequency a student can hear is 20,000 Hz at a wavelength of 1.7 cm. If the highest frequency the instructor can hear is 15,000 Hz; about what wavelength is this in cm?

A. 1.6 cm   C. 2.6 cm
B. 2.3 cm   D. 34.0 cm

84. Suppose the amplitudes of a 15,000 Hz sound wave and a 20,000 Hz sound wave are the same. It is known that the energy in a wave is proportional to the square of the frequency and the square of the amplitude. ($W = Kf^2A^2$). What is the ratio of the energy in the 20,000 Hz wave to the energy of the lower frequency wave?

A. 1.8   C. 6.8
B. 2.4   D. 8.6

85. Some properties of longitudinal waves are similar to those of transverse waves. For example, the speed that both types of waves travel does not usually depend on the frequency. What experimental fact clearly distinguishes longitudinal waves from transverse waves?

A. Longitudinal waves always have longer wavelengths than transverse waves.
B. Transverse waves can be polarized.
C. Transverse waves vibrate parallel to the direction the wave travels.
D. Transverse waves have a higher frequency than longitudinal waves.

86. The students measure the shortest and longest wavelengths of visible light that they can see and find the range to be 400 nm (violet) to about 750 nm (deep red). (1 nm = 10^{-9} m.) They know that light of all wavelengths travels with the same speed, c. The Planck Quantum hypothesis states that the energy of a photon of light is proportional to the frequency, $E = hf$, where h is Planck's Constant. What is the ratio of the energy of 400 nm light to the energy of 750 nm light?

A. 1.88   C. 34.4
B. 2.66   D. 45.6

87. Consider the two sound waves of 20,000 Hz and 15,000 Hz that are heard by the student and instructor. What is the ratio of the speed of sound for the 20,000 Hz wave to the speed of sound for the 15,000 Hz wave?

A. 0.75   C. 1.2
B. 1.0   D. 1.33

Questions 88–95 are independent of any passages and of each other.

88. The electrical repulsive force between two charges of 1 microcoulomb and 2 microcoulombs is 0.54 N. The separation between them is then increased to three times as far. What is the new force between the charges?

A. .03 N   C. .18 N
B. .06 N   D. 1.62 N

89. A piece of copper wire 20 m long has a resistance of 1.2 ohms. Another piece is also 20 m long but has a diameter that is 50% larger. What is the resistance of the larger diameter copper wire in ohms?

A. 0.21 ohms   C. 2.4 ohms
B. 0.53 ohms   D. 2.7 ohms

90. A block of mass 2 kg is connected by a string to a block of mass 0.6 kg. The pair is accelerated by pulling on a string attached to the 2 kg block with an acceleration of 0.2 m/s^2. What is the tension in the string between the two blocks? There is no friction.

A. 0.12 N   C. 0.30 N
B. 0.21 N   D. 0.52 N

91. A proton has a vertically upward velocity in a region where a horizontal magnetic field points due North. What is the direction of the force on the proton?

A. vertically down
B. East, horizontal
C. West, horizontal
D. South, horizontal

92. A car of mass 1000 kg and a small truck of mass 2000 kg crash head-on. Each had a speed of 40 mph at impact. How does the force the truck exerts on the car, F_T, compare to the force the car exerts on the truck, F_C, during the collision?

A. F_T is equal to F_C (and opposite).
B. F_T is one-half of F_C (in same direction).
C. F_T is twice as large as F_C (and opposite).
D. F_T is four times as large as F_C (and opposite).

93. A boat is headed directly across a river 50 m wide in which the current is 1 m/s. The boat's speed in still water is 2 m/s. How long does it take the boat to cross the river?

A. 22.3 s   C. 44.6 s
B. 25 s   D. 50 s

94. A simple pendulum of length L has a period of 2 seconds. What is the period of another pendulum whose length is $4L$?

A. 1 s   C. 4 s
B. 1.41 s   D. 8 s

95. A stretched string is vibrating at a frequency of 120 Hz. Standing waves are set up such that the string of length 80 cm has two "loops" of the standing wave. What is the speed of the wave on the string?

A. 48 m/s   C. 100 m/s
B. 96 m/s   D. 192 m/s

Passage V (Questions 96–105)

Students are given a variety of lenses and optics equipment, such as lens holders, lighted object sources, optical benches, meter sticks and tapes, image screens, and several examples of commercial optical equipment, such as microscopes and telescopes. They are to work in an open-ended optics lab in order to learn the general principles of lenses and the optical devices that can be constructed using lenses.

96. A student is given a short focal length converging lens and a long focal length converging lens. One lens is placed in a holder. A lighted object is placed 18 cm in front of the lens and it is found that a clear image can be focused on a screen placed 36 cm behind the lens. What is the focal length of this lens?

A. 8 cm   C. 27 cm
B. 12 cm   D. 46 cm

97. What magnification is produced by the above lens when the object is 18 cm in front of the lens and the image is 36 cm behind the lens?

   A. 2 ×   C. 4 ×
   B. 3 ×   D. 6 ×

98. A lighted object is placed 6 cm in front of the second lens, which has a focal length of +24 cm. Where is the image and which kind of image is it?

   A. 8 cm in front of the lens; a virtual image
   B. 8 cm behind the lens; a real image
   C. 16 cm in front of the lens; a real image
   D. 16 cm behind the lens; a virtual image

99. The 24 cm focal length lens is used as the objective of a simple refracting telescope and a third converging lens of focal length +8 cm is used as the eyepiece. What is the magnification of this simple refractor?

   A. 0.6 ×   C. 4 ×
   B. 3 ×   D. 6 ×

100. A commercial microscope is examined by the student. The objective is marked 20 × and the eyepiece is marked 10 ×. What power objective should replace the above objective so that the microscope's magnification will be 400 ×?

   A. 5 ×   C. 40 ×
   B. 10 ×   D. 100 ×

101. A lighted object is placed 24 cm in front of a +12 cm focal length lens. The image formed by this lens is the object for a second lens of +24 cm focal length. The second lens is placed 72 cm behind the first lens. Where is the final image with respect to the second lens?

   A. 24 cm in front of #2
   B. 24 cm behind #2
   C. 36 cm in front of #2
   D. 48 cm behind #2

102. A lens of focal length +24 cm is used to view an object placed 12 cm in front of the lens. The object is 5 cm tall. How tall is the image?

   A. 2.5 cm   C. 7.5 cm
   B. 3.3 cm   D. 10 cm

103. A diverging lens of focal length −24 cm is now used with the object 12 cm in front of the lens. How tall is the image if the object is 5 cm tall?

   A. 2.5 cm   C. 8 cm
   B. 3.3 cm   D. 10 cm

104. A nearsighted student cannot see objects clearly unless they are as close as 80 cm (his "far-point"). The image that he sees through his new contact lens is a virtual image because he looks through the lens to see the image. What focal length lenses does he need in order to see very distant objects, such as the stars?

   A. −20 cm   C. −80 cm
   B. −30 cm   D. +40 cm

105. A student uses a lens marked "− 4 D," where D stands for diopters. What is the focal length of this lens in cm?

   A. −0.04 cm   C. −4 cm
   B. −0.25 cm   D. −25 cm

Passage VI (Questions 106–110)

Phases include solid, liquid, and gas. Many materials can exist in any of these depending upon conditions. There is, however, usually a gain or loss of heat in the transition.

106. A mechanical refrigerator is cooled by:

   A. conversion of a liquid to a gas.
   B. conversion of a solid to a liquid.
   C. conversion of a solid to a gas.
   D. conversion of a gas to a solid.

107. The freezing point of a crystalline solid is:

   A. several °C lower than the melting point.
   B. equal to the melting point.
   C. several °C higher than the melting point.
   D. not directly related to the melting point.

108. Transition of a material directly from solid to gas:

   A. is not known.
   B. is known as evaporation.
   C. is known as expiration.
   D. is known as sublimation.

109. Boiling point of a pure liquid is:

A. usually increased by increased pressure.
B. not usually affected by changes in pressure.
C. usually decreased by increased pressure.
D. affected by pressure but in a fairly unpredictable direction.

110. Conversion of oxygen from a gas to a liquid is possible only below −118°C, no matter what pressure is imposed. This temperature is known as the:

A. boiling point.
B. critical temperature.
C. condensation temperature.
D. Clausius temperature.

Passage VII (Questions 111–115)

An enzyme is a special kind of biological catalyst. In many ways it can be considered much as other catalysts.

A series of experiments gave results on the velocity (V) of an enzyme reaction (i.e. rate of formation of products) while keeping the enzyme concentration constant but varying substrate (S). The results were graphed as below:

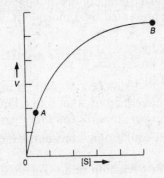

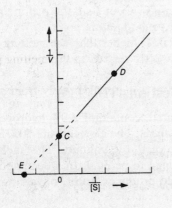

111. Point A is an area where the reaction is _____ order with respect to the substrate.

A. zero   C. second
B. first   D. third

112. Point B is in an area where the reaction is _____ order with respect to the substrate.

A. zero   C. second
B. first   D. third

113. The substrate concentration of point C is:

A. zero.
B. the maximum soluble.
C. infinite.
D. the minimum amount that will give a measurable product.

114. The reciprocal of the ordinate at point C is:

A. the minimum velocity at minimum substrate.
B. the maximum velocity.
C. the minimum velocity at maximum substrate.
D. zero velocity.

115. Considering the two graphs, maximum velocity would be shown (or could be readily computed from):

A. point B.   C. point E.
B. point C.   D. point B or point C.

Passage VIII (Questions 116–120)

By varying the temperature and pressure for Substance X, the following phase diagram is obtained. It indicates the phase(s) that will be found at a variety of temperatures and pressures.

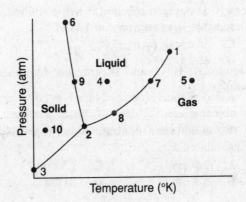

116. Liquid, solid, and gas may be found in equilibrium at the temperature and pressure indicated by:

A. point 1.   C. point 3.
B. point 2.   D. point 4.

117. Starting at a temperature and pressure indicated by point 4 and heating the material without change of pressure, one would reach a phase change at:

A. point 6.   C. point 8.
B. point 7.   D. point 9.

118. Starting at a temperature and pressure indicated by point 10 and increasing the pressure as much as possible without changing temperature, one would:

A. pass through the point where gas, liquid, and solid are in equilibrium.
B. reach a point where solid is in equilibrium with gas.
C. reach a point where solid is in equilibrium with liquid.
D. note no phase change.

119. The critical temperature is indicated at:

A. point 1.   C. point 3.
B. point 2.   D. point 4.

120. The temperature at point 7, at the indicated pressure, is called the:

A. freezing temperature.
B. sublimation temperature.
C. boiling temperature.
D. allotropic temperature.

Passage IX (Questions 121–125)

A newly discovered reaction is being studied. It is concluded that the reaction consists of

$$2A + 3B \rightleftharpoons 3C + 2D$$

(The letters A, B, C, and D represent hypothetical compounds.)

121. The equilibrium constant as written may be calculated as:

A. $\dfrac{[C]^3 \ [D]^2}{[A]^2 \ [B]^3}$

B. $\dfrac{3[C] \ 2[D]}{2[A] \ 3[B]}$

C. $\dfrac{[A]^2 \ [B]^3}{[C]^3 \ [D]^2}$

D. $\dfrac{[C] \ [D]}{[A] \ [B]}$

122. If the equilibrium constant is 0.001:

A. reaction to the right will be favored.
B. reaction to the left will be favored.
C. the reaction rate is fast.
D. the reaction rate is slow.

123. If A, B, and D are gases and C is a solid, the reaction will:

A. be improved toward the right with increased pressure.
B. be improved toward the left with increased pressure.
C. be unaffected by increased pressure.
D. not proceed in either direction in the presence of increased pressure.

124. At standard temperature and pressure, the volume represented by 3 moles of C is about:

A. 22 liters.
B. 45 liters.
C. 67 liters.
D. more than 80 liters.

125. A small equilibrium constant is indicative of:

A. a fast reaction rate.
B. a slow reaction rate.
C. no reaction.
D. none of the above.

Passage X (Questions 126–135)

A liquid is isolated, containing 5.9% hydrogen and 94.1% oxygen by mass. The elements are 50% hydrogen and 50% oxygen by volume. The molecular weight is determined to be 34.0. In a decomposition reaction this liquid produces water, oxygen, and no other products.

126. The empirical formula is:

    A. HO.
    B. H_2O_2.
    C. H_3O_3.
    D. H_3O_4.

127. The molecular formula is:

    A. HO.
    B. H_2O_2.
    C. H_3O_3.
    D. H_3O_4.

128. The balanced equation for the decomposition indicates that one mole of the liquid will produce _____ moles of oxygen.

    A. 0.25
    B. 0.50
    C. 1.0
    D. 2.0

129. The balanced equation for the decomposition indicates that one mole of the liquid will produce _____ moles of water.

    A. 0.25
    B. 0.50
    C. 1.0
    D. 2.0

130. The balanced equation for the decomposition of the liquid indicates the formation of _____ liters of oxygen at S.T.P. from one mole of the liquid.

    A. 1.12
    B. 2.24
    C. 11.2
    D. 22.4

131. The balanced equation for the decomposition of the liquid indicates the formation of _____ g of water from 34 g of the liquid.

    A. 16
    B. 18
    C. 30
    D. 32

132. For an equilibrium reaction at 25°C, the decomposition we have been considering would be _____ by an increase in pressure.

    A. favored
    B. unaffected
    C. adversely affected
    D. affected, but in an unpredictable direction

133. For an equilibrium reaction at 25°C, the decomposition would be _____ by an increase in oxygen without an increase in pressure.

    A. favored
    B. unaffected

C. adversely affected
D. affected, but in an unpredictable direction

134. In the above question, the equilibrium constant would be:

    A. increased.
    B. unaffected.
    C. decreased.
    D. affected, but in an unpredictable direction.

135. The order of the reaction, from information given above, will be definitely

    A. zero.
    B. first.
    C. second.
    D. unpredictable.

Questions 136–142 are independent of any passages and of each other.

136. Catalysts:

    A. are changed and consumed during a reaction.
    B. have virtually no effect on the overall rate of the reaction.
    C. are changed but not consumed during a reaction.
    D. speed up the rate of the reaction.

137. If solution A is less concentrated in dissolved particle content than solution B, then solution B is said to be:

    A. hypertonic.
    B. hypotonic.
    C. isoosmotic.
    D. isotonic.

138. Compared to one mole of oxygen, how many more molecules do two moles of carbon dioxide contain?

    A. 25×10^6
    B. 12.04×10^{46}
    C. 6.02×10^{23}
    D. 12.04×10^{23}

139. Which one of the following acids does not commonly form acid salts?

    A. $HC_2H_3O_2$
    B. H_2SO_4
    C. H_2CO_3
    D. H_3PO_4

140. Which of the statements listed below is false?

    A. An aqueous solution in which $[H^+] > 1 \times 10^{-7}$ is said to be acidic.

    B. Ions are atoms or groups of atoms that have lost or gained one or more electrons.

    C. HCl is a Bronsted acid because it furnishes H^+ ion in solution.

    D. NaOH is called a base because it furnishes Na^+ ions in solution.

141. In the decomposition of $KClO_3$ to generate oxygen gas, MnO_2 is added in order to:

    A. increase the volume of oxygen obtained from the $KClO_3$.

    B. produce oxygen of higher purity.

    C. reduce the temperature at which decomposition of $KClO_3$ takes place.

    D. increase the temperature at which decomposition of $KClO_3$ takes place.

142. The name applied to a substance such as MnO_2 used in the reaction above is a (an):

    A. enzyme.

    B. catalyst.

    C. isotope.

    D. free radical scavenger.

WRITING SAMPLE

2 ESSAYS - TOPICS
60 MINUTES (30 MINUTES/TOPIC)

DIRECTIONS: Your response must be a unified, organized essay; it should contain fully developed, logically constructed paragraphs. Remember quality is more important than length. Before you begin writing, make sure you have read the item carefully and understand what is being asked. Write as legibly as possible. Because your essays will be scored as first-draft compositions, you may cross out and make corrections on your response booklet as necessary. It is not necessary to recopy your essay.

Part 1

Consider this statement:

A wise man sees as much as he ought, not as much as he can.

Montaigne

Write a unified essay in which you perform the following tasks. Explain what the above quotation means. Describe a specific situation in which a wise man sees as much as he can, not as much as he ought. Discuss what you think determines the limits that should and should not be placed on vision.

Part 2

Consider this statement:

There is properly no history; only biography.

Emerson

Write a unified essay in which you perform the following tasks. Explain what you think the above quotation means. Describe a specific situation in which there would, in fact, be history, whether or not there were biography. Discuss what you think determines the relationship between history and biography.

BIOLOGICAL SCIENCES

10 PROBLEM SETS OF 5–10 QUESTIONS EACH
15 PROBLEMS FOLLOWED BY A SINGLE QUESTION
77 QUESTIONS
100 MINUTES

DIRECTIONS: The following questions or incomplete statements are in groups. Preceding each series of questions or statements is a paragraph or a short explanatory statement, a formula or set of formulas, or a definition. Read the written material and then answer the questions or complete the statements. Select the ONE BEST ANSWER for each question and indicate your selection by marking the corresponding letter of your choice on the Answer Form. Eliminate those alternatives you know to be incorrect and then select an answer from among the remaining alternatives.

Passage I (Questions 143–148)

The diagram illustrates a typical neuron, the basic unit of the nervous system, located in a spinal (dorsal root) ganglion. Neurons connect with each other and in that manner an impulse is conducted and transmitted throughout the body. Two types of cell processes are indicated.

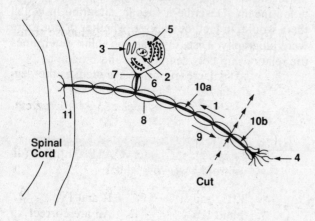

143. An impulse on the skin will be picked up by:

    A. 4.   C. 7.
    B. 6.   D. 10.

144. The genetic material of the cell is located in:

    A. 2.   C. 5.
    B. 3.   D. 7.

145. Protein synthesis is carried out under the direction of:

    A. 3 in 5.   C. 2 in 5.
    B. 2 in 3.   D. 2 in 7.

A person has been in an accident and the physician is conducting a neurological examination. Sensation is lost over several fingers and the examiner fears that a nerve has been cut. Note the cut indication on the diagram preceding question 143.

146. Which process would completely degenerate?

    A. 11.   C. 10a.
    B. 8.   D. 10b.

147. Retrograde degeneration would be visible in:

    A. 2.   C. 6.
    B. 3.   D. 10b.

148. The impulse in the neuron is normally conducted in which direction?

    A. 9.   C. Neither 9 nor 1.
    B. 1.   D. Both 9 and 1.

Passage II (Questions 149–154)

The purpose of these experiments is to illustrate the action of both active and passive driving forces on the absorption of solutions of hemoglobin, Ringer's solution, $MgSO_4$, xylose, and glucose from the lumen of the small intestines *in vivo*.

Fluid can be absorbed from the small intestine even when the luminal solution is isotonic Ringer's. The absence of a net passive driving force for water uptake between lumen and blood indicates that active processes are involved. The active transport is *not* on the water itself but rather on sodium chloride. Active sodium transport from the epithelial cells renders the intercellular spaces sufficiently hypertonic to create osmotic driving forces for water movement out of the lumen.

Glucose is transported from the lumen by means of a specific carrier. The carrier has a site for the sugar and for sodium. It is the sodium gradient across the apical cell membrane that provides the energy for glucose entry. The sodium gradient is maintained by the active extrusion of sodium from the cells. The carrier shows typical saturation kinetics. In the case of glucose, the Km for absorption is 2mM, when sodium levels are 145mM. By contrast, the pentose, xylose, is far less effective as a substrate for this carrier. At the same level of Na, its Km is about 100 mM.

Ions such as Mg^{2+} and SO^{2-}_4, which are poorly absorbed, behave toward the intestinal epithelium almost as if it were a semipermeable membrane. Thus passive osmotic forces play a predominant role in determining the magnitude and direction of fluid movement. A similar statement can be made about intact proteins such as hemoglobin. These are ordinarily impermeable solutes.

By measuring the changes in fluid volume due to the presence of the test substances and by chemically analyzing for changes in the glucose, xylose, and hemoglobin concentration, data on how the *in vivo* intestine treats each substance will be obtained.

Experiment

In two rats, three successive 10 cm segments of intestine are tied off. Injected into the segments of one rat from proximal to distal were solutions of hemoglobin, Ringer's, and $MgSO_4$.

Injected into the segments of rat two from proximal to distal were solutions of xylose, Ringer's, and glucose. After one hour whatever fluid was present in the respective segments was withdrawn, and volumes recorded. Analysis for solutes present were conducted and percentage of absorption and recovery recorded.

149. From the "absorption from the intestine laboratory" when equal volumes of 100 mM of D-glucose or D-xylose are added in isotonic Ringer's solutions to isolated intestinal segments, the following would be expected (Km, glucose 2mM, xylose 100 mM).

   A. Equal volumes would be absorbed in a one-hour incubation.
   B. A greater volume absorbed from the xylose segment than for glucose.
   C. A greater volume absorbed from the glucose segment than for xylose.
   D. No volume change for either.

150. When 1 ml of a 1.8% solution of D-glucose was added to an intestinal segment in isotonic Ring-

er's solution and the total glucose analyzed at one hour, it was found that 1.8 mg was recovered. What percent of the D-glucose injected was absorbed or metabolized?

   A. 1.8%   C. 10%
   B. 1%   D. 90%

151. For the "absorption from the intestine laboratory," when a hemoglobin solution in water was injected into the isolated small intestine, at the end of one hour:

   A. more hemoglobin would be recovered than injected because proteins are secreted into the intestine.
   B. less hemoglobin was recovered because intact proteins are normally absorbed.
   C. less hemoglobin was recovered because bleeding into the intestine would normally occur.
   D. less hemoglobin was recovered because some hemoglobin was adsorbed on the surface of the mucosal lumen.

152. For the "absorption from the intestine laboratory," for injection of D-glucose in isotonic Ringer's solution, inhibition of glucose transport would occur when:

   I. D-galactose was also added to the segment.
   II. sodium ion was replaced by a large cation.
   III. when L-glucose replaced D-glucose.
   IV. when an uncoupler of ATP synthesis (dinitrophenol) was added.

   A. I, II, and III   C. II and IV
   B. I and III   D. All are correct

153. For the "absorption from the intestine laboratory," when 25% $MgSO_4$ was injected into the isolated small intestine, the expected change was:

   A. an increase in volume.
   B. a decrease in volume.
   C. no change in volume.

154. For the "absorption from the intestine laboratory," when a hemoglobin solution in water was injected into the isolated small intestine, the expected change was:

   A. an increase in volume.
   B. a decrease in volume.
   C. no change in volume.

Passage III (Questions 155–161)

The schema of thyroxine formation is outlined below:

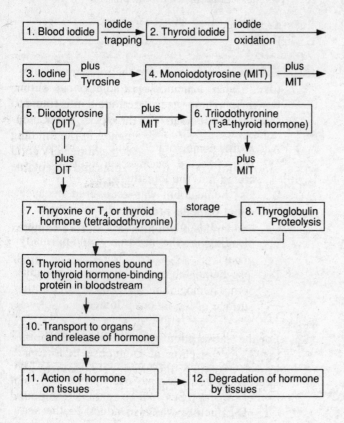

155. Chemically, thyroid hormones are:

  A. iodotyrosines.   C. iodides.
  B. iodothyronines.   D. iodines.

156. In proceeding from compound 3 to compound 4, the amino acid tyrosine is:

  A. oxidized.   C. iodinated.
  B. reduced.   D. synthesized.

157. During transport thyroid hormones are inactive because they are:

  A. in the form of thyroglobulin.
  B. free hormones.
  C. protein-bound.
  D. on red blood cells.

158. Untreated goiter is associated with:

  A. hyperthyroidism.
  B. hypothyroidism.
  C. euthyroidism.
  D. A, B, and C.

159. TSH:

  A. is made up of two peptide chains (alpha and beta).
  B. is released by the hypothalamus.
  C. binds tightly to thyroid binding globulin (TBG).
  D. secretion decreases upon exposure to the cold.

160. Involved in the regulation of the synthesis of thyroid hormone are

  A. availability of iodide ions.
  B. TSH.
  C. negative feedback of circulating T_3 and T_4 at the level of the anterior pituitary (by down regulation of TRH receptors).
  D. all of the above.

161. Which of the following describes the metabolic effect of thyroid hormone?

  A. decreased myocardial beta adrenergic receptors
  B. decreased BMR
  C. increased oxygen consumption
  D. increased plasma cholesterol

Passage IV (Questions 162–166)

The following graph illustrates several phenomena that develop while a muscle is being repetitively stimulated:

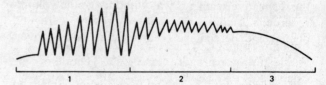

162. In the diagram above, region 1 represents:

  A. summation.
  B. complete or fused tetanus.
  C. repeated identical twitches.
  D. hyperpolarization.

163. What is the most likely cause of the event in region 3?

  A. consumption of ATP stored in the muscle
  B. loss of myosin from the muscle
  C. gradual failure to transmit the stimulus to the contraction apparatus
  D. loss of elasticity within the muscle

---

164. What is the major difference between regions 1 and 2?

  A. Elastic elements have become fully stretched in region 1, but not in region 2.
  B. Elastic elements have become fully stretched in region 2, but not in region 1.
  C. The stimulus strength is greater in region 2.
  D. The stimulus strength is greater in region 1.

165. In the diagram, region 2 represents:

  A. incomplete tetanus.
  B. muscle fatigue.
  C. relaxation.
  D. an absolute refractory period.

166. If a muscle is stimulated to contract, allowed to develop force, but not allowed to shorten, then the contraction is called:

  A. spasmodic.   **C.** tetanic.
  B. isotonic.   **D.** isometric.

Passage V (Questions 167–171)

Epilepsy affects approximately one in 200 people or about 1.2 million persons in the United States alone. Despite pharmacologic treatment, 25% of patients continue to have intermittent seizures, and one-quarter million persons have seizures more frequently than once per month. A form of continuous or recurrent seizures persisting for over 30 minutes is operationally defined as *Status Epilepticus* (SE). SE is associated with an exceptionally high mortality rate of 25%. The incidence of SE is about 250 cases per million population annually.

Seizures are broadly classified as general or partial depending on whether they arise from the entire brain simultaneously or just from a restricted region respectively. They are subclassified on the basis of the presence or absence of associated convulsive activity.

Because of the significance of epilepsy as a public health issue and present inadequacies in drug therapy, better pharmacologic strategies for the treatment of epilepsy are currently being sought. Toward this end, a number of animal models have been developed that can predict the success of new and potentially useful anticonvulsant compounds. These predictions are based on the correlation between the recognized clinical success in treating certain classes of seizures with present anticonvulsants and the degree of efficacy (effectiveness) of these same medications against seizures generated in each of the different animal models.

Class	Generalized			Partial
Subclass	Absence	Tonic-Clonic	Myoclonic	Complex
Convulsive?	No	Yes	Yes	Usually
Animal Model	GABA challenge	Electroshock	Audiogenic mouse	Kindling
First Choice	ESM	PHT	VPA	CBZ
Second Choice	VPA	VPA	PB	PHT
Third Choice				VPA

Abbreviations: CBZ—carbamazepine, ESM—ethosuximide, GABA—gamma amino butyric acid, PB—phenobarbital, PHT—phenytoin, VPA—valproic acid

167. AntiEpp is a new compound that has shown promise in animal seizure models. It is found to have greatest efficacy in the electroshock model and has slightly less efficacy in the kindling model. This predicts that it might be very good in treating ___i___ seizures and acceptable for treating ___ii___ seizures.

	i	ii
A.	generalized convulsive	partial complex
B.	tonic-clonic	no other
C.	tonic-clonic	partial complex
D.	audiogenic mouse	electro shock

168. New compounds are often tested because of chemical similarity to conventional agents. In drug testing, Compound X was found to be effective against the model of absence seizures. It was ineffective in all animal models of other seizure types. Which agent is Compound X probably most similar to?

  A. carbamazepine
  B. ethosuximide
  C. valproic acid
  D. not enough information is available to answer the question

169. The 1990 population of New York City is about 7 million persons. How many persons are statistically likely to suffer from epilepsy?

  A. 3,500 persons   **C.** 35,000 persons
  B. 1,750 persons   **D.** 17,500 persons

170. A patient is found to have been seizing for over an hour. Electrical activity from her brain recorded on an electroencephalogram reveals that the abnormal activity is localized only to a restricted region. The best description of her condition is:

  A. status epilepticus.
  B. generalized status epilepticus.
  C. partial status epilepticus.
  D. partial complex seizure.

171. From information provided in the reading passage, please indicate the approximate number of patients with epilepsy who continue to have seizure at least once per month despite pharmacologic (drug) therapy.

A. 30,000
B. 300,000
C. ¼ million
D. 250,000

Passage VI (Questions 172–179)

Using a syringe containing heparin, fifty milliliters of blood were drawn from a healthy male volunteer. Following centrifugation, the "buffy coat" was removed and a lymphocyte-rich cell population was obtained by sedimentation through 2% Dextran. After washing in 0.9% saline the lymphocytes were placed in cell culture tubes at a concentration of 5×10^6 cells/ml cell culture medium/tube. To one-half of the tubes was added 5 μg of phytohemagglutinin, a substance which causes lymphocytes to undergo mitosis. The other half of the tubes received no phytohemagglutinin. Radioactive tracers for RNA, DNA, and protein synthesis were then added to all tubes and aliquots removed at selected intervals. The following data were obtained:

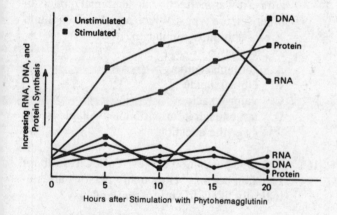

172. The purpose of this experiment was to:

A. determine the role of heparin in blood clotting.
B. determine the sequence of events in cells stimulated to undergo mitosis, and to compare these data to those gathered from unstimulated cells.
C. isolate a pure population of lymphocytes.
D. determine the lifespan of lymphocytes.

173. From these data it can be seen that increased:

A. RNA synthesis precedes increased protein synthesis.
B. DNA synthesis precedes increased protein synthesis.
C. protein synthesis precedes increased RNA synthesis.
D. DNA synthesis precedes increased RNA synthesis.

174. It may also be assumed that:

A. DNA synthesis is dependent on previous RNA synthesis.
B. protein synthesis is dependent on previous DNA synthesis.
C. RNA synthesis is dependent on previous protein synthesis.
D. unstimulated lymphocytes synthesize RNA, DNA, and protein at a low rate.

175. The smallest unit possessing the capability to maintain life and to reproduce is:

A. an organ.
B. a cell.
C. DNA.
D. RNA.

176. Normally, a complete set of chromosomes (2n) is passed on to each daughter cell as a result of:

A. reduction division.
B. mitotic cell division.
C. meiotic cell division.
D. nondisjunction.

177. Messenger RNA receives its instructions from:

A. ribosomes.
B. endoplasmic reticulum.
C. DNA in the nucleus.
D. cytoplasm.

178. During which phase of the mitotic cycle do the two chromatids split apart and start migration toward the poles of the spindle?

A. prophase
B. metaphase
C. anaphase
D. telophase

179. During metaphase of mitosis:

A. there is a dissolution of the chromosomal material.
B. the centrioles with asters are at the opposite poles.
C. the cell membrane starts to reappear.
D. the nuclear membrane disappears.

Passage VII (Questions 180–189)

The liver from a rat was gently homogenized in buffered sucrose solution using a Dounce homogenizer (which does not break most membranous organelles in cells). The homogenate was layered over a sucrose gradient and centrifuged for four hours at 100,000 xg. The sucrose gradient was then collected as a series of fractions. Each fraction was analyzed for DNA concentration, RNA concentration, cytochrome oxidase activity, acid phosphatase activity, and cytochrome P-450 concentration. Concentrations and enzyme activities are given as relative values, with the fraction giving the highest value for each component being shown as 100 and all other values for that component being scaled relative to the highest value.

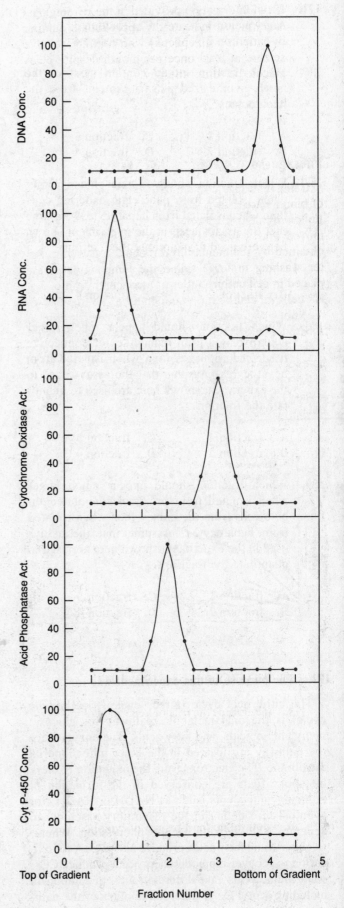

180. Which fraction contains most of the nuclei from the hepatocytes?

A. fraction 1   **C.** fraction 3
B. fraction 2   **D.** fraction 4

181. Which fraction contains most of the mitochonria from the hepatocytes?

A. fraction 1   **C.** fraction 3
B. fraction 2   **D.** fraction 4

182. Which fraction contains most of the rough endoplasmic reticulum from the hepatocytes?

A. fraction 1   **C.** fraction 3
B. fraction 2   **D.** fraction 4

183. Which fraction contains most of the lysosomes from the hepatocytes?

A. fraction 1   **C.** fraction 3
B. fraction 2   **D.** fraction 4

184. Which fraction contains most of the smooth endoplasmic reticulum from the hepatocytes?

A. fraction 1   **C.** fraction 3
B. fraction 2   **D.** fraction 4

185. Which fraction contains most of the Krebs cycle enzymes from the hepatocytes?

A. fraction 1 C. fraction 3
B. fraction 2 D. fraction 4

186. Which fraction should contain most of the newly synthesized plasma proteins from the hepatocytes?

A. fraction 1 C. fraction 3
B. fraction 2 D. fraction 4

187. Which fraction should appear much larger when isolated from pancreatic exocrine cells than when isolated from hepatocytes? Assume that the assays used in the experiment shown here are used to quantitate the fractions.

A. fraction 1 C. fraction 3
B. fraction 2 D. fraction 4

188. Which fraction should appear much larger when isolated from monocytes or connective tissue macrophages than when isolated from hepatocytes? Assume that the assays used in the experiment shown here are used to quantitate the fractions.

A. fraction 1 C. fraction 3
B. fraction 2 D. fraction 4

189. Which fraction should appear much larger when isolated from proximal convoluted tubule cells from the kidney than when isolated from hepatocytes? Assume that the assays used in the experiment shown here are used to quantitate the fractions.

A. fraction 1 C. fraction 3
B. fraction 2 D. fraction 4

Passage VIII (Questions 190–194)

The citric acid cycle (Krebs cycle, tricarboxylic cycle) is the final metabolic pathway for glucose, many amino acids, and fatty acids. The enzymes for the pathway are located in the inner mitochondrial membrane. The electrons from the oxidation of these metabolic fuels are conserved in the formation of reducing equivalents, such as NADH or $FADH_2$ for eventual reoxidation in the respiratory assembly to generate ATP by oxidative phosphorylation. Whereas glucose and fatty acids produce acetyl CoA for oxidation to recover the bond energy and produce CO_2, some amino acids have different routes of catabolism including acetyl CoA, other metabolites of the path-

way, and pyruvate formation. The citric acid cycle can accept metabolites at places other than acetyl CoA and is able to supply metabolites for biosynthesis such as in the synthesis of porphyrins or amino acids. However, net glucose cannot be synthesized from acetyl CoA entering the cycle. The reactions have many similarities such as hydration—dehydration or oxidation, particularly of secondary alcohols to ketone. For every mole of acetyl CoA entering the cycle and condensing with oxaloacetate, 12 moles of ATP and two moles of CO_2 are formed and a mole of oxaloacetate is recovered. The rate of the cycle is controlled by energy levels of the cell at specific enzymatic points including the formation of citric acid and the formation of α-ketoglutarate.

190. For one mole of acetyl CoA entering the Krebs (TCA) cycle (coupled to oxidative phosphorylation):

A. one mole of carbon dioxide and 38 ATP are formed.
B. two moles of carbon dioxide and 38 ATP are formed.
C. two moles of carbon dioxide and 24 ATP are formed.
D. two moles of carbon dioxide and 12 ATP are formed.

191. All of the following are similar pairs of types of reactions starting with pyruvate EXCEPT:

A. isocitrate to oxalosuccinate; malate to oxaloacetate.
B. alpha ketoglutarate to succinyl CoA; acetyl CoA to pyruvate.
C. cis-aconitase to isocitrate; fumarate to malate.
D. pyruvate to acetyl CoA; alpha ketoglutarate to succinyl CoA.

192. The citric acid cycle provides biosynthetic intermediates (net) for the following EXCEPT:

A. acetyl CoA to oxaloacetate.
B. acetyl CoA to malonyl CoA.
C. succinyl CoA to porphyrins.
D. oxaloacetate to aspartate.

193. All of the following are metabolic functions or possible interactions of the tricarboxylic acid cycle EXCEPT:

A. decreased activity when ATP levels are high.

B. control of glycolysis.

C. accepting acetyl CoA from fatty acids, glucose, and some amino acids.

D. net synthesis of glucose occurs from acetyl CoA.

194. All of the following are correct about the citric acid cycle EXCEPT:

A. active in the mature red blood cell in humans.

B. occurs in the mitochondria.

C. provides about 24 ATP/moles of glucose (coupled to ox-phos).

D. when acetyl CoA amount increases it may increase gluconeogenesis from other carbon atoms.

Passage IX (Questions 195–199)

The carbon atom can have four different substituted groups. Because these molecules are not flat, but occupy a three-dimensional shape, they become chiral (handedness, like your right and left hand). The basal molecule that originally all other molecules were compared to was D(+) glyceraldehyde. It has a mirror image L(−) glyceraldehyde with the same chemical and physical properties (with special exceptions) but different biological properties. The D isomer has the OH group on the right side, whereas the L isomer has the OH on the left side. These are enantiomers. The next higher homolog of this aldotriose is an aldotetrose. The family of the aldosugars for trioses and tetroses is shown below. Note that the D tetroses (erythrose and threose) are not entiomers (not mirror images) but are diastereoisomers with different chemical, physical, and biological properties. These D tetroses are also epimers, because they differ only by the configuration around a single carbon atom. The stability of certain stereoforms has allowed them to predominate in nature (D-glucose, for example). The specificity of enzymes allows them to recognize three dimensional stereodifferences. For example, D-glucose and an epimer at the C4 carbon D-galactose. The translation of amino acids in proteins in humans is for the L-form.

D-glyceraldehyde, D-erythrose, D-threose structures

L-glyceraldehyde, L-erythrose, L-threose structures

D-glucose, D-fructose structures

D-mannose, D-galactose structures

195. Amino acids found in humans are usually:

A. optically inactive.

B. of the L-series.

C. of the D-series.

D. a racemic mixture.

196. Carbohydrates in humans (glucose, galactose, fructose, mannose, for example) are usually:

A. optically inactive.

B. of the L-series.

C. of the D-series.

D. a racemic mixture.

197. D-glucose and L-galactose are:

A. epimers.   C. enantiomers.

B. diastereomers.   D. A and B.

198. Epimers of D-glucose include:

A. D-galactose. C. D-fructose.
B. D-mannose.   D. A and B.

199. D-glucose (assume no cyclic structure) has the OH group at _____ carbon as its D indicator.

A. 1   C. 3
B. 2   D. 5

Passage X (Questions 200–204)

The mature human red blood cell is unique in that it has no nucleus and no mitochondria, and has a finite lifetime of 120 days. Its main function is as a carrier of hemoglobin. In fact, the signal for its death is triggered by the loss of hemoglobin function. The red blood cell metabolizes glucose by two pathways with glucose-6-phosphate as the branch point. One direction is the glycolytic pathway to provide energy through substrate level phosphorylation and to produce pyruvate. In order to maintain the glycolytic pathway, the pyruvate is reduced enzymatically using L-lactic dehydrogenase and the coenzyme NADH. The oxidized coenzyme NAD^+ is then used as an electron acceptor in oxidation of 3-phosphoglyceraldehyde in the glycolytic pathway. Lactate leaves the red blood cell and is reoxidized in the liver to pyruvate, which has many fates in metabolism. The second direction for glucose-6-phosphate in metabolism is in the hexose monophosphate pathway (pentose pathway). This pathway produces special reducing equivalents (NADPH) that are used to maintain the red cell membrane, the ferrous ion and molecules, that are the cells' reservoir of -SH groups (glutathione). Drug metabolism frequently requires NADPH so that a deficit in the first enzyme directing this pathway (glucose-6-phosphate dehydrogenase) results in a premature hemolysis of the red blood cell.

200. The end product(s) of catabolism of glucose in the red blood cell by the glycolytic pathway is/are:

A. glucose-6-phosphate.
B. carbon dioxide.
C. acetyl CoA.
D. pyruvate and lactate.

201. The first step in the metabolism of glucose:

A. occurs in the cytoplasm.

B. requires ATP.
C. produces glucose-6-phosphate.
D. all are correct.

202. ATP producing steps in glycolysis include:

A. glucose to glucose-6-phosphate.
B. phosphoenol pyruvate to pyruvate.
C. 1,3 bis phosphoglycerate to 3-phosphoglycerate.
D. B and C.

203. A genetic defect in the red blood cell enzyme glucose-6-phosphate dehydrogenase will result in all of the following EXCEPT:

A. decrease in the formation of NADPH.
B. increase in the hemolysis of red blood cells.
C. failure to reduce pyruvate to lactate.
D. A and B are correct.

204. Glycolysis and the hexose monophosphate shunt:

A. have no common places of interaction.
B. only interface through glucose-6-phosphate.
C. both produce CO_2 in the red blood cell.
D. interact through common intermediates, such as glyceraldehyde-3-phosphate.

DIRECTIONS: Read each passage carefully, study each table, chart or formula, then answer the question following it. Eliminate those choices that you think to be incorrect and mark the letter of your choice on the answer sheet.

EFFECT OF VARIOUS TREATMENTS ON ORGAN WEIGHTS

Treatments	No. of Animals	Body Weight Grams	Organ Weight (mg/100 g Body Weight)		
			Organ 1	Organ 2	Organ 3
Control	8	70	1509 ± 34	223 ± 20	22 ± 0.8
Drug A	8	66	1044 ± 30	87 ± 14	23 ± 1.0
Drug B	8	73	1432 ± 51	224 ± 24	26 ± 0.9
Drug A + B	8	71	1586 ± 68	208 ± 28	25 ± 1.2
Drug C	8	73	1383 ± 80	146 ± 19	31 ± 1.3
Drug B + C	8	65	954 ± 50	61 ± 3	26 ± 2.0

205. The following statements are related to the table above. Based on the information given, select the statement *contradicted by* the information in the table.

A. Causal evaluation of the results leads one to believe that treatment resulted in significant effects.
B. Drugs B and C seem to have acted in an additive manner.

C. The experimenters should have paid closer attention to body weights.

D. Drug C affects all parameters under investigation.

Diet	Losing Weight	Mortality
Balanced Diet	4%	2%
Diet A	90%	74%
Diet A + Vitamin C	84%	72%
Diet A + Vitamin B	4%	2%
Diet A + Vitamin A	88%	76%

Groups of 50 mice were fed the diets listed in the table, and the percentage losing more than 10% of their initial body weight and the percentage mortality after 30 days were recorded.

206. The best conclusion to be drawn from this study is that:

A. diet A is a good reducing diet.
B. diet A lacks B vitamins.
C. vitamin C is not necessary for life.
D. vitamin A is necessary for life.

The epiphyseal cartilage plate is very sensitive to somatotrophin (growth hormone) and, therefore, can be used as an assay for this compound. Species variations exist and other hormones such as estrogen, thyroxine, and several antibiotics also have an effect upon cartilage growth. The assay must be carried out on hypophysectomized animals.

The following experiments were conducted as can be seen from the table:

Test Groups	No. of Animals	Cartilage Growth in μ 1 Injection Daily	Cartilage Growth in μ 2 Injections/Day (½ amount each time)
Control (normal) (saline)	20 (10/injecting group)	100	100
Hypophysectomized (saline)	20	60	60
Hypox + 100 mg STH	20	150	160
Hypox + 300 mg STH	20	180	195
Stressed normal animals (saline)	20	175	190
Hypox & stressed (saline)	20	50	50
Stressed normal + 100 mg STH	20	200	210
Hypox, stressed + 100 mg STH	20	110	120

207. The reason the assay must be carried out on hypophysectomized rats is:

A. just to add another sophisticated method to the experiment.
B. because the pituitary produces its own growth hormone and it might interfere with the assay.

C. to study the pituitary composition of growth hormone.
D. to obtain the animals' own growth hormone.

The following experimental protocol was carried out. Bean seeds were picked for their uniformity and 20 were planted/pot. One hundred percent germination was observed; and when the seedlings were nine days old, the seedlings of uniform growth were selected for treatment with X rays. Four hundred r units/minute were applied at a distance of 30 cm from the object. Seedlings were exposed up to 60 minutes with up to 24,000 r. After exposure, seedlings were placed in a greenhouse and kept at uniform light, temperature, and moisture conditions. Seedlings were measured as indicated in the table.

	CODE I		CODE II
1	From ground to cotyledon (a mark was made on the seedling near the ground with india ink)	A	0 minutes—control
2	Cotyledon to 1st node	B	7.5 minutes—3,000 r
3	Petiole length of 1st leaf	C	15 minutes—6,000 r
4	Midrib of 1st leaf	D	30 minutes—12,000 r
5	From 1st node to tip of the plant (when included)	E	60 minutes—24,000 r

EXPERIMENTAL RESULTS

10 Days

	A	B	C	D	E
1	6.20	6.58	7.30	5.45	4.43
2	2.17	2.16	2.30	1.15	.76
3	.87	1.11	1.10	0.65	.53
4	3.00	3.23	3.02	2.03	1.86
5					

17 Days

	A	B	C	D	E
1	7.08	6.73	8.00	6.99	5.82
2	8.06	7.11	5.36	2.50	1.63
3	4.12	4.50	4.15	2.13	1.70
4	5.44	5.27	5.68	5.33	4.97
5					

33 Days

	A	B	C	D	E
1	7.21	6.73	8.00	7.00	6.05
2	8.07	7.11	5.48	2.65	1.65
3	4.33	4.61	4.86	2.30	1.90
4	5.50	5.50	6.13	5.91	5.25
5	12.56	11.38	5.27		

208. The purpose of this experiment was:

    A. to observe the germination rate.
    B. to check for uniform growth rate
    C. test output and scatter of the X ray machine.
    D. observe X ray effect on growth.

Both sexes carry a complete complement of sex-linked genes. A female, however, with the XX arrangement will only exhibit a recessive gene if she has received it from both parents (a rare event if we are dealing with an uncommon gene of the population); while in the male with the XY arrangement the recessive gene cannot be masked since there is no partner X chromosome and, therefore, a larger number of recessive genes are expressed (examples are hemophilia and color blindness). A man receives his X chromosome from his mother and passes it on to his daughters not his sons. His daughters in this respect are the carriers of his sex-linked traits and their sons will be the affected ones. Let us illustrate with an example. The normal czarina of Russia produced sons suffering from hemophilia, a disease that is caused by a sex-linked recessive gene, h. The more dominant gene, H, produces normal blood clotting. Genotypically, these women must have carried Hh (X_H and X_h). A daughter, depending on the father ($X_H Y$ or $X_h Y$), could have carried $X_H X_h$ or $X_H X_H$ while a son could have been born either with an $X_H Y$ or an $X_h Y$ (hemophilic) chromosomal complement.

209. The following statements are related to the information presented above. Select the statement *supported by* the information given.

    A. A cattle breeder has in a herd a dominant Y-linked trait. A calf sired by a bull carrying this trait is born. The chances of the inheritance of the trait are 50%.
    B. A female calf was born; the chances of exhibiting the trait are zero.
    C. If the sex in the above cross is known, there is no doubt about whether a calf has the trait.
    D. All of the above.

Melanoma tumors were implanted into three strains of mice. Experiments were then performed to determine the types and amounts of host serum antibodies produced against the lipid components of the virus contained in the melanoma cells. The results are summarized in the table below.

Host	Ag A Phenotype	Antilipid Antibody Day 40 Post Implant	Antilipid Antibody Day 60 Post Implant
Strain 1	3/3	4.5 ± 0.3	6.3 ± 1.7
Strain 2	1/3	3.4 ± 0.4	5.5 ± 1.3
Strain 3	1/1	1.3 ± 0.1	1.3 ± 0.3

210. The following statements are related to the information presented above. Select the statement *supported by* the information given.

    A. Strain 1 produced less antilipid antibody at both time periods measured than the other two hosts.
    B. On the basis of this information, Strain 1 animals are less resistant to melanoma-type cancers than either Strain 2 or 3 animals.
    C. All three hosts produced more antibody at 60 days than they did at 40 days.
    D. An Ag A phenotype containing three seems to be related to higher antibody production.

During wound healing, proliferation of cells in epithelial tissues, connective tissues, and vascular tissues occurs in order to fill in and resurface the defect caused by necrotic (dead) tissue. In experimental studies of the cellular kinetics of wound healing, it is often necessary to assess the amount of proliferation in various cell populations. Because cells replicate DNA within 8 to 12 hours before dividing, determination of the frequency of DNA synthesis at a particular time among cells in a population is a good index of the rate of cell division. DNA synthesis can be determined by tagging replicating DNA with radioactive thymidine. By the procedure of autoradiography, the nuclei of cells which have incorporated radioactive thymidine can be identified on histological sections. The percentage of cells labeled with radioactive thymidine is called the labeling index.

The following table includes data on the labeling index of endothelial cells which form the lining of blood vessels.

^{3}H-THYMIDINE INDEX IN WOUND HEALING

Wound Age	Amount of Epidermal Resurfacing	Endothelial Labeling Index
1 day	0%	3.5%
2 days	0%	13.3%
3 days	0-5%	10.5%
6 days	60-70%	5.6%
10 days	90-100%	2.5%

211. The following statements are related to the information presented. Select the statement *not supported by* the information given.

   A. The ^{3}H-thymidine labeling index, and hence the amount of endothelial proliferation, increased before epidermal resurfacing had become evident.
   B. The endothelial labeling index, after 2 days, decreased both with advancing wound age and with advancing surface coverage.
   C. The increased endothelial proliferation at 2 and 3 days led to the formation of new blood vessels, which then induced epidermal resurfacing.
   D. Endothelial proliferation ceases when the wounds are 90–100% resurfaced with epidermis.

Androgen compounds are responsible for maintaining the secondary sex organs and characteristics of organisms. An endocrinology class was divided into 4 groups to conduct a blind experiment and at the end was asked to compare results. Each group received a compound and injected a similar amount. The experimental protocol in male animals was: 1) Unoperated control animals; 2) Unoperated control animals receiving vehicle only; 3) Bilaterally castrated (testes removed) animals; and 4) Bilaterally castrated animals receiving unknown. The results were summarized in table form.

Experimental Groups	Prostate Weight-mg Student Groups				Seminal Vesicle Weight-mg Student Groups			
	1	2	3	4	1	2	3	4
Unoperated Control	33	31	29	34	68	65	63	67
Unoperated Control and Vehicle	31	32	30	31	69	70	65	64
Bilaterally Castrated	10	9	7	8	12	14	10	15
Bilaterally Castrated and Unknown	37	33	28	31	70	64	61	59

212. The following statements are related to the information presented above. Select the statement *supported by* the information given.

   A. The prostate gland is more sensitive than the seminal vesicle to a lack of androgens.
   B. These experiments were properly controlled.
   C. The results obtained are probably not statistically significant.
   D. Bilateral castration removes a major source of sex hormones.

Gerbils were used for this experiment. One group served as a control; one group was thyroidectomized and maintained on 1% calcium gluconate since the parathyroids were probably removed also; one group received daily injections of thyroxin; and one group that was thyroidectomized and maintained as described above also received daily injections of thyroxin. Oxygen was measured in a standard manner. The following were the results.

Groups	Initial Body Weight gm	Final Body Weight gm	Thyroid Gland Weight mg	Liter of O_2 Consumed hour/meter^2
Normal	143	150	5.0	1.54
Hypothyroid	160	174	0.0	0.16
Hyperthyroid	123	120	8.0	7.33
Hypothyroid + thyroxin	164	158	4.9	1.23

213. The following statements are based on the information presented above. Select the statement(s) *consistent with* the information given.

   A. The quantity of heat liberated by an organism as calculated on the basis of respiratory exchange is decreased by deficiencies and elevated by excesses of the active thyroid principle.
   B. After total thyroidectomy, the basal metabolic rate falls to 10% of its normal value.
   C. Hypothyroid animals probably exhibited sluggishness.
   D. All of the above.

A manufacturer is testing a newly designed line of autoclaves that will be marketed. Calibration of timers and temperature controls is critical to insure destruction of bacteria.

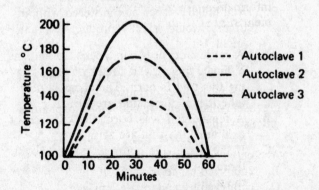

214. Bacteria Z will grow following exposure to temperature below 160°C. Which autoclave will fail to inactivate bacteria Z?

   A. autoclave 1.
   B. autoclave 1 and 2.
   C. autoclave 2 and 3.
   D. autoclave 3.

The pineal complex is implicated in the modulation of reproductive functions of the golden hamster. Surgical removal of the eyes produced atrophy of the testes and seminal vesicles within four to six weeks, and simultaneous pinealectomy prevented the atrophy. In the following experiment the drug MTPH was injected subcutaneously daily for 30 days to learn if there was an enhancement of atrophy. The results are summarized below.

Treatment	Number of Hamsters Treated	Organ Weight (mg/100g body weight)	
		Testes	Seminal Vesicles
Untreated Control	6	2884	722
Blinding	6	1695[a]	396[a]
Pinealectomy	6	2600	544
Blinding, Pinealectomy	6	2580	577
MTPH, No Surgery	6	3069	699
MTPH, Blinding	6	1419[a]	398[a]
MTPH, Pinealectomy	6	2875	591
MTPH, Blinding, Pinealectomy	6	2635	577

[a]($p < 0.05$)

215. The following statements are related to the information presented above. Select the statement *supported by* the information given.

A. Drug MTPH increased the testicular atrophy in blinded hamsters when compared with blinded hamsters not receiving MTPH.
B. Drug MTPH increased the seminal vesicle atrophy in blinded hamsters when compared with blinded hamsters not receiving MTPH.
C. Drug MTPH had no effect on atrophy, either testicular or seminal vesicles.
D. Drug MTPH, when administered without surgery, would affect reproductive organ weight.

216. In the reaction sequence used in breakdown of glycogen in the liver or muscle—glycogen → glucose-1-phosphate→glucose-6-phosphate→ glucose—the first step is:

A. catalyzed by phosphorylase.
B. catalyzed by pepsin.
C. catalyzed by pancreatic amylase.
D. nonenzymatic.

217. A metabolic process that produces energy to convert ADP + phosphate into ATP is the:

A. production of fructose and glucose from sucrose.
B. production of fatty acids and glycerol from triglycerides.
C. production of CO_2 and water from fatty acids.
D. production of steroids from acetate.

218. A negative iodoform test (i.e., no yellow precipitate) will be the result when $NaOH + I_2$ is reacted with:

A. $CH_3-CH-CH_3$
        $|$
        OH

B. $CH_3-C-CH_2-CH_3$
        $\|$
        O

C. $\emptyset-C-CH_3$ (with O double bonded above C)

D. $CH_3-CH_2-CH_2-C=O$ (with H above C)

Phenylamine is cooled to 0°C and treated with HCl and $NaNO_2$. After a few minutes of reaction time cuprous bromide is added, and the solution is heated.

219. The final product would primarily be a (an):

A. azo dye.
B. organometallic compound.
C. monosubstituted benzene containing no metal.
D. disubstituted benzene.

Model Examination D Answer Key

Verbal Reasoning

1. B	14. A	27. B	40. C	53. C
2. B	15. C	28. D	41. A	54. B
3. C	16. A	29. B	42. A	55. A
4. D	17. D	30. B	43. B	56. B
5. D	18. B	31. B	44. B	57. D
6. A	19. C	32. D	45. D	58. D
7. A	20. D	33. C	46. C	59. B
8. C	21. C	34. C	47. C	60. B
9. B	22. D	35. D	48. C	61. C
10. D	23. D	36. D	49. A	62. B
11. D	24. D	37. D	50. B	63. C
12. A	25. D	38. B	51. B	64. C
13. B	26. D	39. C	52. D	65. D

Physical Sciences

66. B	82. C	98. A	113. C	128. B
67. D	83. B	99. B	114. B	129. C
68. A	84. A	100. C	115. D	130. C
69. B	85. B	101. D	116. B	131. B
70. A	86. A	102. D	117. B	132. C
71. C	87. B	103. B	118. D	133. C
72. B	88. B	104. C	119. A	134. B
73. D	89. B	105. D	120. C	135. D
74. B	90. A	106. A	121. A	136. D
75. B	91. C	107. B	122. B	137. A
76. B	92. A	108. D	123. A	138. C
77. C	93. B	109. A	124. C	139. A
78. B	94. C	110. B	125. D	140. D
79. D	95. B	111. B	126. A	141. C
80. D	96. B	112. A	127. B	142. B
81. A	97. A			

Biological Sciences

143. A	159. A	175. B	190. D	205. C
144. A	160. D	176. B	191. B	206. B
145. C	161. C	177. C	192. A	207. B
146. D	162. A	178. C	193. D	208. D
147. A	163. C	179. B	194. A	209. D
148. B	164. B	180. D	195. B	210. D
149. C	165. A	181. C	196. C	211. D
150. D	166. D	182. A	197. B	212. D
151. D	167. C	183. B	198. D	213. D
152. D	168. B	184. A	199. D	214. A
153. A	169. C	185. C	200. D	215. A
154. B	170. C	186. A	201. D	216. A
155. B	171. B	187. A	202. D	217. C
156. C	172. B	188. B	203. C	218. D
157. C	173. A	189. C	204. D	219. C
158. D	174. D			

Explanation of Answers for Model Examination D

VERBAL REASONING

1. **B.** The passage begins by stating that the federal government's role in special education was limited before 1960. It then goes on to highlight the significant laws that have been enacted from 1960 until the passage of P.L. 94–142 in 1975.

2. **B.** Free public education for all handicapped children was brought about in 1975 through the enactment of P.L. 94–142, the Education for All Handicapped Children Act.

3. **C.** Paragraph six explains federal legislation passed in 1970 that was related to the handicapped. Title VI and P.L. 91–230, the Elementary and Secondary Education Assistance Programs Extension, created the Education for the Handicapped Act.

4. **D.** This passage does not describe handicapped conditions.

5. **D.** Eight major mandates of P.L. 94–142 are presented in the later portion of this passage. Answers **A, B,** and **C** represent the first three mandates on the list.

6. **A.** The final paragraph of this passage notes that with the first requirement of P.L. 94–142, early childhood special education became a legal mandate. It states that the downward extension of services will have a significant effect on the young.

7. **A.** According to mandate 5, *prior* public notice and parent involvement is essential in making decisions for educationally handicapped children. **A** is the only case in which parents were informed that something other than regular classroom remediation might be appropriate.

8. **C.** Paragraph one makes it clear that the investigator must focus on the question: "is complainant's job equal in effort and responsibility to that of a male counterpart?" Paragraph seven indicates that the judiciary has not yet endorsed the notion of comparable worth, and the length of employment is not addressed in the reading passage.

9. **B.** Paragraph one makes the point that identical jobs are not necessary because the standard is built on the concept that jobs must be evaluated within a context of substantial equivalency. None of the other statements is supported.

10. **D.** Statements **A** and **B** are not discussed in the passage. Paragraph three contradicts statement **C,** whereas paragraph five implies that Title VII encompasses very broad aspects and reaches beyond the confines of equal wage matters.

11. **D.** Although we might assume that the program of on-the-job training was a positive factor, the law does not address the issue. We could argue that the Department of Labor acted irresponsibly; however, we have no data to substantiate our claim. In the Columbia case, employees were aware of the differences in their positions. Paragraph five supports statement **D** because the court took into consideration the fact that heavy cleaning called for greater effort.

12. **A.** Paragraphs six and seven support statements I, II, and III, however; paragraph seven makes it clear that although the Supreme Court has ruled that Title VII provides a remedy for sex discrimination, the judiciary has not yet endorsed the notion of comparable worth.

13. **B.** Paragraph eight mentions the adverse decision the female guards received during the initial trial, and statement I is supported. It also makes it clear that the appellate court reversed the trial court and held that one could sue even though jobs were not substantially equal; state-

ment III is supported. The paragraph also states that although the Supreme Court did not adopt the concept of comparable worth, it left the door open for further litigation.

14. **A.** Paragraphs nine and ten clearly substantiate statements I, II, and III. Paragraph nine also indicates that the Supreme Court did not indicate how a plaintiff might establish a prima facie case under Title VII, and so statement IV is not supported.

15. **C.** It should be clear to the reader that the issue under consideration is sex discrimination and its resolution.

16. **A.** Paragraph one assigns the skull to Homo sapiens. Man is a vertebrate (subphylum); a mammal (class); Homo is the genus and sapiens is denoted as the species.

17. **D.** Because we are dealing with a fossil, the best answer is an archeologist.

18. **B.** The specimen was found in soil. The fluorine method of dating fossils was developed in 1949 and is based on the fact that buried bones absorb fluorine from the soil, and the amount increases with time.

19. **C.** The older a fossil is, the more fluorine would have been present. A modern jawbone would, on testing, yield a lesser amount of fluorine in comparison to an ancient cranium.

20. **D.** Iron in this case was used to artificially color the mandible to match the cranium.

21. **C.** The last fragment was quite thin; in reality it was chosen by the perpetrator of the hoax (Piltdown Hoax) to duplicate the thinnest part of the first skull.

22. **D.** The passage points out that iron salts are oxidized.

23. **D.** The chromium detected in the jawbone indicates that a dichromate solution was at first used by the forger in an attempt to assist the oxidation of iron salts used to stain the specimens.

24. **D.** There were developments of several methods to study fossils in the 50 years it took to resolve this matter. Although one of the the-

ories proposed was that the missing link was found, the investigation centered on solving the disparity of evidence between the cranium and the jaw. This was a brilliantly devised falsification and no one to date for sure knows who the culprit was.

25. **D.** The first three paragraphs of the passage discuss the material presented in statement I. EUC (end-user computing) is defined in paragraph one, whereas paragraphs two and three describe its strengths and implications for the future. The material presented in statement II, advantages and disadvantages of EUC is presented in paragraphs four and five. The material referred to in statement III, concerning implications of EUC on IS departments and management systems, is pointed out in paragraphs six through eight.

26. **D.** According to the author, statements I, II, and III are the primary reasons for the tremendous growth in end-user computing (EUC). The author presents this information in paragraph two.

27. **B.** In paragraph two, the author states that at the time the passage was written the ratio of white collar workers to computers was about 2:1, but that by the early 1990s this ratio would probably be 1:1.

28. **D.** Each of the three statements is considered to be an advantage of EUC. The author presents the information in paragraph four.

29. **B.** The complexity of successful EUC management is listed as one of its disadvantages. The fifth paragraph of the passage presents this and numerous other disadvantages of EUC.

30. **B.** The sixth paragraph lists the implications of EUC for informationsystems departments. Statement II is the second implication listed.

31. **B.** The two types of basic information center structures are the Canada IBM type and the distributed type. Descriptions of both are given in paragraphs six and seven. The distributed type is seen as the more suitable for managing EUC.

32. **D.** The author concludes the passage by making suggestions for the successful implementation of information centers in companies. Com-

puter (EUC) adoption must be incorporated into a company's overall strategic planning; otherwise it will fail.

33. **C.** Paragraph one indicates that the fiftieth anniversary in the "Promised Land" was celebrated. Also found in paragraph one is the fact that the writer of *Leviticus* had God speak to Moses; there is no evidence in the passage that God ever spoke to Moses. The passage does point out that celebrating is an old practice of mankind, however; there is no comment anywhere to make the reader assume that most celebrations are joyous events.

34. **C.** Statements II and IV are supported by the passage. Paragraph two points out that even with birthdays we call special attention to the "big" years and, the quotation from John Adams leaves no doubt that our Independence Day celebration should be carried out "from this time forward for everyone."

35. **D.** Paragraph three mentions that the inauguration of a new enterprise is always an act of hope and when achievement is history a confident celebration is appropriate. Paragraph four mentions that a celebration is often viewed as the occasion for a new beginning.

36. **D.** Paragraph five indicates that nostalgia, although differently felt, is good for the human spirit. In paragraph four we are told that we usually think that the lives of pioneers are worth emulating and that anniversaries offer us an opportunity to reflect.

37. **D.** Paragraphs seven and eight mention the facts that human pride is a motor of an institutional machine, that we use anniversaries to emphasize legitimacy, and that one cannot ignore the commercial motivation behind celebrations.

38. **B.** The author did use the one hundred fiftieth anniversary of an institution to essentially write a treatise on why we need the act of regular celebrations.

39. **C.** The story cites universal experiences both in myth and in everyday life.

40. **C.** The passage focuses on choice, which, because it is human, is universal.

41. **A.** Because changing or not changing the sail was Theseus's choice, the death of his father resulting from that choice was clearly his responsibility.

42. **A.** The plot itself is a series of choices, one following the other.

43. **B.** The author shows how choices in a myth can be the same choices that anyone can face at any time.

44. **B.** The passage is concerned with the ways in which a character's actions determine his destiny and how major choices lead to other important choices. In Theseus's case, the primary problem is how he will kill the Minotaur.

45. **D.** All the other statements are supported by the passage. It is stated in the passage that caricatures must be based on *fact*.

46. **C.** Statements A, B, and D may be true, but they are not stated in the passage. Statement C is cited as a cause of laughter.

47. **C.** Although the author states A and B, they are not the main point. The passage is set up to lead toward statement C. Statement D is dismissed in the passage.

48. **C.** Statements I and III are stated in the passage to show how caricatures work. Statement II may be true, but it does not indicate *why* caricatures are effective.

49. **A.** The passage does not deal with the possible objections to caricatures stated in B, C, and D. However, A is cited as a danger.

50. **B.** The entire essay deals with the ways in which satirists use exaggeration as a means of communicating their ideas.

51. **B.** The first sentence of the passage identifies aggression as a neurochemical impulse. A, C, and D are contradicted in paragraph one.

52. **D.** B and C are not dealt with in the passage. Lorenz points out specifically that it is *not* the eating enemy, but competition within the species, that poses the greatest threat to an animal species.

53. **C.** According to the passage, there seems to be no other reason for this bickering among one's own, other than the need for stimulation. **A** and **B** are mentioned as the other two basic needs; **D**, structure, is not listed as a need.

54. **B.** The passage identifies the invention of weapons as important in throwing off the natural balance precisely because man possesses the killer instinct without the internal controls or safety devices to limit his use of this instinct.

55. **A.** Hunt's point that man is aggressive without having been programmed as to how he might channel the aggression is a major point on which the author of this passage relies in emphasizing the interdependence of instinct and culture in man's development.

56. **B.** The passage cites a number of ways, many of them perhaps surprising, in which activities of humans can be traced to innate aggression.

57. **D.** Although the essay addresses **A** and **B** specifically, the essay goes far beyond both of these. **D** incorporates both the cultural and the instinctual. The essay addresses the interdependence of the two.

58. **D.** Though one might think, the essay asserts, that people are congested in cities because they like to cooperate, it actually is due to aggressive needs.

59. **B.** The passage states this specifically, and adds that the Shield Soldiers to whom they submitted rendered only token punishment, thus acknowledging the appeasement gesture.

60. **B.** Indirect assessment scores are reliable, so **A** is incorrect. The tests may be biased, but that issue is not addressed in the passage, so **C** is incorrect. **D** is not addressed.

61. **C.** Statement I is contradicted in the passage. Statement II is stated directly. Indirect assessments are an example of a reliable test that is not necessarily valid, so statement III is also correct. Statement IV cannot be true if statement II is true.

62. **B.** Statements **A**, **C**, and **D** are correct, but they do not deal with the idea in reader-response theory that readers bring their own experiences to the reading of a text.

63. **C.** It is the use of a scoring guide, not the particular kind of scoring guide (holistic, primary trait, analytic), that helps increase reliability.

64. **C.** Multiple readings increase the reliability of scores, so **A** is incorrect. **B** and **D** are not addressed in the passage.

65. **D.** The author points out problems with both kinds of testing and does not choose one type as better than the other. The author may agree with **C**, but that is not an evaluation.

PHYSICAL SCIENCES

66. **B.** In the absence of air resistance, both balls have the same vertical acceleration, $g = 9.8$ m/s^2. Because they start from rest at the same height, they will fall equal distances in equal times as shown by the equation $y = \frac{1}{2} gt^2$.

67. **D.** The horizontal velocity of the second ball is $(10$ m/s$)(\cos 30°) = 8.7$ m/s, so it takes it more than 1 s to reach the wall.

68. **A.** The easier way to solve this problem is to equate the work done against friction to the loss of kinetic energy of the masses, i.e.:
$F_f x = \frac{1}{2} mv^2$, where $F_f = \mu N = \mu mg$ where N is the "normal" force (equal to the weight in this case). Solving for $x = v^2/(2 \mu g) = 2$ m for *both* bodies. An alternative solution is to calculate the frictional force and the deceleration. One can then use the equations for uniformly accelerated motion to find the distance. The methods are completely equivalent.

69. **B.** It is possible to calculate the velocities exactly. The initial gravitational potential energy of the block and the ball are converted entirely into kinetic energy at the bottom of the incline. However, part of the kinetic energy of the ball is in the form of rotational kinetic energy about the ball's center of mass. Therefore, at the bottom of the incline, the velocity of the ball's center of mass is less than the linear velocity of the sliding block's center of mass. Understanding this concept, the question can be answered without calculating the velocities. One can do the actual calculations as follows:
   Ball: $mgh = \frac{1}{2} mv^2 + \frac{1}{2} I \omega^2$
where I is the moment of inertia (of a sphere) and ω is the angular velocity. Substituting $I = \frac{2}{5} mr^2$ and $v = r\omega$, one can solve for v.

Ball: $v = \sqrt{(10/7)gh} = 2.646$ m/s.
For the block,
Block: $mgh = \frac{1}{2} mv^2$ and $V = \sqrt{2gh} = 3.13$ m/s.

70. **A.** At the terminal velocity (regardless of the actual terminal velocity), the upward frictional force of air resistance is equal to the weight. $F_f - mg = 0$, because the acceleration is zero.
$F_f = 0.4 \times 9.8 = 3.92$ N.

71. **C.** This is a simple conversion problem. 205 lb $\times$ 1 kg/2.2 lb = 93.2 kg. $W = mg = 913$ N.

72. **B.** The gauge pressure in the foot is higher than the gauge pressure at the level of the aorta. (This is the reason blood pressures are taken with the cuff on the upper arm at the same approximate level as the aorta.) The height difference of 1.35 m creates a "pressure head" causing added pressure, $P_{add} = dgy$, where d is the density of the fluid (blood). Because the added pressure calculated will be in the standard SI units of N/m², the result must be converted to the units of mmHg, using the fact that 1 atmosphere = 1.01×10^5 N/m² = 760 mmHg. Then:
$P = 1050$ kg/m³ $\times 9.8$ m/s² $\times 1.35$ m = 13900 N/m²
  = 13900 N/m² $\times (760$ mmHg/1.01×10^5N/m²) = 105 mmHg. and $P_{total} = 100 + 105 = 205$ mmHg.

73. **D.** This question is a straightforward conversion problem because all the data needed to answer the question is given. The excess intake is 1200 kcal/day or a total of 16800 kcal in two weeks. Then the conversion of this excess intake of energy to a corresponding mass of fat is given by: 16800 kcal/ 9.5 kcal/g = 1700 g.

74. **B.** This question deals with the concept of power as the "rate of doing work"; 1 watt = 1 joule/s. When the metabolic rate is 630 W the student is using 630 joules of energy each second. In 10 minutes (600 s.) the total energy expended is 378,000 joules. The number of liters of oxygen consumed is then obtained by a conversion: # liters = 378,000 joules $\times$ 1 L/20,000 joules = 19 L.

75. **B.** The object (the student) is in static equilibrium. The first law of equilibrium states that the vector sum of the forces acting on the body is zero. In this case, the sum of the upward vertical forces (the scale readings) equals the sum of the downward forces (the student's weight). 90 lb + 100 lb = 190 lb, which is the correct student weight. (The bathroom scales can be set to read zero even with a sturdy board on them.) The second law of equilibrium states that the sum of the counterclockwise torques equals the sum of the clockwise torques. If one takes the axis of rotation to be through the soles of the feet, there will be one counterclockwise torque caused by the force at the head (90 lb) with a lever arm of 1.83 m and one clockwise torque due to the total weight (190) acting down through the center-of-mass at an unknown lever arm, L, measured from the sole of the foot.
90 lb $\times$ 1.83 m $-$ 190 lb $\times L =$
$L = 0.87$m.

76. **B.** The energy of oxidation for fats and oils (9.5 kcal/gm) is given in question 73 above. The desired weight loss of 1 pound of fat corresponds to an energy expenditure of:
0.4545 kg $\times$ 1000 g/kg $\times$ 9.5 kcal/g $\times$ 4185 J/kcal = 1.8×10^7 joules.
500 Watt = 500 joules/sec. So the time required is $t = 1.8 \times 10^7$ joules/(500 joule/sec) = 3.615×10^4 sec = 10 hours.

77. **C.** The voltages of batteries connected in series add. The 6-volt and 12-volt batteries in series are equivalent to an 18-volt battery. Applying Ohm's law, $V = IR$, to the equivalent circuit; the current through the resistor is: $I = V/R = 18$ volts/10 ohm = 1.8 A.

78. **B.** The expression for the equivalent resistance of resistors connected in series is: $R_s = R_1 + R_2 + \ldots . = 4 + 8 = 12$ ohms. We can find the current in this circuit using Ohm's law: $I = V/R_s = 6/12 = 0.5$ A. The power consumed in the *8-ohm resistor* is then found from $P = I^2R = (0.5)^2 \times 8 = 2$ watts. There is additional power consumed in the 4-ohm resistor, of course.

79. **D.** Although this question could be answered in the same manner as the preceding question, one would have to find the individual current through the 8-ohm resistor. It is easier and simpler to note that the full 12 volts is applied across the terminals of the 8-ohm resistor. The power consumed can be found using the expression: $P = IV = (V/R)V = V^2/R$ where we have applied Ohm's law, $V = IR$ to the 8-ohm resistor. Then: $P = 12^2/8 = 18$ watts.

80. **D.** We can find the power from the given information: $P = V^2/R = 18$ W. Power is the "time rate of doing work": (1 W = 1 J/s) $P = E/t$ so that $E = Pt$ where t is the time in seconds. Thus: $E = 18$ joules/s $\times 300$ s $= 5400$ joules.

81. **A.** ($t_i = 20°C$) This heat is generated electrically in the resistor, $H = E = Pt = (V^2/R)t$. Then $m\, C_W\, (t_f - t_i) = (V^2/R)t$. We can solve this expression for t_f, the only unknown. $t_f = 22.6\,°C$.

82. **C.** In any standing wave, the antinodes and nodes always alternate and their separation is always exactly one-quarter wavelength. In this problem, the 25 cm tube length is equal to one-quarter wavelength because the fundamental frequency is the longest wavelength at which resonance can occur. (It is possible for higher frequency resonances to occur at shorter wavelengths so that the tube length will be some odd number of quarter wavelengths.) In this case the wavelength is equal to 4 tube lengths, that is; $\lambda = 1$ m. Then $v = 340$ Hz $\times$ 1 m $= 340$ m/s.

83. **B.** Using the velocity expression: $v = f_1 \lambda_1 =$ 20,000 Hz $\times 1.7 \times 10^{-2}$m $= 340$ m/s. The velocity is nearly the same for any frequency, so that $\lambda_2 = v/f_2 = 2.3 \times 10^{-2}$ m $= 2.3$ cm.

84. **A.** If one simply uses the given expression and takes the ratio of the energies, the constant K and the amplitude squared terms may be cancelled:
$W_{20}/W_{15} = K(20000)^2 A^2/K(15000)^2 A^2 = (20)^2/(15)^2 = 1.8$.

85. **B.** Only transverse waves can be polarized. None of the other answers is true. Longitudinal waves can have either longer or shorter wavelengths and/or frequencies than transverse waves so that **A** and **D** are false. **C** is false because transverse waves, as their name implies, vibrate perpendicularly (transverse) to the direction the wave is traveling.

86. **A.** The quantum of energy for a photon is given, $E = hf$. By substituting for f from the velocity expression, $c = f\lambda$; E may be written as: $E = hc/\lambda$. Then the ratio of energies is $E_{400}/E_{750} = (hc/400)/(hc/750) = 750/400 = 1.88$. (The result illustrates the important fact that short wavelength electromagnetic radiation is more energetic than longer wavelength radia-tion, because the photon energies are *inversely* proportional to the wavelengths.) Notice that when taking the ratio, one does not have to convert nm to m because all the units cancel (as do the constants hc) leaving a pure number for the ratio.

87. **B.** The speed of sound does not depend on either the frequency or the wavelength. It depends on the properties of the air (pressure, temperature, and so on). Thus the speed of sound is the same for both frequencies and the ratio of the speeds is 1.

88. **B.** The fundamental force law for the forces between charged particles is Coulomb's law; $F = kq_1q_2/r^2$, which is an "inverse square law" like the force of gravity. The force then decreases inversely with the square of the separation distance, r. Tripling the separation thus causes the force to decrease to one-ninth of its original value. Thus: 0.54 N/9 = 0.06 N.

89. **B.** The resistance of an "ohmic conductor" depends on the material of which it is composed as well as its geometry. For a wire that is a cylinder, the resistance is proportional to the length and inversely proportional to the cross-sectional area. $R = \vartheta L/A$, where ϑ is the resistivity. The circular cross section has the area of a circle that may be written as $(\pi/4)d^2$ where d is the diameter of the circle. We can take the ratio of the two resistances as follows:
$R_2/R_1 = (\vartheta L/A_2)/(\vartheta L/A_1) = (d_1/d_2)^2$
and $d_2 = 1.5\, d_1$
Then; $R_2 = 1.2$ ohms $\times (1/1.5)^2$.

90. **A.** The key to solving this problem is to isolate the second smaller mass (0.6 kg) in order to show the force(s) acting on it alone. By Newton's second law, the net force on the smaller mass equals the product of the mass and the acceleration, both of which are given.

$F_{net} = ma = 0.6$ kg $\times 0.2$ m/s$^2 = 0.12$ N.

If one makes a simple sketch of the two blocks with the string between, then it is apparent that that the only force acting on the smaller block is the tension in the string. This *is* then the net force and is 0.12 N.

91. **C.** The right-hand screw rule can be used to find the direction of the force. It states that the force vector is perpendicular to the plane of the velocity and magnetic field vectors. The force vector points in the direction a right-hand

screw would advance if turned in the same direction as if one turned the velocity vector toward the B field vector. Thus if one turns the upward pointing velocity vector down toward the horizontal (North) magnetic field vector a right-hand screw turn that direction would advance to the West.

92. **A.** According to Newton's third law the force(s) exerted on the car by the truck is/are *always* equal and opposite to the force(s) exerted on the truck by the car. In fact, this is true regardless of the speeds of the car and truck.

93. **B.** The time the boat takes to cross the river does not depend on the current *if the boat heads directly across.* The boat's velocity across the 50 m width of the river is constant (2 m/s) so that the time can be found from the definition of velocity (as distance/time).

$$t = d/v = 50 \text{ m}/(2 \text{ m/s}) = 25 \text{ s}.$$

94. **C.** The simple pendulum is a simple harmonic oscillator. Its period is proportional to the square root of the length: $T = 2\pi \sqrt{L/g} = C' \sqrt{L}$ where C' is a constant. Setting up the ratio of the periods:

$$T_4/2s = C'(\sqrt{4L})/C'(\sqrt{L}) = \sqrt{4} = 2$$

and $T_4 = 2 \times 2 \text{ s} = 4 \text{ s}.$

95. **B.** For a standing wave on a string, a "loop" length is one-half wavelength (it is the distance between adjacent nodes of the standing wave that are always one-half wavelength apart). The string length of 0.8 m is exactly one wavelength long in this case. The speed of the wave is given by the usual expression:

$$v = f\lambda = 120 \text{ Hz} \times 0.8 \text{ m} = 96 \text{ m/s}.$$

96. **B.** f, p, and q are all positive because the light rays do travel from the object toward the lens and from the lens toward the image point.

$$1/f = 1/18 + 1/36; \quad f = 12 \text{ cm}.$$

97. **A.** The linear magnification is the negative ratio of the image distance to the object distance. $M = -q/p = -36/18 = -2$. The minus sign indicates that the image is inverted and it is 2 times the size of the object. (If q were negative as it might be for a virtual image the magnification would be positive, $-(-q/p)$, which would indicate that the image was upright and not inverted with respect to the object.)

98. **A.** The object is placed inside the focal length (closer to the lens than the focal length). This is the way that one uses a magnifying glass. The image is virtual as shown by the negative image distance; is upright and it is magnified.

$$1/q = 1/f - 1/p = 1/24 - 1/6$$

and $q = -8$ cm. The image is on the same side of the lens as the object (in "front") and can only be seen by looking through the lens at the image.

99. **B.** The magnification of a simple refracting telescope is known as the angular magnification and is given by the ratio of the focal length of the objective to the focal length of the eyepiece:

$$M = f_o/f_e = 3 \text{ X}.$$

100. **C.** For a microscope, the magnification is the product of the magnification of the objective and the magnification of the eyepiece. $M = M_o M_e$

$$M_o = M/M_e = 400/10 = 40\times.$$

101. **D.** This problem is solved by two successive applications of the thin lens formula. One must calculate the object distance for lens #2. Lens #1: $1/q_1 = 1/f_1 - 1/p_1$; $q_1 = 24$ cm (behind #1). For lens #2, $p_2 = 72$ cm $- 24$ m $= 48$ cm (in front of #2). Then $1/q_2 = 1/f_2 - 1/p_2 = 1/24 - 1/48$, and thus $q_2 = +48$ cm (behind #2) The final image is real.

102. **D.** The magnification is the ratio of the image distance, q, to the object distance, p, for a thin lens. $(m = -q/p)$. In order to find the image distance, q, we use the thin lens formula:

$1/f = 1/p + 1/q$, $\quad 1/q = 1/f - 1/p$ or $1/q = 1/24 - 1/12 = -1/24$. Then $q = -24$ cm

and the magnification is: $m = -\left(\dfrac{-24}{12}\right) = +2.$

The image is twice as large as the object, or 10 cm tall. (The plus sign means that this viritual image is upright.)

103. **B.** This problem is done exactly as in the explanation for question 102. This time the focal length $f = -24$ cm so that the image distance is found to be: $1/q = -1/24 - 1/12$ or $q = -8$ cm. The magnification is then equal to: $m = -(-8)/12 = +0.67$ and the image is only 3.3 cm tall. (This image is upright as shown by the plus sign for the magnification. A diverging lens always produces an upright image.)

104. **C.** The very distant objects, such as stars, are effectively an infinite distance away. The thin lens formula, $1/f = 1/p + 1/q$, then yields the result that the image distance is the same as the focal length because $1/p$ is equal to zero for $p =$ infinity. The image must appear at the actual far-point of the eye, that is, at -80 cm (for the virtual image) and thus the required focal length is also -80 cm.

105. **D.** The power in diopters is equal to the reciprocal of the focal length in *meters*. Thus:

$P = 1/f$. Then $f = 1/P = -1/4$ meter $= -0.25$ m or $f = -25$ cm.

106. **A.** The coolant is compressed to form a liquid and becomes warm. The heat is dissipated by a fan. Then the pressure is released from the liquid, allowing its conversion to a gas. This conversion requires heat, the heat of vaporization. It draws heat from surrounding materials.

107. **B.** The transition temperature from solid to liquid should be the same without regard to the direction from which it is approached.

108. **D.** Sublimation is the process of a solid becoming a gas without an intervening liquid.

109. **A.** Increased pressure increases the boiling point.

110. **B.** The critical temperature is the highest temperature at which a gas may be condensed by imposition of high pressure.

111. **B.** Velocity varies in linear fashion with variation of substrate in the area of point A. In this area, the reaction is first order with respect to substrate.

112. **A.** In the area where point B is located, there is no significant change in velocity with a change in substrate. This is zero order with respect to substrate.

113. **C.** At point C the reciprocal substrate concentration is zero, and the substrate concentration would be infinite. Obviously this point cannot be determined by laboratory measurement but must be extrapolated from other data.

114. **B.** The ordinate is reciprocal velocity, and the reciprocal of reciprocal velocity is velocity.

Because this extrapolated point corresponds to the reciprocal of infinite substrate, it also will correspond to the reciprocal of maximum velocity.

115. **D.** Point B represents essentially maximum velocity and point C represents the reciprocal of maximum velocity. The zero order portion of the first graph (encompassing point B) does show some change, and it is somewhat difficult to ascertain at what point maximum velocity has been attained.

116. **B.** The three phases will exist together only at the triple point, point 2.

117. **B.** To raise the temperature without changing the pressure, one would proceed on a horizontal line to the right. Such a line intersects the phase transition line for liquid/gas at point 7.

118. **D.** Proceeding vertically toward the top of the diagram, no phase transition from the existing solid phase is indicated.

119. **A.** No liquid can exist above point 1, regardless of the pressure.

120. **C.** The transition from liquid to gas indicates the boiling temperature at the indicated pressure.

121. **A.** This is the definition of equilibrium constant. Note that the coefficients in the reaction equation become exponents in the equilibrium equation.

122. **B.** When the resultants on the right are written in the numerator, a small number such as this indicates that the reaction as written will be favored to go toward the left.

123. **A.** Five moles of gas are being converted to two moles of gas. Increased pressure will improve reaction toward the right, thus relieving the pressure (Principle of LeChatelier.)

124. **C.** At STP, a mole of any gas occupies 22.4 liters. Three moles times 22.4 liters equals 67.2 liters.

125. **D.** Equilibrium constant indicates the concentrations at equilibrium. It does not deal with the rate in reaching equilibrium.

126. **A.** Knowing the atomic weight of hydrogen as 1.0 and oxygen at 16.0, the simplest proportions are one H and one O. Thus, the empirical formula is HO.

127. **B.** The empirical formula has only a molecular weight of 17.0. Because the true molecular weight is determined as 34.0, the molecular formula must be a multiple, in this case H_2O_2.

128. **B.** $H_2O_2 \rightleftharpoons H_2O + O_2$ (unbalanced)
    Note that we have two hydrogen atoms on each side. However, we have two oxygen atoms on the left side and three on the right. We may try to balance by multiplying H_2O and H_2O_2 by two. We now have
    $$2 H_2O_2 \rightleftharpoons 2 H_2O + O_2$$
    and find that this is balanced. As written, one mole of H_2O_2 will produce only 0.5 mole of O_2.

129. **C.** The balanced equation indicates two moles of H_2O_2 will produce two moles of H_2O or one mole of H_2O_2 will produce one mole of H_2O.

130. **C.** As noted above, one mole of H_2O_2 will produce 0.5 mole of O_2. Because one mole of any gas occupies a volume of 22.4 liters at S.T.P., 0.5 mole will occupy 11.2 liters.

131. **B.**
    $$\begin{array}{cc} 34 & x \\ 2 H_2O_2 \rightleftharpoons 2 H_2O + & O_2 \\ 68 & 36 \end{array}$$

    $$\frac{34}{68} = \frac{x}{36}$$

    $$x = \frac{(36)(34)}{68} = 18.$$

132. **C.** The LeChatelier principle indicates that if a system in equilibrium experiences a change in conditions, chemical reaction will occur to shift the equilibrium and reduce the effect of the changed conditions. Even if reactants and products are all in the gaseous state, there are two moles on the left side and three moles on the right side. Increased pressure would be expected to shift an equilibrium to the left.

133. **C.** If an equilibrium exists, there is an equilibrium constant. Addition of one or more products without changing conditions otherwise will not change the equilibrium constant, but the concentrations of reactants and other products must adjust to maintain the equilibrium constant.

134. **B.** See above. The equilibrium constant would not be affected.

135. **D.** Although it is expected that this would be a first order reaction (rate = k $[H_2O_2]$) it cannot be predicted with certainty. The order of the reaction must be determined on the basis of experimental evidence.

136. **D.** A catalyst is defined as a substance that increases the velocity of a chemical reaction. They are not consumed.

137. **A.** *Hypertonic:* the solution has a higher osmotic pressure than the solution with which it is compared. There is a higher concentration of solute and a lower concentration of solvent. *Hypotonic:* a lower concentration of solute and a higher concentration of solvent are present. *Isotonic:* both solutions have the same osmotic pressure.

138. **C.** One mole of any compound contains 6.02×10^{23} molecules. Two moles of carbon dioxide would contain one mole of molecules more than that contained by one mole of oxygen.

139. **A.** Acid salts are formed by di- and tribasic acids. For example, H_2CO_3 can form the acid salt ($NaHCO_3$) known as sodium hydrogen carbonate or sodium bicarbonate.

140. **D.** NaOH may be called a base because it produces OH^- ions, but it is more properly called a base because it consumes H^+ ions.

141. **C.** The thermal decomposition of $KClO_3$ to produce oxygen will occur if the temperature is sufficiently high. The addition of a catalyst MnO_2 will decrease the activation energy and increase the rate at a lower temperature.

142. **B.** See explanation for question 141.

WRITING SAMPLE
Part 1, Essay

The definition of a wise man generated by this quote hinges on the interpretation of the words "ought" and "can." These words, however, as well as "see," remain ambiguous out of context, thus permitting opposing definitions of a "wise man." If "ought" is taken as a limitation of "can," that is if the wise man sees only what he should or is obliged to see, then the quote takes on overtones of pragmatism. The wise man, or man who would be happy, does not see further than he ought. He sees less than he "can" or could. To see all he is capable of seeing would be unwise, perhaps because seeing all would be painful or would necessitate prying. He could find out more but sees only that which is his business. The wise man limits even his perception to avoid painful realities. On first reading, the quote seems to imply some such limited wisdom, perhaps because the shades of meaning in "ought" and "can" have changed over time. Repulsed by the definition of wisdom generated by this interpretation, one might be driven to reverse the relative magnitude of the terms "ought" and "can." What a wise man ought to see is more than what he can see. He must go beyond what is obvious or visible. The implication here is that the wise man looks beyond or below the surface of perceptible reality. "See" begins to take on shades of meaning akin to "understand" or "infer" beyond superficial perception. The obligation implied by "ought" becomes an obligation to extend rather than an obligation to limit. This second wise man, to be wise, must either dig for more information (things he "ought" to see) or use intuition to understand more than he can see. Without further information on the context of the quote, two possible and opposing wise men remain.

Situations in which the pragmatic position does not apply can be found in psychology. If one believes that unconscious urges or forgotten traumas can have harmful effects on the individual, the wise man might be advised to "see" more than he "can." A man might, for example, have difficulty relating to authority figures who, judging by what he "can" see, restrict him unfairly. If he can "dig down" to or be made to see oedipal impulses underlying the perception of oppression, he may become better able to respond to authority in a prudent, less self-defeating manner. Seeing only what one ought may also have parallels in jurisprudence, where a judge sometimes suppresses information. A decision reached based on the visible, limited facts may then be different (not to mention wrong) from a conclusion based on what one ought to have seen beyond what could be seen. This analogy, if true, argues that if one only attends to what he can see he may be misled. The other wise man, the one who sees more than he "can," may have a less assailable position. Perhaps, the pragmatic wise man is the best example of a situation in which limited wisdom is advisable. It is arguable that seeing too much is painful and potentially harmful. A man might travel to study different cultures only to be more and more sickened by the pain and misery he finds everywhere. One could argue, I suppose, that he would have been wiser, that is happier, less potentially misanthropic, had he limited his vision.

In my mind there are no conditions under which vision or perception or understanding should be limited, if wisdom is the goal. According to the pragmatic reading of the quote, seeing all one can is a mistake, but I would argue limited wisdom is self-contradictory. The truly wise man is one who sees not only all he "can," but what he "ought" as well. In other words, his vision intuits or infers beyond the visible. The wise man and the happy man may inhabit mutually exclusive positions due to the potential pain involved in seeing too far into oneself or others. However, pleasure and the avoidance of pain should not be used as conditions for defining wisdom.

Part 1
Explanation of First Response: 5

The paper focuses on the statement and addresses the three writing tasks. The most difficult task in writing this essay is the first: explaining what Montaigne's quotation actually means. This essay confronts the difficulty squarely, making it clear that one's interpretation of the quotation depends very much on the meanings of the words "ought" and "can." The irony is that "ought" in one sense could be considered a weaker word than "can"; but in another it is stronger. The essay suggests that one must conclude that two entirely different wise men emerge from the quotation depending on the way in which "ought" is defined. Paragraph two, then, moves to the task of providing specific situations in which the two different wise men see as much as they ought and then as much as they should. The example taken from the psychology of unconscious motivation is appropriate and the analogy using judge and jury is particularly imaginative. Finally the essay confronts the ambiguities and paradoxes raised when one considers Montaigne's quotation by taking the stand that a wise man never limits his vision. And ultimately, the essay concludes, wisdom should not be defined in terms simply of pleasure or the avoidance of pain.

This essay provides a sensitive insight into a difficult quotation. The introduction is tightly reasoned; the writing is clear. Paragraph two brings the essay down into the realm of the concrete in its use of unconscious motives and of the judge-jury examples. Because the subject is so highly philosophical, this essay would be strengthened by the use of more concrete details, both in paragraphs one and two. The final paragraph, in which the essay winds down nicely, would especially benefit from a well-chosen concrete illustration. The addition of such specific details would elevate the rating of this essay rating from 5 to 6.

Part 2, Essay

History exists, according to Emerson, only as a document tracing the events of men. Without people, there can be no history. Therefore, history is not a recording of events, but of the men who participated in them. The history of the Cathedral at Chartres does not concern itself primarily with the building, not its stones, its ironworks, its bells. The history of the Cathedral at Chartres focuses on the men who designed and built it, who worshipped and died in it, who tended their flocks in its walls. It is their history, and the history of these men is biography.

If it is true that by definition history is necessarily biography, then the events must take second place to the individuals. After all, biography is typically a document showing how the events have shaped the individual. Is history about the individual? It is not. True, history without the human element is dead, but history enjoys a longer continuum than the life of those it influences, and those influenced by it. History is about eras, thoughts, and ages. The Age of Reason is neither a biography of Rousseau, nor a story with those who believed the tenets as the main characters. It is about the events that took place during the time. History encompasses wars, art, politics, science, and philosophy. No biography can encompass all this. History is a larger container than just the human beings. It must hold many men, many actions, both intended and accidental. History records mistakes, quirks, even coincidences and accidents. So, the history of the Cathedral at Chartres is not about Abbot Sugar or King Louis, it is larger than that. Like the stones, the cathedral's history is longer than the life of man, for the stones live longer than an abbot or king. The space is larger than the area taken up by the bodies it encompasses. It holds many ages of men, their thoughts, errors, treasons, and hopes. No, history cannot be biography, for biography is only a part of history. There are no biographies of stones and ideas, of errors and wars; there are only biographies of men.

But who shaped and stacked the stones? From whom do the errors, ideas, and reasons come? Though one man cannot live as long as a cathedral, the cathedral is nothing but a pile of stones and shards of glass without man and his God to give it meaning. Eras are eras of Man, and the Age of Reason reflects a change of thinking in the minds of man. For if we think of history as biography, we must think of Man as opposed to men. Emerson believed that Man and nature were inextricably entwined. Man and his consciousness were part stone, part God, part evil, part time. Though one man's story cannot be history, Man's story, Man's biography, certainly can, and this story is what we call history. History, then, redefines biography. This definition of biography is not about us as the limited creatures we are as individuals so much as it is about the limitless, encompassing Man as a unified whole. The stones are part of Man, and when labeled as Cathedral and joined to religion, the stones become more of Man. The history of the stones and of the space are then the history of Man, and that, true, is biography.

Part 2
Explanation of Second Response: 5

The essay focuses on the topic defined by Emerson's statement and addresses the three writing tasks. Paragraph one explains Emerson's idea that "there is properly no history; only biography" and illustrates the explanation with a concrete reference to the Cathedral at Chartres. The second paragraph explores in detail the other side of the issue, arguing through historical references that there is, indeed, history independent of biography. The final paragraph presents a balanced consideration of the relation between biography and history, concluding finally that the history of Man, not of men, is biography.

The first section of the essay uses an interesting rhetorical strategy: that of paraphrasing Emerson's statement in such a way that the paraphrases become premises leading to the conclusion that "Therefore, history is not a recording of events, but of the men who participated in them." Some will argue that Emerson's statement is not saying "without people, there can be no history" (the essay's second premise), and thus some will question the foundation of the essay from the beginning. A simple qualifier, such as "perhaps," would strengthen the logic. The second paragraph provides an eloquent defense of the idea that there is indeed history that includes more than biography. It does so by extending the example of the Cathedral at Chartres used in paragraph one and by citing various historical eras and ages. The essay's final paragraph brings the point back to Emerson's assertion and balances it by introducing the concept of the history of Man, a creative solution to the task of exploring the circumstances that determine the relationship between history and biography.

The writing in this essay is clear, and it flows nicely from sentence to sentence. The essay could use a clear transition leading into paragraph two. This is the paragraph that reverses the position explained in paragraph one, and the reader could use help in getting into that position. The essay is rich in concrete details. Especially effective is the extended reference to the Cathedral at Chartres. If this paper had led the reader more smoothly from one task to the next, and if the logic in the first several sentences were tightened, the paper would receive a rating of 6.

BIOLOGICAL SCIENCES

143–148. **(143-B) (144-A) (145-C) (146-D) (147-A) (148-B)** Let us identify the components of the neuron numbered: (2) nucleus with nucleolus, containing the genetic material of the cell and directing the synthetic activity of the cell; (3) Golgi apparatus (zone), the packaging and concentrating area of the cell's secretory activity; (4) dendrites; dendrites are the processes that pick up an impulse and carry it towards the cell body; (5) endoplasmic reticulum (rough in this case—ribosomes are attached), the synthetic machinery of the cell (proteins etc.,); (6) cell membrane, semipermeable and the protector of the cell from its environment; (7) cytoplasm (specifically the area here is called the axon hillock); (8) myelin sheath (Schwann cell covered by its neurilemma, the insulator of the axon); (1) direction of conduction of an impulse; axon (10a) and (10b) conducts impulses away from the dendrites to the function with the dendrites of another neuron. The junction point is known as the synaptic area; the impulse can cross the synapse only from the axon to the dendrite and no backflow is permitted; (11) terminal branches of the axon. In a lesion (cut) the process distal from the cell body would completely degenerate; retrograde degeneration would be detected in the proximal portion and the cell body, however, the proximal portion has the capacity and will regenerate.

149. **C.** Because glucose is absorbed at a faster rate than xylose, due to both passive and active transport, then as the glucose is absorbed, water follows. The transport system for glucose is working maximally as indicated by the initial concentration of glucose being 50 times the apparent K_m of transport.

150. **D.** A 1.8% solution contains 1.8 g/100 ml of solution. This is 1,800 mg/100 ml, which is 18 mg/ml. For the recovery of 1.8 mg, this represents $(1.8/18 \times 100)$ a 10% recovery meaning that 90% has been metabolized or transported out of the lumen of the intestine.

151. **D.** Hemoglobin is a large (64,000 MW) molecule. Because the gut was ligated below the pancreas and proteolytic enzymes present were washed out, no digestion of the protein could occur. Large molecules are not readily transported across cell membranes. Due to the vast surface area of the small intestine with its many microvilli, some of the protein would be adsorbed on this surface and visible through the heme prosthetic group color.

152. **D.** All are correct. I. D-galactose is transported by the same carrier as glucose, therefore, by addition of galactose, a competition for transport between glucose and galactose occurs. II. The transport carrier is sodium ion selective. A larger cation, while having the appropriate charges, does not fit the selective carrier. III. The carrier is specific for the D-glucose; L-glucose would be transported by passive diffusion only. IV. Because the carrier is an energy requiring process, by limiting the supply of ATP, the transport is decreased.

153. **A.** A 25% solution of $MgSO_4$ is hypertonic. Neither Mg nor SO_4 ions are readily transported so the net effect is a water flow into the lumen becoming an isotonic solution.

154. **B.** Hemoglobin is not absorbed and an aqueous solution is not isotonic. Assuming that the hemoglobin is not ionized, a 0.3 M solution would have to have $64,000 \times 0.3$ g/liter. This solution must be hypotonic, which can be only modified by water flow out of the lumen.

155–157. **(155-B) (156-C) (157-C)** The answers can be found in the flow diagram of the question. Thyroid hormones (T_3 and T_4) are iodothyronines. The union of iodine and tyrosine is called iodination, and the active thyroid principal is protein-bound during transport to the target organs.

158. **D.** Hyperthyroidism, hypothyroidism and euthyroidism can be associated with goiter. In hyperthyroidism, thyroxin is released into the bloodstream at a rate exceeding needs. BMR accelerates resulting in rapid pulse and respiration, increased appetite with concomitant weight loss, nervousness, and protruding eyes. If not treated, goiter and thyroid exhaustion can occur; treatment involves antithyroid drugs or thyroidectomy. The opposite, hypothyroidism, exhibits a gland that cannot meet

secretory demands; the body's metabolic rate is depressed and symptoms are the reverse of the above cited. When hypothyroidism occurs during childhood, a cretin is the result; mental retardation and stunted growth are features. Treatment requires administration of thyroid hormone. Goiter simply means enlargement of the gland and can be present in the normal (euthyroid) state.

159. **A.** Thyroid stimulating hormone produced by the basophils of the anterior pituitary is a glycoprotein made up of two peptide chains (alpha and beta). Certain regions of the hypothalamus have a neuroendocrine function because neurosecretory cells release hormones that affect anterior pituitary function. TRH secreted by the hypothalamus reaches the pituitary via the hypophyseal-portal circulation and elicits TSH production. Thyroxin binds to TBG. Exposure to cold would elicit a compensatory increase in BMR and, hence, thyroid activity.

160. **D.** Also see explanations for questions 158 and 159. Control of thyroid principal is via the pituitary. TSH stimulates the thyroid to produce thyroxin; its release is related to levels in the bloodstream. Low levels increase TSH and thyroxin release, but as levels rise to normal and above, further production and release of TSH is curtailed and thyroxin production falls. This feedback system maintains balance.

161. **C.** See explanations for questions 158–160.

162. **A.** The effect of repeated close-spaced stimuli is that a summation occurs: each contraction is somewhat larger than the preceding one.

163. **C.** ATP continues to be supplied in adequate amounts, even during the period of loss of contraction ability (fatigue). Some link between the stimulating event and the responding event (sliding of actins over myosins), however, gradually becomes less efficient.

164. **B.** During the summation period each new stimulus arrives before the preceding twitch can reach the relaxation period, and elastic elements in the muscle become stretched without rebounding to their original shape. The muscle eventually reaches a steady state of nearly full contraction (region 2), when all elastic elements are fully stretched.

165. **A.** When a volley of stimuli is applied to a muscle, each succeeding stimulus may arrive before the muscle can completely relax from the contraction caused by the preceding stimulus. The result is summation, an increased strength of contraction. If the frequency of stimulation is very fast, individual contractions fuse and the muscle smoothly and fully contracts. This is a tetanus.

166. **D.** The word contraction refers to those processes that are manifested externally by either a shortening of a muscle or by tension development in a muscle. If the muscle length is held constant, the contraction is referred to as an isometric contraction. In an isometric contraction, the passive tension remains constant with the active tension being added to it to produce the total tension of the muscle. If the muscle shortens during contraction, it is called an isotonic contraction and the total tension remains constant.

167. **C.** The drug most closely resembles PHT (phenytoin) in terms of its high efficacy in the electroshock model of tonic-clonic seizures and its adequate efficacy in the kindling model of partial complex seizures. **A,** though not completely incorrect, is not the best answer. PHT, the drug this experimental agent AntiEpp acts most like, is not effective in the audiogenic mouse model of myoclonic seizures, which is also a form of generalized convulsive seizures. **D** is also incorrect for this reason. The better answer is C.

168. **B.** Ethosuximide is the only drug that is exclusively effective against the animal model of absence seizures. **A** is incorrect because carbamazepine has highest efficacy in the kindling model and in partial complex seizures. **C** is incorrect because valproic acid shows some degree of efficacy in all seizure models and the corresponding clinical conditions. Again, Compound X, like ethosuximide, shows efficacy only against the GABA challenge model of absence seizures. Given the premise that investigational compounds are selected in part because of a chemical nature similar to presently used compounds, there is enough information to respond that this agent is "probably most similar" to ethosuximide. So **D** is also incorrect.

169. **C.** It is stated that 1 in 200 persons suffer from epilepsy in the United States and that

there are 7 million persons in New York City. Thus, the correct answer can be derived as follows:

$$\frac{1}{200} = \frac{X}{7,000,000} \text{ or rearranging,}$$

$$X = \frac{(7,000,000)\,(1)}{200} \text{ or } X = 35,000$$

This can be calculated more rapidly in your head realizing that:

$$\frac{1}{200} = \frac{.5}{100} = \frac{5}{1,000} = \frac{50}{10,000} = \frac{500}{100,000} =$$

$$\frac{5,000}{1,000,000} \text{ or } \frac{35,000}{7,000,000}$$

A or **D** reflect a mathematical mistake. **B** is the probable number of yearly deaths from status epilepticus.

170. **C.** Status epilepticus is defined in the first paragraph of the passage as a seizure that persists for over 30 minutes. A partial seizure emanates from a restricted region. This woman's seizure is described as having lasted for "over an hour" and was observed on the electroencephalogram as "localized only to a restricted region." Thus, "partial status epilepticus" is the *best* answer. **A**, status epilepticus is correct but does not fully describe the patient's condition. Neither does partial complex seizure (**D**). Finally, generalized seizures, you are told, arise from the entire brain simultaneously. Again, this woman's seizure is restricted or partial. For this reason, **B** is incorrect.

171. **B.** The reading passage states that there are approximately 1.2 million persons with epilepsy in the United States. It also indicates that 25% of patients with epilepsy continue to have seizures at least once per month. So, the correct answer is generated by taking 25% of 1.2 million, or

$$0.25 \times 1,200,000 = 300,000$$

A, 30,000 represents a mathematical mistake. So does **D**, 250,000. **C**, ¼ million, is just another way of saying 250,000 and is also incorrect.

172. **B.** It is the purpose of this experiment to determine the sequence of events in cells stimulated to undergo mitosis, and to compare the data to those gathered from unstimulated cells.

173. **A.** Analysis of the graphs clearly shows that RNA synthesis precedes increased protein synthesis; at around 17 hours they are equal and RNA continues to drop, whereas protein synthesis increases.

174. **D.** It is safe to assume that unstimulated lymphocytes synthesize RNA, DNA, and protein at a low rate. One of the premier functions of DNA is the production of RNA; most RNA is produced in the nucleus. DNA determines and acts as a template for RNA synthesis. With the help of a transcription enzyme (RNA polymerase), a complimentary RNA strand is produced; once produced it moves into the cytoplasm.

175. **B.** The cell is the basic unit of structure and function and the basis of all life; all cells come from preexisting cells.

176. **B.** A complete set of chromosomes ($2n$) is passed on to each daughter cell as a result of mitotic cell division. Cells that are produced mitotically are genetically alike.

177. **C.** Messenger RNA (mRNA) from the nucleus brings the coded message for protein synthesis to ribosomes in the cytoplasm.

178. **C.** Mitosis is divided into:
   (1) prophase—chromosomes become distinct and nucleoli disappear; centrioles, asters, and spindle appear; nuclear membrane disappears.
   (2) metaphase—chromosomes move to equator of cell.
   (3) anaphase—the two chromatids split apart and start migration toward the poles of the spindle, and the spindle loses its definition.
   (4) telophase—chromosomes lengthen and become less distinct and nucleoli reappear.
   (5) interphase—cell growth, protein + DNA synthesis, and chromosomes duplicate.

179. **B.** During metaphase of mitosis, the centrioles with asters are at the opposite poles; the chromosomes move to the equator of the cell. Also see explanation for question 178.

180. **D.** Nuclei have the highest DNA concentration among cellular organelles. The DNA in fraction 3 is in mitochondria.

181. **C.** Cytochrome oxidase is the enzyme complex that transfers electrons from the mitochondrial electron transport chain to oxygen and is therefore located in mitochondria.

182. **A.** Most of the RNA found in a mature cell is ribosomal RNA, and the cytoplasmic ribosomal RNA in a hepatocyte should occur in a mixture of free ribosomes and rough endoplasmic reticulum. Because only one peak of RNA occurred at the top of the gradient, fraction 1 must contain both free and membrane-bound ribosomes and therefore contains the rough endoplasmic reticulum. The RNA in fraction 3 probably represents ribosomes in mitochondria. The RNA in fraction 4 is probably partially assembled ribosomes in the nucleoli in the nuclei.

183. **B.** Acid phosphatase is a lysosomal enzyme and occurred only in fraction 2 among the choices.

184. **A.** Cytochrome P-450 is involved in detoxification reactions in smooth endoplasmic reticulum and only occurred in fraction 1 among the choices.

185. **C.** Krebs cycle enzymes are located in the mitochondria and should therefore occur in the same fractions that contain cytochrome oxidase activity.

186. **A.** Plasma proteins are secreted proteins and therefore should be made on the rough endoplasmic reticulum in fraction 1.

187. **A.** A cell that secretes large amounts of protein (such as a pancreatic exocrine cell) should contain large arrays of rough endoplasmic reticulum, which would increase fraction 1. Secretory granules could increase fraction 2 or fraction 3, but the assays used would not detect pancreatic enzymes or their contribution to a fraction.

188. **B.** Phagocytic cells, such as monocytes or macrophages, contain large numbers of lysosomes that would contribute to the acid phosphatase activity measured in fraction 2.

189. **C.** Proximal convoluted tubule lining cells contain large numbers of mitochondria that supply the large amounts of energy needed to support the active transport used for resorption of solutes from urine. High numbers of mitochondria should increase fraction 3.

190. **D.** Two moles of carbon dioxide formed and 12 ATP formed per mole of acetyl CoA. The reactions produce three moles of NADH and one mole of $FADH_2$. Reoxidation of these coenzymes in the respiratory assembly will produce three ATP/NADH and two ATP/$FADH_2$. The remaining one ATP is a substrate level phosphorylation of GDP to GTP by succinyl CoA. GTP can phosphorylate ADP to ATP.

191. **B.** The reaction acetyl CoA to pyruvate does not occur. This is one of the reasons that we cannot make (net) glucose from acetyl CoA. Choice **D** shows two very similar reactions of oxidative decarboxylation. The same coenzymes, mechanism, and release of CO_2 occur. Choice **A** indicates both oxidations of a secondary alcohol. The product, oxalosuccinate, spontaneously decarboxylates due to the instability of the keto acid formed to yield alpha ketoglutarate. Choice **C** indicates both hydration reactions.

192. **A.** For the citric acid cycle to function, as acetyl CoA is catabolized it reacts with oxaloacetate to form citrate. In specific reactions, CO_2 is lost and oxaloacetate is regenerated. Oxaloacetate may be considered catalytic for the cycle. Oxaloacetate plus acetyl CoA forms 2 CO_2 and oxaloacetate. **B** is a true statement in that the synthesis of fatty acids in the cytoplasm occurs through this step. **C** is also true because the first step in the synthesis of the porphyrin ring (heme) occurs from succinyl CoA. The last two choices are also true because transamination from these keto acids (using some other amino acids as the amino group donor) results in the formation of the specific amino shown.

193. **D.** Net synthesis of glucose does not take place because the reaction pyruvate to acetyl CoA is not reversible under physiological conditions and also because for every acetyl CoA condensing with oxaloacetate, 2 CO_2 is formed. Choice **A** is true because specific enzymes of the pathway are inhibited by high levels of ATP (citrate synthase) or stimulated by low levels of ADP (isocitrate dehydrogenase). Choice **B** is correct. One control of the glycolytic pathway has citrate as a negative effector (phosphofructokinase). Choice **C** is a true statement. The citric acid cycle is the final metabolic pathway for many metabolites.

194. **A.** The red blood cell (mature RBC) does not contain mitochondria where the citric acid cycle takes place; see **B**. Choice **C** is true; for every acetyl CoA (two per glucose mole) 12 ATP are formed. Substrate level phosphorylation (GTP + ADP to ATP + GDP) form one and reoxidation of reducing equivalents in oxidative phosphorylation forms 11 ATP. When acetyl CoA levels are high, several things can happen: (1) the citric acid cycle may be maximal (depends on ATP needs); (2) fatty acids may be synthesized; (3) ketone bodies may be formed; (4) gluconeogenesis is stimulated because the enzyme pyruvate carboxylase requires high levels to activate it for the synthesis of net oxaloacetate from pyruvate and CO_2. Eventually glucose may be formed anew from the pyruvate (gluconeogenesis).

195. **B.** L-amino acids are those coded for translation into proteins. D-amino acids are rare, although found in some bacteria. All of the amino acids with one exception, glycine, are optically active. This is a physical property that molecules may have when they are chiral.

196. **C.** In contrast to the amino acids, all of the main carbohydrates are of the D configuration. Notable exceptions are some L sugars found in blood group glycoproteins, such as L-fucose.

197. **B.** Diastereomers (diastereo-isomers) are not mirror images (enantiomers) and have different chemical, physical, and biological properties. If the question had asked D-glucose and D-galactose, the answer would be **D**. That is, they are both epimers and diastereomers.

198. **D.** D-galactose is an epimer at C4 of glucose, and D-mannose is an epimer at C2 of glucose. D-fructose is a keto hexose and has similar OH configuration to D-glucose at C atoms 3, 4, 5.

199. **D.** The structure below contrasts D-glyceraldehyde to D-glucose. It is as if the three carbon atom difference were by addition to the C-1 of glyceraldehyde.

200. **D.** Pyruvate is formed from the high energy compound phosphoenolpyruvate catalyzed by the enzyme pyruvate kinase. As NADH builds up from an earlier step, the keto acid pyruvate is reduced to the hydroxy-acid lactate. Choice **A** is the first product formed in all cells that metabolize glucose. Carbon dioxide (**B**) is not produced in the glycolytic pathway. Acetyl CoA (**C**) is formed in mitochondria from pyruvate by the pyruvate dehydrogenase complex.

201. **D.** The glycolytic pathway takes place in the cytoplasm. The first step, glucose to glucose-6-phosphate, is catalyzed by a kinase and uses ATP to phosphorylate glucose.

202. **D.** Choice A requires ATP, whereas **B** and **C** are substrate level phosphorylations (ADP + high energy phosphate to give ATP).

203. **C.** The enzyme glucose-6-phosphate dehydrogenase, the first enzyme in the hexosemonophosphate shunt, catalyzes the oxidation to 6-phosphogluconate and the reduction of $NADP^+$ to NADPH. Red cell lysis occurs for a number of different reasons, including changes in hemoglobin, such as the oxidation of ferrous ion to ferric ion (which does not carry oxygen). Failure to maintain a reduced cell membrane results in a cell that does not fit through capillaries. Pyruvate is reduced to lactate by NADH.

204. **D.** After the formation of pentose phosphate, further catabolism produces common intermediates, such as glyceraldehyde-3-P, and fructose-6-phosphate provide an interchange between these two pathways. Only the hexose monophosphate shunt produces carbon dioxide in the red blood cell. This occurs by oxidation of 6-phosphogluconate to reduce $NADP^+$. The oxidized product is decarboxylated to a pentose phosphate and carbon dioxide. Another name for the hexose monophosphate shunt is the pentose pathway.

205. **C.** Except for statement **C,** all of the others are supported by the evidence. To infer that the experimenters should have paid closer attention to body weights is not supported because the greatest difference between the six groups (8 animals/group) was 8 grams, organ weights were corrected for body weight, and organ weights/g body weight do not appear to vary with body weight.

206. **B.** This study was designed to determine what vitamins were missing from diet A. The data indicated that diet A lacked the B vitamins. Thiamine (B_1) is essential for the proper functioning of the nervous system; deficiency will result in beriberi. Riboflavin (B_2) converts tryptophan to nicotinic acid; general problems with vision, skin, coordination, and growth can occur. In the experiment, the difference between the percentage losing weight and percentage mortality within each group is best explained by individual variation among mice within each group.

207. **B.** Acidophils (alpha cells) of the pituitary secrete somatotropic hormone (STH, growth hormone), which stimulates generalized body growth. Hypersecretion before ossification is complete results in giantism, whereas thereafter, acromegaly is the consequence. Hyposecretion leads to dwarfism. Our assay had to be conducted on hypophysectomized rats because the pituitary produces growth hormone that might interfere with the assay.

208. **D.** The purpose of this experiment was to observe X ray effect on growth. X rays can be lethal; they are used in combination with chemotherapy to treat certain malignant growths. The table also shows that plants exposed to 24,000 r units exhibit a marked effect; growth from the cotyledon to the first node was greatly decreased. This was the part most affected; the midrib lengths were not affected.

209. **D.** Because the Y-chromosome always passes from father to son, all male offspring (half of the total, on average) have the father's Y-chromosome. If the gene is dominant, all males will exhibit the trait. Female offspring could not, because they get the father's X-chromosome, not the Y.

210. **D.** Melanoma is a malignancy. The data shows that an Ag A phenotype containing three seems to be related to higher antibody production. If one possesses a 1/3 Ag A phenotype the mouse resulting from a cross of Strain with one of Strain 3 would probably be a bette antibody producer than a sibling having a 1/ Ag A phenotype. Statements **A** and **C** are clearly contradicted by the data, whereas statement **B** is neither contradicted nor supported.

211. **D.** Statement **C** is neither supported nor contradicted by the data. Statement **D** is contradicted by the evidence because even after 90-100% resurfacing, an endothelial labeling index of 2.5% is exhibited. Statements **A** and **B** are supported by the information presented.

212. **D.** The actions of LH and FSH in the male on the testes are to promote androgen secretion and spermatogenesis. Androgenic actions of testosterone are: (1) maintenance of secondary sex organs; (2) promotion of secondary sex characteristics (size of genitalia, voice, muscle development, and hair distribution); (3) normal development of body growth and psychological balance. The statement (**D**) that bilateral castration removes a major source of sex hormones is clearly the only one supported by the experiment; all others are contradicted.

213. **D.** Thyroid hormone controls the rate of metabolism, growth, maturation, and differentiation of the organism, and it influences nervous system activity. All the statements are consistent with the information and are true concerning thyroid activity. The quantity of heat liberated is decreased by deficiencies and elevated by excesses of thyroxin; after thyroidectomy the basal metabolic rate drops, and animals probably exhibit sluggishness and slight obesity.

214. **A.** It is obvious that because bacteria Z could grow following exposure to temperatures below 160°C, it cannot be destroyed in autoclave 1.

215. **A.** The testes of blinded hamsters weighed 1695 mg/100 g of body weight if no MTPH was given. Application of MTPH reduced the weight to 1419 mg/100 g, indicating increased atrophy.

216. **A.** Conversion of glycogen to glucose-1 phosphate is catalyzed by the enzyme, phosphorylase. Pancreatic amylase is usually not in

contact with glycogen (except dietary glycogen); in any case it would not catalyze the formation of glucose-1-phosphate.

217. **C.** Production of glucose and fructose from sucrose and production of fatty acids and glycerol from triglycerides are both simple hydrolytic reactions in which essentially no energy is gained or lost. Production of steroids from acetate (as is true with most synthetic reactions) requires energy input. Production of CO_2 and water from fatty acids yields large amounts of energy.

218. **D.** A yellow precipitate of iodoform is produced in this reaction with methyl ketones, alcohols that may be oxidized to methyl ketones, or acetaldehyde.

219. **C.** We have described conditions for the formation of a diazonium salt and then replacement of the diazonium salt by Br to produce monobromobenzene. (The replacement is known as the Sandmeyer reaction). The intermediate diazonium salt is often unstable at room temperature, so a lower temperature is used.

Appendix

LOGARITHMS AND EXPONENTS

Logarithms

The logarithm of any number is the exponent of the power to which 10 must be raised to produce the number. The logarithm X of the number N to the base 10 is the exponent of the power to which 10 must be raised to give N (for example, $\log_{10} N = X$). Logarithms consist of two parts. First, there is the "characteristic," which is determined by the position of the first significant figure of the number in relation to the decimal point. If we count leftwards from the decimal point as positive and rightwards as negative, the characteristic is equal to the count ending at the right of the first significant figure. Thus, the characteristic of the logarithm of 2340 is 3, and of 0.00234 is -3. Second, there is the "mantissa." It is always positive, is found in logarithm tables, and depends only on the sequence of significant figures. Thus, the mantissa for the two numbers is the same, namely 0.3692. The logarithm of a number is the sum of the characteristic and the mantissa. Thus, $\log 2340 = 3.3692$ while $\log 0.00234 = -3 + 0.3692 = -2.6308$.

The logarithms of the whole integers 1 to 10 are given below.

$\log 1.0 = 0.000$	$\log 6.0 = 0.778$
$\log 2.0 = 0.301$	$\log 7.0 = 0.845$
$\log 3.0 = 0.477$	$\log 8.0 = 0.903$
$\log 4.0 = 0.602$	$\log 9.0 = 0.954$
$\log 5.0 = 0.699$	$\log 10.0 = 1.000$

Useful Rules in Handling Logarithms

1. The logarithm of a product is equal to the sum of the logarithms of the factors:

$$\log ab = \log a + \log b$$

(Check this out by solving for $\log 6$, using $\log 2 + \log 3$.)

2. The logarithm of a fraction is equal to the logarithm of the numerator minus the logarithm of the denominator:

$$\log \frac{a}{b} = \log a - \log b$$

Example:

$$\log \frac{10}{2} = \log 10 - \log 2 = \log 5$$

How about log 2.5? The answer from the log tables is 0.398.

3. The logarithm of the reciprocal of a number is the negative logarithm of the number:

$$\log \frac{1}{a} = \log 1 - \log a$$

Since $\log 1 = 0$, then

$$\log \frac{1}{a} = -\log a$$

Equally,

$$\log \frac{1}{2} = -\log 2 = -0.301$$

4. The logarithm of a number raised to a power is the logarithm of the number multiplied by the power:

$$\log a^b = b \log a$$

$$\log 2^2 = 0.603$$

Exponents

It is convenient to express large numbers as 10^x, where x represents the number of places that the decimal must be moved to place it after the first significant figure. This also represents $10 \cdot 10$ for x times. For example, 1,000,000 may be expressed as 1×10^6; 3663 as 3.663×10^3; and so on. To multiply, the exponents are added, but coefficients are multiplied. To divide, the exponents are subtracted, but coefficients are divided.

Multiplying: $(1 \times 10^x) \cdot (1 \times 10^y) = 1 \times 10^{x+y}$

$(4 \times 10^2) \cdot (2 \times 10^3) = 8 \times 10^5$

Dividing: $(1 \times 10^x) \div (1 \times 10^y) = 1 \times 10^{x-y}$

$(4 \times 10^2) \div (2 \times 10^3) = 2 \times 10^{-1}$

Numbers less than 1 are 10^{-x}. For example, 0.000001 is 1×10^{-6}.

Multiplying: $(1 \times 10^{-x}) \cdot (1 \times 10^{-y}) = 1 \times 10^{-(x+y)}$

$(4 \times 10^{-2}) \cdot (2 \times 10^{-3}) = 8 \times 10^{-5}$

A large number multiplied by a small number:

$$(4 \times 10^{-2})(2 \times 10^3) = 8 \times 10^1$$

(Logarithms and Exponents are reproduced through the courtesy of Dr. Richard B. Brandt, Dept. of Biochemistry, MCV, VCU, Richmond, Virginia, 23298).

Table of Common Logarithms

Numbers	0	1	2	3	4	5	6	7	8	9
10	0000	0043	0086	0128	0170	0212	0253	0294	0334	0374
11	0414	0453	0492	0531	0569	0607	0645	0682	0719	0755
12	0792	0828	0864	0899	0934	0969	1004	1038	1072	1106
13	1139	1173	1206	1239	1271	1303	1335	1367	1399	1430
14	1461	1492	1523	1553	1584	1614	1644	1673	1703	1732
15	1761	1790	1818	1847	1875	1903	1931	1959	1987	2014
16	2041	2068	2095	2122	2148	2175	2201	2227	2253	2279
17	2304	2330	2355	2380	2405	2430	2455	2480	2504	2529
18	2553	2577	2601	2625	2648	2672	2695	2718	2742	2765
19	2788	2810	2833	2856	2878	2900	2923	2945	2967	2989
20	3010	3032	3054	3075	3096	3118	3139	3160	3181	3201
21	3222	3243	3263	3284	3304	3324	3345	3365	3385	3404
22	3424	3444	3464	3483	3502	3522	3541	3560	3579	3598
23	3617	3636	3655	3674	3692	3711	3729	3747	3766	3784
24	3802	3820	3838	3856	3874	3892	3909	3927	3945	3962
25	3979	3997	4014	4031	4048	4065	4082	4099	4116	4133
26	4150	4166	4183	4200	4216	4232	4249	4265	4281	4298
27	4314	4330	4346	4362	4378	4393	4409	4425	4440	4456
28	4472	4487	4502	4518	4533	4548	4564	4579	4594	4609
29	4624	4639	4654	4669	4683	4698	4713	4728	4742	4757
30	4771	4786	4800	4814	4829	4843	4857	4871	4886	4900
31	4914	4928	4942	4955	4969	4983	4997	5011	5024	5038
32	5051	5065	5079	5092	5105	5119	5132	5145	5159	5172
33	5185	5198	5211	5224	5237	5250	5263	5276	5289	5302
34	5315	5328	5340	5353	5366	5378	5391	5403	5416	5428
35	5441	5453	5465	5478	5490	5502	5514	5527	5539	5551
36	5563	5575	5587	5599	5611	5623	5635	5647	5658	5670
37	5682	5694	5705	5717	5729	5740	5752	5763	5775	5786
38	5798	5809	5821	5832	5843	5855	5866	5877	5888	5899
39	5911	5922	5933	5944	5955	5966	5977	5988	5999	6010
40	6021	6031	6042	6053	6064	6075	6085	6096	6107	6117
41	6128	6138	6149	6160	6170	6180	6191	6201	6212	6222
42	6232	6243	6253	6263	6274	6284	6294	6304	6314	6325
43	6335	6345	6355	6365	6375	6385	6395	6405	6415	6425
44	6435	6444	6454	6464	6474	6484	6493	6503	6513	6522
45	6532	6542	6551	6561	6571	6580	6590	6599	6609	6618
46	6628	6637	6646	6656	6665	6675	6684	6693	6702	6712
47	6721	6730	6739	6749	6758	6767	6776	6785	6794	6803
48	6812	6821	6830	6839	6848	6857	6866	6875	6884	6893
49	6902	6911	6920	6928	6937	6946	6955	6964	6972	6981
50	6990	6998	7007	7016	7024	7033	7042	7050	7059	7067
51	7076	7084	7093	7101	7110	7118	7126	7135	7143	7152
52	7160	7168	7177	7185	7193	7202	7210	7218	7226	7235
53	7243	7251	7259	7267	7275	7284	7292	7300	7308	7316
54	7324	7332	7340	7348	7356	7364	7372	7380	7388	7396

Numbers	0	1	2	3	4	5	6	7	8	9
55	7404	7412	7419	7427	7435	7443	7451	7459	7466	7474
56	7482	7490	7497	7505	7513	7520	7528	7536	7543	7551
57	7559	7566	7574	7582	7589	7597	7604	7612	7619	7627
58	7634	7642	7649	7657	7664	7672	7679	7686	7694	7701
59	7709	7716	7723	7731	7738	7745	7752	7760	7767	7774
60	7782	7789	7796	7803	7810	7818	7825	7832	7839	7846
61	7853	7860	7868	7875	7882	7889	7896	7903	7910	7917
62	7924	7931	7938	7945	7952	7959	7966	7937	7980	7987
63	7993	8000	8007	8014	8021	8028	8035	8041	8048	8055
64	8062	8069	8075	8082	8089	8096	8102	8109	8116	8122
65	8129	8136	8142	8149	8156	8162	8169	8176	8182	8189
66	8195	8202	8209	8215	8222	8228	8235	8241	8248	8254
67	8261	8267	8274	8280	8287	8293	8299	8306	8312	8319
68	8325	8331	8338	8344	8351	8357	8363	8370	8376	8382
69	8388	8395	8401	8407	8414	8420	8426	8432	8439	8445
70	8451	8457	8463	8470	8476	8482	8488	8494	8500	8506
71	8513	8519	8525	8531	8537	8543	8549	8555	8561	8567
72	8573	8579	8585	8591	8597	8603	8609	8615	8621	8627
73	8633	8639	8645	8651	8657	8663	8669	8675	8681	8686
74	8692	8698	8704	8710	8716	8722	8727	8733	8739	8745
75	8751	8756	8762	8768	8774	8779	8785	8791	8797	8802
76	8808	8814	8820	8825	8831	8837	8842	8848	8854	8859
77	8865	8871	8876	8882	8887	8893	8899	8904	8910	8915
78	8921	8927	8932	8938	8943	8949	8954	8960	8965	8971
79	8976	8982	8987	8993	8998	9004	9009	9015	9020	9025
80	9031	9036	9042	9047	9053	9058	9063	9069	9074	9079
81	9085	9090	9096	9101	9106	9112	9117	9122	9128	9133
82	9138	9143	9149	9154	9159	9165	9170	9175	9180	9186
83	9191	9196	9201	9206	9212	9217	9222	9227	9232	9238
84	9243	9248	9253	9258	9263	9269	9274	9279	9284	9289
85	9294	9299	9304	9309	9315	9320	9325	9330	9335	9340
86	9345	9350	9355	9360	9365	9370	9375	9380	9385	9390
87	9395	9400	9405	9410	9415	9420	9425	9430	9435	9440
88	9445	9450	9455	9460	9465	9469	9474	9479	9484	9489
89	9494	9499	9504	9509	9513	9518	9523	9528	9533	9538
90	9542	9547	9552	9557	9562	9566	9571	9576	9581	9586
91	9590	9595	9600	9605	9609	9614	9619	9624	9628	9633
92	9638	9643	9647	9652	9657	9661	9666	9671	9675	9680
93	9685	9689	9694	9699	9703	9708	9713	9717	9722	9727
94	9731	9736	9741	9745	9750	9754	9759	9763	9768	9773
95	9777	9782	9786	9791	9795	9800	9805	9809	9814	9818
96	9823	9827	9832	9836	9841	9845	9850	9854	9859	9863
97	9868	9872	9877	9881	9886	9890	9894	9899	9903	9908
98	9912	9917	9921	9926	9930	9934	9939	9943	9948	9952
99	9956	9961	9965	9969	9974	9978	9983	9987	9991	9996

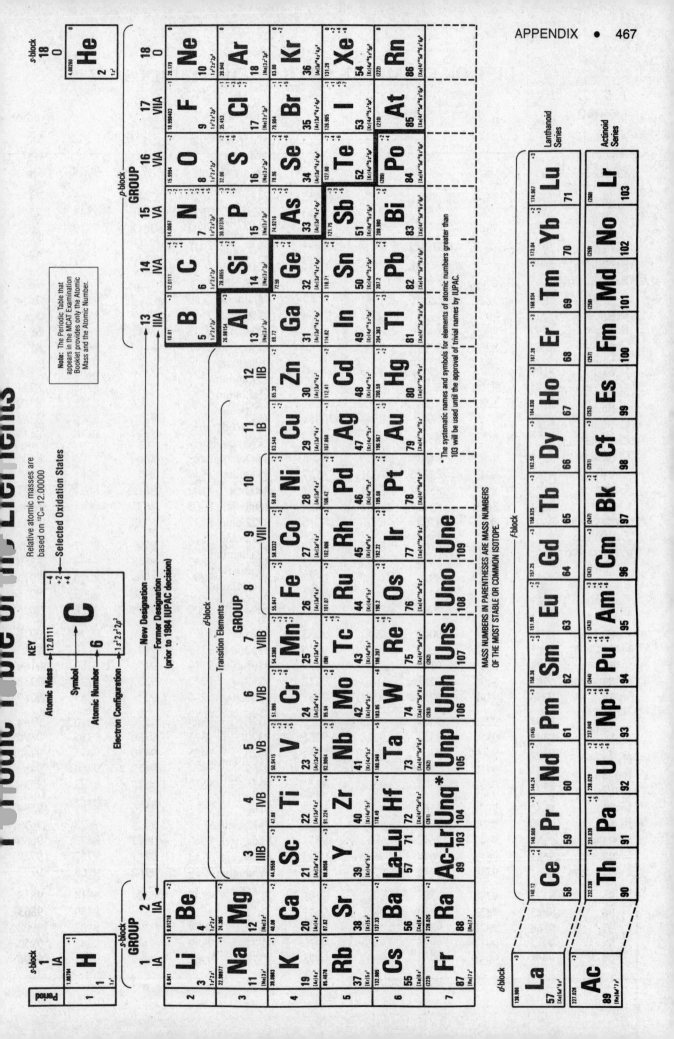

Periodic Table of the Elements

LIST OF ELEMENTS WITH THEIR SYMBOLS

Element	Symbol	Element	Symbol
Actinium	Ac	Mendelevium	Md
Aluminum	Al	Mercury	Hg
Americium	Am	Molybdenum	Mo
Antimony	Sb	Neodymium	Nd
Argon	Ar	Neon	Ne
Arsenic	As	Neptunium	Np
Astatine	At	Nickel	Ni
Barium	Ba	Niobium	Nb
Berkelium	Bk	Nitrogen	N
Beryllium	Be	Nobelium	No
Bismuth	Bi	Osmium	Os
Boron	B	Oxygen	O
Bromine	Br	Palladium	Pd
Cadmium	Cd	Phosphorus	P
Calcium	Ca	Platinum	Pt
Californium	Cf	Plutonium	Pu
Carbon	C	Polonium	Po
Cerium	Ce	Potassium	K
Cesium	Cs	Praseodymium	Pr
Chlorine	Cl	Promethium	Pm
Chromium	Cr	Protactinium	Pa
Cobalt	Co	Radium	Ra
Copper	Cu	Radon	Rn
Curium	Cm	Rhenium	Re
Dysprosium	Dy	Rhodium	Rh
Einsteinium	Es	Rubidium	Rb
Element 106		Ruthenium	Ru
Erbium	Er	Samarium	Sm
Europium	Eu	Scandium	Sc
Fermium	Fm	Selenium	Se
Fluorine	F	Silicon	Si
Francium	Fr	Silver	Ag
Gadolinium	Gd	Sodium	Na
Gallium	Ga	Strontium	Sr
Germanium	Ge	Sulfur	S
Gold	Au	Tantalum	Ta
Hafnium	Hf	Technetium	Tc
Helium	He	Tellurium	Te
Holmium	Ho	Terbium	Tb
Hydrogen	H	Thallium	Tl
Indium	In	Thorium	Th
Iodine	I	Thulium	Tm
Iridium	Ir	Tin	Sn
Iron	Fe	Titanium	Ti
Krypton	Kr	Tungsten	W
Lanthanum	La	Uranium	U
Lawrencium	Lr	Vanadium	V
Lead	Pb	Xenon	Xe
Lithium	Li	Ytterbium	Yb
Lutetium	Lu	Yttrium	Y
Magnesium	Mg	Zinc	Zn
Manganese	Mn	Zirconium	Zr

REFERENCE TABLES FOR CHEMISTRY

PHYSICAL CONSTANTS AND CONVERSION FACTORS

Name	Symbol	Value(s)	Units
Angstrom unit	Å	1×10^{-10} m	meter
Avogadro number	N_A	6.02×10^{23} per mol	
Charge of electron	e	1.60×10^{-19} C	coulomb
Electron volt	eV	1.60×10^{-19} J	joule
Speed of light	c	3.00×10^8 m/s	meters/second
Planck's constant	h	6.63×10^{-34} J·s	joule-second
		1.58×10^{-37} kcal·s	kilocalorie-second
Universal gas constant	R	0.0821 L·atm/mol·K	liter-atmosphere/mole-kelvin
		1.98 cal/mol·K	calories/mole-kelvin
		8.31 J/mol·K	joules/mole-kelvin
Atomic mass unit	μ(amu)	1.66×10^{-24} g	gram
Volume standard, liter	L	1×10^3 cm^3 = 1 dm^3	cubic centimeters, cubic decimeter
Standard pressure, atmosphere	atm	101.3 kPa	kilopascals
		760 mmHg	millimeters of mercury
		760 torr	torr
Heat equivalent, kilocalorie	kcal	4.18×10^3 J	joules

Physical Constants for H$_2$O

Molal freezing point depression . . . . 1.86°C
Molal boiling point elevation . . . . 0.52°C
Heat of fusion . . . . 79.72 cal/g
Heat of vaporization . . . . 539.4 cal/g

STANDARD UNITS

Symbol	Name	Quantity
m	meter	length
kg	kilogram	mass
Pa	pascal	pressure
K	kelvin	thermodynamic temperature
mol	mole	amount of substance
J	joule	energy, work, quantity of heat
s	second	time
C	coulomb	quantity of electricity
V	volt	electric potential, potential difference
L	liter	volume

Selected Prefixes

Factor	Prefix	Symbol
10^6	mega	M
10^3	kilo	k
10^{-1}	deci	d
10^{-2}	centi	c
10^{-3}	milli	m
10^{-6}	micro	μ
10^{-9}	nano	n

RELATIVE STRENGTHS OF ACIDS IN AQUEOUS SOLUTION AT 1 atm AND 298 K

Conjugate Pairs		K_a
ACID	BASE	
$HI = H^+ + I^-$		very large
$HBr = H^+ + Br^-$		very large
$HCl = H^+ + Cl^-$		very large
$HNO_3 = H^+ + NO_3^-$		very large
$H_2SO_4 = H^+ + HSO_4^-$		large
$H_2O + SO_2 = H^+ + HSO_3^-$		1.5×10^{-2}
$HSO_4^- = H^+ + SO_4^{2-}$		1.2×10^{-2}
$H_3PO_4 = H^+ + H_2PO_4^-$		7.5×10^{-3}
$Fe(H_2O)_6^{3+} = H^+ + Fe(H_2O)_5(OH)^{2+}$		8.9×10^{-4}
$HNO_2 = H^+ + NO_2^-$		4.6×10^{-4}
$HF = H^+ + F^-$		3.5×10^{-4}
$Cr(H_2O)_6^{3+} = H^+ + Cr(H_2O)_5(OH)^{2+}$		1.0×10^{-4}
$CH_3COOH = H^+ + CH_3COO^-$		1.8×10^{-5}
$Al(H_2O)_6^{3+} = H^+ + Al(H_2O)_5(OH)^{2+}$		1.1×10^{-5}
$H_2O + CO_2 = H^+ + HCO_3^-$		4.3×10^{-7}
$HSO_3^- = H^+ + SO_3^{2-}$		1.1×10^{-7}
$H_2S = H^+ + HS^-$		9.5×10^{-8}
$H_2PO_4^- = H^+ + HPO_4^{2-}$		6.2×10^{-8}
$NH_4^+ = H^+ + NH_3$		5.7×10^{-10}
$HCO_3^- = H^+ + CO_3^{2-}$		5.6×10^{-11}
$HPO_4^{2-} = H^+ + PO_4^{3-}$		2.2×10^{-13}
$HS^- = H^+ + S^{2-}$		1.3×10^{-14}
$H_2O = H^+ + OH^-$		1.0×10^{-14}

Note: $H^+(aq) = H_3O^+$

Sample equation: $HI + H_2O = H_3O^+ + I^-$

CONSTANTS FOR VARIOUS EQUILIBRIA AT 1 atm AND 298 K

$H_2O(\ell) = H^+(aq) + OH^-(aq)$	$K_w = 1.0 \times 10^{-14}$
$H_2O(\ell) + H_2O(\ell) = H_3O^+(aq) + OH^-(aq)$	$K_w = 1.0 \times 10^{-14}$
$CH_3COO^-(aq) + H_2O(\ell) = CH_3COOH(aq) + OH^-(aq)$	$K_b = 5.6 \times 10^{-10}$
$Na^+F^-(aq) + H_2O(\ell) = Na^+(OH)^- + HF(aq)$	$K_b = 1.5 \times 10^{-11}$
$NH_3(aq) + H_2O(\ell) = NH_4^+(aq) + OH^-(aq)$	$K_b = 1.8 \times 10^{-5}$
$CO_3^{2-}(aq) + H_2O(\ell) = HCO_3^-(aq) + OH^-(aq)$	$K_b = 1.8 \times 10^{-4}$
$Ag(NH_3)_2^+(aq) = Ag^+(aq) + 2NH_3(aq)$	$K_{eq} = 8.9 \times 10^{-8}$
$N_2(g) + 3H_2(g) = 2NH_3(g)$	$K_{eq} = 6.7 \times 10^5$
$H_2(g) + I_2(g) = 2HI(g)$	$K_{eq} = 3.5 \times 10^{-1}$

Compound	K_{sp}	Compound	K_{sp}
AgBr	5.0×10^{-13}	Li_2CO_3	2.5×10^{-2}
AgCl	1.8×10^{-10}	$PbCl_2$	1.6×10^{-5}
Ag_2CrO_4	1.1×10^{-12}	$PbCO_3$	7.4×10^{-14}
AgI	8.3×10^{-17}	$PbCrO_4$	2.8×10^{-13}
$BaSO_4$	1.1×10^{-10}	PbI_2	7.1×10^{-9}
$CaSO_4$	9.1×10^{-6}	$ZnCO_3$	1.4×10^{-11}

STANDARD ENERGIES OF FORMATION OF COMPOUNDS AT 1 atm AND 298 K

Compound	Heat (Enthalpy) of Formation* kcal/mol ($\triangle H_f^\circ$)	Free Energy of Formation* kcal/mol ($\triangle G_f^\circ$)
Aluminum oxide $Al_2O_3(s)$	−400.5	−378.2
Ammonia $NH_3(g)$	−11.0	−3.9
Barium sulfate $BaSo_4(s)$	−352.1	−325.6
Calcium hydroxide $Ca(OH)_2(s)$	−235.7	−214.8
Carbon dioxide $CO_2(g)$	−94.1	−94.3
Carbon monoxide $CO(g)$	−26.4	−32.8
Copper (II) sulfate $CuSO_4(s)$	−184.4	−158.2
Ethane $C_2H_6(g)$	−20.2	−7.9
Ethene (ethylene) $C_2H_4(g)$	12.5	16.3
Ethyne (acetylene) $C_2H_2(g)$	54.2	50.0
Hydrogen fluoride $HF(g)$	−64.8	−65.3
Hydrogen iodide $HI(g)$	6.3	0.4
Iodine chloride $ICl(g)$	4.3	−1.3
Lead (II) oxide $PbO(s)$	−51.5	−45.0
Magnesium oxide $MgO(s)$	−143.8	−136.1
Nitrogen (II) oxide $NO(g)$	21.6	20.7
Nitrogen (IV) oxide $NO_2(g)$	7.9	12.3
Potassium chloride $KCl(s)$	−104.4	−97.8
Sodium chloride $NaCl(s)$	−98.3	−91.8
Sulfur dioxide $SO_2(g)$	−70.9	−71.7
Water $H_2O(g)$	−57.8	−54.6
Water $H_2O(\ell)$	−68.3	−56.7

*Minus sign indicates an exothermic reaction.

Sample equations:

$2Al(s) + \frac{3}{2} O_2(g) \rightarrow Al_2O_3(s) + 400.5 \text{ kcal}$

$2Al(s) + \frac{3}{2} O_2(g) \rightarrow Al_2O_3(s) \quad \triangle H = -400.5 \text{ kcal/mol}$

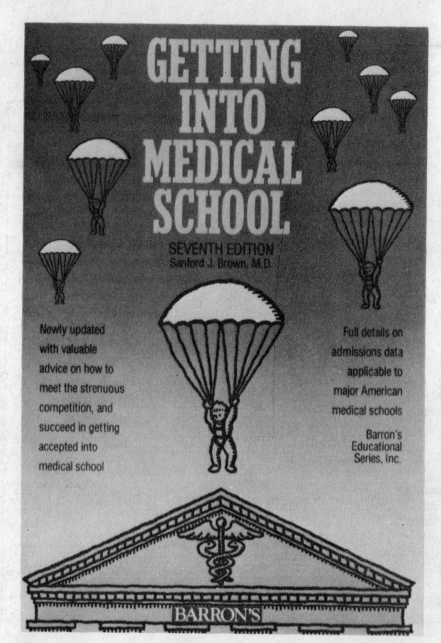
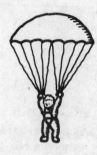

GETTING INTO MEDICAL SCHOOL

SEVENTH EDITION
Sanford J. Brown, M.D.

Newly updated with valuable advice on how to meet the strenuous competition, and succeed in getting accepted into medical school

Full details on admissions data applicable to major American medical schools

Barron's Educational Series, Inc.

BARRON'S

"Majoring in a non-science will probably raise your overall GPA and put you in a more advantageous position when seeking admission..."

"Apart from their annual pilgrimage to a medical school (a trip which you can more profitably make on your own), the value of [premedical clubs] is dubious..."

"The premedical adviser holds no degree or certification for the job, is not licensed, and is not subject to peer review. The adviser is only as good as personal interest and involvement allow."

The hardest obstacle to overcome in becoming a physician is getting admitted to a medical school. This book cuts through the official jargon and tells you exactly what you really need to do to be accepted. How to choose a college and a major field of study, how to avoid the "Premed Syndrome," how to cope with the MCAT, when, where, and how to apply to medical school, and how to deal with rejections. With a directory of AMA-approved medical schools.

$9.95 Canada $13.95